MOOD DISORDERS

recognition and treatment

Edited by

Peter R Joyce and Philip B Mitchell

UNSW PRESS

A UNSW Press book

Published by
The University of New South Wales Press Ltd
University of New South Wales
Sydney NSW 2052
AUSTRALIA
www.unswpress.com.au

First published 2004

National Library of Australia
Cataloguing-in-Publication entry
Mood disorders : recognition and treatment.

Includes index.
ISBN 0 86840 447 0.

1. Affective disorders - Diagnosis. 2. Affective disorders - Treatment. I. Joyce, Peter R. II. Mitchell, Philip B.

616.8527

Cover design Di Quick
Printer Ligare

CONTENTS

FOREWORD

It came as a surprise to most physicians of my acquaintance that mood disorders already contribute so much to human misery. It is greater than many of the diseases that carry higher profile and prestige in calls for research in medicine. The final chapter of this outstanding multi-author volume reviews how this has been quantified and why it so important. The previous 39 chapters review where we are in addressing the personal, medical and social challenges that mood disorders present.

The emphasis on a scientific approach to psychiatry is explicit in this volume – and it is vital that it should be. Perhaps too often psychiatry has regarded its illnesses as so complex that a multiplicity of competing views can be afforded equal status. Hence, a biological, a social, a psychodynamic or a family 'view' may develop mutually exclusive explanations of the same phenomenon. And the explanations may acquire a defining professional identity for the people who hold them. A scientific approach can protect us from factionalism, as well as ignorance. By science is simply meant reliable knowledge, rather than anecdote. Such knowledge is essentially unitary and harmonising. It is often just such knowledge that patients seek from their doctors about their illness – how long it will last, whether it will recur, whether it runs in families and what the best treatment is. Science is underpinned by the principle that if an approach is wrong, then it will be found out by our inability to replicate results and failure to move on to more fruitful hypotheses. Scientific ideas are falsifiable; anecdote and personal experience are not.

Reliable knowledge about any natural phenomenon increases as more effort is expended on primary research. During the past century, medicine has generally been transformed by just such a scientific approach in almost every specialty. Arguably, psychiatrists, despite a basic medical training, have been the slowest to adopt science wholeheartedly, perhaps because emotion, thinking and behaviour have been slow to yield to scientific enquiry. That situation is rapidly changing and psychiatry must fully embrace the neuroscience revolution of the past two decades in the interests of our patients and their families. The promise of science relates to what is sometimes disparaged as the medical model in psychiatry. But a medical model implies a unifying scientific discipline, not an exclusive reliance on medicines. Furthermore, too often, criticism of the medical model is little better than a criticism of doctors – a dislike of the cut of our collective jib. By all means replace doctors with someone better, but let them still thirst for reliable knowledge.

This is a timely volume because there are grounds for cautious optimism around some of the scientific developments that seem most critical for improving clinical care. We understand much more about the genetic and environmental causes of depression. We have accumulated almost two decades of experience using new drugs for depression that are based on heuristically useful models of psychotropic action and that have a lower burden of side effects. We are starting to see new medicines, and new research into bipolar disorder, shamefully neglected as a research area for too long. We have a better understanding of how to use talking treatments. There are considerable problems still in understanding mood disorders in childhood, but the issue is now recognised. All the key areas for clinical understanding have seen significant advances since the last edition of this book, and the complete revision reflects this progress. Peter Joyce and Philip Mitchell have done a remarkable job of assembling so much information so rapidly and effectively. They and their colleagues deserve the gratitude of all who read or simply dip into this book.

Guy Goodwin
University Department of Psychiatry
Warneford Hospital
Oxford, UK

PREFACE

Bipolar disorder and depression are major causes of disease burden. This book contains accessible accounts of our current understanding of mood disorders from senior Australian and New Zealand academics and clinicians, or from individuals with strong links to these two countries. Since the 1960s, Australian and New Zealand researchers have made major contributions to our knowledge of these conditions. The book is aimed primarily at psychiatric registrars and psychiatrists, but we believe it will also be highly relevant to clinical psychologists, mental health nurses, mental health professionals, general practitioners, and medical and health science students. We also hope that the book will be read by individuals, and their families, who suffer from and live with mood disorders.

This book begins with descriptions of depression and mania, with frequent quotations from individuals who have experienced these mood states. This is followed by a description of how bipolar disorder affects an individual's life. Subsequent chapters present the symptomatology and diagnosis of mood disorders from the more conventional clinician's perspective. Further chapters highlight mood disorders at the different stages of life, the links of mood disorders with other mental and physical disorders, our understanding of the aetiology of mood disorders, the treatments for mood disorders, and a range of other important areas.

We wish to thank all the authors for their contributions to this book. We would especially like to acknowledge the extensive work of Judith Stone, who undertook all the initial editing. We would also like to acknowledge Mary Halbmeyer from the University of New South Wales Press for her efforts in the publication of this book.

Peter R Joyce and Philip B Mitchell

LIST OF CONTRIBUTORS

Maria Aslam
Medical Student
University of New South Wales
Sydney, New South Wales, Australia

Jillian Ball
BA, MA(ClinPsych), PhD
Conjoint Lecturer
University of New South Wales;
Research Psychologist, Prince of Wales Hospital
Randwick, New South Wales, Australia

Caroline J. Bell
BM BCh, MD, MRCPsych
Senior Lecturer
Department of Psychological Medicine
Christchurch School of Medicine and Health Sciences
University of Otago
Christchurch, New Zealand

Tracey V. Barnfield
MA(Hons), DipClinPsych, MNZCCP
Senior Clinical Psychologist and Lecturer in Clinical Psychology
Wellington School of Medicine and Health Sciences
University of Otago
Wellington, New Zealand

Michael Berk
MB BCh, MMed(Psych), FF(Psych), FRANZCP, PhD
Professor of Psychiatry
Barwon Health and Geelong Clinic
The University of Melbourne
Victoria, Australia

Philip M. Boyce
LRCP, MRCS, MB BS, FRANZCP, MD, Dip.Psychotherapy
Professor of Psychiatry
Westmead Hospital
Sydney, New South Wales;
Professor and Head
Discipline of Psychological Medicine
Faculty of Medicine
The University of Sydney
New South Wales, Australia

Philip M.J. Brinded
MB BS, FRANZCP
Clinical Associate Professor
Department of Psychological Medicine
Christchurch School of Medicine & Health Sciences
University of Otago;
Chair of Clinical Directors and Director of Adult Mental Health Services
Canterbury District Health Board
Christchurch, New Zealand

Graham D. Burrows, AO, KCSJ
BSc, MB ChB, DPM, MD, FRANZCP, FRCPsych, MRACMA, DipMHlthSc(Clinical Hypnosis), FACham
Professor
University of Melbourne
Austin Health
Heidelberg, Victoria, Australia

Gerard J. Byrne
BSc(Med), MB BS, PhD, FRANZCP
Associate Professor of Geriatric Psychiatry
Department of Psychiatry
School of Medicine
The University of Queensland
Brisbane, Queensland, Australia

Janet D. Carter
BA(Hons), MA(Dist), DipClinPsych, PhD
Research Fellow
Clinical Research Unit
Department of Psychological Medicine
Christchurch School of Medicine and Health Sciences
University of Otago
Christchurch, New Zealand

Neil Cole
BA, LLB
Barrister and Solicitor
Supreme Court of Victoria;
Head of Depression Awareness Research Project

Mental Health Research Institute of Victoria
Melbourne, Victoria, Australia

John T. Condon
MB BS, MD, Dip Psychotherapy, FRANZCP
Professor of Psychiatry
Flinders University of South Australia
Flinders Medical Centre
Bedford Park, South Australia.

Marie T. Crowe
BA, MNurs, PhD, RPN
Senior Lecturer in Mental Health Nursing
Department of Psychological Medicine
Christchurch School of Medicine and Health Sciences
University of Otago
Christchurch, New Zealand

Tracey A. Davenport
BA(Hons), GCM
Senior Research Psychologist
School of Psychiatry
University of New South Wales
New South Wales, Australia

Brian Dean
MSc, PhD, CBIOL, FI BIOL
Head
The Rebecca L. Cooper Research Laboratories
The Mental Health Research Institute of Victoria
Melbourne, Victoria, Australia

Mark J.A. Earthrowl
BM, MRCPsych
Clinical Head and Consultant Forensic Psychiatrist
Canterbury Regional Forensic Service
Canterbury District Health Board
Christchurch, New Zealand

Peter M. Ellis
MA, BM BCh, PhD, FRANZCP
Professor of Psychological Medicine
Wellington School of Medicine and Health Sciences
University of Otago
Wellington, New Zealand

Peter Gallagher
BSc(Hons), MPhil
Research Associate
School of Neurology, Neurobiology and Psychiatry
University of Newcastle upon Tyne
United Kingdom

Robert D. Goldney
MB BS, MD, FRCPsych, FRANZCP
Professor of Psychiatry
The University of Adelaide
The Adelaide Clinic
Gilberton, South Australia

Sarah E. Gordon
BSc, LLB, MBHL
Managing Director
Case Consulting Ltd
New Zealand

Philip L. Hazell
BMedSc, MB ChB, PhD, FRANZCP, Cert. Accred. Child Psychiatry (RANZCP)
Conjoint Professor of Child and Adolescent Psychiatry
University of Newcastle
New South Wales, Australia

Ian B. Hickie
MD, FRANZCP
Professor of Psychiatry and Executive Director
Brain and Mind Research Institute
The University of Sydney
New South Wales, Australia
Sean D. Hood
MB BS, MSc, FRANZCP
Senior Lecturer
School of Psychiatry and Clinical Neurosciences
University of Western Australia
Perth, Australia

Gordon F.S. Johnson
MB BS, DPM , FRCPsych, FRANZCP
Emeritus Professor of Psychiatry
University of Sydney;
Director
Mood Disorders Unit
Northside Clinic
Sydney, New South Wales, Australia

Jennifer Jordan
DipClinPsych, MA(Psychology), MNZCCP
Research Fellow
Department of Psychological Medicine and Health Sciences
Christchurch School of Medicine and Health Sciences
University of Otago
New Zealand

Anthony F. Jorm
BA, GDipComp, MPsych, PhD, DSc, FASSA
Professor and Director
Centre for Mental Health Research
Australian National University
Canberra, Australia

Peter R. Joyce
BSc, MB ChB, PhD, FRANZCP
Professor and Head of Department of Psychological Medicine
Christchurch School of Medicine and Health Sciences
University of Otago
Christchurch, New Zealand

Claire M. Kelly
BA(Hons)
PhD Student, Epidemiology
Centre for Mental Health Research
Australian National University
Canberra, Australia
Martin A. Kennedy
BSc(Hons), PhD
Health Research Council of New Zealand
Senior Research Fellow
Department of Pathology
Christchurch School of Medicine and Health Sciences
University of Otago
Christchurch, New Zealand

Kylie King
Medical Student
University of New South Wales
Sydney, Australia

Suzanne E. Luty
BM BS, FPCert DRCOG, PhD, FRANZCP
Senior Lecturer
Department of Psychological Medicine
Christchurch School of Medicine and Health Sciences
University of Otago
Christchurch, New Zealand

Gin S. Malhi
MB ChB, BSc, FRANZCP, MRCPsych
Senior Lecturer
School of Psychiatry
University of New South Wales;
Prince of Wales Hospital
Randwick, New South Wales, Australia.

Graham Martin
MD, MB BS, FRANZCP, DPM, Cert. Child & Adolescent Psych.,
RANZCP
Professor of Child and Adolescent Psychiatry
The University of Queensland
Herston, Queensland, Australia

Virginia V.W. McIntosh
BA(Hons), PhD, DipClinPsych
Scientific Officer and Clinical Psychologist
Department of Psychological Medicine
Christchurch School of Medicine and Health Sciences
University of Otago
Christchurch, New Zealand
Janice M. McKenzie
MB ChB, FRCP, FRANZCP
Senior Lecturer
Department of Psychological Medicine
Christchurch School of Medicine and Health Sciences
University of Otago
Christchurch, New Zealand

Philip B. Mitchell
MB BS, MD, FRANZCP, FRCPsych
Professor and Head of the School of Psychiatry
University of New South Wales
Prince of Wales Hospital
Randwick, New South Wales, Australia

Stephanie Moor
MB ChB, MRCPsych
Senior Lecturer in Child and Adolescent Psychiatry
Department of Psychological Medicine
Christchurch School of Medicine and Health Sciences
University of Otago
Christchurch, New Zealand

Roger T. Mulder
MB ChB, PhD, FRANZCP
Professor
Department of Psychological Medicine
Christchurch School of Medicine and Health Sciences
University of Otago
Christchurch, New Zealand

Trevor R. Norman
BSc(Hons), PhD
Associate Professor
University of Melbourne
Austin Health
Heidelberg, Victoria, Australia

James S. Olver
MB BS, FRANZCP, MPM, MD,

DipMHlthSc(Hypnosis)
University of Melbourne
Austin Health
Heidelberg, Victoria, Australia

Jane E. O'Malley
BA, MA, PhD, RCN
Senior Lecturer in
Mental Health Nursing
Department of Psychological
Medicine
Christchurch School of
Medicine and Health Sciences
University of Otago
Christchurch, New Zealand

Gordon Parker
MB BS, FRANZCP, MD, PhD, DSc
Professor
School of Psychiatry;
Executive Director
Black Dog Institute
Prince of Wales Hospital
Randwick, New South Wales, Australia

Eugene S. Paykel
MD, FRCP, FRCPsych, FMedSci
Emeritus Professor of Psychiatry
University of Cambridge
Cambridge
United Kingdom

Dr Richard Porter
MB BS, MD, MA, DipObst, MRCPsych
Senior Lecturer
Department of Psychological Medicine
Christchurch School of Medicine and
Health Sciences
University of Otago
Christchurch, New Zealand

Geraldine R. Rogers
BSc, PhD
Research Fellow
Department of Pathology
Christchurch School of Medicine and
Health Sciences
University of Otago
Christchurch, New Zealand

Elizabeth Scarr
BSc(Hons), PhD
Senior Research Officer
The Rebecca L. Cooper Research
Laboratories
The Mental Health Research
Institute of Victoria
Victoria, Australia

Peter R Schofield
BScAgr, PhD, DSc
Director
Neurobiology Research Program;
National Health and Medical Research
Council Senior Principal Research Fellow;
Professor of Medicine and Professor of
Biotechnology
Garvan Institute of Medical Research
Sydney, New South Wales, Australia

Isaac Schweitzer
MB BS, MD, FRANZCP
Healthscope Chair of Psychiatry
The Melbourne Clinic
Department of Psychiatry
University of Melbourne
Victoria, Australia

J. Douglas Sellman
MB ChB, PhD, FRANZCP, FAChAM
Associate Professor and Director
National Addiction Centre
Department of Psychological Medicine
Christchurch School of Medicine and
Health Sciences
University of Otago
Christchurch, New Zealand

Suresh Sundram
MB BS, MMed, PhD, FRANZCP
Head Molecular Psychopharmacology
Mental Health Research Institute of
Victoria
Melbourne, Victoria, Australia

Patrick F. Sullivan
BS, MD, FRANZCP
Professor
Departments of Genetics, Psychiatry and
Epidemiology
University of North Carolina
Chapel Hill, North Carolina, United States
of America

John W. G. Tiller
MD, MB ChB, BSc, DPM, FRACP,
FRANZCP, CertChildPsychiatry (RANZCP)
Professor of Psychiatry
University of Melbourne
Albert Road Clinic
Melbourne, Victoria, Australia

Fraser C. Todd
MB ChB, FRANZCP, FACham
Senior Lecturer
National Addiction Centre
Department of Psychological Medicine

Christchurch School of Medicine and Health Sciences
University of Otago
Christchurch, New Zealand

Virginia Tuckwell
BA BiolSci, MSc
Research Fellow
The Melbourne Clinic
Department of Psychiatry
University of Melbourne
Victoria, Australia

William G.A. Watkins
MB ChB, MRCPsych, MRCP, MRCP(Can), DipChildPsych, FRANZCP
Senior Lecturer Child and Adolescent Psychiatry
Department of Psychological Medicine
Christchurch School of Medicine & Health Sciences
University of Otago
Christchurch, New Zealand

Kay A. Wilhelm
MB BS, MD, RANZCP
Clinical Associate Professor of Psychiatry
Faculty of Medicine;
Consultant Psychiatrist
Black Dog Institute, University of New South Wales;
Senior Staff Specialist Consultation Liaison Psychiatry
St Vincent's Hospital
Sydney, New South Wales, Australia

SECTION

I

The Experience of Mood Disturbance

CHAPTER 1

BEYOND DESCRIPTION

Pete M Ellis and
Sarah E Gordon

I see no value in my having been depressed. It is a dreadful scourge which has caused me terrible pain, caused my first wife much distress and my children much unhappiness. It is a disease, no question of that, and one which like all the others demands to be understood and relieved. Yes, of course I have learned who my true friends are and who can stay by me in my worst times – but that is no justification for what is a dreadful scourge. It does help to know there are others and that slowly people, including doctors, are beginning to learn something about it. But it has been around an awfully long time, a lot of people are suffering and it is about bloody time we took it seriously.

Milligan and Clare (1994)

I am a middle-aged Maori woman who has a good job, who has raised a family and enjoys life. From time to time I become depressed and need access to mental health services. Many thousands of women are like me. *Tangata whaiora* needs are not just to do with a diagnosis or clinical treatment. They are to do with our lives, about regaining our self-esteem, about getting a job and about somewhere safe to live, just like anyone else. You see, our illness is only one part of our life.

Tawhai (1999)

This volume offers descriptions of depressive illness from the viewpoint of the observing clinician. As such, there is an emphasis on depression being described according to the impersonal, operationally defined terms of the *Diagnostic and Statistical Manual of Mental Disorders* (DSM-IV) and the *International Classification of Diseases* (ICD-10). This chapter attempts to offer some insights into this condition, through extended quotations from people who have written of their personal experiences. Interestingly, these are often from people suffering from bipolar disorder. This may reflect the association between creativity and this disorder, as many of these descriptions are from prominent writers, or perhaps experiencing such extremes of mood lends itself to more comparative reflection.

Several authors have written of the difficulty they have in conveying their experience of depression to others. William Styron (1992), the prize-winning novelist, wrote:

> Depression is a disorder of mood, so mysteriously painful and elusive in the way that it becomes known to the self – to the mediating intellect – as to verge close to being beyond description. It thus remains nearly incomprehensible to those who have not experienced it in its extreme mode, although the gloom, 'the blues' which people go through occasionally and associate with the general hassle of everyday existence are of such prevalence that they do give many individuals a hint of the illness in its catastrophic form.

In contrast, Spike Milligan emphasised the difficulty for others to truly appreciate the pain of depression and its qualitatively different nature from that of the common and familiar emotion of despondency in this discussion with Anthony Clare (Milligan and Clare 1994):

> Clare: But most people get depressed.
>
> Milligan: Not to the extent that a neurotic does. You can tell it. It's the mere fact that you've never been this side of the emotional fence. I can tell that you've never been this deep down yourself. I can tell it. Difficult to describe.
>
> Clare: Why is it so difficult to describe?
>
> Milligan: It's invisible. There's no written diagrams. It's an abstract, it's a sensation, and if you ask people to paint it most depressives will draw black. Have you noticed that? Black paintings all over the place, so we know that it has no colour for a start.

The eminent physician Moran Campbell, who suffered from bipolar disorder, also echoed this view, but emphasised the anergia and lassitude of depression as the most difficult aspects for others to understand. In his memoirs (Campbell 1988), he wrote:

> To those who have never been really depressed it is probably easier to understand the sadness, the greyness, the hopelessness, and the thoughts of suicide than to sympathise with the lack of energy or drive, the overwhelming inertia. To me, however, the lack of energy is the

> bigger problem and I cannot over-emphasise this dissociation between the mood of depression and the lassitude of depression. I can reason intellectually about the sad things and see that I am unreasonable but I cannot do anything about the inertia. There is a limit to the extent to which one can 'pull oneself together' when even washing and dressing become major tasks. Even if I can make the effort I do whatever I do slowly and badly. There are, however, discrepancies in that generalisation. When I am depressed I may have difficulty in changing my clothes but I can still function quite well in such demanding activities as lecturing. This paradox hinges on the need for initiative in the one activity and not in the other. I have a contract to give the lecture and the programme for it – getting there, arranging the slides, etc – takes over. Any initiative would have to be to arrange not to give the lecture and taking that step would be even more distressing. On the other hand, I have no contract to change my clothes. Most of life's activities are closer to changing clothes than to lecturing so that difficulties of coping with these activities are very pervasive ...
>
> I realise that all normal people are from time to time 'bugged' by not wanting to be bothered by such trivia as changing their clothes. Agreed. The difficulty I find when depressed is quantitative, not qualitative. It is like walking through soft sand or deep snow. I get slower and slower and just want to lie down; but then doing nothing rouses the angst. An ironical consequence of this lack of energy is that I do things long before they need to be done because of my fear that, if I wait, I will not be able to do them at all.

Sylvia Plath, in her book *The Bell Jar* (1971), provided a further graphic description of this sense of lassitude:

> I hadn't washed my hair for three weeks ...
>
> I hadn't slept for seven nights.
>
> My mother told me I must have slept, it was impossible not to sleep in all that time, but if I slept, it was with my eyes wide open, for I had followed the green, luminous course of the second hand and the minute hand and the hour hand of the bedside clock through their circles and semicircles, every night for seven nights, without missing a second, or a minute, or an hour.
>
> The reason I hadn't washed my clothes or my hair was because it seemed so silly.
>
> I saw the days of the year stretching ahead of me like a series of bright, white boxes, and separating one box from another was sleep, like a black shade, only for me, the long perspective of shades that set off one box from the next had suddenly snapped, and I could see day after day glaring ahead of me like a white, broad, infinitely desolate avenue.
>
> It seemed silly to wash one day when I would only have to wash again the next.
>
> It made me tired just to think of it.
>
> I wanted to do everything once and for all and be through with it.
>
> Quoted in Goodwin and Jamison (1990)

It is salutary to recall that one of the earliest descriptions of depression appears to be in the book of Job in the Bible. Satan robbed Job of all his family, his possessions and his health. Covered with sores, Job found himself on a dunghill, where he gave long monologues about his condition and his suffering. He clearly describes his torment by the familiar symptoms of depression (Job 3:20–30:9):

> Why is light given to him that is in misery, and life to the bitter in soul, who long for death, but it comes not, and dig for it more than for hid treasures; who rejoice exceedingly, and are glad, when they find the grave?
>
> When I lie down I say: When shall I arise? But the night is long, and I am full of tossing until the dawn ...
>
> My days are swifter than a weaver's shuttle, and come to their end without hope.
>
> ... so I am allotted months of emptiness, and nights of misery are apportioned to me.
>
> My spirit is broken, my days are extinct, the grave is ready for me.
>
> Surely there are mockers about me ...
>
> He has made me a byword of the peoples, and I am one before whom men spit.
>
> Terrors are turned upon me; my honour is pursued as by the wind and my prosperity has passed away like a cloud. And now my soul is poured out within me; days of affliction have taken hold of me. The night racks my bones, and the pain that gnaws me takes no rest. With violence it seizes my garment; it binds me about like the collar of my tunic. God has cast me into the mire, and I have become like dust and ashes.

A profound sense of alienation from one's usual self was well described by the Austrian composer Hugo Wolf (1891), and echoed by Spike Milligan:

> Since then I have led, truly, the existence of a frog and not even that of a living one, but that of a galvanised frog. To be sure, I appear at times merry and in good heart, talk, too, before others quite reasonably, and it looks as if I felt, too, God knows how well within my skin; yet the soul maintains its deathly sleep and the heart bleeds from a thousand wounds.
>
> Wolf (1891)

> I have got so low that I have asked to be hospitalised and for deep narcosis. I cannot stand being awake. The pain is too much. I have had thoughts of suicide. I get depressed that I am old. Something has happened to me – this vital spark has stopped burning – I go to a dinner table now and I don't say a word, just sit there like a dodo. Normally I am the centre of attention, keep the conversation going – so that is depressing in itself. It's like another person taking over, very strange. The most important thing I say is 'good evening' and then I go quiet and other people will talk. It must be a bit unbalanced at the table with me just sitting there dead-silent.
>
> Milligan and Clare (1994)

William Styron echoed this sense of being taken over by another person, and described feeling as if he was accompanied by a second self:

> a wraithlike observer who, not sharing the dementia of his double, is able to watch with dispassionate curiosity as his companion struggles against the oncoming disaster, or decides to embrace it. There is a theatrical quality about all this, and during the next several days, as I went about stolidly preparing for extinction, I couldn't shake off a sense of melodrama – a melodrama in which I, the victim-to-be of self-murder, was both the solitary actor and lone member of the audience.

John Custance (1952), British writer and former naval intelligence officer, described the cognitive clouding of depression and changed perception of his world in these extracts:

> I seem to be in perpetual fog and darkness. I cannot get my mind to work; instead of associations 'clicking into place' everything is inextricable jumble; instead of seeming to grasp a whole, it seems to remain tied to the actual consciousness of the moment. The whole world of my thoughts is hopelessly divided into incomprehensible watertight compartments. I could not feel more ignorant, undecided or inefficient. It is appallingly difficult to concentrate, and writing is pain and grief to me.
>
> I was utterly miserable and wanted to die, but my fears, troubles and worries were of normal human mischances which might happen to anybody. I feared poverty, failure in life, inability to educate my children, making my wife miserable, losing her, ending up in the gutter as the most revolting type of beggar and so on. My fears had in fact become so overpowering as to appear to me like certainties, but they were only earthly, human fears. Beyond the ridge bordering this ordinary universe of common human experience unending horrors awaited me. But I did not know; I had not crossed it, at any rate in that direction.
>
> Quoted in Goodwin and Jamison (1990)

Depression can directly affect a wide range of physiological functions of the body, including gastrointestinal and menstrual functioning. The following account describes this in relation to pregnancy and delivery:

> I always tell people that when I am sick my whole body shuts down. It wasn't until the later stage of my first pregnancy that I could actually provide 'proof'. During my pregnancy, I remained on my medication until two weeks prior to the due date, upon which I began a scheduled withdrawal programme. A couple of days into the withdrawal I started to become depressed. Ten days into the withdrawal, my physical responses to later stage pregnancy (Braxton Hicks contractions, early lactation) had ceased. This was confirmed by the obstetricians and a fetal tocograph. Unless my mental health was addressed, the professionals anticipated that I would have no chance at a natural labour. As a result, my medication was reintroduced. Within five days I started to feel better and my labour began, naturally, ten days after the reinstatement of the medication.

Depression can also affect the degree of pain and concern associated with a physical condition. The eighteenth-century Swiss physician and writer Johann Georg Zimmerman, who attended both the Russian and Prussian royal courts, suffered from an inguinal hernia and also depression. He described these conditions in a letter to a friend:

> Now my dearest and best friend, I would like to ask you for a good advice. I'm suffering all torments of the deepest melancholia. This is the result of the constant swelling of the abdomen, the immense fear accompanied with it, the constant pulling, tearing and burning in my right testicle which has been swollen for 5 years, the similar sensations and the extreme weakness in both legs and arms, and most of all the inexpressible effort I have to force myself to make, if after the first hour of the day I have to write a letter, read a page or make a visit. The effect of all this is that nothing in the world gives me joy anymore, that I feel alarmed about all work, and that all in all I fear everything, that I don't hope for anything good for myself, expect the worst of everything, and with the exception of one very dear house, I shy away and flee all people.
>
> Quoted in Goodwin and Jamison (1990)

Zimmerman described a reversal of the usual diurnal pattern of mood, as did Styron (1992):

> The mornings themselves were becoming bad now as I wandered about lethargic, following my synthetic sleep, but afternoons were still the worst, beginning about three o'clock, when I'd feel the horror, like some poisonous fogbank, roll in upon my mind, forcing me into bed. There I would lie for as long as six hours, stuporous and virtually paralysed, gazing at the ceiling and waiting for that moment of evening when, mysteriously, the crucifixion would ease up just enough to allow me to force down some food and then, like an automaton, seek an hour or two of sleep again.

Styron referred to synthetic sleep, and this is often a consideration in managing the effects of depression:

> One thing that few people understand about depression is that it can affect both the waking and the sleeping states. While asleep, the troubled subconscious continues to torment the individual through abstract nightmarish depictions of the waking torture. At times the only respite from this full-time horror can be the induction of 'synthetic' sleep. I don't know why it is referred to as 'sleep' because the use of sedatives doesn't result in a pleasant state of restful slumber. In reality it shuts down both the conscious and subconscious – it switches off the mechanics of the mind. Rather than providing the individual with an eight hour period of restorative REM, it simply provides the individual with a small period of respite from the torture. And that can be valuable. In some respects, sedation was my only relief for a long time. I would take the pills and within twenty minutes I would know that there would be no more for a good two hours. Of course, now looking back, I can see that the sedation saved me from the more permanent and final form of respite, that being suicide.

Loss has long been considered a key issue in depression. Styron discussed this at some length:

> Loss in all its manifestations is the touchstone of depression ... I felt loss at every hand. The loss of self-esteem is a celebrated symptom, and my own sense of self had all but disappeared along with my self-reliance. This loss can quickly degenerate into dependence, and from dependence into infantile dread. One dreads the loss of all things, all people close and dear. There is an acute fear of abandonment. Being alone in the house, even for a moment, caused me exquisite panic and trepidation.
>
> Of the images recollected from that time the most bizarre and discomfiting remains the one of me, age four and a half, tagging through a market after my long-suffering wife; not for an instant could I let out of my sight the endlessly patient soul who had become a nanny, mommy, comforter, priestess, and most importantly, confidante – a counsellor of rock-like centrality to my existence whose wisdom far exceeded that of Dr Gold.
>
> ... There is no doubt that as one nears the penultimate depths of depression – which is to say just before the stage when one begins to act out one's suicide instead of being a mere contemplator of it – the acute sense of loss is connected with a knowledge of life slipping away at accelerated speed. One develops fierce attachments. Ludicrous things – my reading glasses, a handkerchief, a certain writing instrument – become the object of my demented possessiveness. Each momentary misplacement filled me with a frenzied dismay, each item being the tactile reminder of a world soon to be obliterated.

Whereas Styron described his extensive rumination and plans for suicide, others act more impulsively and others again, such as Campbell (1988), are inhibited by the effect of their intended suicide:

> Ironically, the inertia of depression makes killing myself very difficult because I just cannot think of a way to kill myself painlessly without making a mess of my body and without distressing the family. The risk I fear is suddenly being faced with the opportunity to kill myself on the spur of the moment.

For some, depression is part of a bipolar illness. This description by Kay Jamison of her own illness raises aspects of the unpleasant and frightening dysphoria of mania, its associated amnesia, the damage caused by these episodes to relationships, finances and occupation, the shame, the fear of recurrence and the lack of certainty about the sufferer's true identity. These and other issues are discussed in more detail elsewhere in this book:

> There is a particular kind of pain, elation, loneliness, and terror involved in this kind of madness. When you're high it's tremendous. The ideas and feelings are fast and frequent like shooting stars and you follow them until you find better and brighter ones. Shyness goes, the right word and gestures are suddenly there. The power to seduce and captivate others a felt certainty. There are interests found in uninteresting people. Sensuality is pervasive and the desire to seduce and be seduced irresistible. Feelings of ease, intensity, power, well-being, financial omnipotence, and euphoria now pervade one's marrow. But, somewhere, this changes. The fast ideas are far too fast and there are

> far too many; overwhelming confusion replaces clarity. Memory goes. Humour and absorption on friends' faces are replaced by fear and concern. Everything previously moving with the grain is now against – you are irritable, angry, uncontrollable, and enmeshed totally in the blackest caves of the mind. You never knew those caves were there. It will never end. Madness carves its own reality. It goes on and on and finally there are only others, recollections of your behaviour – your bizarre, frenetic, aimless behaviours – for mania has at least some grace in partly obliterating memories. What then, after the medications, psychiatrist, despair, depression, and overdose? All those incredible feelings to sort through. Who is being too polite to say what? Who knows what? What did I do? Why? And most hauntingly, when will it happen again? Then, too, are the annoyances – medicine to take, resent, forget, take, resent, and forget, but always to take. Credit cards revoked, bounced cheques to cover, explanations due at work, apologies to make, intermittent memories of vague men (what did I do?) friendships gone or drained, a ruined marriage. And always, when will it happen again? Which of my feelings are real? Which of the me's is me? The wild, impulsive, chaotic, energetic and crazy one? Or the shy, withdrawn, desperate, suicidal, doomed and tired one? Probably a bit of both, hopefully much that is neither. Virginia Woolf, in her dives and climbs, said it all: 'How far do our feelings take their colour from the dive underground? I mean, what is the reality of any feeling?'
>
> Jamison (1995)

People who have had repeated protracted depressions or unstable bipolar disorder often complain of their difficulty identifying their 'normal' mood state, and sense of true self.

The lack of obvious evidence of illness with depression is a particular difficulty, leading to expectations that people with the condition should be able to manage their lives as usual, without any of the allowances afforded those with more obvious conditions. Styron (1992) used the term walking wounded to describe people suffering from depression:

> For in virtually any other serious sickness, a patient who felt similar devastation would be lying flat in bed, possibly sedated and hooked up on tubes and wires of life-support systems, but at the very least in a posture of repose and in an isolated setting. His invalidism would be necessary, unquestioned and honourably attained. However, the sufferer from depression has no such option and therefore finds himself, like a walking casualty of war, thrust into the most intolerable social and family situations. There he must, despite the anguish devouring his brain, present a face approximating the one that is associated with ordinary events and companionship. He must try to utter small talk, and be responsive to questions, and knowingly nod and frown and, God help him, smile. But it is a fierce trial attempting to speak a few simple words.

On recovery from depression, there may be an unspoken conspiracy by both the person recovered from depression and those around them to avoid discussing what happened during that period, to the extent that the person may come to doubt the reality of their original experience, as described here by Custance (1952). This may lead the individual to underestimate the benefit of relapse prevention measures:

> But once I get out of a mental hospital all this changes. I find myself in a totally different 'atmosphere'. I cannot, however hard I try, get even my most intimate relatives and friends to understand or take any interest in what may or may not have happened to me during my 'madness'. Gradually the vividness of my memory fades; like my relatives, I try to put the whole experience out of my mind, and in fact it does to a certain extent disappear into 'lower levels of my Unconsciousness'. Then I find myself genuinely wondering whether these memories so far as they are conscious at all, are not 'delusions', 'hallucinations', as unreal as the actual technical hallucination I know I have had ...
>
> Others strive to come to terms with the experience and integrate it into their concept of self, even identifying some positive aspects of the experience. For me, 'recovery' is living with an absence of symptoms but with constant medication and self-monitoring. I could never say I was lucky or privileged to experience depression. However, learning to survive with depression has taught me some valuable 'life' lessons. I still consider my initial years working to survive as the time of my life that I have worked harder than any other so I suppose it taught me a good work ethic. Above all else, I think I learnt about human vulnerability which has meant I place the utmost value on those aspects of life that we often, at a young age at least, take for granted – family, friends, good health and a state of being that enables you to nurture and enjoy those things.
>
> Quoted in Goodwin and Jamison (1990)

In recent years, there has been a reconsideration of terms such as *treatment response* and *treatment outcome*. It has been increasingly recognised that outcomes can be, and should be, seen from several different perspectives. The concept of recovery, as envisaged by the Mental Health Commission of New Zealand, is the ability to live well in the presence or absence of one's mental illness, with *living well* defined by the person with the mental illness. Part of this process involves affected people taking charge of their lives for themselves, as indicated in the following extracts:

> Depression is never the same – in each episode there is always something different. It gives you strength, it gives you knowledge. But the people around you have to be aware that just because you've been depressed before doesn't mean you know what to do. All I can do is ask my friends and family to support me and to help and when I don't need help to let me get on with it and not be too protective.
>
> Emma (1999)

> Now, if I felt that I wasn't having a good day I would be less inclined to stick my head under the pillow. I have more strategies. I believe that finding someone and talking to them is helpful, and being open about what's wrong with me rather than trying to hide it. I think the shame

> and the guilt stuff is really crippling because that's the stuff that puts you to bed and puts your head under the pillow and you don't want to see anybody. Now I can say, 'Look, I'm not feeling so good today. Can I come and talk to you or can I just come and be with you?' I would never have been able to do that years ago. I can remember sitting in the bath sobbing, and I had a flatmate who was very very good to me and I didn't speak to her for a week. I just completely withdrew. But I don't see it as a good way for me any more. I know it's hard sometimes not to withdraw but I've got to actually make the effort to talk.
>
> Cummings (1999)

> Sometimes I feel, 'Here I am again. Why am I not in control?' Every time you think you're getting it right, you punish yourself severely if you get to that bad place again. One of my recovery messages for myself is that if you do get there again, you mustn't punish yourself for that. That just makes it worse. There are no good things about being there, but it's a real thing and it's me. It's part of who I am.
>
> I have a history of investigation in my recovery. Trying to record what I thought the problem was, looking for reasons, as well as solutions. One thing I used to do was blame. I'd blame my boyfriend or whoever was around me – 'it's because he doesn't tell me he loves me enough' or something. Then after the psychiatrist told me about neurotransmissions, it was their fault. Then I decided it was the contraceptive pill's fault. It was all because of hormones. At one point, I thought it was a post-natal depression. Then I decided it might have been because of things that happened a long, long time ago when I was a kid. There was an event that happened when I was nine years old on the beach, and it did have a very profound effect on me. So I thought it was that for a while. Then I looked at some other men in my life and thought it's all their fault. Now I'm way past all that blaming. It might be a mixture of all those things or it might be none of those things. It doesn't really matter. All of those things had an impact on who I am and what my life is. The blaming thing is not helpful. It's not why I am depressed that matters, it's how I deal with it.
>
> Thompson (1999)

> I have all these protections that I use. If I am going somewhere, I make sure that I am not going to expose myself to something that I know is not going to be good for me, or good for my health. I like to plan things and I like things to go to plan. If they don't go to plan I go to pieces, so I have to be in control of that plan and other people just have to understand that.
>
> Tawhai (1999)

On recovery, there is sometimes consideration of the risks of inheritance, particularly with bipolar disorder. This involves not only a decision whether or not to have children but also a sense of guilt that one may have passed on 'defective' genes. Joshua Logan (1976) described a discussion with his first wife:

> I asked her if she wanted to have children with me.
> She said no.
> I asked her why, but she refused to answer ... she would never have children by me, and that I should know why. I looked at her blankly, and she added:
> 'I have no wish to bring insane children into this world.'

Not uncommonly, relatives, particularly children, of a depressed person will be concerned about the risk of developing the same disorder, particularly if they identify closely with that parent. Indeed, they can be so sensitised to the features of a depressive illness that they may fear that relatively minor symptoms reflect more serious problems, and present with fear of depression rather than depression itself. Sadly for some, their fears will eventually be realised.

Any description of the experience of depression would be incomplete without some reference to the process of treatment. Styron (1992) described the sense of asylum he experienced in hospital, after a protracted and unsuccessful period of outpatient treatment:

> ... in fact, the hospital was my salvation, and it is something of a paradox that in this austere place with its locked and wired doors and desolate green hallways – ambulances screeching night and day ten floors below – I found the repose, the assuagement of the tempest in my brain, that I was unable to find in my quiet farmhouse.
> This is partly the result of sequestration, of safety, of being removed to a world in which the urge to pick up a knife and plunge it into one's own breast disappeared in the newfound knowledge, quickly apparent even to the depressive's fuzzy brain, that the knife with which he is attempting to cut his dreadful Swiss steak is bendable plastic. But the hospital also offers the mild, oddly gratifying trauma of sudden stabilisation – a transfer out of the too familiar surroundings of home, where all is anxiety and discord, into an orderly and benign detention where one's only duty is to try to get well. For me, the real healers were seclusion and time.

Many people experience suboptimal (and worse) treatment for their depression. There are many reasons for this, which will not be explored here. Styron offered a caustic but pertinent account of several aspects of his own treatment, which highlights an understandable resentment of rigid adherence to a particular model of treatment irrespective of the needs, wishes or interests of those directed to receive this:

> Our class was run by a delirious young woman with a fixed, indefatigable smile, who was plainly trained at a school offering courses in Teaching Art to the Mentally Ill; not even a teacher of very young retarded children could have been compelled to bestow, without deliberate instruction, such orchestrated chuckles and coos ... she would tell us to make drawings of themes that we ourselves had chosen. For example: My House. In humiliated rage I obeyed, drawing a square, with a door and four cross-eyed windows, a chimney on top issuing forth a curlicue of smoke. She showered me with praise.

However, it is perhaps more valuable to stress what patients have found useful, and the final two extracts offer some guidance on this:

> I remember sitting in your office a hundred times during those grim months and each time thinking, what on earth can he say that will make me feel better or keep me alive? Well, there never was anything you could say, that's the funny thing. It was all the stupid, desperately optimistic, condescending things you didn't say that kept me alive; all the compassion and warmth I felt from you that could not have been said; all the intelligence, competence, and time you put into it; and your granite belief that mine was a life worth living. You were terribly direct which was terribly important, and you were willing to admit the limits of your understanding and treatments when you were wrong. Most difficult to put into words but in many ways the essence of everything. You taught me that the road from suicide to life is cold and colder and colder still, but – with steely effort, the grace of God, and an inevitable break in the weather – that I could make it.
>
> Patient's account to Goodwin and Jamison (1990)

In her book *Beyond All Reason*, Morag Coate (1964) said:

> Living as a patient in a mental hospital is an illuminating way of discovering what doctors are like and what their work can mean. The psychiatrists who are most concerned about their patients must suffer much stress and many disappointments, but they might well be warmed to know the tributes paid to them in those night-time discussions that they never hear …
>
> Because the doctors cared, and one of them still believed in me when I believed in nothing, I have survived to tell this tale. It is not only the doctors who perform hazardous operations or give life saving drugs in obvious emergencies who hold the scales at times between life and death. To sit quietly in a consulting room and talk to someone would not appear to the general public as a heroic or dramatic thing to do. In medicine there are many different ways of saving lives. This is one of them.
>
> Quoted in Goodwin and Jamison (1990)

REFERENCES

Campbell MEJ (1988) *Not Always on the Level*. London: The Memoir Club.

Cummings P (1999). In Leibrich J (ed), *A Gift of Stories*. Wellington: University of Otago Press/Mental Health Commission.

Emma (1999) In *The Sun Will Shine Again: Stories of survival and optimism in the face of mental illness*. Wellington: Schizophrenia Fellowship, p. 17.

Goodwin FK, Jamison KR (1990) *Manic–Depressive Illness*. New York: Oxford University Press.

Jamison KR (1995) *An Unquiet Mind. A memoir of moods and madness*. New York: Alfred A Knopf.

Logan J (1976) *Josh: My Up and Down, In and Out Life*. New York: Delacorte Press.

Milligan S, Clare A (1994) *Depression and How to Survive it*. London: Arrow.

Styron W (1992) *Darkness Visible. A memoir of madness*. New York, NY: Random House.

Tawhai S (1999) In Leibrich J (ed), *A Gift of Stories*. Wellington: University of Otago Press/Mental Health Commission, p. 54.

Thompson T (1999) In Leibrich J (ed), *A Gift of Stories*. Wellington: University of Otago Press/Mental Health Commission, p. 54.

CHAPTER 2

SURVIVING BIPOLAR DISORDER

Neil Cole and
Suresh Sundrum

Before discussing the topic of surviving bipolar disorder, it is probably wise to discuss the term *surviving*, for it should be something one can talk about in the past tense. It is, however, not quite that simple. Surviving a mental illness is ongoing – it is not as if one has recovered or is recovering. Surviving bipolar, or any illness for that matter, suggests there is something fatal about the illness. Although there is that side to the illness (with a very high rate of suicide), it is also about surviving the illness per se. This means to come through the harsher elements of it and, after diagnosis, being able to live a relatively stable life conscious of the vagaries of the illness, including its medications, symptoms and treatment. It is also about enduring the isolation one feels from others who are well, who go on living oblivious to the fact that you might be going through a phase of not caring whether you go on, or the opposite feeling that they can't keep up with you.

That I survived is in some ways a mystery to me, for they were truly some of the more difficult times of my life. At the same time, I did fulfil a very productive life, was married, had young children and was a Member of Parliament. My life was not as productive as it should have been, but it was none the less quite productive. The consequences of the illness were all too apparent once diagnosed, including separation, failed career as a Member of Parliament, and financial difficulties. The parliamentary career was to dissolve after diagnosis; however, many of my problems were set in train much earlier.

Once I had been diagnosed, stigma became an issue. Although it did not worry me to have the illness, I knew it would be problematic once people knew. From a career point of view, it could be used against me. This did not particularly worry me because, in a sense, there is always something that will be used against you in politics. Moreover, I felt no shame at having the illness. It was probably more difficult within my marriage and friendships because when I did explain it to people, they didn't have any understanding of the illness. Comments like 'we didn't think you had anything wrong with you' or 'we all have our ups and downs' were common and frustrating.

This was much worse with my wife. I at least had some conception of what I was doing and what was illness or not. It was much more difficult for her to sort out whether a behaviour was illness-related or just me. It became vital that she be given information as to what symptoms she could expect to see in me and to understand that this was an illness, not just me being difficult or impossible to live with. It was even harder for my young sons, who had little conception of why I would behave unusually or say odd things when I was either manic or depressed, and then change again. The effect of delayed diagnosis on both my marriage and my children cannot be underestimated, and the lack of information from my previous treating doctors once I was diagnosed is difficult to understand now. This information needn't be exhaustive but simply explaining that my symptoms, especially my libido, were a function of my illness and as difficult to control as, say, pain is would have been helpful for my wife and our marriage. I don't know how the effect on my children could have been lessened, unless things were patiently explained to them by their mother or me, or even by a health care professional, but we didn't know how to do it and the doctors seem to have forgotten our children.

The symptoms of the illness were multiple and marked. They included an unstoppable flight of ideas. These were particularly bad at night and made it hard to sleep, or coexisted with insomnia – I would lie awake with thoughts racing so fast I couldn't remember them. Lack of sleep was a constant problem: a couple of hours a night, sometimes none. Libido issues were a major problem. For the manic person the libido drives them; it's insatiable and leads to a lack of sexual inhibition. The desire to achieve sexual satisfaction is so overwhelming it is difficult to concentrate on anything else. Trying to resist or stop it is, as I said, almost as difficult as trying to stop a bad pain – almost impossible.

Excessive spending, or spending without regard to the consequences of your actions, is one of the most peculiar aspects of the illness and most pronounced. It is not just the amount of money spent but also the manner. Including a total lack of appreciation of how much money a person has. This is coupled with a belief that there is no shortage of money, or that somehow the money issue will sort itself out.

One can become very irritable when manic. Agitated as well as aggressive, coupled with intolerance of other people's views. My mind was moving so fast, I was talking very quickly and emphatically. It was infuriating when people would disagree, didn't understand me or seemingly couldn't keep up. This was exacerbated by the flight of ideas that I had, which were always numerous, quite good sometimes, even brilliant, original and worthy of consideration, yet just as often ill considered and foolhardy. Very often, my brilliant ideas were ephemeral. Pursuing one idea one day as if there was no tomorrow, then not even considering it the next makes you look unstable and erratic.

This irritability always seemed justified to me. It was other people who couldn't keep up. The intensity of the irritability paralleled my mania and was inverse to my self-control or self-monitoring. It was enormously difficult to keep under check and would seep out even in situations or with people where it was unjustified or inappropriate. Because it can be such a destructive symptom, I now constantly monitor myself for signs of it, which of course is a fraught exercise as irritation and annoyance are inevitable features of all our lives. Not only does a person with bipolar have to experience and deal with irritation, he or she also has to worry that it may be a sign of impending relapse.

All of this came with a sense of grandiosity – somehow believing that I was more important than others, that I was, or potentially was, a great person. There wasn't much I couldn't do, including becoming a Minister. While this was possible, it was poorly motivated: namely, to promote myself publicly.

I was imbued with an elevated feeling that there was nothing or very little that could stop me. Others would feel how uplifted I was and they would, particularly the not so strong, be buoyed by my energy, drive and commitment. During these periods I had an abundance of energy when not preoccupied, and even when preoccupied with high sexual drive, could be very productive. Disastrous in a relationship, because if your partner can't keep up there is a tendency to say, 'if you don't like it, leave'. At work I would often make excessive phone calls to people, pushing the wonderful ideas that I had. One tends to be a bit open and honest about things, which invariably leads to becoming vulnerable.

During these high phases, I was often very sensitive, particularly to taste. Occasionally I would have a glass of red wine at lunch. The taste of it was so nice that I wanted to have more. Then I started to believe I was becoming an alcoholic because it was so nice to drink. So I gave up drinking. I drank very little, never at night and only sometimes at lunchtime. However, this was my reaction and the feeling was very real that I was starting to like it too much.

I've been lucky in being able to regulate my alcohol intake and not being involved with illicit drugs. The impact these have had in acquaintances in triggering or worsening episodes of both mania and depression both by themselves and by decreasing compliance with treatment, the financial cost and, most importantly, the burden on family, work and social life have created havoc. I know one person whose early symptom of mania is a taste for heroin, a drug he experimented with as a young man. Now in his 40s, his previous two manic episodes have seen him lose his marriage and then his house in trying to pay for his habit without resorting to crime. When well, he stops and reflects upon the devastation it has caused. Since he started seeing a psychiatrist, his next manic episode saw him spend only $600 on heroin, and he didn't use at all for the most recent episode. This indicates the importance of recognising substance abuse as a symptom and getting in early and effective treatment.

There are things that are common to both manic and depressive phases. I have already mentioned the alienating effect on relationships and alcohol and drugs, but two that don't get thought of much are sleep and stress. For me, both manic and depressive phases are almost heralded by poor sleep, the difference being that in the manic phase I don't want to or feel the need to sleep, whereas when depressed it seems like an impossible goal and even when I do sleep it is never enough or refreshing. Too often the doctor considers sleep problems secondary, that somehow they will resolve once the episode has resolved. In fact, I find that aggressively dealing with the sleep problems not only shortens the episode but lessens the distress and suffering associated with the episode. Doctors, rather than ignoring or dismissing sleep difficulties, should see them (at least for some people) as an early warning sign and an opportunity for early intervention. The other similar aspect to both types of episodes is the role of stress. Every kind of stress – financial, family, relationship, social or occupational – can play its part in triggering off an episode, either manic or depressive. I am wary of engaging in stressful situations for fear of the effect it will have on my mental health. This is an important preventive strategy, but it also limits what I feel I want to take on, especially work and relationships.

When I was depressed, the symptoms were the exact opposite. One time I was so hit by inertia all I could do was sit in a beanbag, with no energy, watch television and eat chocolate. I believed there was no point in living and had an all-prevailing sense of hopelessness about me. Everything lacks meaning and despondency takes over. I used to feel I'll be 50 in fifteen years time; I'll have to go through this for another fifteen years, what's the point? There didn't seem any point in doing so and the pain of continuing seemed too great to have to put up with for that long. My appetite subsided except for food that gave me instant gratification, particularly sweet things. Together with the feeling of hopelessness came a lack of interest in things that normally I was very interested in. I didn't care about my football team, my partner, my job. This lack of interest made me very dismissive of things. Things that were once important weren't anymore. What was quite rightly important to other people wasn't to me. We all get things out of perspective from time to time; my problem was throwing everything out because I didn't care and lacked interest. My libido also subsided for months on end. After a while of not caring about anything, I would start to have suicidal thoughts. These were pervasive and made it very hard to think about anything else. Sometimes they would include the way it might be done, other times it was just a feeling of: one could die now and be content with that. The feeling is just overwhelming, although it isn't just about suicide per se, but that feeling that death could be a good thing because it would end it all. Other times, and quite often, I would have the opposite feeling of anxiety about dying. That I was going to die one day, I was getting older and it wasn't far away. While these contradictory feelings would overcome me, one thing remained constant – my children. The thought of leaving them, no matter how depressed

I was, was so hurtful that it became my reason for living. Equally, when I was anxious, it was them I thought about and was most scared of leaving.

While depressed, I could become very self-centred. My feelings of uselessness and bleakness would dominate my conversations and the topic of conversation would always be my view of the world or the state of things. Often as not, I would phone people and tell them how I was feeling. At the same time, for whatever reason, seeing the dark side of things could also mean seeing people's plight and understanding their problems. There was an increase in sensitivity to other people's problems: not only could I be very sympathetic, they could also make me more depressed. Part of depression is the ability to see things other people cannot see, or to see them in a way that other people can't or don't want to.

Then there was the utter loneliness. The feeling of being alone in a crowded room is one of the most frightening of all. Worse still is when you are alone and lonely. Then there was another state of fearing being alone. The thought that you knew you had to be by yourself and to be so scared of that.

Through all of this, your judgment becomes flawed. Fear of being alone makes you seek out people. This is a problem because you are vulnerable: vulnerable because you are beholden to people whose company you want. If, on top of this, you are obsessed, not capable of thinking rationally and scared of not having company, then you do imprudent things and agree to do things you shouldn't.

After 10 years on lithium, I would have to give it credit for being the single biggest reason for my surviving and living a relatively normal and happy life. It took away almost immediately any problems with high libido, spending, relaxed my fast thought process, slowed down my talking, and even allowed me to sit still for prolonged periods. The flight of ideas changed dramatically. Although I had many ideas before that used to race through my head, once I went onto lithium the thoughts didn't go, they just did not race through my head at such a fast rate. This led to a dramatic change in my life for the first time I became very interested in creative writing. After lithium I began writing, first comedy sketches then plays. My mind became channelled towards writing plays more as a hobby, although a time-consuming one, and as a way of occupying my mind with something that was interesting and fulfilling. That I could now concentrate for prolonged periods made a big difference to my life. It is hard to explain the feeling of being able to sit and write for prolonged periods and not feel the need to make a phone call; to get up and go for a walk; to go and talk to someone.

There have still been times when I was high. However, certain things that were there before lithium are gone and do not seem to be recurring for me. In fact, these days any signs of being high are usually readily identifiable. Feeling unusually happy, not being able to sleep at all, wanting to clean everything out of my house. As part of my survival mechanism, I do not carry credit cards and I try to tie my money up so I cannot get to it quickly. For some people it can be wise to see a financial counsellor who can suggest other ways of tying up money so that in a manic phase the person doesn't blow away their house or superannuation.

The antidepressants, on the other hand, have done a lot to restore my mood. The difference between being depressed and not is quite stark. For me, antidepressants have been able to reverse my mood state so much that if all the symptoms of depression described above applied they would go with the antidepressants. Not all antidepressants worked for me – it was a process of trial and error. However, once the right one was struck, it made a profound difference.

One of the problems with antidepressants is that they can have side effects. For me, lack of sleep has been a problem. It can be extremely frustrating not being able to sleep, particularly when it drags on over many nights without respite. Sexual dysfunction can also occur with some antidepressants. Antidepressants can lower libido quite substantially, an unfortunate consequence given it is one of the symptoms of depression that the drug is trying to counteract.

Complying with medication has never been a real problem for me. There have been few side effects from taking lithium. In the early days, this caused a tremor in my hands. I put on weight; however, this was, I think, mostly due to increased fluid intake because lithium tends to make you thirsty. My mouth gets very dry sometimes. Sometimes, of course, the dosage has to be increased and this can make you very thirsty.

Balancing the medications is always difficult. To know if you are going high and to perhaps change your medication is not as simple as it might sound. Often you don't know you are high, or of an elevated mood. You think that you are just a little happier or the house does need to be cleaned out. It is why it is so important to see a psychiatrist on a regular basis, to discuss mood variations, be monitored in general and to have someone to talk through what has been happening. Only then would the medication be varied up or down.

Over the years, my illness has become like a companion. It never leaves. Mood variations, by definition, are not constant. They move up and down! Sometimes they are a disorder; most of the time they are not. Living with the constant thought that if you are happy you might be high or if you are down and despondent it might be depression or just daily life stress is not easy. It is also not impossible. However, it is always there.

The mere fact that each morning and each night you have to take medication is a reminder of the illness. It can be a good reminder of course, because it reminds you what a difference the medication has made to your life. It can also make you think about where you are at that moment in yourself.

Over the years, matters have arisen in dealing with doctors that I wished had been done differently or better. The most important was the lack of information that was given to my wife and what we should have said to the children about my illness. The second was developing a set of early warning signs that I was in imminent danger of relapsing either into a manic or depressive episode. As I've stated, for me disturbed sleep and irritation are good pointers; for others it may be increasing drug use, spending too much, or thinking about death. It is going to be different for each person and it can be very hard for that person or his or her family to work out by themselves.

Rather than working it out over many episodes, it would have saved a lot of trouble if we'd been made aware that there is a similarity or signature to the episodes. Both my wife and I being aware of it might have enabled us to get treatment for me started or adjusted earlier. Even if such a description is modified over time, it is of tremendous benefit, more so if combined with a plan as to how to access treatment immediately. The last thing is that it's hard enough to get in to see a psychiatrist, let alone find one. I've been fortunate in that my psychiatrist of recent times has been accessible. I know, however, how much easier it is if there is regular contact between the psychiatrist and the GP. If the GP has some confidence and knowledge in recognising symptoms and signs of relapse and then adjusting medication it makes life so much easier, but is entirely dependent on the GP and the psychiatrist communicating.

Since diagnosis, there have been significant changes in my life. Being treated has meant the illness doesn't dominate my life as it did before diagnosis, even though I didn't know it. It meant that, even though the treatment wasn't perfect, I was and am being treated. It is possible to live a comfortable life without the all-pervasive symptoms of a mental illness. There are still many issues and times when I feel much worse than others; however, the difference is stark. It is possible to live a full life and do most things that most other people do.

Perhaps the biggest single issue in surviving bipolar is that it is ongoing, it's chronic. Medications work and are getting better. They only work if the mood swings are adequately monitored. They only work if you have a life plan for handling day-to-day matters and long-term goals. I don't carry credit cards because of the risk of using them imprudently while high. I keep my house free of clutter so it doesn't make me anxious and annoyed that I have to throw everything out. This doesn't mean I haven't or don't go high, rather they are defence mechanisms against the extremes of the illness. However, on top of this, it is necessary to address the issue itself if I do go high by knowing the signs and speaking to my psychiatrist on the phone or at her office. It is like having a work plan, or a plan of action. That's why the illness is always with me in a sense – one has to be planning ahead and on guard for changes in mood.

I have been diagnosed for 10 years now. When my psychiatrist told me I was manic–depressive I didn't know what it was. It has taken me many years to learn a lot about the illness. I've been hospitalised once for three weeks and have had bouts of mania and depression. Mostly depression. The illness isn't as pervasive, but it's not going away. We learn to live with it. We survive it.

SECTION

II

Phenomenology and Classification

CHAPTER 3

THE ASSESSMENT AND CLASSIFICATION OF DEPRESSION

Peter R Joyce

The core symptomatology of depression or melancholia has been recognised for thousands of years, and classical descriptions are easily recognised today (Jackson 1986). Many of the best descriptions of depression are provided by articulate individuals from all walks of life who report their own experiences (Styron 1990; Jamison 1995). Depression has been recognised across cultures, and can also be recognised in species other than humans. Studies in primates strongly suggest that depression is not a uniquely human disorder.

Although depression and mania are classified as *mood disorders*, or affective disorders, in the World Health Organization's *International Classification of Diseases* (ICD) and in the American Psychiatric Association's *Diagnostic and Statistical Manual of Mental Disorders* (DSM), it is not clear that *mood*, or affect, is the primary or fundamental pathological change. In both depression and mania, the sadness or depressed mood and the elation or euphoria may be epiphenomena of more fundamental psychopathological changes in energy, motivation or activation. Many patients with depression admit to loss of enjoyment, pleasure, energy and motivation and disturbed sleep, appetite and concentration, but do not acknowledge sadness or depressed mood. Similarly, many patients with mania do not experience euphoria or elation.

In DSM-IV, the necessary symptomatology for a major depressive episode is a period of at least 2 weeks during which there is either a depressed mood or a loss of interest or pleasure in most activities, and at least four additional symptoms from a list of changes in appetite or weight, disturbed sleep, altered psychomotor activity, decreased energy, feelings of worthlessness or guilt, impaired concentration, thinking or decisiveness, and recurrent thoughts of death or suicidal ideation or behaviour. All symptoms must be present most of the day, most days, for at least 2 weeks, and be associated with significant distress or impairment. However, impairment may include superficially normal functioning but an increased effort is required to carry on with normal activities. Typically, an individual continues to work, but personal, family and leisure activities largely cease. The DSM-IV criteria for a major depressive episode are shown in Box 3.1

BOX 3.1

THE DSM-IV CRITERIA FOR MAJOR DEPRESSIVE EPISODE

A Five (or more) of the following symptoms have been present during the same two week period and represent a change from previous functioning; at least one of the symptoms is either (1) depressed mood or (2) loss of interest or pleasure.

Note: Do not include symptoms that are clearly due to a general medical condition, or mood-incongruent delusions or hallucinations.

1. depressed mood most of the day, nearly every day, as indicated by either subjective report (e.g., feels sad or empty) or observation made by others (e.g., appears tearful)
2. markedly diminished interest or pleasure in all, or almost all, activities most of the day, nearly every day (as indicated by either subjective account or observation made by others)
3. significant weight loss when not dieting or weight gain (e.g., a change of more than 5% of body weight in a month), or decrease or increase in appetite nearly every day
4. insomnia or hypersomnia nearly every day
5. psychomotor agitation or retardation nearly every day (observable by others, not merely subjective feelings of restlessness or being slowed down)
6. fatigue or loss of energy nearly every day
7. feelings of worthlessness or excessive or inappropriate guilt (which may be delusional) nearly every day (not merely self-reproach or guilt about being sick)
8. diminished ability to think or concentrate, or indecisiveness, nearly every day (either by subjective account or as observed by others)
9. recurrent thoughts of death (not just fear of dying), recurrent suicidal ideation without a specific plan, or a suicide attempt or a specific plan for committing suicide.

B The symptoms do not meet criteria for a Mixed Episode.

C The symptoms cause clinically significant distress or impairment in social, occupational, or other important areas of functioning.

D The symptoms are not due to the direct physiological effects of a substance (e.g., a drug of abuse, a medication) or a general medical condition (e.g., hypothyroidism).

E The symptoms are not better accounted for by Bereavement, i.e., after the loss of a loved one, the symptoms persist for longer than 2 months or are characterized by marked functional impairment, morbid preoccupation with worthlessness, suicidal ideation, psychotic symptoms or psychomotor retardation.

SOURCE Reprinted with permission from the *Diagnostic and Statistical Manual of Mental Disorders*, Fourth Edition, Text Revision. Copyright American Psychiatric Association 2000.

After a major depressive episode has been recognised and diagnosed, it should be further indicated as to whether it is an episode within a bipolar disorder or whether it is a major (unipolar, or non-bipolar) depressive disorder. The episode should also be specified by severity (mild, moderate, severe without psychotic features, severe with psychotic features), and whether it is current or in partial or full remission. Additional specifiers for a major depressive episode include melancholic features, atypical features, catatonic features, chronic, with post-partum onset or seasonal pattern. Before discussing current criteria for these subtypes of depression, it is useful to consider the history of depression diagnosis and the objectives of any classification system.

RELIABILITY, VALIDITY AND UTILITY OF CLASSIFICATIONS

The purpose of any classification system is to assist clinical practice. A system will be useful if different clinicians and consumers can use terms and definitions consistently and reliably. To achieve reliability, explicit definitions (criteria) have been in widespread use since the 1970s, and were formally incorporated into diagnostic systems (DSM-III) in 1980 by the American Psychiatric Association, and later by the World Health Organization in ICD-10. For a diagnostic system to assist clinical practice, reliability is but the first step; ultimately, diagnostic systems must be valid and have utility (Kendell and Jablensky 2003). In most instances, this means that the diagnosis should give us information about aetiology, pathophysiology, prognosis or treatment. Although a diagnosis of major depressive disorder provides clinicians with some information, such as increased familial risk of depression, increased likelihood of future depressive symptoms, increased risk of suicidal behaviour and likelihood of improvement with a range of antidepressant drugs and psychological therapies, the boundaries of major depression (which include five symptom criteria, 14 days' duration and functional impairment) have little empirical support. Thus, DSM-IV major depression may be a diagnostic convention imposed on a continuum of depressive symptoms (Kendler and Gardner 1998).

DSM-IV defines *dysthymia* as a depressive disorder with a duration of at least 2 years. However, most patients who meet criteria for dysthymia have at some stage in their depression history also met criteria for a major depressive episode. Given the lack of empirical support for a major depressive episode, the boundaries of this with dysthymia are also problematic. Thus, it is most useful to consider major depressive episodes and dysthymia as conventions that relate to number of depressive symptoms and chronicity, and that identify a broad and heterogeneous syndrome of depression. This syndrome may be better represented as a continuum, rather than as a discrete category (Angst and Merikangas 2001), although clinicians are likely to continue to find that a categorical system has greater utility (Kendell and Jablensky 2003).

Historically, the greatest debate in the classification of depression has not been about the boundaries of major depression, but whether depression is a unitary syndrome or whether there are two or more disorders of differing aetiologies and responses to treatment that constitute the broader depressive syndrome. The binary view of depression held that *endogenous*, or *melancholic*, depression is a distinct entity to other (for example, *neurotic*, or *reactive*) depressions, and has a different aetiology and response to treatment. At the extreme, it was considered that melancholic depressions were associated with a family history of depression, adequate premorbid personality functioning, absence of life events as precipitating factors, a good response to tricyclic antidepressants (or electroconvulsive therapy) and a poor response to psychotherapies. Conversely, neurotic depression was associated with an interplay of personality vulnerability and adverse life events, a poorer response to antidepressants (or to electroconvulsive therapy) and a better response to psychotherapies. Although some people continue to adhere strongly to the view that melancholic depression is a distinct entity (Parker 2000; Roth 2001), most do not consider that the data are sufficiently convincing that melancholia is such a distinct entity, although they are reluctant to discard the concept completely as it has some limited clinical utility and validity (Rush and Weissenburger 1994). The inconsistency of the data supporting the distinctiveness, or otherwise, of melancholia is compounded by the lack of consensus on the essential clinical features for this diagnosis and the lack of agreement between varying definitions of melancholia (Davidson et al. 1988; Joyce et al. 2002). In clinical studies, melancholic depression is consistently more severe than non-melancholic depression. Kendler (1997), in a population-based twin study, found that melancholic major depression is a quantitatively more severe form of depression, but is not aetiologically distinct from non-melancholic depression.

If a classification system were to be based partially on distinct aetiologies, then currently the most distinct aetiological factors are vascular risk factors for some late onset depressive and bipolar disorders (Hickie et al. 2001; Cassidy and Carroll 2002). By contrast, most adolescent and adult onset depressive disorders probably arise from an interaction of genetics, temperament, personality, early life experiences and recent life events (Kendler et al. 2002). Contrary to expectations, individuals with a genetic loading for depression experience more life events before the onset of depressive episodes, rather than fewer, as was predicted by the old binary model of depression (McGuffin et al. 1988). However, Kendler et al. (2001) have suggested that depressive episodes which occur with little provocation arise either from many previous depressive episodes or by high genetic risk.

Currently, the best-validated depressive subtypes arise from data on treatment response. Depression with delusions has a very poor response to tricyclic antidepressants but a satisfactory response to combined tricyclic antidepressant plus antipsychotic drug or to electroconvulsive therapy (Spiker and Kupfer 1988). Preliminary reports with serotonin reuptake inhibitor antidepressants have challenged the historical evidence that antidepressants alone have a low probability of achieving remission in psychotic depression (Gatti et al. 1996). There are additional lines of evidence to support the concept of psychotic depression as a distinct subtype, including a very high rate of activation of the hypothalamic–pituitary–adrenal axis, altered patterns of cerebrospinal fluid and plasma dopamine and noradrenaline and their metabolites, distinct clinical features such as absence of diurnal variation, distinctive sleep electroencephalogram, distinct neurocognitive deficits and increased mortality (Jeste et al. 1996; Nelson and Davis 1997; Vythilingam et al. 2003).

The other depressive subtype with a distinct treatment response is *atypical* depression. The DSM-IV criteria include reactivity of mood, reversed vegetative sleep and appetite symptoms (that is, hypersomnia and hyperphagia) and a personality vulnerability to interpersonal rejection. These criteria may not be the optimal ones, and do not show a strong internal consistency (Parker et al. 2002), but they do identify depressed patients with a poor response to tricyclic antidepressants but a good response to monoamine oxidase inhibitors (Stewart et al. 1989). Depressed patients with atypical features probably respond to selective serotonin reuptake inhibitors (Pande et al. 1996; Joyce et al. In press), although the New York group who did the pioneering work on atypical depression have data that question the superior efficacy of selective serotonin reuptake inhibitors (McGrath et al. 2000).

Over recent years, an emerging area of debate has been the expansion of the *bipolar spectrum* concept (see Chapter 6). The relevance of this to debates about the classification of depression is that the bipolar–unipolar dichotomy has usually taken precedence over subtypes of unipolar depression and there are minimal data on subtypes of bipolar depression. With the expansion of the bipolar spectrum concept, the subtypes of depression will need further re-examination in the light of the changing bipolar–unipolar distinction.

DSM-IV SUBTYPES OF DEPRESSION

In DSM-IV, the first step in classification is to make the diagnosis of a major depressive episode. Based upon a history of hypomania or mania, the distinction is then made between bipolar disorder (including bipolar II disorder or bipolar disorder not otherwise specified) and major (unipolar) depression. The depressive episode (regardless of the bipolar or unipolar distinction) may then be specified.

It is unfortunate that DSM-IV has combined severity (mild, moderate, severe) with psychotic features (severe with mood-congruent psychotic features, severe with mood-incongruent psychotic features), as this implies that all psychotic depressions are severe. In clinical practice this is not inevitable, and there are depressed patients with psychotic features whose depressive symptoms are only mild or moderate. Winokur (1984) has suggested that the vulnerability to develop psychotic features while depressed is inherited independently of any vulnerability to depression. Recent studies raise the possibility that genetic polymorphisms of dopamine ß-hydroxylase influence the probability of *paranoid ideation* in depression (Wood et al. 2002) or under the influence of cocaine (Cubells et al. 2000), rather than psychotic features just being an aspect of severity.

Specifiers in DSM-IV also include whether this is a first or recurrent episode of depression, whether there is a seasonal pattern to recurrent depressions, whether there was a post-partum onset, and whether it is chronic (longer than 2 years' duration). Boxes 3.2 and 3.3 list the DSM-IV criteria for the melancholic and atypical depression specifiers.

BOX 3.2

DSM-IV CRITERIA FOR MELANCHOLIC FEATURES SPECIFIER

Specify if:

With Melancholic Features (can be applied to the current or most recent Major Depressive Episode in Major Depressive Disorder and to a Major Depressive Episode in Bipolar I or Bipolar II Disorder only if it is the most recent type of mood episode).

A Either of the following, occurring during the most severe period of the current episode:
   1 loss of pleasure in all, or almost all, activities
   2 lack of reactivity to usually pleasurable stimuli (does not feel much better, even temporarily, when something good happens).

B Three (or more) of the following:
   1 distinct quality of depressed mood (i.e., the depressed mood is experienced as distinctly different from the kind of feeling experienced after the death of a loved one)
   2 depression regularly worse in the morning
   3 early morning wakening (at least 2 hours before usual time of awakening)
   4 marked psychomotor retardation or agitation
   5 significant anorexia or weight loss
   6 excessive or inappropriate guilt.

BOX 3.3

DSM-IV CRITERIA FOR ATYPICAL FEATURES SPECIFIER

Specify if:

With Atypical Features (can be applied when these features predominate during the most recent 2 weeks of a Major Depressive Episode in Major Depressive Disorder or in Bipolar I or Bipolar II Disorder when the Major Depressive Episode is the most recent type of mood episode, or when these features predominate during the most recent 2 years of Dysthymic Disorder).

A Mood reactivity (i.e., mood brightens in response to actual or potential positive events).

B Two (or more) of the following features:
   1 significant weight gain or increase in appetite
   2 hypersomnia
   3 leaden paralysis (i.e., heavy, leaden feelings in arms or legs)
   4 long-standing pattern of interpersonal rejection sensitivity (not limited to episodes of mood disturbance) that results in significant social or occupational impairment.

C Criteria are not met for With Melancholic Features or with Catatonic Features during the same episode.

OTHER FEATURES OF DEPRESSION

The depressive symptomatology described in DSM-IV and ICD-10 covers only that used in these conventional diagnostic systems, and should not be seen as the full range of phenomena observed in depressive disorders. Although the phenomena used in DSM-IV are routinely enquired about in clinical practice, there is remarkably little systematic research on the wider range of depressive phenomena.

Depressed patients usually exhibit changes in social relationships, especially avoidance, withdrawal, irritability and interpersonal sensitivity. Thus, some depressed patients report not answering the telephone, not answering the door and even hiding from possible visitors. Patients may describe crossing the street to avoid meeting old friends and keeping out of sight if they anticipate seeing someone they know. Within relationships, there may not be only a loss of sexual interest and performance but a withdrawal from intimacy. Sometimes, family and friends are on the receiving end of the irritability and anger that is often symptomatic of depression. Sometimes family are confused by the good appearance a depressed patient presents to strangers, while the family see the irritability, lethargy and anhedonia. With close friends, there are often mixed feelings, in that patients are offended if friends do not make contact but then wish they would leave after just a short time during a visit. In hospital, it is often advisable to suggest that friends and family make frequent but short visits. Some patients, when depressed, may become more dependent, others become jealous, even to the extent of the jealousy being delusional.

In hypomania and mania perceptions may be sharpened, whereas in depression perception may be dulled. Depressed patients may therefore dress in dull clothes, or even neglect their appearance. Whereas manic patients may prefer open spaces and open windows and doors, depressed patients may feel more comfortable in smaller rooms, may draw the curtains, avoid sunlight and wish to hide away.

Anxiety symptoms, including panic attacks, phobias, obsessions and compulsions, are frequently seen in depressed patients. Sometimes these may clearly predate the onset of the depressive episode, but in other cases they emerge simultaneously with the depressive symptoms. Occasionally, depressed patients may report a decrease in obsessions or compulsions during a depressive episode, as if the anhedonia and lethargy of the depression overrides the usual need to undertake the compulsive behaviours. Eating disorder symptomatology may also predate or develop during a depressive episode. Sometimes patients with a depression during which they overeat present to eating disorder services because of their craving, bingeing and concern about body image and shape.

Somatoform phenomenology, including pain, conversion symptoms and hypochondria, are relatively common in depression. In primary care, many depressed patients present with their somatic symptoms and only upon enquiry report the traditional depressive symptoms. Conversely, some who present with clear depressive symptoms may reveal their somatic symptoms or hypochondriacal concerns only with careful questioning.

Although changes in appetite and weight are widely expected during depressive episodes, there may also be a wide range of other gastrointestinal symptoms, including lack of taste, foul taste, foul mouth or body odour, dry mouth, nausea, diarrhoea or constipation. During treatment, the interpretation of diarrhoea or constipation symptoms can be further complicated because of the effects of antidepressants and other medications on gastrointestinal function. The overlap of depression with irritable bowel syndrome requires more research.

Changes in skin and hair may occur during depression, and these are not just because of self-neglect. Skin disorders, notably acne in young people, may be markedly exacerbated by depression. Often the skin becomes more oily, dry or red. Hair may lose its vitality and become dull and flat during depressive episodes.

Changes in the cardiovascular system have been noted in depression, although the best documentation has been in patients with bipolar disorder studied across mood episodes (Lovett Doust et al. 1980). Blood clotting may vary across mood episodes (Ho-Yen et al. 1983). Lithium pharmacokinetics may vary with mood state, with higher plasma levels observed during depression and lower levels during mania (Kukopulos et al. 1985). Many depressed patients show changes in acute phase plasma proteins, inflammatory and immunological parameters (Kronfol and Remick 2000). Similarly, there are extremely well documented changes in the neuroendocrine system, especially in the hypothalamic–pituitary–adrenal and hypothalamic–pituitary–thyroid axes (Pariante and Miller 2001; Bauer et al. 2002; Gold et al. 2002). There are also reports of mood-dependent neurological symptoms, such as tardive dyskinesia. (Changes in neurocognitive functioning are also well described in depression and are discussed in Chapter 12.)

Not all the changes that occur during depressive episodes should automatically be interpreted as pathological. For instance, during depression, patients may perceive the world more accurately, and are certainly able to more accurately assess negative threats. Euthymia may involve the ability to selectively disregard real but negative threats to the integrity of the individual.

ASSESSMENT OF DEPRESSION

The most important tool in the assessment of depression (and bipolar disorder) is obtaining a good psychiatric history. This needs to include not only a history of the current episode but also a history of past mood episodes and symptoms. A comprehensive history would also include information about family history, developmental history, personality functioning, physical disease history, alcohol and drug use and relevant comorbid mental disorders. Often an adequate history requires a history not just from the patient but also from family or friends. The need for history from others is especially important in children, individuals from cultures different from the interviewer's, individuals with intellectual impairment, the severely affectively ill, and may be very important in bipolar patients (especially when in a manic phase of illness). Even in patients able to give a good history of their own illness, it is important to understand that in a single interview some phenomena may well be missed or underestimated. For instance, in one interview, obtaining a history of a past hypomanic episode is relevant, but failing to elicit a past hypomanic episode does not rule out a bipolar diagnosis. In other terms, the reliability for a diagnosis of hypomania based on one interview is low, but this is because the sensitivity rather than the specificity is low (Rice et al. 1986).

In obtaining the history of the current depressive episode, it is necessary to enquire about the onset of symptoms (abrupt onset of symptoms is more common in bipolar disorder), the duration of symptoms, the severity of the episode, the type of symptoms (for example, melancholic, atypical, psychotic) and to assess risk, especially of suicide. It is also necessary to enquire about the life context of the patient at the time of onset of an episode and to ascertain whether particular life events occurred in the months before onset or after the onset of the current depressive episode. Historical evidence of bipolarity is also of importance, as this may influence decisions about management.

RECOGNITION AND NON-RECOGNITION OF DEPRESSION

The key to the recognition and diagnosis of a depressive episode is for the interviewing clinician to have a high index of suspicion for depression and to ensure that the appropriate questions are asked. Studies in primary care across countries have consistently shown that about half of the people with a current major depressive episode are not recognised as such. A variety of factors, apart from too low an index of suspicion, contribute to the non-recognition of depressive disorders in both primary care and mental health services. In primary care settings, it is clear that if patients present with somatic complaints (for example, pain, sleep disturbance) then the probability that a depressive episode will be diagnosed is considerably less than when patients present with psychological complaints.

Another common issue associated with the non-diagnosis (rather than non-recognition) of depressive episodes is the fallacy of *understandability*. In these situations, it is recognised that a patient has some depressive symptoms but, because of presumptions about causes, the symptoms are not carefully enquired about and, as they are deemed understandable, are presumed not to justify a diagnosis of major depression. This happens both in the context of adverse life circumstances (for example, complicated grief) and in the presence of physical illness, where it may be taken to be normal to be depressed. For example, after a stroke, depressive symptoms are dismissed with a statement such as, 'Well, wouldn't you be depressed if you had had a stroke?'. Research to date does not support understandability as a useful factor in determining what treatment should be offered to a patient suffering from a depressive episode; much more important are the duration, severity and type of depressive symptoms.

Another situation where the fallacy of understandability leads to the non-diagnosis of depression is when either the patient or clinician concludes that the current difficulties are a direct result of some childhood factor such as sexual abuse. Although childhood sexual abuse is a risk factor for depression, there are many factors in the aetiology of depression, and selectively focusing on single risk factors and not diagnosing a current depressive episode is usually associated with deficient care being provided for the patient.

Yet another factor that is associated with a failure to diagnose depression is when patients have a comorbid axis I or axis II mental disorder. Just because major complaints focus on eating disorder psychopathology or anxiety symptoms does not mean a depressive disorder is not the principal, or at least a comorbid, diagnosis. Note, however, that depressive symptoms in the context of alcohol dependence are more likely to be substance-induced than an independent mood disorder. Perhaps of greater concern is the non-diagnosis of depression when patients have, or are considered to have, a personality disorder. In this situation, judgmental opinion that the primary psychopathology is a personality disorder (especially borderline or antisocial personality disorders) too often leads to a neglect or dismissal of the depressive symptomatology.

RATING SCALES FOR DEPRESSION

In the assessment of depressed patients, or for epidemiological or genetic studies, various structured interviews have been developed for making a depressive diagnosis. Such interviews include the Structured Clinical Interview for DSM (Spitzer et al. 1992), the Structured Clinical Assessment for Neuropsychiatry, the Composite International Diagnostic Interview and the Diagnostic Interview Schedule.

In clinical studies, it is also usual to use rating scales for the severity of depression, and these can be repeated over the course of treatment. Clinical trial guidelines recommend the use of at least one clinician-rated scale, with the two most commonly used scales being the Hamilton Depression Rating Scale and the Montgomery Asberg Depression Rating Scale. It is often useful to also use self-report questionnaires, such as the Beck Depression Inventory or the 90-item Hopkins Symptom Checklist.

CONCLUSION

Depressive disorders have been recognised for thousands of years, across cultures and in non-human species. The essential features, including social withdrawal, anhedonia, loss of motivation and fatigue, are widely recognised. DSM-IV and ICD-10 have imposed a diagnostic convention on a continuum of depressive symptomatology, and this convention has widespread acceptance and utility. However, major depression is almost certainly a heterogeneous syndrome, and ignoring this heterogeneity has not advanced research into depression, or towards understanding its aetiology or treatment. Appropriate use of depression specifiers and subtypes such as psychotic, atypical and melancholia provide additional useful information for clinicians; however, areas of controversy remain for all these subtypes.

REFERENCES

Angst J, Merikangas KR (2001) Multi-dimensional criteria for the diagnosis of depression. *Journal of Affective Disorders* 62:7-15.

Bauer M, Heinz A, Whybrow PC (2002) Thyroid hormones, serotonin and mood: Of synergy and significance in the adult brain. *Molecular Psychiatry* 7:140-56.

Cassidy F, Carroll BJ (2002) Vascular risk factors in late onset mania. *Psychological Medicine* 32:359-62.

Cubells JF, Kranzler HR, McCance-Katz E, Anderson GM, Malison RT, Price LH, et al. (2000) A haplotype at the DBH locus, associated with low plasma dopamine beta-hydroxylase activity, also associates with cocaine-induced paranoia. *Molecular Psychiatry* 5:56-63.

Davidson J, Woodbury MA, Pelton S, Krishnan R (1988) A study of depressive typologies using grade of membership analysis. *Psychological Medicine* 18:179-89.

Gatti F, Bellini L, Gasperini M, Perez J, Zanardi R, Smeraldi E (1996) Fluvoxamine alone in the treatment of delusional depression. *American Journal of Psychiatry* 153:414-16.

Gold PW, Drevets WC, Charney DS (2002) New insights into the role of cortisol and the glucocorticoid receptor in severe depression. *Biological Psychiatry* 52:381-85.

Hickie IB, Scott E, Naismith S, Ward PB, Turner K, Parker G, et al. (2001) Late-onset depression: Genetic, vascular and clinical contributions. *Psychological Medicine* 31:1403-12.

Ho-Yen DO, Kay DSG, Henderson R, Todd AS, Naylor GJ (1983) Factor VIII-related antigen and procoagulant activity in manic–depressive patients. *Journal of Affective Disorders* 5:209-13.

Jackson SW (1986) *Melancholia and Depression from Hippocratic Times to Modern Times*. New Haven, CT: Yale University Press.

Jamison KR (1995) *An Unquiet Mind. A memoir of moods and madness*. New York: Alfred A Knopf.

Jeste DV, Heaton SC, Paulsen JS, Ercoli L, Harris J, Heaton RK (1996) Clinical and neuropsychological comparison of psychotic depression with nonpsychotic depression and schizophrenia. *American Journal of Psychiatry* 153:490-96.

Joyce PR, Mulder RT, McKenzie JM, Luty SE, Cloninger CR (In press) Atypical depression, atypical temperament and a differential antidepressant response to fluoxetine and nortriptyline. *Depression and Anxiety*.

Joyce PR, Mulder RT, Luty SE, McKenzie JM, Sullivan PF, Abbott RM, et al. (2002) Melancholia: Definitions, risk factors, personality, neuroendocrine markers and differential antidepressant response. *Australian and New Zealand Journal of Psychiatry* 36:376-83.

Kendell RE, Jablensky A (2003) Distinguishing between the validity and utility of psychiatric diagnoses. *American Journal of Psychiatry* 160:4-12.

Kendler KS (1997) The diagnostic validity of melancholic major depression in a population-based sample of female twins. *Archives of General Psychiatry* 54:299-304.

Kendler KS, Gardner CO, Jnr (1998) Boundaries of major depression: An evaluation of DSM-IV criteria. *American Journal of Psychiatry* 155:172-77.

Kendler KS, Thornton LM, Gardner CO (2001) Genetic risk, number of previous depressive episodes, and stressful life events in predicting onset of major depression. *American Journal of Psychiatry* 158:582-86.

Kendler KS, Gardner CO, Prescott CA (2002) Toward a comprehensive developmental model for major depression in women. *American Journal of Psychiatry* 159:1133-45.

Kronfol Z, Remick DG (2000) Cytokines and the brain: Implications for clinical psychiatry. *American Journal of Psychiatry* 157:683-94.

Kukopulos A, Minnai G, Muller-Oerlinghausen B (1985) The influence of mania and depression on the pharmacokinetics of lithium: A longitudinal single-case study. *Journal of Affective Disorders* 8:159-66.

Lovett Doust JW, Munro A, Christie H (1980) Vascular correlates of circular type manic–depressive disorder. *Biological Psychiatry* 15:741-48.

McGrath PJ, Stewart JW, Janal MN, Petkova E, Quitkin FM, Klein DF (2000) A placebo-controlled study of fluoxetine versus imipramine in the acute treatment of atypical depression. *American Journal of Psychiatry* 157:344-50.

McGuffin P, Katz R, Bebbington P (1988) The Camberwell Collaborative Depression Study. III. Depression and adversity in the relatives of depressed probands. *British Journal of Psychiatry* 152:775-82.
Nelson JC, Davis JM (1997) DST studies in psychotic depression: A meta-analysis. *American Journal of Psychiatry* 154:1497-503.
Pande AC, Birkett M, Fechner-Bates S, Haskett RF, Greden JF (1996) Fluoxetine versus phenelzine in atypical depression. *Biological Psychiatry* 40:1017-20.
Pariante CM, Miller AH (2001) Glucocorticoid receptors in major depression: Relevance to pathophysiology and treatment. *Biological Psychiatry* 49:391-404.
Parker G (2000) Classifying depression: Should paradigms lost be regained? *American Journal of Psychiatry* 157:1195-203.
Parker G, Roy K, Mitchell P, Wilhelm K, Malhi G, Hadzi-Pavlovic D (2002) Atypical depression: A reappraisal. *American Journal of Psychiatry* 159:1470-79.
Rice JP, McDonald-Scott P, Endicott J, Coryell W, Grove WM, Kelller MB, et al. (1986) The stability of diagnosis with an application to bipolar II disorder. *Psychiatry Research* 19:285-96.
Roth M (2001) Unitary or binary nature of classification of depressive illness and its implications for the scope of manic depressive disorder. *Journal of Affective Disorders* 64:1-18.
Rush AJ, Weissenburger JE (1994) Melancholic symptom features and DSM-IV. *American Journal of Psychiatry* 151:489-98.
Spiker DG, Kupfer DJ (1988) Placebo response rates in psychotic and nonpsychotic depression. *Journal of Affective Disorders* 14:21-3.
Spitzer RL, Williams JB, Gibbon M, First MB (1992) The Structured Clinical Interview for DSM-III-R (SCID): I. History, rationale, and description. *Archives of General Psychiatry* 49:624-29.
Stewart JW, McGrath PJ, Quitkin FM, Harrison W, Markowitz J, Wager SG, et al. (1989) Relevance of DSM-III depressive subtype and chronicity of antidepressant efficacy in atypical depression: Differential response to phenelzine, imipramine, and placebo. *Archives of General Psychiatry* 46:1080-7.
Styron W (1990) *Darkness Visible. A memoir of madness*. New York: Random House.
Vythilingam M, Chen J, Bremner JD, Mazure CM, Maciejewski PK, Nelson JC (2003) Psychotic depression and mortality. *American Journal of Psychiatry* 160:574-76.
Winokur G (1984) Psychosis in bipolar and unipolar affective illness with special reference to schizo-affective disorder. *British Journal of Psychiatry* 145:236-42.
Wood JG, Joyce PR, Miller AL, Mulder RT, Kennedy MA (2002) A polymorphism in the dopamine beta-hydroxylase gene is associated with 'paranoid ideation' in patients with major depression. *Biological Psychiatry* 51:365-69.

CHAPTER 4

SUBTYPING THE DEPRESSIVE DISORDERS

Gordon Parker

It is human nature to attempt to classify, or *type*, things, usually by looking for shared features and thus making pattern analyses. Such a process is progressively developed, reflecting maturation. For instance, a child may recognise a 'car', later enrich the description by size ('big car') and colour ('red car'), before mastering precise subtyping ('that's a Mercedes SLK 230 Kompressor'). Greater specification and sophistication of pattern analysis has obvious advantages. If asked by the police to describe the get-away car, nominating model specifics and number plate is of greater assistance than merely observing a 'major car'. Similarly, the classification of the depressive disorders can be simple or sophisticated.

The simple binary subtyping model has a long history. In Corinthians, St Paul (Altschule 1967) is said to have distinguished two types of depression, one 'from God' (reflecting its seemingly inexplicable onset and severity) and the other 'of the world' (seemingly explicable by salient life event stresses). While subsequent commentators, particularly European psychiatrists, enriched the clinical descriptions and argued for multiple depressive subtypes, variants of that binary view had significant currency until early in the twentieth century, at that time contrasting *endogenous/psychotic* and *reactive/neurotic* types. This simple dichotomous subtyping system had some utility in that people with *endogenous depression* appeared to have certain biological *endogeneity* symptoms (for example, non-reactive mood, early morning wakening, appetite and weight loss) over-represented, a stronger genetic contribution, an aetiology relating more to biological than to psychosocial determinants (leading to a search for laboratory tests such as the dexamethasone suppression test), to show a minimal response to placebo, and to be more likely to respond to physical treatments.

However, and as detailed elsewhere (Boyce and Hadzi-Pavlovic 1996), the then Medical Superintendent of the Maudsley Hospital, Mapother, offered a challenge in 1926, arguing that there really were no practical differences between those two broad depressive conditions with regard to cause, prognosis or treatment. His argument for a unitarian view (that there is just one type of depression that varies dimensionally) started an intense unitary–binary debate which occupied the next 50 years. Despite numerous multivariate analyses and other arguments, the binarians had failed to produce sufficiently convincing evidence by the end of the 1970s – when the revisionist and influential *Diagnostic and Statistical Manual of Mental Disorders*, third edition (DSM-III) model, was being developed.

The reasons for the binarians failing to prove their case are several. First, their multivariate analyses most commonly involved principal components or factor analysis, methods that identify dimensions rather than categories, and which more likely separated anxiety from depression, rather than identifying two putative depressive subtypes. Second, there was over-inclusion of a range of non-discriminatory clinical features – an issue now detailed. The distinguished Australian psychiatrist Sir Aubrey Lewis (1934) closely studied sixty-one people with depression, and concluded that he could find no qualitative distinctions. Subsequently, Kiloh and Garside (1977) extracted data on fifty-eight variables from Lewis's published works, analysed the dataset and argued that their own statistical approach identified two depressive types. We subsequently undertook latent class analyses of the same dataset (Parker and Hadzi-Pavlovic 1993). When we included all forty-two clinical features assessed by Lewis, a unimodal distribution of scores was created, supporting a single-class depression model. However, when we refined the analysis to fourteen items that we held a priori to be strong putative markers of separate subtypes, a distinct bimodal distribution favouring two depressive classes (qua melancholic and non-melancholic) was demonstrated. Such analyses suggest that negative studies failing to demonstrate support for the binarian view may have obscured the solution by including too many non-differentiating items. Third, the binarian view failed because it, like the unitarian view, is overly simplistic. If *depression* can exist as a disease, a disorder and a syndrome, as well as being a normal response to life vicissitudes, why should we expect that a single model should operate or be all-explanatory?

As noted, the introduction of DSM-III in 1980, with its non-aetiological, criterion-based model, effectively snuffed out a subtyping paradigm for the depressive disorders. Its intrinsic model dimensionalised the depressive disorders (major versus minor), as well as dimensionalising duration, persistence and recurrence features. Subsequently, terms and diagnoses such as *subsyndromal* and *subclinical* have extended the dimensional concept. Even more recently, *spectrum* and *continuum* models have been articulated, whereby the mood disorders (not merely depression) are dimensionalised and viewed as ranging from psychotic depression through major and minor depression, as well as mixed states, to an opposing bipolar pole. Such dimensional models are reductionist and simplistic, oversimplifying and compromising clinical management. Thus, some clinicians operate to a facile maxim of electroconvulsive therapy (ECT) for severe depression, antidepressant drug for moderate depression, and psychotherapy for mild depression.

In operation, the DSM dimensional approach creates pseudo-categories along a dimensional continuum. Over time, *major depression* (the central construct) has been reified as an entity when, in reality, it is a pseudo-entity. It has also proven remarkably unhelpful for researchers and for clinicians, as now overviewed.

First, a term such as *major depression* lacks intrinsic logic. If I go to a dermatologist and have a brown blotch inspected, I will not feel particularly informed to hear that it is a major or minor blotch. I want to know whether it is a melanoma or a freckle. Kendell (1989) has argued that the division of *the pox* into smallpox, and the separation of *the dropsy* into cardiac and renal-induced conditions allowed medicine to progress on a more rational basis, respecting subtyping, aetiology, prognosis and differential treatment strategies. Similarly, practitioners would not regard a diagnosis based on severity of pain as being profound, but would seek to pursue features of the pain as a marker of disorder and cause, so as to shape rational and relevant interventions.

Second, despite major depression being the principal depressive diagnosis studied in the past 20 years (whether in treatment or investigatory studies), results have been distinctly sterile. This is best illustrated in the efficacy studies for major depression, where antidepressant drug trials have generated the largest database existing in psychiatry. Meta-analyses of treatments for major depression inform us (Parker et al. 2003) that all old and new antidepressants show equal efficacy (intra-class and inter-class) and that response rates for differing drugs are equivalent to psychotherapies such as cognitive behaviour therapy (CBT), counselling, St John's wort and even bibliotherapy (reading about depression in books). Such 'results' principally reflect interventions being tested as universal treatments, and the heterogeneity of quite varying expressions of depression being conglomerated into major depression (with the consequent washout of treatment-specificity effects). An additional confounder reflects the high responsivity of the depressive disorders in subjects in drug trials, whether subjects are receiving antidepressant medication or placebo, making separation of antidepressant drug and placebo difficult. For example, analysis of drug trial data submitted over the past decade to the US Food and Drug Administration (for the approval of new antidepressants) has shown that, in most trials, the antidepressant drug has not separated from placebo (Kirsch et al. 2003). Thus, our efficacy database (which is based on a dimensional model) does little to inform clinical practice.

Results of meta-analyses also lead to an *equipotency of treatment* interpretation, where everyone is a winner, as all therapists (whether using drugs, CBT or charisma) can claim that their treatment is effective. Further, it promotes the *affective fallacy*, a literary term used to describe the error of evaluating work by its effects on the reader rather than considering the integral strength of the work itself. This leads to the bizarre situation where the practitioner's discipline or preference of treatment modality, rather than the disorder characteristics, determines management. Thus, an individual with depression type X is highly likely to receive antidepressant medication if consulting a general practitioner, CBT from a psychologist, counselling from a counsellor, hypnotherapy from a hypnotherapist and crystal therapy from a woman wearing a caftan. We need to recognise and challenge the roulette therapy consequences of current classificatory systems.

The above argues for the rejection of the unitarian dimensional model, principally on grounds of logic and misinformation. The difficulty then is how best to model the depressive disorders, with the risk being that every individual with an interest in this field is likely to have his/her own idiosyncratic model. Ours is now offered for consideration.

We propose a three-class hierarchical model (Parker 2000). The central component is a mood disorder, ubiquitous to each depressive class, but (overall) increasingly severe as one moves from non-melancholic to melancholic and to psychotic depression. We then argue (Parker and Hadzi-Pavlovic 1996; Parker 2000) that the division between non-melancholic and melancholic depression is provided by a class-specific feature – psychomotor disturbance (operationalised as involving a central cognitive processing component together with either motor retardation or agitation)–and best rated by clinical observation. The distinction between melancholic and psychotic depression is provided by the additional specific component of psychotic features in the latter, although psychomotor disturbance is (generally) also more severe than in melancholic depression.

This subtyping, hierarchical model therefore defines and allows the clinical separation of two specific classes – psychotic and melancholic depression. It does not, however, define non-melancholic depression. Instead, it models non-melancholic depression as a heterogeneous residual class comprising multiple disorders, leading to this class lacking any specific clinical features and therefore requiring a differing model for definition, as considered shortly.

Our models include functional underpinnings (Malhi et al. 2003), and here we impute the progressive recruitment of differing neurotransmitters as the three tiers are ascended. This model allows the pathogenesis of the more biological melancholic and psychotic depressive disorders to be pursued. For example, we have detailed how we impute disruption to certain fronto-subcortical neural networks as relevant to *functional* and *structural* expressions of melancholia (Austin and Mitchell 1996), a model not dissimilar to one for Parkinson's disease.

Perhaps more importantly, marked treatment differentials are observable across the three classes. For example, meta-analyses (Parker et al. 1992) of physical treatments for psychotic depression identify a 25 per cent response to antidepressant alone, 33 per cent to antipsychotic drug alone and 80 per cent to their combination, the last akin to the response to ECT. For melancholic depression, we have demonstrated a gradient, most distinct in older patients, whereby the broader-action antidepressants have much greater efficacy than the narrow-action antidepressants (Parker 2002). This model has major treatment implications, and respects the clinical observation that the selective serotonin reuptake inhibitors (SSRIs) are not always as effective as the dual-action antidepressants in people with melancholic depression, which, in turn, may not always be as effective as the broader-action tricyclic and monoamine oxidase inhibitor drugs.

In the past few years we have attempted to model the non-melancholic depressive disorders, and have argued that this heterogeneous residue of conditions is best conceptualised dimensionally, but here weighting the effects of life events and predisposing temperament or personality, rather than severity. Two life-event-weighted classes have long been proposed: a reactive or adjustment depression, and a chronic situational depression. Broad contrasting patterns argue for differential management approaches.

Our analyses suggest that a pure reactive depressive disorder is rare in clinical populations, while common in community and general practice settings (Parker et al. 1998). In essence, this reflects reactive depression's closeness to *normal* depression where, in response to the vicissitudes of life, most people become depressed – but experience a spontaneous remission in hours or days. Generally, such individuals are highly primed to respond to an empathic, comprehensive and commonsense assessment, with such conditions further activating their propensity to spontaneous remission. In clinical psychiatric practice, such states are rare because there are usually additional disorder-propagating factors, whether related to the nature of the stressful event or to the individual's personality or to additional biological factors. The high responsivity of such disorders ensures that the capacity of any additional therapeutic component to improve effectiveness above nonspecific clinical strengths is slight, partially explaining in this group the lack of differentiation of antidepressants from placebo in recent drug efficacy studies.

We conceptualise the more chronic *situational* depressions as akin to a *learned helplessness* model, whereby severe and ongoing social factors (for example, a dysfunctional marriage and the inability to escape) cause the individual to lose drive, motivation, and to become depressed. Here, there is an argument for social engineering, whereby a lever might be applied to causal and propagating factors (although this is generally difficult in practice). Here, SSRI medication may frequently be helpful, less by solving or resolving the social problem and more by decreasing the individual's worrying about the issue, so that such patients often report that, while their problems are still present, they are 'swimming rather than sinking'.

Turning to the personality contribution, it is illuminating to see a series of studies that occurred in the two decades prior to DSM-III, as overviewed by Roth and Barnes (1981), and in which there was impressive consensus in results. In essence, after excluding the more biological disorders, those studies suggested subgroups of non-melancholic depressed subjects with (a) a primary anxiety disorder, (b) an irritable/hostile personality style, or (c) a formal personality disorder.

We have attempted to determine how far dimensions of personality may be pursued to provide a clinically meaningful model in terms of having diagnostic and treatment implications (Parker et al. 1998; Parker and Roy 2002). In particular, we have pursued a spectrum model which allows that differing neurobiological processes shape temperament and personality which, in turn, following exposure to a severe or salient stressful event, shape the surface pattern clinical feature. For example, we have demonstrated that people who have a personality style of *anxious worrying* and who tend to worry, go quiet and cry by themselves when stressed are highly likely to develop a clinical pattern of *anxious depression*. By contrast, those who also have high trait anxiety but who, under stress, tend to externalise the anxiety are more likely to present with an *irritable depression* pattern. The latter are generally pleasant people who express (when depressed) some guilt about how they are being snappy or crabby with family members. We therefore distinguish them from those revealing a surface pattern of *hostile depression*, in which the temperament or personality style is more weighted to cluster B volatile and self-centred characteristics, and thus we argue against viewing irritable depression and hostile depression as synonymous constructs.

We have further modelled *atypical depression* (Parker et al. 2002) as another spectrum concept, but at some considerable variance from its present DSM-IV status. We have found that such individuals are more likely to have a personality style of interpersonal sensitivity making them more sensitive to perceived or actual rejection. Further, we have argued that some of the surface markers of their depression (for example, hypersomnia and hyperphagia) may not be depressive 'symptoms' but more related to homeostatic mechanisms, whereby the excessive sleep and craving for certain foods rich in L-tryptophan have restitutive potential.

This subtyping model has key treatment implications. For instance, those with an overall style of *emotional dysregulation* (that is, anxious worrying or irritable depression) are highly likely to benefit from SSRI medication, as this 'regulates' their predispositional personality style. Those with a hostile depression have a low response rate to any medication and poor compliance with treatment, findings that argue for a quite differing therapeutic paradigm.

Other salient personality dimensions have treatment implications. Thus, we have reviewed evidence suggesting that those who are introverted or have an *avoidant* temperament style are not only at distinctly greater risk of non-melancholic depression, but may benefit preferentially from a behavioural therapy approach. Those with a *perfectionist* personality style are less likely to get depressed (perhaps reflecting their need to control their life and not expose themselves to depressogenic events) but, if they do get depressed, do poorly with most interventions. For those with a personality disorder, and who often are viewed by clinicians as having a *characterological self-blaming* style, evidence of specifically effective treatments is difficult to find; hardly surprising when many such individuals have been recipients of developmental deprivation or abuse, and often lack coping strengths. Such data arguing for some specificity between disorder type and treatment approach are at variance with a dimensional approach to modelling the depressive disorders.

The dimensional model should embarrass the profession. A simple binary or dichotomous model has a range of intrinsic limitations, particularly in providing minimal information about the residual, less biological conditions. We therefore favour a mix-and-match model, arguing that there are certain more categorical depressive subtypes (psychotic and melancholic depression) that can be operationally defined and diagnosed. We then model the non-melancholic disorders by dimensionally weighting the relevance of life event stress and personality style. We suggest that there is sufficient indicative treatment specificity data to support the overall model, and that the model respects the pattern analysis of clinical observation and offers a more logical 'horses for courses' approach to the management of depressive disorders. We continue to argue for the progressive development of a matrix whereby knowledge is accrued and respected when it demonstrates that certain depressive disorders are differentially responsive to differing treatments.

ACKNOWLEDGMENTS

My thanks to Kerrie Eyers and Yvonne Foy for manuscript preparation.

REFERENCES

Altschule MD (1967) The two kinds of depression according to St. Paul. *British Journal of Psychiatry* 113:779-80.

Austin MP, Mitchell P (1996) Melancholia as a neurological disorder. In Parker G, Hadzi-Pavlovic D (eds), *Melancholia: A disorder of movement and mood. A phenomenological and neurobiological review.* New York: Cambridge University Press, pp. 223-36.

Boyce P, Hadzi-Pavlovic D (1996) Some historical aspects. In Parker G, Hadzi-Pavlovic D (eds), *Melancholia: A disorder of movement and mood. A phenomenological and neurobiological review.* New York: Cambridge University Press, pp. 9-19.

Kendell RE (1989) Clinical validity. In Robins LN, Barrett JE (eds), *The Validity of Psychiatric Diagnosis.* New York: Raven Press, pp. 305-23.

Kiloh LG, Garside RF (1977) Depression: A multivariate study of Sir Aubrey Lewis's data on melancholia. *Australian and New Zealand Journal of Psychiatry* 11:149-56.

Kirsch I, Moore TJ, Scoboria A, Nicholls S (2003) The Emperor's new drugs: An analysis of antidepressant medication data submitted to the US Food and Drug Administration. *Prevention and Treatment* 5:1-11.

Lewis A (1934) Melancholia: A clinical survey of depressive states. *Journal of Mental Science* 80:277-378.

Malhi GS, Parker GB, Greenwood J (2003) Structural and functional models of depression: From sub-types to substrates. *(Submitted).*

Parker G (2000) Classifying depression: Should paradigms lost be regained? *American Journal of Psychiatry* 157:1195-203.

—— (2002) Differential effectiveness of newer and older antidepressants appears mediated by an age effect on the phenotypic expression of depression. *Acta Psychiatrica Scandinavica* 106:168-70.

Parker G, Hadzi-Pavlovic D (1993) Old data, new interpretation: A re-analysis of Sir Aubrey Lewis' M.D. thesis. *Psychological Medicine* 23:859-70.

—— (eds) (1996) *Melancholia: A disorder of movement and mood. A phenomenological and neurobiological review.* New York: Cambridge University Press.

Parker G, Roy K (2002) Examining the utility of a temperament model for modelling non-melancholic depression. *Acta Psychiatrica Scandinavica* 106:54-61.

Parker G, Roy K, Eyers K (2003) Cognitive behavior therapy for depression? Choose horses for courses. *American Journal of Psychiatry* 160:825-34.

Parker G, Roy K, Hadzi-Pavlovic D, Pedic F (1992) Psychotic (delusional) depression:

A meta-analysis of physical treatments. *Journal of Affective Disorders* 24:17-24.
Parker G, Roy K, Mitchell P, Wilhelm K, Malhi G, Hadzi-Pavlovic D (2002) Atypical depression: A reappraisal. *American Journal of Psychiatry* 159:1470-9.
Parker G, Hadzi-Pavlovic D, Roussos J, Wilhelm K, Mitchell P, Austin MP, et al. (1998) Non-melancholic depression: The contribution of personality, anxiety and life events to subclassification. *Psychological Medicine* 28:1209-19.
Roth M, Barnes TRE (1981) The classification of affective disorders: A synthesis of old and new concepts. *Comprehensive Psychiatry* 22:54-77.

CHAPTER 5

SYMPTOMATOLOGY AND DIAGNOSIS OF BIPOLAR DISORDER

Philip B Mitchell,
Kylie King and
Maria Aslam

Bipolar disorder in its classic form is usually considered a distinctive condition, readily distinguished from other mental illnesses. Despite this, it is increasingly apparent that the diagnosis is often delayed or missed. This concerning state of affairs was highlighted by a recent survey undertaken by the United States National Depressive and Manic–Depressive Association (Hirschfeld et al. 2003). That study found that, although one-third of patients sought help within 1 year of illness onset, a further one-third waited at least 10 years before seeking help. Sixty-nine per cent reported having been misdiagnosed before the appropriate diagnosis, with those misdiagnosed receiving a mean of 3.5 other diagnoses and having consulted four medical practitioners in the process. The most common misdiagnosis was unipolar depression (60 per cent), followed by anxiety disorder (26 per cent), schizophrenia (18 per cent), borderline or antisocial personality disorder (17 per cent), alcohol or substance abuse or dependence (16 per cent), and schizoaffective disorder (11 per cent). Women were more likely to be misdiagnosed with depression, and men with schizophrenia.

Respondents to the survey who were misdiagnosed believed that the most common reason was a lack of understanding of the illness by the health care professional concerned (60 per cent). Twenty-eight per cent attributed misdiagnosis to their own failure to report all symptoms. More than a third of those who were initially misdiagnosed did not receive a correct diagnosis for ten or more years after seeking treatment.

HISTORICAL OVERVIEW

The earliest descriptions of mania and melancholia can be traced to the classical Greek medical writers. Although Hippocrates was the first to specifically describe mania and melancholia, Aretaeus of Cappadocia is generally credited with the recognition of the coexistence of mania and melancholia in the same patient over a lifetime:

> The development of a mania is really a worsening of the disease (melancholia) rather than a change into another disease ... In most of them (melancholics) the sadness became better after various lengths of time and changed into happiness; the patients then developed a mania.

Nineteenth century France was a turning point for the contemporary concept of bipolar disorder. Based on the longitudinal observations of patients, Jeanne-Pierre Falret defined *la folie circulaire* as a separate nosological entity involving the sequential change between mania and melancholia with intermediate intervals of varying length (Falret 1851).

Emil Kraepelin was responsible for the next major advance in the classification of bipolar disorder. He established the dichotomy between *dementia praecox*, a chronic deteriorating psychotic illness and the episodic *manic–depressive insanity* (Kraepelin 1896). However, Kraepelin's unitary concept of manic–depressive insanity was controversial, as it eliminated the separation between what we now term unipolar depression and bipolar disorders. The actual term *bipolar disorder* was coined by the German psychiatrist Leonhard (1957).

ACUTE EPISODES: MANIA, BIPOLAR DEPRESSION AND MIXED EPISODES

Symptomatology of mania

CLINICAL DESCRIPTIONS

> Nothing is more addictive than the high of a manic euphoria. Once you have tasted that soaring, exhilarating, invincible, phantasmagorical feeling of 'IT'S GREAT TO BE ME! I CAN DO ANYTHING!', once you've experienced the rush of your mind in overdrive, the creativity pouring through it, the connectivity of burgeoning lateral thinking, the ridiculous ease of witty repartee, the unutterable knowledge of your own immensity, your own infinity, then life without another mania is a dreary prospect indeed.
>
> Margo Orum (1996)

Most diagnostic systems distinguish between *hypomania* and *mania*, with the disturbance in hypomania generally not severe enough to 'cause marked impairment in social or occupational functioning or to require hospitalisation'. Mania is often also characterised by delusions or hallucinations. As it can be difficult to distinguish between the concepts clinically, the generic term *mania* will be used in this chapter to encompass both terms. The formal distinguishing criteria for hypomania and mania from the fourth edition of the *Diagnostic and Statistical Manual of Mental Disorders* (DSM-IV) are detailed in Boxes 5.1 and 5.2.

BOX 5.1

DSM-IV CRITERIA FOR HYPOMANIC EPISODE

A A distinct period of persistently elevated, expansive, or irritable mood, lasting throughout at least 4 days, that is clearly different from the usual non-depressed mood.

B During the period of mood disturbance, three (or more) of the following symptoms have persisted (four if the mood is only irritable) and have been present to a significant degree:

1 inflated self-esteem or grandiosity, decreased need for sleep (e.g., feels rested after only 3 hours of sleep)

2 more talkative than usual or pressure to keep talking

3 flight of ideas or subjective experience that thoughts are racing

4 distractibility (i.e., attention too easily drawn to unimportant or irrelevant external stimuli)

5 increase in goal-directed activity (either socially, at work or school, or sexually) or psychomotor agitation

6 excessive involvement in pleasurable activities that have a high potential for painful consequences (e.g., engaging in unrestrained buying sprees, sexual indiscretions, or foolish business investments).

C The episode is associated with an unequivocal change in functioning that is uncharacteristic of the person when not symptomatic.

D The disturbance in mood and the change in functioning are observable by others.

E The episode is not severe enough to cause marked impairment in social or occupational functioning, or to necessitate hospitalization, and there are not psychotic features.

F The symptoms are not due to the direct physiological effects of a substance (e.g., a drug of abuse, a medication, or other treatment) or a general medical condition (e.g., hyperthyroidism).

SOURCE Reprinted with permission from *Diagnostic and Statistical Manual of Mental Disorders*, Fourth Edition, Text Revision. Copyright American Psychiatric Association 2000.

BOX 5.2

DSM-IV CRITERIA FOR MANIC EPISODE

A A distinct period of abnormally and persistently elevated, expansive, or irritable mood, lasting at least 1 week (or any duration of hospitalisation if necessary).

B During the period of mood disturbance, three (or more) of the following symptoms have persisted (four if the mood is only irritable) and have been present to a significant degree:

1 inflated self-esteem or grandiosity

2 decreased need for sleep (e.g., feels rested after only 3 hours of sleep)

3 more talkative than usual or pressure to keep talking

4 flight of ideas or subjective experience that thoughts are racing

5 distractibility (i.e., attention too easily drawn to unimportant or irrelevant external stimuli)

6 increase in goal-directed activity (either socially, at work or school, or sexually) or psychomotor agitation

7 excessive involvement in pleasurable activities that have a high potential for painful consequences (e.g., engaging in unrestrained buying sprees, sexual indiscretions, or foolish business investments).

C The symptoms do not meet criteria for a Mixed Episode.

D The mood disturbance is sufficiently severe to caused marked impairment in occupational functioning or in usual social activities or relationships with others, or to necessitate hospitalization to prevent harm to self or others, or there are psychotic features.

E The symptoms are not due to the direct physiological effects of a substance (e.g., a drug of abuse, a medication, or other treatment) or a general medical condition (e.g. hyperthyroidism).

SOURCE Reprinted with permission from *Diagnostic and Statistical Manual of Mental Disorders*, Fourth Edition, Text Revision. Copyright American Psychiatric Association 2000.

The clinical picture of mania is usually distinctive. The key criterion is the mood disturbance, most usually elevated (euphoric to grandiose), although sometimes irritability or irascibility may dominate. In conjunction with expansiveness, the manic patient will tend to dominate the clinical interaction, often being genuinely entertaining. Associated disinhibition promotes frank self-disclosure or intrusiveness towards others. Judgment is impaired, leading for example to disastrous business decisions. Concurrently, creativity is often increased (occasionally constructively), libido enhanced, and the individual may spend large amounts of money and socialise extensively. Manic patients talk more and more rapidly, while their conversation (like much of their activity) is distinctly distractible. They appear pressured to keep talking, often evidencing flight of ideas. They sleep less, but do not complain about any effects of sleep deprivation. They tend to dress colourfully and see the world differently. Delusions, and more rarely hallucinations, if present, are usually mood-congruent, consistent with the inflated self-esteem and identity.

It is unfortunate that traditional clinical teaching often portrays the stereotypical manic patient as displaying grandiose delusions or severely disturbed behaviour. Although such patients do represent the severe pole of the condition, they certainly do not reflect the most common presentations. Most manic patients are not psychotic. The central change in thinking is a markedly exaggerated and inflated opinion of the individual's abilities and capacities. This distorted thinking flows from the pathologically elevated mood – the primary dysfunction of mania (although irritability usually lies just below the surface). The impaired judgment that derives from this distorted thinking results in poor decision-making, which may have serious ramifications. For example, the businessman who is manic may make unwise investments or embark upon unrealistic schemes. Spending is often excessive. Old relationships may be disrupted or new relationships formed, leading to significant remorse once the mania resolves. Insight is invariably lost early, usually within hours or days of the commencement of the manic episode.

Most manic patients become much busier than normal, but their busyness is not productive. Rather it is disorganised and poorly focused, with usually nothing of substance being achieved. Another reflection of the increase in energy associated with manic episodes is a reduced need for sleep.

Affected individuals may go for days without sleep, or require only several hours of sleep per night, after which they awake feeling refreshed.

Increased talkativeness is also common and may manifest in frequent inappropriate use of the telephone, often at inconvenient hours of the night. The specific abnormalities of thought form are pressure of speech and flight of ideas, which are accompanied by the subjective experience of racing thoughts. As the severity of an episode increases, patients may develop psychotic experiences not dissimilar to those seen in schizophrenia. Hallucinations – usually auditory, but sometimes visual – may occur. Both the delusions and hallucinations are less complex and systematised than those of schizophrenia. The usual themes are grandiosity or persecution.

KRAEPELIN'S CATEGORIES OF MANIA Kraepelin categorised mania on the basis of severity, describing the following subgroups: hypomania (periods of pathologically elevated mood without delusions), mania (pathologically elevated mood with transient psychotic experiences), delusional mania (fixed delusions and/or hallucinations), and delirious mania (the distractibility and impaired concentration is so severe that the episode mimics delirium).

QUANTITATIVE STUDIES OF THE PHENOMENOLOGY OF MANIA There have been several multivariate studies examining for factors or components of mania. In the most significant of these, Cassidy et al. (1998) reported five significant factors: dysphoric symptoms (such as depressed mood, lability, guilt, anxiety and suicidal thoughts), psychomotor acceleration, psychosis, increased hedonic function, and irritable aggression.

Symptomatology of bipolar depression

> Mania is sickness for one's friends, depression for one's self. Both are chemical. In depression, one wakes, is happy for about two minutes, probably less, and fades into the dread of the day. Nothing will happen, but you know twelve hours will pass before you are back in bed and sheltering your consciousness in dreams, or nothing. It isn't danger; it's not an accomplishment. I don't think it a visitation of the angels but a weakening in the blood.
>
> Robert Lowell

> Surprisingly little has been done to describe quantitatively the clinical features of bipolar depression per se.
>
> Goodwin and Jamison (1990, p. 42)

Episodes of depression are less obvious to others than periods of mania, and thus may not be adequately recognised or addressed. Some patients do not experience their depression as an abnormal mood but rather as reduced energy or motivation.

There has been increasing interest in the phenomenology of bipolar depression, particularly in view of a recent resurgence of interest in therapeutics for this phase of the condition. If distinctive features for bipolar depression were able to be demonstrated in comparison to unipolar depression, there would be potential clinical utility in assisting diagnosis in complex scenarios such as first onset depressive episodes, depressed patients with an ambiguous past history of hypomania or mania, or the apparent unipolar depressed patient with a family history of bipolar disorder.

There have been relatively few methodologically rigorous studies of the phenomenology of bipolar depression. In this chapter we focus on two recent publications from our group in Sydney. Reviews of the broader literature are available in Mitchell et al. (1992, 2001) and Mitchell and Sengoz (1996). Our particular research interest has been in the comparative phenomenology of bipolar depression and major depressive disorder (unipolar depression).

In the first of these papers (Parker et al. 2000), we focused on the relative prevalence of melancholic syndromes in bipolar and unipolar depression. This study used three large depressive datasets recruited over a fifteen-year period. These datasets comprised eighty-three bipolar disorder and 904 unipolar patients assessed in detail while depressed. *Melancholia* was defined using several diagnostic systems (DSM-III, DSM-III-R or DSM-IV; CORE-I or CORE-II; and operationalised clinical diagnoses). We found that subjects with bipolar disorder were significantly more likely than unipolar patients to be diagnosed as melancholic by each of the DSM (69 versus 37 per cent), CORE (59 versus 33 per cent) and clinical (70 versus 29 per cent) systems. Furthermore, after logistic regression, bipolar depressed patients were significantly more likely to demonstrate psychomotor disturbance and pathological guilt.

In the second paper (Mitchell et al. 2001), we undertook a fine-grained analysis of the more recent (third) of these datasets. The aim of this study was to identify particular symptomatic differences between bipolar and unipolar depressed patients. The sample comprised 270 inpatients and outpatients with a current DSM-IV major depressive episode. Thirty-nine of the patients had DSM-IV bipolar I disorder.

These bipolar depressed patients were compared with thirty-nine unipolar depressed subjects matched for age, sex and the presence or absence of DSM-IV melancholia. Although there was no difference in severity of depression (assessed by the Hamilton Rating Scale for Depression), subjects with bipolar depression were significantly more likely to have had a past psychotic depressive episode. With regard to current symptomatology, they were more likely to report worthlessness, anhedonia, restlessness, leaden paralysis and hypersomnia. Conversely, they were less likely to manifest tearfulness, anxiety and the tendency to blame others. The most striking differences, however, were observed in the objective features of depressive psychomotor disturbance as rated by the CORE scale (this is an eighteen-item scale with subscales for retardation, agitation and non-interactiveness, the latter being a proxy for cognitive dysfunction). Bipolar patients were less emotionally reactive, had a greater delay in responding verbally, and demonstrated more slowed movement. There were no differences in agitation items. Bipolar patients scored higher on both the retardation subscale and total CORE score.

These findings suggested features with potential clinical utility for diagnosing bipolar depression, wich we have described as a *bipolar depression signature*. These features are:

- signs of psychomotor retardation
- melancholic symptoms such as worthlessness, unvarying mood and marked anhedonia
- *atypical* depressive symptoms such as hypersomnia and leaden paralysis
- a past history of psychotic depression
- the absence of anxiety, initial insomnia, the tendency to blame others and tearfulness.

Although we acknowledge that these features are group means and not pathognomonic of bipolar depression, they do provide the clinician with a useful shortlist that should alert one to the possibility of bipolar disorder. Furthermore, they are consistent with traditional clinical descriptions (Goodwin and Jamison 1990).

Other bipolar depressive presentations which we have not examined formally (but consider not uncommon alternative manifestations of bipolar depression) include anergia and lethargy without prominent subjective mood symptoms; and otherwise standard depressive syndromes, but with an *emptiness* or *lack* of emotions.

Our studies have focused on depressed subjects with bipolar I disorder. The Italian researcher Benazzi has undertaken similar studies with bipolar II depressed patients, predominantly in a private practice outpatient context. Benazzi (2003) has also reported an increased prevalence of atypical features in bipolar II compared with unipolar depressed patients; but he found no difference in rates of psychomotor retardation (Benazzi 2002). This suggests both commonalities and distinctions between bipolar I and II depression.

Symptomatology of mixed episodes

Although occasional symptoms of depression are not uncommon during mania, some patients have profound levels of depression. Such episodes are variously termed *dysphoric mania*, *mixed episodes* or *mixed affective states*. Mixed episodes appear to be biologically distinct, being associated with high rates of cortisol non-suppression after dexamethasone, and responding preferentially to valproate rather than lithium.

While the formal DSM-IV definition (see Box 5.3) requires the concurrent presence of both manic and depressed syndromes, quantitative studies suggest that mania plus at least two of six dysphoric symptoms (such as depressed mood, anhedonia, guilt, suicide, fatigue and anxiety) is a more valid definition (Cassidy et al. 2000).

BOX 5.3

DSM-IV CRITERIA FOR MIXED EPISODE

A The criteria are met both for a Manic Episode and for a Major Depressive Episode (except for duration) nearly every day during at least a 1-week period.

B The mood disturbance is sufficiently severe to cause marked impairment in occupational functioning or in usual social activities or relationships with others, or to necessitate hospitalization to prevent harm to self or others, or there are psychotic features.

C The symptoms are not due to the direct physiological effects of a substance (e.g., a drug of abuse, a medication, or other treatment) or a general medical condition (e.g., hyperthyroidism).

SOURCE Reprinted with permission from *Diagnostic and Statistical Manual of Mental Disorders*, Fourth Edition, Text Revision. Copyright American Psychiatric Association 2000.

LIFETIME BIPOLAR DISORDER DIAGNOSES

Bipolar I and bipolar II disorders

Dunner and Fieve (1974) were the first to distinguish between distinct bipolar I and bipolar II disorders. Bipolar I was defined by manic periods, which are severely disruptive and/or require hospitalisation, and often accompanied by psychotic features. Bipolar II patients have periods of hypomania, with the periods of abnormally elevated mood not being as disruptive or requiring hospitalisation. Such patients are not psychotic.

Epidemiological studies of the prevalence of bipolar II disorder vary. Some studies suggest that bipolar I and II disorders are equally common, while others have demonstrated that bipolar II is the more common phenotype (Benazzi and Akiskal 2003).

The distinction of bipolar II from bipolar I disorder is supported by data on the prior course of illness, characteristics of the index episode and familial aggregation of patients with this illness (Endicott et al. 1985). Formal studies have demonstrated good inter-rater reliability for bipolar II disorder when patients are interviewed by experienced psychiatrists (Simpson et al. 2002).

Rapid-cycling pattern

This is defined as the occurrence of four or more episodes of mania or depression in a 12-month period. At any one time, about 25–50 per cent of patients have rapid cycling pattern, but for individual patients this may change with time. Although no obvious cause is usually apparent, rapid cycling may occasionally be due to either antidepressants or hypothyroidism.

Seasonal affective pattern

A small proportion of bipolar disorder patients experience depression during the winter months and hypomania in spring or autumn. Though well described in Western Europe and the United States, this appears to be less common in Australia, where there are less extreme differences in daylight hours between the seasons.

Unipolar mania

Research has shown unipolar mania to be a relatively uncommon presentation. Leonhard (1957) reported the rate of 'pure' mania as 9 per cent in his group. Others such as Winokur et al. (1969) all found the rate to be less than 5 per cent in their samples, and recommended its incorporation under the rubric of *bipolar disorder* in view of the shared genetic diathesis and similar response to treatments such as lithium. Recently Yazici et al. (2001) have reopened the question of recognition of unipolar mania as a distinct entity.

It is interesting to note that unipolar mania has been reported to be more prevalent in non-Western countries such as Indonesia, Nigeria, China and the Caribbean, where rates of up to 30 per cent of pure mania have been reported. It is unclear whether the discrepancy between findings in the West and other countries are due to true differences or differing diagnostic criteria.

THE DIAGNOSTIC BOUNDARIES OF BIPOLAR DISORDER

The classic bipolar I disorder syndrome has been referred to recently by Ketter as 'Cade's disease' (Ghaemi et al. 2002), in recognition of John Cade's seminal discovery of the effect of lithium in the treatment of mania. Bipolar disorder often has overlapping symptomatology, or contested boundaries, with other psychiatric disorders (Blacker and Tsuang 1992), and is often comorbid with conditions such as anxiety and substance abuse. It is this overlap that may account for at least some of the frequently delayed or mistaken diagnoses of this condition referred to previously. The comorbidity of bipolar disorder with anxiety and substance abuse is addressed in Chapters 24 and 25.

Relevant differential diagnoses include schizophrenia, schizoaffective disorder, personality disorder, cyclothymia and a number of organic determinants of secondary mania (which should be suspected particularly in late onset manic presentations). Secondary mania is dealt with in Chapter 8.

Schizophrenia versus bipolar disorder

Bipolar disorder patients are frequently misdiagnosed as having schizophrenia at their first presentation (Joyce 1984). Although in some cases this may be due to poor diagnostic practice, there are often mixed schizophrenic and manic features at the first presentation, suggesting that the illness is not fully 'crystallised' at that point. It may therefore be necessary to be cautious about the diagnosis of a first episode of acute psychosis, and to wait for the diagnosis to become apparent over time.

Most research has continued to support Kraepelin's dichotomy of manic–depressive insanity (bipolar disorder) and dementia praecox (schizophrenia). Experienced clinicians have no difficulty distinguishing schizophrenia from bipolar disorder in the classic forms; the diagnostic difficulty occurs in the not infrequent atypical or hybrid presentations. Most familial data suggest separate inheritance for the two disorders (Goodwin and Jamison 1990), though authorities such as Berrettini (2000) have contested this. Therapeutic response distinguishes between the entities to some extent. The benefit of treatment with lithium is markedly decreased in patients with schizophrenia; on the other hand, atypical antipsychotics are clearly effective in both disorders. Structural abnormalities are more frequently observed in patients with schizophrenia. In general, the current classification criteria are reliable over time, as patients remain within their respective category with low rates of diagnostic crossover. However, it must be conceded that some patients initially diagnosed on several occasions with schizophrenia ultimately manifest as undoubtedly having bipolar disorder (Daniels et al. 2003). Overall, these findings imply that the two diseases are in fact two separate entities. Others contest this, conceptualising these two presentations as reflective of a continuum of psychosis, or as varying manifestations of a unitary psychotic disorder (McGorry 1991).

Schizoaffective disorder versus bipolar disorder

The term *schizoaffective disorder* describes patients with a hybrid syndrome manifesting with features of schizophrenia and mania and/or depression. It is maintained in the DSM-IV as a separate category with bipolar and depressed forms (see Box 5.4). The Research Diagnostic Criteria nosology distinguishes between manic and depressed types of schizoaffective disorder, with the former being more closely related to bipolar disorder and the latter to schizophrenia. Schizoaffective disorder has a course and outcome between those of schizophrenia and bipolar disorder (Angst 1986). Additionally, findings from family studies of schizoaffective disorder are not clear-cut. In families of a proband with schizoaffective disorder (bipolar type), there is a modest increase in the occurrence of bipolar disorder but an even greater increase in the occurrence of schizophrenia (Kendler et al. 1986). Furthermore, patients with schizoaffective disorder respond to lithium, but not to the same extent as those with bipolar disorder (Levitt and Tsuang 1988). Biological studies have yet to demonstrate replicable differences separating schizoaffective disorder from the other two major psychotic disorders. Thus, schizoaffective disorder appears either to be an atypical manifestation of bipolar disorder or schizophrenia or to represent one manifestation of a continuum between these two illnesses.

BOX 5.4

DSM-IV CRITERIA FOR SCHIZOAFFECTIVE DISORDER

A An uninterrupted period of illness during which, at some time, there is either a major depressive episode, a manic episode, or a mixed episode concurrent with symptoms that meet criterion A for schizophrenia.

B During the same period of illness, there have been delusions or hallucinations for at least 2 weeks in the absence of prominent mood symptoms.

C Symptoms that meet criteria for a mood episode are present for a substantial portion of the total duration of the active and residual periods of the illness.

D The disturbance is not due to the direct physiological effects of a substance (e.g., a drug of abuse, a medication) or a general medical condition.

Specify type:

Bipolar type if the disturbance includes a manic or a mixed episode (or a manic or mixed episode and major depressive episodes)

Depressive type if the disturbance only includes major depressive episodes

SOURCE Reprinted with permission from *Diagnostic and Statistical Manual of Mental Disorders*, Fourth Edition, Text Revision. Copyright American Psychiatric Association 2000.

Personality disorders versus bipolar disorder

The relationship of bipolar disorder and the cluster B personality disorders, particularly borderline personality disorder, remains controversial. The overlap of symptoms has caused investigators to question whether personality disorders merely co-occur with bipolar disorder and other mood disorders, or whether borderline personality disorder may in fact be a variant of mood disorders (McGlashan 1983). There is frequent clinical difficulty distinguishing bipolar disorder from the cluster B personality disorders, as those with borderline personality disorder often demonstrate affective instability, impulsivity and transient psychosis. People with histrionic personality disorder frequently manifest with flamboyance, emotional shifts and low frustration tolerance. Subjects with narcissistic personality disorder can display grandiosity (Blacker and Tsuang 1992). Furthermore, these personality disorders often overlap. One study that attempted to distinguish between bipolar disorder and borderline personality disorder found that borderline patients could be differentiated by temperament and character deviation (Atre-Vaidya and Hussain 1999). It is possible that personality disorders can mimic bipolar disorder, especially when they coexist with substance abuse; they may also contribute to the development of bipolar disorder by unmasking latent symptoms (Blacker and Tsuang 1992).

Cyclothymic disorder versus bipolar disorder

Cyclothymia is regarded as either a mild form of bipolar disorder or a personality style predisposing to its development. In the DSM-IV definition (see Box 5.5), cyclothymic disorder is conceptualised as a syndrome that resembles hypomania and/or depression; the symptoms are fewer and lesser in severity, duration or pervasiveness and do not meet the full criteria for either diagnosis. It is a dimensional diagnosis, which covers the territory between normal personality characteristics (depressive and hyperthymic temperaments) and mild bipolar disorder.

Although it is a widely held view that bipolar disorder and cyclothymia exist on a continuum, the exact nature of the relationship between the two conditions has not been elucidated. A prospective study by Akiskal et al. (1977) verified that many patients with bipolar disorder have a history of antecedent cyclothymia. Those authors also reported a substantial incidence of hypomania in cyclothymic patients being treated with antidepressants. In addition, nearly all family studies support cyclothymia and bipolar disorder having a shared genetic predisposition. There are increased rates of cyclothymia in families of patients with bipolar disorder and vice versa (Weissman et al. 1984). Patients with cyclothymia have also been reported to respond to treatment with lithium (Akiskal et al. 1977; Baldessarini 1985).

BOX 5.5

DSM-IV CRITERIA FOR CYCLOTHYMIC DISORDER

A For at least 2 years, the presence of numerous periods with hypomanic symptoms and numerous periods with depressive symptoms that do not meet criteria for a major depressive episode. Note: In children and adolescents, the duration must be at least 1 year.

B During the above 2-year period (1 year in children and adolescents), the person has not been without the symptoms in criterion A for more than 2 months at a time.

C No major depressive episode, manic, or missed episode has been present during the first 2 years of the disturbance.

The soft bipolar spectrum

The concept of the *soft bipolar spectrum* was first proposed by Akiskal and Mallya (1987). The hard bipolar disorder phenotype includes psychotic and non-psychotic bipolar I, whereas the soft spectrum incorporates a broad conceptualisation of bipolar II (including cyclothymic temperament as an alternative to hypomania) and further overlapping subsyndromal manifestations. Akiskal and Pinto (2000) label such subsyndromal presentations as bipolar III disorders, including recurrent depression arising from a hyperthymic temperamental background, and/or a bipolar family history. These authors have gone on to describe an 'evolving spectrum of bipolar disorders':

- bipolar $^{1}/_{2}$ (schizobipolar disorder)
- bipolar I (manic–depressive illness)
- bipolar I$^{1}/_{2}$ (depression with protracted hypomania)
- bipolar II (depression with spontaneous discrete hypomanic episodes of less than 4 days' duration)
- bipolar II$^{1}/_{2}$ (depression superimposed on cyclothymic temperament)
- bipolar III (depression plus hypomania occurring solely in association with antidepressant or other somatic treatment)
- bipolar III$^{1}/_{2}$ (depression imposed on hyperthymic temperament)
- bipolar IV (depression superimposed on a hyperthymic temperament).

Angst et al. (2003) have reported that at least 11 per cent of the general population has such a broad presentation of bipolar II disorder, and a further 13 per cent has features consistent with of bipolar III disorder, suggesting that about a quarter of the community suffer from the soft bipolar spectrum. Such propositions have not been accepted uncritically by the field. One of the strongest protagonists of the opposing viewpoint has been Baldessarini (2000), who has voiced concern over the 'trivialisation' of the core concept of bipolar disorder, particularly as contemporary research of the narrow paradigm has led to major advances in mechanistic understanding and increasingly effective therapeutics.

CONCLUSION

While there is clear consensus about the definition of the core syndromes of bipolar I and II disorder, the broader concept of the soft bipolar spectrum remains controversial. Despite this, patients with bipolar I and II disorder are often incorrectly diagnosed for prolonged periods. A sophisticated diagnostic appraisal needs to consider both the overlap boundaries with other mental illnesses and the frequent comorbidity with substance abuse and anxiety.

REFERENCES

Akiskal HS, Mallya G (1987) Criteria for the 'soft' bipolar spectrum: Treatment implications. *Psychopharmacology Bulletin* 23:68-73.

Akiskal HS, Pinto O (2000) The soft bipolar spectrum: Footnotes to Kraepelin on the interface of hypomania, temperament and depression. In Marneros A, Angst J (eds), *Bipolar Disorders: 100 years after manic depressive insanity*. London: Kluwer Academic Publishers, pp. 37-62.
Akiskal HS, Djenderedjian AM, Rosenthal RH, Khani MK (1977) Cyclothymic disorder: Validating criteria for inclusion in the bipolar affective group. *American Journal of Psychiatry* 134:1227-33.
Angst J (1986) The course of schizoaffective disorders. In Maneros A, Tsuang MT (eds), *Schizoaffective Psychoses*. Berlin: Springer-Verlag.
Angst J, Gamma A, Benazzi F, Ajdacic V, Eich D, Rossler W (2003) Toward a re-definition of subthreshold bipolarity: Epidemiology and proposed criteria for bipolar-II, minor bipolar disorders and hypomania. *Journal of Affective Disorders* 73:133-46.
Atre-Vaidya N, Hussain SM (1999) Borderline personality disorder and bipolar mood disorder: Two distinct disorders or a continuum? *Journal of Nervous and Mental Disease* 187:313-15.
Baldessarini RJ (1985) *Chemotherapy in Psychiatry: Principles and practice*. Cambridge, MA: Harvard University Press.
—— (2000) A plea for integrity of the bipolar disorder concept. *Bipolar Disorders* 2:3-7.
Benazzi F (2002) Psychomotor changes in melancholic and atypical depression: Unipolar and bipolar-II subtypes. *Psychiatry Research* 112:211-20.
—— (2003) Clinical differences between bipolar II depression and unipolar major depressive disorder: Lack of an effect of age. *Journal of Affective Disorders* 75:191-5.
Benazzi F, Akiskal HS (2003) Refining the evaluation of bipolar II: Beyond the strict SCID-CV guidelines for hypomania. *Journal of Affective Disorders* 73:33-8.
Berrettini WH (2000) Are schizophrenic and bipolar disorders related? A review of family and molecular studies. *Biological Psychiatry* 48:531-8.
Blacker D, Tsuang MT (1992) Contested boundaries of bipolar disorder and the limits of categorical diagnosis in psychiatry. *American Journal of Psychiatry* 149:1473-83.
Cassidy F, Forest K, Murry E, Carroll BJ (1998) A factor analysis of the signs and symptoms of mania. *Archives of General Psychiatry* 55:27-32.
Cassidy F, Ahearn E, Murry E, Forest K, Carroll BJ (2000) Diagnostic depressive symptoms of the mixed bipolar episode. *Psychological Medicine* 30:403-11.
Daniels BA, Kirkby KC, Mitchell P, Hay D, Bowling A (2003) Heterogeneity of admission history among patients with bipolar disorder. *Journal of Affective Disorders* 75:163-70.
Dunner DL, Fieve RR (1974) Clinical factors in lithium carbonate prophylaxis failure. *Archives of General Psychiatry* 30:229-33.
Endicott J, Nee J, Andreasen N, Clayton P, Keller M, Coryell W (1985) Bipolar II. Combine or keep separate? *Journal of Affective Disorders* 8:17-28.
Falret JP (1851) De la folie circulaire ou forme de maladie mentale caracterisee par l'alternative rguliere de la manie et de la melancholie. *Bullet de l'Academie Nationale de Medecine (Paris)*.
Ghaemi SN, Ko JY, Goodwin FK (2002) 'Cade's disease' and beyond: Misdiagnosis, antidepressant use, and a proposed definition for bipolar spectrum disorder. *Canadian Journal of Psychiatry* 47:125-34.
Goodwin FK, Jamison KR (1990) *Manic–Depressive Illness*. New York: Oxford University Press.
Hirschfeld RM, Lewis L, Vornik LA (2003) Perceptions and impact of bipolar disorder: How far have we really come? Results of the national depressive and manic–depressive association 2000 survey of individuals with bipolar disorder. *Journal of Clinical Psychiatry* 64:161-74.
Joyce PR (1984) Age of onset in bipolar affective disorder and misdiagnosis as schizophrenia. *Psychological Medicine* 14:145-9.
Kendler KS, Gruenberg AM, Tsuang MT (1986) A DSM-III family study of the non-schizophrenic psychotic disorders. *American Journal of Psychiatry* 143:1098-105.
Kraepelin E (1896) *Psychiatrie 5*. Auflage, Leipzig: Barth.

Leonhard K (1957) The classification of endogenous psychoses. In Robins E (ed), *Aufteilung der Endogenen Psychosenm*, 1 ed. Berlin: Akademie-Verlag.
Levitt JJ, Tsuang MT (1988) The heterogeneity of schizoaffective disorder: Implications for treatment. *American Journal of Psychiatry* 145:926-36.
McGlashan TH (1983) The borderline syndrome. II. Is it a variant of schizophrenia or affective disorder? *Archives of General Psychiatry* 40:1319-23.
McGorry PD (1991) Paradigm failure in functional psychosis: Review and implications. *Australian and New Zealand Journal of Psychiatry* 25:43-55.
Mitchell P, Sengoz A (1996) Phenotypical expression of melancholia contrasted for those with bipolar and unipolar illness courses. In Parker G, Hadzi-Pavlovic D (eds), *Melancholia: A disorder of movement and mood*. New York: Cambridge University Press, pp. 172-8.
Mitchell P, Parker G, Jamieson K, Wilhelm K, Hickie I, Brodaty H, et al. (1992) Are there any differences between bipolar and unipolar melancholia? *Journal of Affective Disorders* 25:97-105.
Mitchell PB, Wilhelm K, Parker G, Austin MP, Rutgers P, Malhi GS (2001) The clinical features of bipolar depression: A comparison with matched major depressive disorder patients. *Journal of Clinical Psychiatry* 62:212-16.
Orum M (1996) *Fairytales in Reality: My victory over manic depression*. Melbourne: Pan Macmillan Australia.
Parker G, Roy K, Wilhelm K, Mitchell P, Hadzi-Pavlovic D (2000) The nature of bipolar depression: Implications for the definition of melancholia. *Journal of Affective Disorders* 59:217-24.
Simpson SG, McMahon FJ, McInnis MG, MacKinnon DF, Edwin D, Folstein SE, et al. (2002) Diagnostic reliability of bipolar II disorder. *Archives of General Psychiatry* 59:736-40.
Weissman MM, Gershon ES, Kidd KK, Prusoff BA, Leckman JF, Dibble E, et al. (1984) Psychiatric disorders in the relatives of probands with affective disorders. The Yale University–National Institute of Mental Health Collaborative Study. *Archives of General Psychiatry* 41:13-21.
Winokur G, Clayton PJ, Reich T (1969) *Manic Depressive Illness*. St Louis: CV Mosby.
Yazici O, Kora K, Ucok A, Saylan M, Ozdemir O, Kiziltan E, et al. (2001) Unipolar mania: A distinct disorder? (research report). *Journal of Affective Disorders* 71:97-103.

CHAPTER 6

THE BIPOLAR SPECTRUM

Michael Berk
and Gin S Malhi

Diagnosis is a critical part of the treatment process. Psychiatry is hampered by the absence of any pathophysiological validation of diagnostic categories or their boundaries. Although current practice has adopted a categorical approach as opposed to a dimensional approach, we should proceed with caution. In the remainder of medicine, symptoms are a core part of diagnosis of disorders of known aetiology and pathogenesis. However, individual disorders have protean manifestations and many disorders frequently have common symptoms. A diagnostic system that relies principally on phenomenology, as is the case in psychiatry, is extremely unlikely to reflect pathology if and when it is found. It would be akin to diagnosing cough, dyspnoea or chest pain as 'disorders' without access to any diagnostic markers. In psychiatry the clinical picture is even more complex, as there are almost no pathognomonic symptoms, with most symptoms or symptom complexes occurring across a range of diagnoses. The most specific syndrome in psychiatry is perhaps mania, which means that diagnoses that stem from this are possibly easier to establish.

The *bipolar spectrum* can be conceptualised in several dimensions:

- unipolar through cyclothymia and bipolar II disorder to bipolar I disorder
- bipolar disorder through schizoaffective disorder to schizophrenia
- bipolar disorder and the personality disorders, particularly borderline personality.

This highlights a further difficulty when relying on a phenomenology-based diagnostic system that lacks definitive markers. Hence the need to invoke the concept of a spectrum, which in itself identifies the tensions between a categorical diagnostic system and a dimensional one.

Despite this complexity, and perhaps even more so because of it, the need for accurate and appropriate diagnosis remains. Clearly, diagnosis is a core predictor of outcome, and determines treatment. This is important in all psychiatric disorders, but is of particular significance in bipolar disorder, as some treatments (for example, antidepressants) can exacerbate bipolar disorder by inducing mania or precipitating rapid cycling. Hence, distinguishing unipolar and bipolar depression is of utmost importance but not readily achieved. In clinical practice, many patients present with symptom profiles that span the major depression and bipolar disorder diagnostic categories of the *Diagnostic and Statistical Manual of Mental Disorders*, fourth edition (DSM-IV). The same applies to the depression–anxiety spectrum; however, overlapping treatments between anxiety and depressive disorders make diagnostic distinction less critical than when considering unipolar and bipolar disorder, where often quite different therapeutic approaches are necessary.

Classical descriptions of bipolar disorder originate from the work of Kraepelin and Kretshmer, who described affective states spanning a continuum of severity that included individuals with low-grade affective manifestations that fluctuated over time. Indeed, the unipolar–bipolar continuum has a long history, conceptualised and reformulated by Edda Neele, Leonhard, Perris, Angst and Winokur among others (Akiskal 2002). Fieve et al. (1976) attempted to bridge unipolar and bipolar disorder by creating an intermediary construct, bipolar II. This they defined by the occurrence of manic episodes of insufficient severity to require hospitalisation, termed hypomania. Bipolar III disorder was added later to describe patients who became manic or hypomanic because of antidepressant therapy.

EPIDEMIOLOGY

The bipolar spectrum occupies a prominent place in the epidemiology of psychiatric illnesses (Lopez-Ibor 1990). Bipolar I disorder occurs in between 0.4 and 1.7 per cent of the population, on a par with schizophrenia. Milder forms of the illness are more common, with cyclothymia seen in some 5–6 per cent of the population and hypomania in 3–5 per cent. Thus the total bipolar spectrum includes some 3–7 per cent of the population (Akiskal 1999) and, applying a broad definition of the spectrum, Angst and colleagues reported a 10.9 per cent prevalence (Angst et al. 2003).

Part of the reason for this is that the spectrum is also thought to include subthreshold cases. Interestingly, the original Epidemiological Catchment Area study (Robins et al. 1984) found rates of bipolar I disorder of 0.8 per cent and of hypomania of 0.5 per cent. However, reanalysis of the data to include subthreshold cases among the sample of 18 252 subjects suggests that 5.1 per cent have subthreshold manic symptoms, increasing the total bipolar spectrum to 6.4 per cent. Individuals within the spectrum show greater levels of marital disruption, health service utilisation, need for welfare and disability benefits, and suicidal behaviour, suggesting significant morbidity and *caseness* in this group (Judd and Akiskal 2003).

The clinical picture often begins in adolescence, or occasionally pre-adolescence, with the mean age of onset around 18 years of age. However, many individuals do not enter formal treatment at this stage. To some extent this is understandable, as the diagnosis is difficult to make with certainty – initial misdiagnoses include unipolar depression, adjustment disorder, or borderline personality disorder. It is not uncommon for the illness to start with mild mood swings, with the illness then progressively worsening as the amplitude or the frequency increases until threshold symptoms are reached (Angst 1998). Of note, a 10-year follow-up of childhood depression found that 33.3 per cent later met criteria for bipolar I and that 15.3 per cent met criteria for bipolar II disorder (Geller et al. 2001). A prospective study also found that 12.5 per cent of people who initially had a diagnosis of unipolar disorder later were assessed as having bipolar disorder, with bipolar II pattern being more common than bipolar I (Akiskal et al. 1995). A cohort of depressed and anxious subjects followed up in primary care (Manning et al. 1998) was also found to have high levels of bipolar disorder (30 per cent), predominantly bipolar II. High rates of occupational, leisure and relationship dysfunction are common in bipolar II, more so than in either bipolar I or unipolar disorder (Coryell et al. 1985).

DIAGNOSIS

According to DSM-IV, diagnosis of bipolar II disorder necessitates the presence or history of one or more major depressive episode and the presence or history of at least one hypomanic episode. The latter has to be of at least 4 days' duration and involve an observable change of functioning in the absence of marked impairment or psychosis. Three of the following are required:

- inflated self-esteem or grandiosity
- decreased need for sleep
- talkativeness or pressure of speech
- flight of ideas or racing thoughts
- distractibility
- increased goal-directed activity
- excess pleasure-seeking behaviour.

The DSM-IV 4-day duration requirement is not concordant with epidemiological studies, which suggest a modal duration of 1–3 days or 2 days. Finally, it is important to note that, for a diagnosis of bipolar II, at no time can the individual have experienced a manic episode.

Clearly, the distinction between bipolar I and II is somewhat arbitrary and quite contentious; however, to complicate matters further there are also several subsyndromal bipolar disorders. Bipolar III disorder is defined as hypomania secondary to pharmacotherapy. The implication being that there is perhaps an innate propensity in these individuals towards bipolarity that is triggered by pharmacological challenge. Interestingly, antidepressant-induced hypomania has a similar outcome to spontaneous hypomania, and a pattern of positive family history of bipolarity similar to that with bipolar I disorder, although family history is present in only 15 per cent of patients. Furthermore, hyperthymic, dysthymic or cyclothymic premorbid temperaments are not infrequent. However, these conditions, also described as *persistent temperamental dysregulations* (Akiskal 1994), are contentious and not recognised by DSM-IV, and hence are grouped together as bipolar disorder not otherwise specified (Cassano et al. 1992). Their mean age of onset is 14 years.

Rapid cycling, technically the occurrence of four or more episodes of depression or mania/hypomania over 12 months, is strongly associated with bipolar II diagnosis, is more common in females (Endicott 1998) and confers a risk of suicide. Both antidepressants and substance abuse are implicated in its development, and thyroid disorders and abnormalities of seizure threshold may also be risk factors. Indeed there is some evidence that rapid cycling bipolar disorder responds better to anticonvulsants than to lithium (Ferrier et al. 2001).

Clinically, it is not uncommon for patients with bipolar disorder to present with repeated depressive episodes and therefore be erroneously diagnosed as having a unipolar depressive disorder. Usually this is only corrected when they have a manic or hypomanic episode. These individuals are called *converters*, and this phenomenon occurs in between 10.7 and 27.4 per cent of unipolar depressed patients. Converters tend to have a more tempestuous course with shorter periods of wellness, a history of temperamental instability, a younger age of onset, an unstable interpersonal and occupational history, and postnatal episodes. Therefore, clinical features such as these occurring in a patient presenting with depression should raise suspicions regarding bipolarity (Goodwin and Jamison 1990; Ferrier et al. 2001). Other factors reported as predicting bipolarity in patients presenting with depression are an early age of onset, a family history of bipolarity, a premorbid hyperthymic personality, the occurrence of atypical depressive features, psychotic episodes, post-partum depression, antidepressant-induced mania or hypomania, antidepressant wear-off and antidepressant non-response (Ghaemi et al. 2001).

The presence of agitated mania-like symptoms in a depressive episode is also considered a possible reason for inclusion in the bipolar spectrum. In subjects with unipolar diagnoses, the presence of features such as flight of ideas, aggression, increased social contact, racing thoughts and irritability is thought to constitute a manic mixed state, and hence form part of the bipolar spectrum.

Consequently, Ghaemi and colleagues have proposed a definition of the bipolar spectrum based on the clinical clues in the history (Boxes 6.1 and 6.2) and Akiskal and Pinto have proposed a detailed system of classification (Box 6.3).

BOX 6.1

BIPOLARITY: CLUES IN THE HISTORY

1. Recurrent major depressive episodes (>3)
2. Early age of onset of major depressive episode (age <25 years)
3. Family history of bipolar disorder in first-degree relative
4. Hyperthymic personality (at baseline, non-depressed state)
5. Atypical depressive symptoms (DSM-IV criteria)
6. Brief major depressive episodes (on average, <3 months)
7. Psychotic major depressive episodes
8. Post-partum depression
9. Antidepressant-induced mania or hypomania
10. Antidepressant 'wear-off' (acute but not prophylactic response)
11. Lack of response to ≥3 adequate antidepressant treatment trials

SOURCE Ghaemi et al. (2002).

BOX 6.2

A PROPOSED DEFINITION OF BIPOLAR SPECTRUM DISORDER

A At least one major depressive episode.

B No spontaneous hypomanic or manic episodes.

C Either of the following, plus at least 2 items from criterion D, or both of the following plus 1 item from criterion D:

1. A family history of bipolar disorder in a first-degree relative
2. Antidepressant-induced mania or hypomania.

D If no items from criterion C are present, 6 of the following 9 criteria are needed:

1. Hyperthymic personality (at baseline, non-depressive state)
2. Recurrent major depressive episodes (>3)
3. Brief major depressive episodes (on average, <3 months)
4. Atypical depressive symptoms (DSM-IV criteria)
5. Psychotic major depressive episodes
6. Early age of onset of major depressive episode (age <25)
7. Post-partum depression
8. Antidepressant 'wear-off' (acute but not prophylactic response)
9. Lack of response to ≥3 antidepressant treatment trials.

SOURCE Ghaemi et al. (2002).

BOX 6.3

CLASSIFICATION OF THE BIPOLAR SPECTRUM

Bipolar $^{1}/_{2}$	Schizobipolar
Bipolar I	Mania with or without depression
Bipolar I$^{1}/_{2}$	Protracted hypomania with depression
Bipolar II	Depression with hypomania
Bipolar II$^{1}/_{2}$	Depression with cyclothymia
Bipolar III	Depression with hypomania associated with antidepressants
Bipolar III$^{1}/_{2}$	Depressive and hypomanic swings associated with stimulants
Bipolar IV	Depression with hyperthymic temperament

SOURCE Akiskal and Pinto (1999).

CLINICAL PRESENTATION

The presentation of bipolar spectrum disorders is invariably that of depression. Bipolar I disorder often presents with mania; the other end of the spectrum does so far less often. Other reasons for presentation include sleep disturbance, anxiety and comorbidity with, for example, substance abuse.

The bipolar spectrum is far more prevalent in primary care settings than previously appreciated. In a cohort of 108 patients followed longitudinally with anxiety or depression in primary care, 26 per cent had bipolar disorder. Of those with bipolar disorder, most had bipolar II rather than bipolar I disorder (Manning et al. 1997). The French EPIDEP study, which sought out bipolar II patients in a cohort of outpatients with depression, found a 40 per cent incidence of bipolar II disorder, compared with a rate of 22 per cent at primary assessment. The figures in this study reflect both the difficulty in primary evaluation of this group of patients and the frequency of the disorder in practice. The benefit of a longitudinal perspective is emphasised by the fact that the rate of diagnosis increases with the period of follow-up (Hantouche et al. 1998). In a corroborative study, a third of depressed patients in a series of 405 patients belonged to the bipolar spectrum. Similarly, 37 per cent of people who present after a first manic or hypomanic episode attract a unipolar diagnosis. Of those subsequently prescribed antidepressants, 55 per cent subsequently developed mania or hypomania, and 23 per cent developed rapid cycling (Ghaemi et al. 2000).

In the community, the gap between the onset of symptoms and diagnosis can be as long as a decade (Lewis 2001). In a community study, only 19.8 per cent of individuals with a positive screen for bipolar I or II disorder received a diagnosis of bipolar disorder, while 31.2 per cent received a unipolar diagnosis. Untreated or inappropriately treated symptoms lead to periods of extended morbidity and contribute to long-term destabilisation of mood through inappropriate interventions. Appropriate and early diagnosis is therefore essential to optimise clinical outcomes.

GENETICS OF THE SPECTRUM

A familial aggregation of the bipolar spectrum would suggest its diagnostic validity, as mood disorders tend to have a familial clustering. Furthermore, while bipolar disorders are clearly found in families of probands with bipolar disorder, so too are a range of other mood disorders. It is this finding that has perhaps played a dominant role in the conceptualisation of the spectrum (Akiskal 2002). The identification of specific genes that may confer susceptibility is currently an area of intense investigation. In a recent review, the rate of bipolar disorder in relatives of probands with bipolar disorder was about 7 per cent, with a higher proportion (10 per cent) having unipolar disorder (Malhi et al. 2000). This is double the population risk of about 5 per cent and suggests an aetiological relationship between the two phenotypes. Twin and adoption studies suggest that this risk is genetic rather than environmental, that the penetrance of the genetic factors is less than 100 per cent, and that genetic traits have variable expression in terms of phenomenology. This is complicated by the likelihood that bipolar disorder displays genetic heterogeneity and that its expression is non-Mendelian, like that of many other illnesses such as hypertension or cancer.

Studies of bipolar II disorder have similarly shown that, although bipolar II disorder is the most common phenotype in relatives of probands with the disorder, higher than expected rates of other mood disorders have been found (Coryell et al. 1984). Phenomenological heterogeneity is found in most genetic studies (DePaulo et al. 1990; Sadovnick et al. 1994).

In contrast, studies of schizoaffective disorder have found mixed results. Broadly, the findings suggest that the depressive subtype of schizoaffective disorder is more related to schizophrenia, and the manic subtype is more related to bipolar disorder. However, although early studies reported that bipolar disorder was no more common in families of subjects with schizophrenia than the general population, and vice versa, recent data are more ambivalent (Erlenmeyer-Kimling et al. 1997). Other genetic studies have shown overlapping genetic vulnerability of bipolar disorder with alcohol and other substance abuse and panic disorder (Winokur et al. 1998).

CLINICAL FEATURES

Differentiating clinical features would be of value in defining the bipolar spectrum. Empirically, the bipolar spectrum midpoint is best represented by bipolar II disorder. Several clinical features vary across bipolar I disorder, bipolar II disorder and unipolar disorder. Whereas in unipolar disorder there is a well-documented female preponderance and bipolar I disorder tends to display equivalent sex ratios, bipolar II disorder seems to occupy an intermediate position (Benazzi 1999; Canceil et al. 1999), although it is important to note that some studies report no clear sex separation (Hendrick et al. 2000). Generally, the age of onset of bipolar II disorder is reported as being earlier than that of unipolar disorder (Angst 1986) and either similar to (McMahon et al. 1994; Judd et al. 2003) or later than that of bipolar I disorder (Gershon 1990). There is also a suggestion that bipolar II disorder with atypical depression may start earlier than the non-atypical pattern of illness.

A high risk of suicide is consistently reported in studies of bipolar disorder. Suicide risk may be greatest in the mixed phase of the disorder (Tondo et al. 1999). Particularly high rates of suicide have been associated with bipolar II disorder, perhaps partly because mixed states are reported as being more common in bipolar II disorder (Benazzi 2001). Interestingly, in most but not all studies, depression severity is similar in bipolar II and unipolar depression and both appear to have similar rates of melancholia. Rates of hospitalisation are lower in bipolar II than in bipolar I patients, and psychotic symptoms are less common in bipolar II disorder (Vieta et al. 1997; Baldessarini et al. 1999; Benazzi 2000b).

Atypical features such as hypersomnia, hyperphagia, marked fatigue and rejection sensitivity are common in bipolar II disorder, more so than unipolar disorder, and especially in females; however, mood reactivity is usually preserved (Rihmer et al. 1995; Perugi et al. 1998; Benazzi 2000a, c; Benazzi and Rihmer 2000). Similarly, psychomotor retardation is reportedly more common in bipolar than unipolar disorder (Kupfer et al. 1988), and bipolar disorder, both types I and II, is associated with higher rates of substance abuse than in the general population. However, bipolar II patients have higher rates of comorbid anxiety, in particular social and simple phobias, and may have a more recurrent pattern than bipolar I disorder, with more hypomanic and depressive episodes than bipolar I patients (Judd et al. 2003), although illness episodes may be shorter. In contrast, unipolar patients have a longer illness, with shorter cycles, a greater number of overall episodes, and lower rates of recovery and more chronic outcome compared with bipolar II subjects (Angst 1986). Interestingly, a key distinguishing feature of bipolar as opposed to unipolar disorder appears to be the acute onset and abrupt offset of episodes (Angst 1986; Akiskal 1996). Seasonal associations are also well recognised, with bipolar I disorder often having onset of mania in spring and autumn and depression in summer and winter, while bipolar II disorder is linked to summer and winter births and depression in spring and summer (Vieta et al. 1997).

PERSONALITY

The role of personality within the various manifestations of the bipolar spectrum is complex, and a review of the research pertaining to this area presents conflicting findings. The most consistent finding is that there are more borderline features in bipolar disorder. In patients with diagnoses of borderline personality diagnoses, 66 per cent have comorbid affective diagnoses (Akiskal et al. 1985), with bipolar II disorder being particularly over-represented (Koenigsberg et al. 2002). In one group of borderline patients, the rate of bipolarity was 69 per cent (Deltito et al. 2001) and patients also had family histories more similar to bipolar than control subjects. Furthermore, there are many affective symptoms in the borderline rubric, to the extent that some authors suggest that a subgroup of patients with borderline symptoms may represent ultra-rapid or mixed phase bipolar spectrum patients (Akiskal

1994). The symptoms of mood lability, impulsivity and interpersonal sensitivity are related to bipolar spectrum pathology, and it has been argued that the construct of borderline personality disorder is better conceptualised as part of the bipolar spectrum. In addition, it is argued that this formulation presents patients with borderline personality disorder as being more amenable to psychological and pharmacological interventions geared to their temperamental attributes.

Further supportive evidence for the relationship between bipolar spectrum and borderline personality comes from reports that this group responds to mood stabilisers such as valproate (Hollander et al. 2001), lamotrigine (Pinto and Akiskal 1998) and atypical antipsychotics such as olanzapine (Zanarini and Frankenburg 2001). Although it is true that differing disorders can respond to similar agents, the pattern of overlap is certainly suggestive. Furthermore, it has also been noted that individuals diagnosed as being borderline during episodes of mood disturbance do not usually have a prior diagnosis of personality disorder. Finally, treatment of the bipolar spectrum disorder is often associated with resolution of elements within the personality domain.

TREATMENT

Antidepressant trial data in bipolar disorder are scant. Although there is some evidence of the utility of antidepressants in the acute treatment of bipolar depression, there is no good evidence of their utility in prophylaxis. In a review of seven published trials of long-term antidepressant treatment, Ghaemi (2002) concluded that no antidepressant proved to be more effective than lithium alone. Furthermore, antidepressant treatment carried clear risks of induction of mania and rapid cycling (Wehr et al. 1988). This risk is somewhat exaggerated, but still illustrates the importance of accurately differentiating unipolar and bipolar spectrum disorders.

Short-term studies of antidepressants in bipolar II disorder have been published. Fluoxetine was reported as efficacious in a short-term controlled trial. Switch rates of 2 per cent were described. Venlafaxine was reported as effective in a 6-week study (Amsterdam and Garcia-Espana 2000). Tranylcypromine was shown to be superior to imipramine in a trial of anergic bipolar I and II patients. Lower switch rates in bipolar II than bipolar I disorder were described (Himmelhoch et al. 1991). Open label data suggest utility of bupropion in bipolar II depression (Haykal and Akiskal 1990). Data on the long-term effects of antidepressant therapy on the course of bipolar II disorder do not yet exist.

There are some early data that point to the efficacy of lithium in bipolar II disorder (Fieve et al. 1976), and lithium's prophylactic effects with regard to suicide have also been noted. The discontinuation risk of lithium is thought to be slightly lower in bipolar II than in bipolar I disorder (Baldessarini et al. 1999), and the probability of remaining depression-free after 2 years of taking lithium ranged from 42 to 55 per cent in a trial of bipolar II patients (Peselow et al. 1982). A greater response to lithium in classical bipolar I disorder, and of carbamazepine in a mixed group of people with bipolar II and bipolar not otherwise specified, is described (Greil and Kleindienst 1999).

In a mixed cohort of refractory bipolar I and II patients, open data with valproate combined with antidepressants suggested efficacy, although the study cohort did include subjects with mania, rapid cycling and depression (Schaff et al. 1993). A positive series in adolescent bipolar II disorder with lithium, valproate and carbamazepine has been described (Kowatch et al. 2000). Low-dose valproate (125–500 mg) has been claimed to be efficacious in a small trial of cyclothymia and rapid cycling (Jacobsen 1993).

In a trial of rapid-cycling bipolar disorder, greater efficacy of lamotrigine was seen in bipolar II than bipolar I patients (Calabrese et al. 2000). In a randomised, placebo-controlled trial, lamotrigine plus fluoxetine was superior to fluoxetine and placebo in a group of patients with resistant depression, including both bipolar II and unipolar patients (Barbosa et al. 2003).

CONCLUSION

There are significant differences between bipolar I and II disorders, supporting the view that they are separate conditions, albeit overlapping clinically to an extent. The bipolar II spectrum is the most common form. Clear phenomenological similarities tie the two of them to a similar root, with bipolar I being more severe and bipolar II being perhaps more recurrent and chronic a disorder. There is also the suggestion that the two disorders are related in an affective liability threshold model of aetiology – a possibility that compounds the hope that definitive genetic and molecular markers will demarcate their boundaries.

However, clinically, the necessity for diagnostic clarity remains and there are clear imperatives for making the correct diagnosis. The therapeutic approaches for the unipolar and bipolar spectrums are forever diverging, and therefore the early diagnosis and institution of appropriate management strategies is critical. All this underscores the need for an increased evidence base in these severe and highly prevalent disorders. The starting point should perhaps be the consistent adoption of a suitable classification system.

REFERENCES

Akiskal HS (1994) The temperamental borders of affective disorders. *Acta Psychiatrica Scandinavica. Supplementum* 379:32-7.

—— (1996) The prevalent clinical spectrum of bipolar disorders: Beyond DSM-IV. *Journal of Clinical Psychopharmacology* 16 (2 Suppl 1):4S-14S.

—— (1999) Bipolarity: Beyond classic mania. *Psychiatric Clinics of North America* 22:517-703.

—— (2002) The bipolar spectrum – the shaping of a new paradigm in psychiatry. *Current Psychiatry Reports* 4:1-3.

Akiskal HS, Pinto O (1999) The evolving bipolar spectrum: Prototypes I, II, III and IV. *Psychiatric Clinics of North America* 22:517-34.

Akiskal HS, Chen SE, Davis GC, Puzantian VR, Kashgarian M, Bolinger JM (1985) Borderline: An adjective in search of a noun. *Journal of Clinical Psychiatry* 46:41-8.

Akiskal HS, Maser JD, Zeller PJ, Endicott J, Coryell W, Keller M, et al. (1995) Switching from 'unipolar' to bipolar II. An 11-year prospective study of clinical and temperamental predictors in 559 patients. *Archives of General Psychiatry* 52:114-23.

Amsterdam JD, Garcia-Espana F (2000) Venlafaxine monotherapy in women with bipolar II and unipolar major depression. *Journal of Affective Disorders* 59:225-59.

Angst J (1986) The course of affective disorders. *Psychopathology* 19 Suppl 2:47-52.

—— (1998) The emerging epidemiology of hypomania and bipolar II disorder. *Journal of Affective Disorders* 50:143-51.

Angst J, Gamma A, Benazzi F, Ajdacic V, Eich D, Rossler W (2003) Toward a re-definition of subthreshold bipolarity: Epidemiology and proposed criteria for bipolar-II, minor bipolar disorders and hypomania. *Journal of Affective Disorders* 73:133-46.

Baldessarini RJ, Tondo L, Hennen J (1999) Effects of lithium treatment and its discontinuation on suicidal behavior in bipolar manic–depressive disorders. *Journal of Clinical Psychiatry* 60 Suppl 2:77-84.

Barbosa L, Berk M, Vorster M (2003) A double-blind, randomised placebo controlled trial of augmentation with lamotrigine or placebo in patients concomitantly treated with fluoxetine for resistant major depressive episodes. *Journal of Clinical Psychiatry* 64: 403-7.

Benazzi F (1999) Bipolar II disorder is common among depressed outpatients. *Psychiatry and Clinical Neurosciences* 53:607-9.

—— (2000a) Bipolar II depression with melancholic features. *Annals of Clinical Psychiatry* 12:29-33.

—— (2000b) Atypical bipolar II depression compared with atypical unipolar depression and nonatypical bipolar II depression. *Psychopathology* 33:100-2.

—— (2000c) Depression with DSM-IV atypical features: A marker for bipolar II disorder. *European Archives of Psychiatry and Clinical Neuroscience* 250:53-5.

—— (2001) Depressive mixed state: Testing different definitions. *Psychiatry and Clinical Neurosciences* 55:647-52.

Benazzi F, Rihmer Z (2000) Sensitivity and specificity of DSM-IV atypical features for bipolar II disorder diagnosis. *Psychiatry Research* 93:257-62.

Calabrese JR, Suppes T, Bowden CL, Sachs GS, Swann AC, McElroy SL, et al. (2000) A double-blind, placebo-controlled, prophylaxis study of lamotrigine in rapid-cycling bipolar disorder. Lamictal 614 Study Group. *Journal of Clinical Psychiatry* 61:841-50.

Canceil O, Bouzid R, Olie JP, Loo H, Poirier MF (1999) First clinical episode of bipolar disorders: A study within a population of bipolar I and bipolar II French patients. *Encephale* 25:523-7.

Cassano GB, Akiskal HS, Savino M, Musetti L, Perugi G (1992) Proposed subtypes of bipolar II and related disorders: With hypomanic episodes (or cyclothymia) and with hyperthymic temperament. *Journal of Affective Disorders* 26:127-40.

Coryell W, Endicott J, Andreasen N, Keller M (1985) Bipolar I, bipolar II, and nonbipolar major depression among the relatives of affectively ill probands. *American Journal of Psychiatry* 142:817-21.

Coryell W, Endicott J, Reich T, Andreasen N, Keller M (1984) A family study of bipolar II disorder. *British Journal of Psychiatry* 145:49-54.

Deltito J, Martin L, Riefkohl J, Austria B, Kissilenko A, Corless C, Morse P (2001) Do patients with borderline personality disorder belong to the bipolar spectrum? *Journal of Affective Disorders* 67:221-8.

DePaulo JR, Simpson SG, Gayle JO, Folstein SE (1990) Bipolar II disorder in six sisters. *Journal of Affective Disorders* 19:259-64.

Endicott J (1998) Gender similarities and differences in the course of depression. *Journal of Gender Specific Medicine* 1:40-3.

Erlenmeyer-Kimling L, Adamo UH, Rock D, Roberts SA, Bassett AS, Squires-Wheeler E, et al. (1997) The New York High-Risk Project. Prevalence and comorbidity of axis I disorders in offspring of schizophrenic parents at 25-year follow-up. *Archives of General Psychiatry* 54:1096-102.

Ferrier IN, MacMillan IC, Young AH (2001) The search for the wandering thymostat:

A review of some developments in bipolar disorder research. *British Journal of Psychiatry. Supplement* 41:s103-6.

Fieve RR, Kumbaraci T, Dunner DL (1976) Lithium prophylaxis of depression in bipolar I, bipolar II, and unipolar patients. *American Journal of Psychiatry* 133:925-9.

Geller B, Zimerman B, Williams M, Bolhofner K, Craney JL (2001) Bipolar disorder at prospective follow-up of adults who had prepubertal major depressive disorder. *American Journal of Psychiatry* 158:125-7.

Gershon ES (1990) Genetics. In Goodwin FK, Jamison KR (eds), *Manic Depressive Illness*. Oxford University Press, pp. 373-401.

Ghaemi SN, Boiman EE, Goodwin FK (2000) Diagnosing bipolar disorder and the effect of antidepressants: A naturalistic study. *Journal of Clinical Psychiatry* 61:804-0; quiz 09.

Ghaemi SN, Ko YJ, Goodwin FK (2001) The bipolar spectrum and the antidepressant view of the world. *Journal of Psychiatric Practice* 7:287-97.

Ghaemi SN, Ko JY, Goodwin FK (2002) 'Cade's disease' and beyond: Misdiagnosis, antidepressant use, and a proposed definition for bipolar spectrum disorder. *Canadian Journal of Psychiatry* 47:125-34.

Goodwin FK, Jamison KR (1990) *Manic–Depressive Illness*. New York: Oxford University Press.

Greil W, Kleindienst N (1999) Lithium versus carbamazepine in the maintenance treatment of bipolar II disorder and bipolar disorder not otherwise specified. *International Clinical Psychopharmacology* 14:283-5.

Hantouche EG, Akiskal HS, Lancrenon S, Allilaire JF, Sechter D, Azorin JM, et al. (1998) Systematic clinical methodology for validating bipolar-II disorder: Data in mid-stream from a French national multi-site study (EPIDEP). *Journal of Affective Disorders* 50:163-73.

Haykal RF, Akiskal HS (1990) Bupropion as a promising approach to rapid cycling bipolar II patients. *Journal of Clinical Psychiatry* 51:450-5.

Hendrick V, Altshuler LL, Gitlin MJ, Delrahim S, Hammen C (2000) Gender and bipolar illness. *Journal of Clinical Psychiatry* 61:393-6.

Himmelhoch JM, Thase ME, Mallinger AG, Houck P (1991) Tranylcypromine versus imipramine in anergic bipolar depression. *American Journal of Psychiatry* 148:910-16.

Hirschfeld RM, Calabrese JR, Weissman MM, Reed M, Davies MA, Frye MA, et al. (2003) Screening for bipolar disorder in the community. *Journal of Clinical Psychiatry* 64:53-9.

Hollander E, Allen A, Lopez RP, Bienstock CA, Grossman R, Siever LJ, et al. (2001) A preliminary double-blind, placebo-controlled trial of divalproex sodium in borderline personality disorder. *Journal of Clinical Psychiatry* 62:199-203.

Jacobsen FM (1993) Low-dose valproate: A new treatment for cyclothymia, mild rapid cycling disorders, and premenstrual syndrome. *Journal of Clinical Psychiatry* 54:229-34.

Judd LL, Akiskal HS (2003) The prevalence and disability of bipolar spectrum disorders in the US population: Re-analysis of the ECA database taking into account subthreshold cases. *Journal of Affective Disorders* 73:123-31.

Judd LL, Akiskal HS, Schettler PJ, Coryell W, Maser JD, Rice JA, et al. (2003) The comparative clinical phenotype and long term longitudinal episode course of bipolar I and II: A clinical spectrum or distinct disorders? *Journal of Affective Disorders* 73:19-32.

Koenigsberg HW, Harvey PD, Mitropoulou V, Schmeidler J, New AS, Goodman M, et al. (2002) Characterizing affective instability in borderline personality disorder. *American Journal of Psychiatry* 159:784-8.

Kowatch RA, Suppes T, Carmody TJ, Bucci JP, Hume JH, Kromelis M, et al. (2000) Effect size of lithium, divalproex sodium, and carbamazepine in children and adolescents with bipolar disorder. *Journal of the American Academy of Child and Adolescent Psychiatry* 39:713-20.

Kupfer DJ, Carpenter LL, Frank E (1988) Is bipolar II a unique disorder? *Comprehensive Psychiatry* 29:228-36.
Lewis L (2001) The use of surveys as an advocacy tool. *Fourth International Conference on Bipolar Disorder*. Pittsburgh, USA, 14–16 June.
Lopez-Ibor JJ (1990) The spectrum of mood disorders. *Journal of Clinical Psychiatry* 51 Suppl:62-4.
Malhi GS, Moore J, McGuffin P (2000) The genetics of major depressive disorder. *Current Psychiatry Reports* 2:165-9.
Manning JS, Connor PD, Sahai A (1998) The bipolar spectrum: A review of current concepts and implications for the management of depression in primary care. *Archives of Family Medicine* 7:63-71.
Manning JS, Haykal RF, Connor PD, Akiskal HS (1997) On the nature of depressive and anxious states in a family practice setting: The high prevalence of bipolar II and related disorders in a cohort followed longitudinally. *Comprehensive Psychiatry* 38:102-8.
McMahon FJ, Stine OC, Chase GA, Meyers DA, Simpson SG, DePaulo JR, Jnr (1994) Influence of clinical subtype, sex, and lineality on age at onset of major affective disorder in a family sample. *American Journal of Psychiatry* 151:210-15.
Perugi G, Akiskal HS, Gemignani A, Pfanner C, Presta S, Milanfranchi A, et al. (1998) Episodic course in obsessive-compulsive disorder. *European Archives of Psychiatry and Clinical Neuroscience* 248:240-4.
Peselow ED, Dunner DL, Fieve RR, Deutsch SI, Rubinstein ME (1982) Age of onset of affective illness. *Psychiatria Clinica* 15:124-32.
Pinto OC, Akiskal HS (1998) Lamotrigine as a promising approach to borderline personality: An open case series without concurrent DSM-IV major mood disorder. *Journal of Affective Disorders* 51:333-43.
Rihmer Z, Rutz W, Pihlgren H (1995) Depression and suicide on Gotland. An intensive study of all suicides before and after a depression-training programme for general practitioners. *Journal of Affective Disorders* 35:147-52.
Robins LN, Helzer JE, Weissman MM, Orvaschel H, Gruenberg E, Burke JD, Jr, et al. (1984) Lifetime prevalence of specific psychiatric disorders in three sites. *Archives of General Psychiatry* 41:949-58.
Sadovnick AD, Remick RA, Lam RW, Zis AP, Yee IM, Huggins MJ, et al. (1994) Mood Disorder Service Genetic Database: Morbidity risks for mood disorders in 3,942 first-degree relatives of 671 index cases with single depression, recurrent depression, bipolar I, or bipolar II. *American Journal of Medical Genetics* 54:132-40.
Schaff MR, Fawcett J, Zajecka JM (1993) Divalproex sodium in the treatment of refractory affective disorders. *Journal of Clinical Psychiatry* 54:380-4.
Tondo L, Baldessarini R, Hennen J, Minnai G, Salis P, Scamonatti L, et al. (1999) Suicide attempts in major affective disorder patients with comorbid substance use disorders. *Journal of Clinical Psychiatry* 60 Suppl 2:63-9.
Vieta E, Benabarre A, Colom F, Gasto C, Nieto E, Otero A, et al. (1997) Suicidal behavior in bipolar I and bipolar II disorder. *Journal of Nervous and Mental Disease* 185:407-9.
Wehr TA, Sack DA, Rosenthal NE, Cowdry RW (1988) Rapid cycling affective disorder: Contributing factors and treatment responses in 51 patients. *American Journal of Psychiatry* 145:179-84.
Winokur G, Turvey C, Akiskal H, Coryell W, Solomon D, Leon AC, et al. (1998) Alcoholism and drug abuse in three groups – bipolar I, unipolars and their acquaintances. *Journal of Affective Disorders* 50:81-9.
Zanarini MC, Frankenburg FR (2001) Olanzapine treatment of female borderline personality disorder patients: A double-blind, placebo-controlled pilot study. *Journal of Clinical Psychiatry* 62:849-54.

SECTION

III

Aetiology and Pathophysiology

CHAPTER 7

THE GENETIC EPIDEMIOLOGY OF MAJOR DEPRESSION

Patrick F Sullivan

A question that often arises in the clinical management of major depression is: 'Doctor, why am I depressed?'. For the empirically minded, this is a deceptively tricky and even frustrating question. The weighty phrases *multifactorial aetiology* and *bio-psycho-social model* have certainly been uttered by many psychiatrists and often appear to address the patient's concerns. However, what do these terms really mean? How indeed do people come to have major depression? How can the literature inform clinical practice regarding the aetiology of major depression?

The purpose of this chapter is to review what is known about the causes of major depression with reference to the approaches of genetic epidemiology. Genetic epidemiology investigates the interaction of genetic and environmental risk factors influencing the development of familial conditions like major depression (Plomin et al. 1997). It also represents a shift in the conceptualisation of causative factors in its attempt to determine the relative contributions of genetic and environmental factors (Thomas 2000). Traditional epidemiological studies have tended to focus on environmental sources of causation to the neglect of genetic aetiological factors. Traditional genetic studies have tended to focus on genetic sources of causation at the expense of environmental aetiological factors. Genetic epidemiology attempts to address the question of the extent to which the relevant aetiological factors are due to genetic influences (nature) and to what extent due to environmental influences (nurture). Instead of asking 'nature or nurture', a genetic epidemiologist would ask 'to what extent nature and to what extent nurture'.

THE EPIDEMIOLOGY OF MAJOR DEPRESSION

It is useful briefly to review the epidemiology of major depression. The lifetime prevalence of major depression has been investigated in random community samples in various countries. Although the findings of individual studies vary considerably as a function of the diagnostic instrument and criteria used to define major depression, the lifetime prevalence of major depression appears to be on the order of 10–20 per cent (Weissman et al. 1993a) and may be particularly high in New Zealand (Wells et al. 1989). In other words, about one in every five or ten adults is likely to experience an episode of major depression at some point in their lifetime. Of those who report an episode of major depression in their lifetime, about half had been depressed in the 6 months prior to interview.

Major depression is associated with considerable mortality, morbidity (greater than a number of common chronic medical conditions), and tends to be a chronic or recurring illness. By 2020, major depression is projected to become the second leading cause of disability worldwide (Murray and Lopez 1996). Only a minority of individuals with major depression receive any form of treatment, despite the availability of effective psychological and pharmacological interventions.

SOCIODEMOGRAPHIC RISK FACTORS FOR MAJOR DEPRESSION

Traditional epidemiological studies have identified some sociodemographic risk factors for major depression. Being female has been shown to be a risk factor for major depression in several studies, with women having about twice the risk men have (Weissman et al. 1993a). Age cohort effects appear to influence the risk of major depression, with increased risk in younger age cohorts.

With regard to background or childhood events, the presence of intrafamilial sexual abuse, extended parental separations, and a poorer perceived parental relationship appear to increase the risk of major depression. However, parental death does not seem to be a potent risk factor for major depression.

Recent life circumstances appear to be associated with major depression. For example, lacking social supports, marital status (separated, divorced, or widowed), and adverse or stressful recent life events have been linked to major depression.

Of relevance to this chapter is the consistent finding that a positive family history is a risk factor for major depression (Weissman 1987).

THE APPROACH OF GENETIC EPIDEMIOLOGY

If a disorder has been shown to be *familial* (that is, it runs in families), the next step is to attempt to understand why. To what extent is the familial clustering of a disorder due to biological inheritance and to what extent due to environmental factors to which members of a family tend to be exposed? The answer to this question has important implications for attempts to understand the causes of disorders like major depression, as well as for attempts to fashion rational primary preventive efforts. For example, if a disorder is largely genetically determined (for example, Huntington's disease), then understanding its aetiology will probably involve molecular genetics. If a disorder is largely due to environmental exposures (for example, smoking and lung cancer), then preventive efforts will necessarily involve breaking the appropriate causal chain.

Genetic epidemiological studies that attempt to address these issues in humans are typically of three designs: family, adoption, and twin studies.

In *family studies*, the relatives of probands with and without a certain trait are systematically studied to determine whether the trait in question is familial. The approach is essentially that of the familiar case–control design, with cases defined by the presence of major depression, controls by its absence, and with the presence of major depression in immediate relatives as a putative risk factor. The demonstration that a disorder is familial is often viewed as an important first step, as disorders that do not run in families are unlikely to have a genetic basis. However, family studies are unable to separate genetic influences from environmental risk factors that run in families. To delineate nature and nurture, different types of studies are needed.

Adoption studies are a social experiment. Individuals born to one set of parents are raised separately by unrelated parents. Genetic effects are revealed by the degree of resemblance between adoptees and their biological parents and environmental effects by the resemblance between adoptees and their adoptive parents. In theory, adoption studies are an elegant way to tease apart the influences of genetic and environmental factors.

Two assumptions potentially limit the validity of adoption studies. The first assumption is the issue of *representativeness*: if biological and adoptive parents are not representative, then attempting to generalise results from an adoption study to other individuals may not be appropriate. Indeed, participation in adoption does not appear to be a random process, as adoptive parents are often somewhat older and desire an adoptive child because of infertility. Biological parents in the past tended to relinquish children for adoption because of social attitudes about illegitimacy. As illegitimacy is now far less of a concern in most industrialised countries, the purpose of adoption has shifted to situations where the biological parents have severely neglected or abused a child or where a parent is deemed incapable of appropriate care (for example, in the case of a severe mental illness). The second assumption is whether genetic and environmental influences are relatively unrelated. If genetic and environmental factors are highly correlated, then the adoption design is essentially a family study and uninformative.

The literature suggests that participation in adoption is not a random process and therefore generalising results from an adoption study must be done cautiously. However, the second assumption appears to be reasonable, as only small correlations between the relevant genetic and environmental factors have been found.

Twin studies compare the degree of similarity between *monozygotic* and *dizygotic* twin pairs. Monozygotic twins are assumed to be genetically identical, whereas dizygotic twins are non-identical siblings from the same pregnancy. By comparing the resemblance of monozygotic twin pairs for a trait with the resemblance of dizygotic twin pairs, genetic and environmental effects can be separated. In addition, the latter can be further partitioned into shared and unshared environmental effects. *Shared environment*, also known as familial environment, refers to the environmental variables to which both members of a twin pair are exposed. Examples of shared environmental effects are certain aspects of the uterine environment before birth (for example, maternal illness or infection), familial variables (for example, parental socioeconomic status or divorce), and the culture in which the twins live. *Unshared environment*, also known as individual-specific environment, refers to the environmental variables to which one member of a twin pair is uniquely exposed. Examples of unshared environmental effects are certain aspects of the uterine environment before birth (for example, differences in placental blood flow), individual relationships with parents, siblings, or peers, and experiencing specific events (for example, some form of trauma). Unshared environmental effects usually also include measurement error; the importance of this technical point is discussed below.

The validity of the twin design rests upon several assumptions, particularly the *equal environment assumption* (that exposure to the relevant environmental variables is no greater in monozygotic twins than in dizygotic twins). Although this assumption continues to receive empirical support, that twins are known to have higher rates of perinatal and birth complications and the unusual nature of the twin relationship itself may limit the unqualified generalisability of results from these studies.

An important point to bear in mind for results of both adoption and twin studies is that the terms *genetic effects* and *environmental effects* are latent variables. Latent variables are not measured or observed directly, but rather are inferred from measurements on individuals who are part of certain sorts of relationship (such as twin pairs or those involved with adoption). Furthermore, these latent variables attempt to explain the variation within a group of individuals.

Suppose we have interviewed a large number of twins and have carefully determined whether each person has ever had a major depressive episode. Although we would expect a significant minority of these individuals to have had a depressive episode, this would clearly not be the case for all subjects. Thus, individuals vary in regard to the presence of lifetime major depression. As these individuals are pairs of twins, we are able to understand more about the reasons underlying the observed variation in the presence of lifetime depression. Specifically, we can determine the percentage of the observed variation due to genetic, shared environmental, and unshared environmental effects.

For example, for the liability to developing major depression, suppose that 50 per cent of the variation is due to genetic effects, none to shared environmental effects, and the remaining 50 per cent to unshared environmental effects. These findings suggest that half the variation for major depression is under genetic control, half is due to factors specific to one sibling and not another, and that familial and cultural variables common across siblings are unimportant. Although such findings might clarify our understanding of the causes of major depression, they leave many important questions unanswered. As these effects are defined with reference to groups rather than individuals, from a clinical perspective, how do such results translate to a particular patient? Which genes are responsible for the genetic variation? Precisely how and where do these genes exert their effects? What are the important environmental variables? Why is shared environment so unimportant?

STUDIES OF THE GENETIC EPIDEMIOLOGY OF MAJOR DEPRESSION

Following the above introduction to the general approach of genetic epidemiology, the next step is to review what is known about the genetic epidemiology of major depression. The following is distilled from a recent meta-analysis (Sullivan et al. 2000).

Family studies

Five family studies of major depression have demonstrated its familiality–the tendency for major depression to run in families (Tsuang et al. 1980; Gershon et al. 1982; Weissman et al. 1984; Maier et al. 1993; Weissman et al. 1993b). In comparison to the relatives of normal controls, the immediate relatives of people with major depression are more likely to be afflicted with major depression. A recent meta-analysis calculated the odds ratio for this relationship to be 2.84 (95% CI, 2.31–3.49).

Many of these studies have been particularly well conducted with large samples, superior methodology, and careful attention to the process by which diagnoses are determined. However, with rare exceptions, depressed people were recruited from psychiatric treatment settings, which could bias the results if treatment-seeking itself runs in families. For example, it seems plausible that people who become depressed would be more likely to recognise their depression and to seek psychiatric treatment if they had a relative who had been treated for depression (particularly if the treatment had been successful). If treatment-seeking runs in families, the finding that major depression is familial (in clinical samples) could merely be an artefact. Both studies that have assessed this issue agree that this bias exists; one suggests that its magnitude is quite modest and the other that its magnitude is substantial.

Major depression appears to be a familial disorder. Although there is some concern that such results are artefactual, the weight of the available evidence appears to support this conclusion.

Twin studies

Six twin studies have investigated major depression (Kendler et al. 1995a; McGuffin et al. 1996; Lyons et al. 1998; Bierut et al. 1999; Kendler et al. 2000). A recent meta-analysis determined that the familial aggregation of major depression was due to genetic effects (heritability in liability 37%; 95% CI, 31%–42%). Shared environmental effects were minimal (0%; 95% CI, 0%–5%) and individual-specific environmental effects were substantial (63%; 95% CI, 58%–67%).

Unshared environment also includes measurement error. Even when carefully done, the assessment of lifetime major depression is not particularly reliable; if the same questions about lifetime major depression are asked on different occasions, the answers often differ. Accounting for measurement error often increases the heritability of major depression. The principal weaknesses of the available studies pertain to the twin design itself. Although the assumptions behind the twin methods appear to be reasonable, the unusual nature of the twin relationship may hinder the generalisation of these results.

Adoption studies

Two of three published adoption studies provide support for genetic effects on major depression (von Knorring et al. 1983; Cadoret et al. 1985; Wender et al. 1986). The adoption design is a fairly compelling social experiment. However, the existing adoption studies all have at least one critical weakness. In particular, none has used direct interviews with a representative sample of adoptees.

Conclusion

Major depression is a familial disorder and its familiality mostly or entirely results from genetic influences. Environmental influences specific to an individual are also aetiologically significant. Major depression is a complex disorder that does not result from genetic or environmental influences alone, but rather from both. These findings are notably consistent across samples and methodologies and are likely to be generally applicable conclusions.

To the extent that the results from twin studies generalise to singletons, genetic factors may be highly important. It is very interesting that shared environmental factors appear to be so unimportant – familial factors such as general parental style and background demographic variables appear to be unrelated to the aetiology of major depression. These findings represent a serious challenge to social learning theory and notions of *vertical transmission* of disorders from parent to child via social learning. This is not to say that family factors are unimportant; for example, the parent–child relationship appears to be quite specific (rather than general) and such unshared environmental factors may be very relevant.

These results are important, but many unanswered questions remain. The entities of genetic and unshared environmental effects are latent, aggregate variables. To understand the aetiology of major depression, we need to learn more about the specific genes and environmental forces involved. In addition, it is important to remember that these variables are derived from large groups of people; we need to know more about how they apply to individuals, as this is the focus of clinical practice.

COMORBIDITY

Major depression has been observed to occur in conjunction with other psychiatric disorders at greater than chance rates. Lifetime anxiety disorders, childhood conduct disorder, and alcohol abuse or dependence are associated with the lifetime risk of a major depressive episode. The co-occurrence of major depression with these other psychiatric conditions appears to be accentuated in clinical samples.

There are many unresolved questions regarding the concept of *comorbidity*. For example, it is unclear whether major depression that occurs alone is aetiologically similar to or distinct from major depression that occurs in individuals who had or who have another psychiatric condition. In addition, the influence of historical or current comorbid conditions on the temporal course of major depression is as yet unresolved.

Some authors have posited that, from a genetic perspective, there is a heritable *general neurotic factor* that mediates risk of depression and other comorbid conditions (Andrews et al. 1990). Other authors hold that independent genetic factors are fundamental to the observed comorbidity (Kendler et al. 1995b). At present, this matter is unresolved.

AN AETIOLOGICAL MODEL OF MAJOR DEPRESSION

The accumulated evidence concerning the aetiology of major depression suggests that it is a complex disorder. A mix of genetic and environmental factors appears to be involved in determining the liability to lifetime major depression. This conclusion is probably what is meant when reference is made to the *multifactorial* or *bio-psychosocial* aetiology of major depression. However, these explanations remain vague and unspecified.

Kendler and colleagues have published an interesting paper in which they attempted to develop an empirical model that combined and ranked genetic and environmental risk factors for major depression (Kendler et al. 1993). It is important to note that this model attempted to predict new episodes of major depression over about a 2-year period rather than lifetime major depression.

Kendler and colleagues studied 680 pairs of female twins three times over 30 months. The model included the interactions among a considerable number of variables, which included traumatic experiences, genetic factors, personality variables, and interpersonal stressors. Their exploratory model enjoyed a fair degree of success, as it was able to account for 50 per cent of the variation in developing major depression. In addition, the model could rank the relative strength of the predictors independently of one another. Strong predictors were recent stressful life events, genetic risk factors, past history of major depression, and neuroticism. Predictors of intermediate strength were recent life difficulties, parental warmth, and lifetime traumas. Modest predictors were social support and parental loss.

Although this model was clearly preliminary, it seems to be a sensible and clinically useful model concerning the interaction and relative importance of these variables. It assigned some meaning to the obfuscating terms *multifactorial* and *bio-psychosocial* and added a sense of order to the multitude of variables (such as stressful life events, family history, past history, and personality) thought important in the genesis of major depression.

It is important to note that this model has limitations. First, it was only partially successful; although one can argue that accounting for 50 per cent of the variance in any psychiatric variable is impressive, it is still far short of the ultimate mark. Second, this model attempted to predict new episodes of major depression; it is plausible that factors that influence the onset or the first episode of major depression are different from the factors that influence subsequent episodes. Third, the genetic variable used was crude (a history of major depression in a co-twin); genetic factors might appear more important than this model indicates if a more sophisticated measure of genetic risk were used.

Finally, it is important to state a caution. Even when there is overwhelming evidence that some human trait or medical disorder is heritable, such findings must not be equated with certain risk. Genetic determinism and similar fatalistic interpretations of the evidence are inappropriate for a variety of reasons. Perhaps the most important finding of studies of this sort is that both nature and nurture are important. Even when an individual carries a strong genetic predisposition, the ultimate expression of that predisposition is influenced by many factors – biology, environment, personal choices and chance are certainly all involved.

CONCLUSION

What of the question posed in the introductory paragraphs: what are the implications of the existing research on the genetic epidemiology of major depression for clinical practice?

First, these results provide strong support for the validity of the entity of major depression. The clear implication of family genetic factors in the aetiology of major depression combined with evidence about course, treatment outcome, morbidity and mortality strongly supports the validity of major depression as a disorder and as a significant public health problem.

Second, both genetic and environmental factors are important in the aetiology of major depression. The understanding of precisely what these terms mean is as yet elusive. As the field matures, perhaps a more sophisticated understanding will be forthcoming.

Finally, the above points could certainly be applied to the clinical management of individuals with major depression. Many individuals afflicted with major depression believe their symptoms to be their own fault, resulting from moral weakness, some past event, or improper attitude. The available data suggest that such assumptions are generally simplistic and may be frankly incorrect. Applying the findings from the genetic epidemiology literature to the clinical management of major depression can be very helpful in relieving the patient from undue self-blame and framing the appropriate treatment goals.

ACKNOWLEDGMENTS

PFS was supported by grants MH-59160, AI-38429, NS-41483 and CA-85739 from the United States National Institutes of Health.

REFERENCES

Andrews G, Stewart G, Morris-Yates A, Holt P, Henderson S (1990) Evidence for a general neurotic syndrome. *British Journal of Psychiatry* 157:6-12.

Bierut LJ, Heath AC, Bucholz KK, Dinwiddie SH, Madden PAF, Statham DJ, et al. (1999) Major depressive disorder in a community-based twin sample: Are there different genetic and environmental contributions for men and women? *Archives of General Psychiatry* 56:557-63.

Cadoret RJ, O'Gorman TW, Heywood E, Troughton E (1985) Genetic and environmental factors in major depression. *Journal of Affective Disorders* 9:155-64.

Gershon ES, Hamovit J, Guroff JJ, Dibble E, Leckman JF, Sceery W, et al. (1982) A family study of schizoaffective, bipolar I, bipolar II, unipolar, and normal control probands. *Archives of General Psychiatry* 39:1157-67.

Kendler KS, Gardner CO, Prescott CA (2000) Corrections to two prior published articles. *Archives of General Psychiatry* 57:94-5.

Kendler KS, Pedersen NL, Neale MC, Mathe AA (1995a) A pilot Swedish twin study of affective illness including hospital- and population-ascertained subsamples: Results of model fitting. *Behavior Genetics* 25:217-32.

Kendler KS, Kessler RC, Neale MC, Heath AC, Eaves LJ (1993) The prediction of major depression in women: Toward an integrated etiologic model. *American Journal of Psychiatry* 150:1139-48.

Kendler KS, Walters EE, Neale MC, Kessler RC, Heath AC, Eaves LJ (1995b) The structure of the genetic and environmental risk factors for six major psychiatric disorders in women. Phobia, generalized anxiety disorder, panic disorder, bulimia, major depression, and alcoholism. *Archives of General Psychiatry* 52:374-83.

Lyons MJ, Eisen SA, Goldberg J, True W, Lin N, Meyer JM, et al. (1998) A registry-based twin study of depression in men. *Archives of General Psychiatry* 55:468-72.

Maier W, Lichtermann D, Minges J, Hallmayer J, Heun R, Benkert O, et al. (1993) Continuity and discontinuity of affective disorders and schizophrenia. Results of a controlled family study. *Archives of General Psychiatry* 50:871-83.

McGuffin P, Katz R, Watkins S, Rutherford J (1996) A hospital-based twin register of the heritability of DSM-IV unipolar depression. *Archives of General Psychiatry* 53:129-36.

Murray CJL, Lopez AD (1996) Evidence-based health policy – Lessons from the Global Burden of Disease Study. *Science* 274:740-3.

Plomin R, DeFries JC, McClearn GE, Rutter M (1997) *Behavioral Genetics*, 3rd edn. New York: W.H. Freeman and Company.

Sullivan PF, Neale MC, Kendler KS (2000) Genetic epidemiology of major depression: Review and meta-analysis. *American Journal of Psychiatry* 157:1552-62.

Thomas DR (2000) Genetic epidemiology with a capital 'E'. *Genetic Epidemiology* 19:289-300.

Tsuang MT, Winokur G, Crowe RR (1980) Morbidity risks of schizophrenia and affective disorders among first degree relatives of patients with schizophrenia, mania, depression and surgical conditions. *British Journal of Psychiatry* 137:497-504.

von Knorring AL, Cloninger CR, Bohman M, Sigvardsson S (1983) An adoption study of depressive disorders and substance abuse. *Archives of General Psychiatry* 40:943-50.

Weissman MM (1987) Advances in psychiatric epidemiology: Rates and risks for major depression. *American Journal of Public Health* 77:445-51.

Weissman MM, Bland R, Joyce PR, Newman S, Wells JE, Wittchen HU (1993a) Sex differences in rates of depression: Cross-national perspectives. *Journal of Affective Disorders* 29:77-84.

Weissman MM, Wickramaratne P, Adams PB, Lish JD, Horwath E, Charney D, et al. (1993b) The relationship between panic disorder and major depression. A new family study. *Archives of General Psychiatry* 50:767-80.

Weissman MM, Gershon ES, Kidd KK, Prusoff BA, Leckman JF, Dibble E, et al. (1984) Psychiatric disorders in the relatives of probands with affective disorders. The Yale

University–National Institute of Mental Health Collaborative Study. *Archives of General Psychiatry* 41:13-21.

Wells JE, Bushnell JA, Hornblow AR, Joyce PR, Oakley-Browne MA (1989) Christchurch Psychiatric Epidemiology Study, Part I: Methodology and lifetime prevalence for specific psychiatric disorders. *Australian and New Zealand Journal of Psychiatry* 23:315-26.

Wender PH, Kety SS, Rosenthal D, Schulsinger F, Ortmann J, Lunde I (1986) Psychiatric disorders in the biological and adoptive families of adopted individuals with affective disorders. *Archives of General Psychiatry* 43:923-9.

CHAPTER 8

AETIOLOGY AND PATHOPHYSIOLOGY OF BIPOLAR DISORDER

Philip B Mitchell
and Peter R Schofield

At present, we have no specific knowledge of the presumed abnormal molecular processes causing bipolar disorder. There is no doubt, however, that this is a strongly biological and frequently inherited disorder. The interaction of this genetic diathesis with environmental insults such as stressful life events or substance abuse is a common pathway to the ultimate expression of the clinical phenotype.

This chapter focuses on genetic and pharmacological investigations into the mechanisms causing bipolar disorder. Brain imaging and neuropathological studies are dealt with in Chapters 11 and 13. Comorbidity of bipolar disorder with substance use is discussed in Chapter 24.

HISTORICAL WRITINGS

Although *mania* is an old term, originally connoting a broad range of psychotic disorders with overactivity or aggressive behaviour, it undoubtedly always included patients currently described by that rubric. The earliest 'explanation' of the cause of mania was probably that of Hippocrates, who ascribed this condition to an excess of yellow bile. In the first century, Aretaeus of Cappadocia believed that mania was due to an inflammation of the brain caused by heat from the heart. Such classical descriptions probably influenced the sixteenth century French medical academic Fontanon:

> This disease [mania] occurs when the brain suffers either by itself or by reason of sympathetic reaction. It occurs sometimes solely from the warmer intemperatura of the brain without a harmful humor, and this is like what happens in drunkenness. It occasionally arises from stinging and warm humors, such as yellow bile, attacking the brain and stimulating it along with its membranes. It sometimes even originates in incorrupt blood, which may even be temperate but which harms the brain by its quantity alone.

Reflecting the increasing scientific understanding of the late nineteenth century, Henry Maudsley surmised:

> Joy and grief evidently lie very near one another in the region of molecular physics; a very little difference of motion makes the difference between the one and the other. No wonder then that melancholy and mania alternate with each other in the same case or are so mixed that it is hard to say which name ought to be used.

This observation of Maudsley was astute, as any causative explanation must account for the propensity to swings of both mania and depression. Hitherto many studies and hypotheses have only addressed the causes or correlates of mania or depression per se.

GENETIC STUDIES

The firmest and most consistently replicated evidence for aetiological factors in bipolar disorder is that of genetic origins (Craddock and Jones 1999). While the specific genetic defect or defects are still elusive, there is no doubting the strongly inherited nature of the condition. The following discussion reviews the evidence for this.

Evidence for the familial tendency of bipolar disorder

The first step in investigating the genetics of a disorder is to demonstrate familiality. Bipolar disorder is clearly more prevalent in the first-degree relatives of bipolar probands, with rates of 1.5 to 14.5 per cent compared with 0.2 to 1.3 per cent in controls (Andreasen et al. 1987). For families of bipolar I probands, there appear to be increased rates of both bipolar I and bipolar II disorders. First-degree relatives of people with bipolar disorder have a risk of seven times the population rate for developing this condition. Unipolar depression definitely occurs more frequently in these pedigrees, with rates of 7.8 to 22.8 per cent, higher than the rates of 4.6 to 5.9 per cent found in control pedigrees. Overall, first-degree relatives have about twice the risk of the general community for developing depression. Two of these studies have also examined rates of cyclothymia, suggesting that this is also increased – with morbid risks of 2.6 to 3.0 per cent compared with up to 0.8 per cent in controls.

In summary, rates of mood disorder are clearly increased in the families of bipolar disorder probands, with rates of 7.8 to 30.8 per cent compared with 4.8 to 6.3 per cent in control pedigrees. These figures indicate a strong familial, and therefore possibly genetic, diathesis to a spectrum of mood disorders in such families. This spectrum appears to include at least bipolar disorder, unipolar depression and schizoaffective disorder (bipolar type), and possibly cyclothymia.

Twin studies

Unlike family studies, a review of twin studies cannot assemble a large amount of data on bipolar disorder alone. Most investigations have examined heterogeneous groups of unipolar and bipolar subjects. The seminal studies, notably those carried out in Scandinavia and the United Kingdom, have recruited from systematically collected twin and psychiatric registers.

Three of the larger studies warrant particular attention. Bertelsen et al. (1977) interviewed 133 twins from 220 potential cases identified through the Danish Psychiatric Twin Register. This study demonstrated a gradient of heritability declining from bipolar disorder with manic episodes (bipolar I: 0.77), through bipolar disorder with hypomania (bipolar II: 0.68) to unipolar disorder (0.41 for three or more episodes and 0.22 for less than three episodes). This strongly supports the concept of bipolar disorder as a biological disorder, principally genetic in aetiology, with less severe depressive disorders as correspondingly less genetically and more environmentally determined.

Bertelsen and colleagues also examined the extent to which polarity 'breeds true'. Of thirty-two concordant monozygotic pairs, fourteen were concordant for bipolar disorder and eleven for unipolar disorder. They demonstrated that the seven pairs in which one twin had unipolar depression and the other bipolar disorder was significantly fewer than would be predicted if both disorders shared the same genotype. This finding is in contrast with the familial aggregation data, which suggest that unipolar depression and bipolar disorder are on an inherited continuum of affective illness.

Torgersen (1986) undertook a similar register-based study of Norwegian twins. Like Bertelsen's group, Torgersen found a decreasing gradient of heritability from bipolar disorder, through psychotic major depression, nonpsychotic major depression to dysthymic disorder and depressive adjustment disorder.

In the largest and most recent twin study, McGuffin et al. (2003) studied sixty-seven twin pairs in which the proband had bipolar disorder (thirty monozygotic and thirty-seven dizygotic), and 177 twin pairs where the proband had depression (sixty-eight monozygotic and 109 dizygotic). They found 67 per cent concordance in monozygotic twins and 19 per cent in dizygotic twins, estimating the heritability of bipolar disorder to be 85–89 per cent. Furthermore, their data were not consistent with the proposition that depression is merely a less severe manifestation of the same genetic vulnerability. There was, however, substantial genetic overlap between bipolar disorder and unipolar depression, interpreted by the authors as indicative of a correlated liability model.

Adoption studies

Adoption studies of mood disorders, although limited in number, provide another means to assess the genetic contribution to disease aetiology. Only two studies have specifically examined bipolar disorder, and the total sample sizes are small.

Mendlewicz and Rainer (1977) carried out the first adoption study of bipolar disorder. The probands were twenty-nine adoptees ascertained from medical records of outpatient and inpatient clinics. Psychopathology in their biological and adoptive parents was compared with that of (1) parents of bipolar individuals who were not adopted, (2) biological and adoptive parents of healthy adoptees, and (3) parents of individuals who had contracted poliomyelitis in childhood or adolescence.

They found an excess of psychopathology in the biological parents of affected adoptees compared with their adoptive parents. Similar levels of psychopathology were found in the biological parents of non-affected adoptees and non-adoptees. Although the total incidence of psychopathology was slightly greater for the biological parents of normal adoptees than in their adoptive parents, this was due to cases of alcoholism and sociopathy rather than mood disorders. Parents of children with poliomyelitis were found to have the same level of disorder as adoptive parents, indicating the comparability of adoptive parents of affected children to other parents raising an ill child.

Mendlewicz and Rainer found that the cases of unipolar depression in biological parents almost always preceded the occurrence of bipolar disorder in their children, while always following it in adoptive parents. They speculated that cases of unipolar depression in adoptive parents might be reactive and less severe forms of the disorder. This study supported the notion that familial aggregation of bipolar disorder is the result of genetic rather than social transmission.

Wender et al. (1986) carried out a study in which seventy-one adoptees with a history of mood disorder were individually matched with a control adoptee on the basis of sex, age, time spent with biological mother, age at transfer and socioeconomic status of the adoptive parents. Psychiatric histories of relatives were accessible by the cross-matching of Danish population registries and psychiatric records. An excess of bipolar and unipolar depression was found in the biological relatives of affected compared with control adoptees. This difference was not maintained for neurotic depression and *affect reaction*. No significant differences were found between the two groups for adoptive relatives. Thus, like Mendlewicz and Rainer's study, this study supports a genetic basis for mood disorders, particularly in severe forms.

The few studies involved makes the identification of trends impossible. Nevertheless, the only study using a homogeneous group of probands (Mendlewicz and Rainer 1977) found strong evidence for genetic effects. Similar results were obtained by Wender et al. (1986) when comparison was restricted to severe disorders. In this light, the results may be seen as supporting the results of family and twin studies.

The Human Genome Project

Completion of the human genome sequence has now demonstrated that humans possess about 30 000 protein-coding genes, fewer than earlier estimations of around 100 000 (Lander et al. 2001; Venter et al. 2001; Mattick

2003). The Human Genome Project was established in 1990 with the goal of analysing the structure of human DNA and determining the location of each of these genes. This enormous undertaking provided detailed physical maps of the human genome (all the genetic material in human chromosomes), and provided markers for specific regions of the genome to be used to potentially identify sites of abnormality for the more than 4000 human diseases with genetic origins, such as bipolar disorder. Most importantly, this project has provided the actual sequence of the approximately three billion base pairs of DNA.

It is also now apparent that only about 1.5 per cent of the human genome codes for protein. Non-protein-coding RNAs are thought to represent 50–75 per cent of all transcripts in humans. Although the function of this enormous output is currently poorly understood, it seems likely that it plays a critical regulatory role during development. It is possible that abnormalities in this regulatory architecture (which controls patterns and amounts of protein) may be responsible for mental illness, rather than abnormalities of protein-coding regions themselves (Mattick 2003).

Identifying disease genes

Genes that are physically distant on chromosomes are not predictably co-inherited, because of the process of recombination. Conversely, genes that are situated close to each other are more likely to be co-inherited. Therefore, if a particular polymorphism (or structural variant) of a gene is always co-inherited with a particular polymorphism of another gene, it is indicative that these two genes are physically proximate. That is, they are *linked*.

A gene is linked to a disease when it can be demonstrated that a particular polymorphism occurs more frequently than expected by chance in people with the particular illness. This can be investigated in a family by linkage studies; between siblings by sib-pair analyses; or in populations by association studies (linkage disequilibrium). If a gene is found to be linked to a disease, that does not necessarily indicate that it is the disease gene, but it means that the disease gene is nearby in that particular chromosomal region. Pedigree linkage analyses allow identification of disease genes neighbouring the marker gene; linkage disequilibrium provides high power for identifying disease genes of small effect close to the marker gene.

The provision of detailed physical maps and sequencing from the Human Genome Project and other similar research has allowed the capacity to test for linkage to most of the human genome. It is now possible to routinely undertake *genome scans*, testing for linkage genes at least 10 cM (centimorgans) apart (a *centimorgan* is a measure of rates of recombination, and is roughly equivalent to one million base pairs). If linkage is found, that indicates that the disease gene is in that region. More detailed mapping (1–2 cM) can be undertaken to eventually isolate the genetic region more accurately. The process of *positional cloning* is then used to identify the actual gene and disease-causing variant.

These developments mean that there is now a practical reality to the identification of genes for disease even when no known defect or pathology is known. Linked genes can be cloned, their amino acid structure identified, and eventually their function determined. Examples are the genes for Huntington's chorea and Duchenne's muscular dystrophy. Such genes may or may not have been previously recognised – for example, since it is estimated that half of all genes are expressed in the brain, and less than 20 per cent of known genes have clearly defined biological functions, a very large number of genes expressed in the human brain are of an unknown structure or function.

The definitive test of the involvement of a particular gene in a Mendelian or monogenic disorder is the demonstration of a mutation of that gene only in people with the condition, while for complex genetic disorders, such as the mental illnesses, susceptibility gene variants will be overly represented in the disease population. The identification of particular causal mutations is now a feasible technical procedure, and the identification of susceptibility alleles is beginning to meet with experimental success.

Mode of inheritance of bipolar disorder

Most psychiatric conditions do not demonstrate Mendelian patterns of inheritance such as the autosomal dominant inheritance of Huntington's chorea. Even categorically defined disorders such as schizophrenia and bipolar disorder are considered to be *non-Mendelian*, or complex, genetic disorders, for which there is an interaction between a number of genes and environmental factors. Other complex traits in medicine include cardiac disease, epilepsy, asthma and hypertension. Current thinking is that the *functional psychoses* such as bipolar disorder are *oligogenic*, that is, they are caused by the epistasis (or interaction) of a small number of genes, some of which may be of small effect, and others of large effect. It is thought that few (if any) families have illness due to one single major gene. Indeed, if this were the case, it would be expected that pedigrees with dominantly inherited illness (with a likely early age of onset) had been identified, as has been the case for the Mendelian forms of early onset Alzheimer's disease and early onset breast cancer.

Linkage studies in bipolar disorder

Although there is undoubted evidence for significant genetic transmission of bipolar disorder, the specific abnormal genes involved remain to be identified. Since the initial unreplicated report of linkage of this condition to genes on the short arm of chromosome 11 (region 11p15) in a large Amish family by Egeland and colleagues in 1987, there have many further linkage studies.

There have been two major approaches to linkage studies using DNA markers. The first is *genome scanning*: the systematic analysis of linkage of multiple markers which are selected to ensure an overall covering of the entire genome. There are now several published genome scans of bipolar disorder, though fewer than in other conditions such as schizophrenia. As yet, there are no well-replicated susceptibility genes or regions for bipolar disorder. An important recent development has been the first published meta-analysis of genome scans for this condition (Segurado et al. 2003). This study used eighteen genome screen datasets, including 2437 individuals with bipolar disorder, schizoaffective disorder or recurrent depression. No region achieved genome-wide statistical significance. The most significant findings were on chromosomes 9p, 10q and 14q. In the current largest single pedigree sample (that of the NIMH Genetics Initiative), which comprises 250 pedigrees (Dick et al. 2003), genome-wide significant linkage was found on chromosomes 17q and 6q.

An alternative (though to some extent overlapping) strategy is the *candidate gene* approach, which investigates the linkage of specific genes (for example, receptor or enzyme genes) that may have theoretical relevance to the particular disease of interest. Various candidate genes of interest in bipolar disorder have been reported recently. A number of studies have found the gene for brain-derived neurotrophic factor to be associated with susceptibility to bipolar disorder (Neves-Pereira et al. 2002). Hattori et al. (2003) have reported that polymorphisms at the *G72/G30* gene locus on chromosome 13q were associated with bipolar disorder in two independent pedigree series. Intriguingly, this replicated an initial identification of the role of the *G72/G30* locus in schizophrenia, consistent with the thesis of Berrettini (2000), who has proposed a close genetic relationship between these two conditions. Finally, in a very recent report using lymphoblastoid cells collected from bipolar disorder twins, Kakiuchi et al. (2003) have identified *XBPI* (a pivotal gene in the endoplasmic reticulum stress response) as contributing to the genetic risk for bipolar disorder. However, as with earlier candidate gene analyses, the critical factor in assessing the relevance of each of these recent exciting reports will be replication in large independent cohorts.

A complementary approach to candidate gene identification has recently become available through the use of gene expression or profiling studies. A recent study by Tkachev et al. (2003) has highlighted the power of these molecular biological techniques in evaluating disease mechanisms using post mortem brain tissue. That group examined gene expression using differential display, quantitative PCR and microarray analysis. They found a reduction of key oligodendrocyte-related and myelin-related genes in both bipolar disorder and schizophrenia, suggesting the possibility of common causative and pathophysiological pathways.

Progress in the field has been inhibited by the lack of replicated findings from both genome scan and candidate gene analyses. Clearly, larger pedigree collections are needed to confirm findings of linkage in disparate samples. Also, alternative means of testing for linkage, such as using *endophenotypes* (simpler physiological markers which underlie the complex clinical phenotype), have been proposed, although well-validated biological abnormalities are lacking from this illness. One recent promising candidate comes from the report of slow binocular rivalry in bipolar disorder patients (Miller et al. 2003).

There are major benefits that will arise from the ultimate identification of susceptibility genes for bipolar disorder. Apart from elucidating mechanisms of illness and the nature of the interaction between genes and environment, it will allow for the development of aetiologically targeted pharmaceutical therapies, and a rational classification system (Craddock and Jones 1999).

HINTS FROM NATURE: SECONDARY MANIA AND BIPOLAR DISORDER

Do *experiments of nature* reveal any hints about the aetiology of bipolar disorder? Since the seminal review of the syndrome of secondary mania by Krauthammer and Klerman in 1978, a slow stream of case reports has continued to appear. However, it must be acknowledged that the proportion of manic episodes due to identifiable organic factors has always been considered low.

Drug-induced mania

Medications that induce mania in a considerable proportion of patients include antidepressants, prednisone, adrenocorticotrophic hormone or cortisone, L-dopa, bromocriptine, iproniazid and baclofen. Almost half of such medication-induced manic episodes occur within the first week of treatment.

Endocrine dysfunction

THYROID DYSFUNCTION Although hyperactivity is not uncommon in hyperthyroid patients, there have only been a few reports of frank mania. Intriguingly, there have been also reports of hypomania apparently related to hypothyroidism. Hypothyroidism has also been reported to occur at an increased prevalence in patients with rapid-cycling bipolar disorder.

HYPOTHALAMIC–PITUITARY–ADRENAL AXIS DYSFUNCTION Hypomania may be caused by excessive endogenous steroids, as well as excessive exogenous steroids (as discussed above).

Neurological disorders

BRAIN INJURY DUE TO CEREBROVASCULAR DISEASE AND CLOSED HEAD INJURY There have been few reports associating brain injury with hypomania, compared with the relatively large number of reports of depression in such patients. However, despite the infrequency of such reports, there has been some consistency in linking mania with right hemisphere lesions, and in particular those located in basal temporal regions. Robinson's group at Johns Hopkins Hospital in Baltimore has reported a significantly greater frequency of right hemisphere injury associated with the limbic system (specifically in the orbitofrontal and basal temporal cortices, the head of the caudate and the thalamus) in patients developing secondary mania, compared with those developing major depression. Furthermore, this research group has suggested that risk factors for mania in people with brain injuries include a family history of bipolar disorder and anterior subcortical atrophy. They have identified possible anatomical locations of lesions in patients who developed typical recurrent bipolar disorder, as opposed to a single manic episode, finding that bipolar disorder patients had subcortical lesions (mainly of the right head of the caudate and right thalamus) whereas patients with single episodes of mania had high frequencies of cortical involvement (mainly right orbitofrontal and basal temporal cortices).

EPILEPSY There has been interest in the association between epilepsy (in particular, complex partial seizures) and psychosis since the original report of Flor-Henry. Although most descriptions have suggested an association between epilepsy and schizophrenia, recent reports have suggested that mania may also occur at an increased prevalence in patients with complex partial seizures.

OTHER NEUROLOGICAL DISORDERS Both single episodes of mania and recurrent bipolar disorder have been associated with a large variety of neurological dysfunctions. These have included limbic arteriovenous malformations, idiopathic dystonia, multiple sclerosis, cerebral sarcoidosis involving the limbic system, subarachnoid haemorrhage, right frontal arteriovenous malformations, acoustic neuromas and pericallosal arterial ectasia. Recent reports have indicated that olfactory groove meningiomas frequently present with psychiatric manifestations, particularly mania (Turazzi et al. 1999).

Late onset mania

Various studies have suggested an increased prevalence of neurological disorders in people with late onset mania. These studies have consistently found a reduced incidence of a family history of bipolar disorder or other psychiatric disorders in such patients, particularly in men. Recent research has indicted that late onset mania is also associated with an increased mortality rate compared with both depressed and non-mood-disordered controls.

Infections

Although the original reports on secondary mania suggested an association between a range of different infections and secondary mania, more recent publications have focused upon a possible association with HIV/AIDS. These accounts, of patients with both AIDS and AIDS-related complex, have suggested that these disorders may lead to a syndrome indistinguishable from the idiopathic functional mania. It has been estimated that manic syndromes are found in 8 per cent of patients with AIDS. In a sample of patients who became manic, those who had a previous history of mood disorders presented with mania later in the course of HIV infection, and had a higher prevalence of comorbid dementia than those with previous mood disturbance.

SIGNAL TRANSDUCTION PATHWAYS

Some recent hypotheses on the aetiology of bipolar disorder have been stimulated by basic research findings on the effects of lithium (Pilcher 2003) and valproate on intracellular signal transduction pathways (Manji and Lenox 2000). Such a general conceptual approach to further understanding of mechanisms underlying bipolar disorder was eloquently articulated by John Cade back in 1970:

> That lithium, a single inorganic ion, can reverse a major psychotic reaction must have, quite apart from its substantial therapeutic value, profound theoretical significance in unravelling the mystery of the so-called functional psychoses. It must be regarded as a major research tool.

Phosphoinositide system

Phosphoinositides are lipids within the cell membrane. Their breakdown pathway, which leads to intracellular calcium release, comprises one of the major intracellular *second messenger* systems. Lithium inhibits several of the enzymes involved in phosphoinositide metabolism and the generation of free inositol – particularly the enzyme inositol monophosphatase (Berridge et al. 1989). This action leads to reduced inositol production, which in turn leads to lower levels of phosphoinositides, with a resulting slowing of this second messenger system. The action of lithium on the phosphoinositide system may explain two notable features of this medication: (1) why it has little effect on normal individuals, and (2) why it has no substantial effect on peripheral tissues. The effect of lithium would be expected to be proportional to the demand for inositol. Neurones operating normally turn over little inositol; hence the effect of lithium would be minimal. However, pathologically increased lipid turnover (as may be occurring in mania) would lead to a greater demand for inositol; hence, the effect of enzyme blockade would be more pronounced. Thus, lithium may have the effect of normalising abnormally activated cells. Furthermore, lithium would be expected to be specific to the central nervous system (CNS), as cells outside the CNS can easily use plasma-accessible inositol and do not rely on recycling of intracellular stores. Cells within the CNS, on the other hand, depend on recycled intracellular inositol, as little plasma inositol crosses the blood–brain barrier. This postulated theory for the mechanism of action of lithium implies that an accelerated turnover of inositol lipids occurs in bipolar disorder. A related alternative theory is that lithium acts via reduced protein kinase C activity, which results in reduced phosphorylation of physiologically important phosphoproteins such as MARCKS (Manji and Lenox 2000).

Williams et al. (2002) showed that lithium, carbamazepine and valproic acid all inhibit the collapse of sensory neuron growth cones and increase growth cone area. These effects do not depend on GSK-3 (see below) or histone deacetylase inhibition. Williams et al. showed that inositol is able to reverse the effects of the drugs on growth cones, again supporting the role of inositol depletion in bipolar pathogenesis. In addition, they showed that the development of the slime mould *Dictyostelium* is sensitive to lithium and to valproic acid, but that deletion of the prolyl oligopeptidase gene, which regulates inositol metabolism, removes this sensitivity. Inhibitors of prolyl oligopeptidase were also shown to reverse the drug effects on sensory neuron growth cone area and collapse.

Calcium

The significant role of intracellular calcium in the phosphoinositide second messenger system has been discussed already. A potential aetiological role of calcium in bipolar disorder has been suggested by a number of studies. Mainly originating from Dubovsky's group in Colorado, these studies have demonstrated consistent findings of increased platelet and lymphocyte intracellular calcium, and increased red blood cell calcium ATPase activity in both mania and bipolar depression. While such findings in peripheral blood cells may not correlate with brain calcium function, the findings nonetheless indicate the value of further research into calcium activity in this disorder.

Guanine nucleotide binding proteins

There has been considerable interest in the role of guanine nucleotide binding proteins (G proteins) in both the mechanism of action of lithium and the aetiology of bipolar disorder. G proteins are present within all cells, in which they act as *coupling* agents between receptors in the cell membrane and internal second messenger systems such as adenylyl cyclase and the phosphoinositide system. Each G protein comprises three subunits (α, β, γ), of which the (? form has been most researched. There is a large family of G proteins, including stimulatory (Gs) and inhibitory (Gi) types.

The effect of lithium upon G proteins was first reported by Avissar et al. (1988). They found that this medication reduces Gs function in rat tissue. Other investigators have subsequently confirmed this basic action of lithium on Gs. In 1991, lithium was found to decrease platelet Gαi function in human subjects. Such reports of lithium affecting Gs and Gi function have understandably stimulated interest in a potential role of abnormal G proteins in the pathogenesis of bipolar disorder itself. In 1991, it was reported that G proteins are hyperfunctional in the leukocytes of untreated manic patients. In the same year, Young et al. (1991) from Canada reported on a post mortem study of bipolar and control subjects, finding significantly increased levels of Gαs in the cerebral cortex. In 1994, Young et al. investigated G protein expression in the leukocytes of unmedicated depressed bipolar and unipolar patients. Although G protein concentrations were no different from controls in the unipolar patients, both Gαs and Gδ levels were increased in the leukocytes of the bipolar depressed group.

Manji and Mitchell also demonstrated higher levels of Gα in peripheral blood cells of bipolar disorder patients. And Mitchell et al. (1997) found higher levels of Gα, in both bipolar I and bipolar II patients. Significantly, however, this abnormality was found in euthymic bipolar patients irrespective of treatment, suggesting that the dysfunction represented a trait abnormality. This contention was consistent with the finding of a strong trend towards higher Gαs levels in peripheral cells of lithium-treated euthymic bipolar affective patients (Manji et al. 1995), although Avissar et al. (1997) reported these findings to be state-dependent but not trait-dependent. While these findings would suggest an inherited vulnerability, two specific genetic studies examining Gαs in bipolar pedigrees have excluded linkage (Gejman et al. 1993). The reason for this apparent discrepancy is unclear, but it may indicate that the abnormally elevated G protein expression in bipolar affective patients is secondary to some other regulatory factor (genetic or circulating). Overall, however, these studies suggest that abnormal G proteins may play a central role in the pathophysiology of this enigmatic disorder.

Glycogen-synthase kinase-3 (GSK-3)

In 1996, Klein et al. reported that lithium inhibits activity of the enzyme glycogen-synthase kinase-3 (GSK-3). This action may be the mediating process in the action of lithium in increasing grey matter volume, by prompting production of new neurones. Lithium also appears to be neuroprotective (Hashimoto et al. 2002).

CONCEPTUAL MODELS OF THE AETIOLOGY OF BIPOLAR DISORDER

There have been few attempts to develop comprehensive conceptual models for the aetiology or pathophysiology of bipolar disorder. Here we discuss a number of pharmacological and functional models. Other models based on neuropathological and brain injury findings are discussed elsewhere in the relevant chapters.

Mandell and Knapp (1976) have proposed that the essential dysfunction was an 'inordinate degree of proneness to phase coherence and emergent self-organisation across levels in cooperative brain systems'. The authors went on to propose that 'high coherence leads to macroscopic oscillations, increased tendency to order in response to perturbation, and close juxtaposition of regions of phase transitions to bifurcations and turbulence'. They suggested that lithium may act to 'uncouple this pathological degree of molecular cooperativity'.

Using a functional dimensional approach, Carroll et al. (1994) suggested that this condition may be best understood as due to disturbances in central pleasure-reward and pain mechanisms, as well as psychomotor regulation. Carroll went on to propose specific neuroanatomical and neurotransmitter substrates for these functional dimensions.

In recent years, other conceptual models have been developed in response to the increased understanding of intracellular signal transduction mechanisms and the action of lithium on these. Wachtel (1990) has proposed a functional imbalance between intracellular signalling systems in bipolar disorder. This theory was based on the findings that lithium, at therapeutic concentrations, alters the availability of metabolites of both the adenylyl cyclase (cAMP) and the phosphoinositide IP3/DAG second messenger systems. Lithium would work in depression by deamplifying overactive phospholipase C – restoring balance between the systems and dampening cAMP-activated signals. Mania would result from relative hyperactivity of cAMP-mediated cellular responses due to increased activity of the adenylyl cyclase system.

Schreiber and Avissar (1991) have hypothesised that a primary disturbance of G protein activity may be the biological basis for bipolar disorder. They have proposed that a hyperfunctioning G protein, by its effects on the balance of second messenger systems and hence the state of intracellular phosphorylation, could lead to a catastrophically unstable dynamic system analogous to the affective shifts suffered by bipolar patients. The recent series of reports of increased Gαs levels in patients with bipolar disorder is consistent with this theory.

A physiological model has been proposed by Pettigrew and Miller on the basis of their observation of a trait-dependent slow perceptual alternation in binocular rivalry in euthymic patients with bipolar disorder (Miller et al. 2003). They speculate that such 'stuck' switching mechanisms may be indicative of a genetically determined dysfunction of the brain oscillators that control rates of interhemispheric switching.

CONCLUSION

Although at present the defective molecular underpinnings of bipolar disorder are poorly understood, recent major advances in molecular genetic technologies and increasing understanding of the pharmacological action of the mood stabilisers provide optimism that significant insight into the aetiological mechanisms will develop in the coming decade. Such knowledge will undoubtedly revolutionise the treatment and diagnosis of this disabling condition.

REFERENCES

Andreasen NC, Rice J, Endicott J, Coryell W, Grove WM, Reich T (1987) Familial rates of affective disorder. A report from the National Institute of Mental Health Collaborative Study. *Archives of General Psychiatry* 44:461-9.

Avissar S, Schreiber G, Danon A, Belmaker RH (1988) Lithium inhibits adrenergic and cholinergic increases in GTP binding in rat cortex. *Nature* 331:440-2.

Avissar S, Nechamkin Y, Barki-Harrington L, Roitman G, Schreiber G (1997) Differential G protein measures in mononuclear leukocytes of patients with bipolar mood disorder are state dependent. *Journal of Affective Disorders* 43:85-93.

Berrettini WH (2000) Are schizophrenic and bipolar disorders related? A review of family and molecular studies. *Biological Psychiatry* 48:531-8.

Berridge MJ, Downes CP, Hanley MR (1989) Neural and developmental actions of lithium: A unifying hypothesis. *Cell* 59:411-19.

Bertelsen A, Harvald B, Hauge M (1977) A Danish twin study of manic–depressive disorders. *British Journal of Psychiatry* 130:330-51.

Cade J (1949) Lithium salts in the treatment of psychotic excitement. *Medical Journal of Australia* 2:349-52.

Carroll BJ (1994) Brain mechanisms in manic depression. *Clinical Chemistry* 40:303-8.

Craddock N, Jones I (1999) Genetics of bipolar disorder. In Hyman SE (ed), *The Science of Mental Health*. New York: Routledge, pp. 29-38.

Dick DM, Foroud T, Flury L, Bowman ES, Miller MJ, Rau NL, et al. (2003) Genomewide linkage analyses of bipolar disorder: A new sample of 250 pedigrees from the National Institute of Mental Health Genetics Initiative. *American Journal of Human Genetics* 73:107-14.

Gejman PV, Martinez M, Cao Q, Friedman E, Berrettini WH, Goldin LR, et al. (1993) Linkage analysis of fifty-seven microsatellite loci to bipolar disorder. *Neuropsychopharmacology* 9:31-40.

Hashimoto R, Hough C, Nakazawa T, Yamamoto T, Chuang DM (2002) Lithium protection against glutamate excitotoxicity in rat cerebral cortical neurons: Involvement of NMDA receptor inhibition possibly by decreasing NR2B tyrosine phosphorylation. *Journal of Neurochemistry* 80:589-97.

Hattori E, Liu C, Badner JA, Bonner TI, Christian SL, Maheshwari M, et al. (2003) Polymorphisms at the G72/G30 gene locus, on 13q33, are associated with bipolar disorder in two independent pedigree series. *American Journal of Human Genetics* 72:1131-40.

Kakiuchi C, Iwamoto K, Ishiwata M, Bundo M, Kasahara T, Kusumi I, et al. (2003) Impaired feedback regulation of XBP1 as a genetic risk factor for bipolar disorder. *Nature Genetics* 35:171-5.

Klein PS, Melton DA (1996) A molecular mechanism for the effect of lithium on development. *Proceedings of the National Academy of Sciences of the United States of America* 93:8455-9.

Krauthammer C, Klerman GL (1978) Secondary mania: Manic syndromes associated with antecedent physical illness or drugs. *Archives of General Psychiatry* 35:1333-9.

Lander ES, Linton LM, Birren B, Nusbaum C, Zody MC, Baldwin J, et al. (2001) Initial sequencing and analysis of the human genome. *Nature* 409:860-921.

Mandell AJ, Knapp S (1976) A neurobiological model for the symmetrical prophylactic action of lithium in bipolar affective disorder. *Pharmakopsychiatrie Neuro-Psychopharmakologie* 9:116-26.
Manji HK, Lenox RH (2000) Signaling: Cellular insights into the pathophysiology of bipolar disorder. *Biological Psychiatry* 48:518-30.
Manji HK, Chen G, Shimon H, Hsiao JK, Potter WZ, Belmaker RH (1995) Guanine nucleotide-binding proteins in bipolar affective disorder. Effects of long-term lithium treatment. *Archives of General Psychiatry* 52:135-44.
Mattick JS (2003) The human genome and the future of medicine. *Medical Journal of Australia* 179:212-16.
McGuffin P, Rijsdijk F, Andrew M, Sham P, Katz R, Cardno A (2003) The heritability of bipolar affective disorder and the genetic relationship to unipolar depression. *Archives of General Psychiatry* 60:497-502.
Mendlewicz J, Rainer JD (1977) Adoption study supporting genetic transmission in manic–depressive illness. *Nature* 268:327-9.
Miller SM, Gynther BD, Heslop KR, Liu GB, Mitchell PB, Ngo TT, et al. (2003) Slow binocular rivalry in bipolar disorder. *Psychological Medicine* 33:683-92.
Mitchell PB, Manji HK, Chen G, Jolkovsky L, Smith-Jackson E, Denicoff K, et al. (1997) High levels of Gs alpha in platelets of euthymic patients with bipolar affective disorder. *American Journal of Psychiatry* 154:218-23.
Neves-Pereira M, Mundo E, Muglia P, King N, Macciardi F, Kennedy JL (2002) The brain-derived neurotrophic factor gene confers susceptibility to bipolar disorder: Evidence from a family-based association study. *American Journal of Human Genetics* 71:651-5.
Pilcher HR (2003) Drug research: The ups and downs of lithium. *Nature* 425:118-20.
Schreiber G, Avissar S (1991) Lithium sensitive G protein hyperfunction: A dynamic model for the pathogenesis of bipolar affective disorder. *Medical Hypotheses* 35:237-43.
Segurado R, Detera-Wadleigh SD, Levinson DF, Lewis CM, Gill M, Nurnberger JI, Jr, et al. (2003) Genome scan meta-analysis of schizophrenia and bipolar disorder. Part III: Bipolar disorder. *American Journal of Human Genetics* 73:49-62.
Tkachev D, Mimmack ML, Ryan MM, Wayland M, Freeman T, Jones PB, et al. (2003) Oligodendrocyte dysfunction in schizophrenia and bipolar disorder. *Lancet* 362:798-805.
Torgersen S (1986) Genetic factors in moderately severe and mild affective disorders. *Archives of General Psychiatry* 43:222-6.
Turazzi S, Cristofori L, Gambin R, Bricolo A (1999) The pterional approach for the microsurgical removal of olfactory groove meningiomas. *Neurosurgery* 45:821-5.
Venter JC, Adams MD, Myers EW, Li PW, Mural RJ, Sutton GG, et al. (2001) The sequence of the human genome. *Science* 291:1304-51.
Wachtel H (1990) The second-messenger dysbalance hypothesis of affective disorders. *Pharmacopsychiatry* 23:27-32.
Wender PH, Kety SS, Rosenthal D, Schulsinger F, Ortmann J, Lunde I (1986) Psychiatric disorders in the biological and adoptive families of adopted individuals with affective disorders. *Archives of General Psychiatry* 43:923-9.
Williams RS, Cheng L, Mudge AW, Harwood AJ (2002) A common mechanism of action for three mood-stabilizing drugs. *Nature* 417:292-5.
Young LT, Li PP, Kish SJ, Siu KP, Warsh JJ (1991) Postmortem cerebral cortex Gs alpha-subunit levels are elevated in bipolar affective disorder. *Brain Research* 553:323-6.
Young LT, Li PP, Kamble A, Siu KP, Warsh JJ (1994) Mononuclear leukocyte levels of G proteins in depressed patients with bipolar disorder or major depressive disorder. *American Journal of Psychiatry* 151:594-6.

CHAPTER 9

PSYCHOSOCIAL STRESS AND DEPRESSION

Eugene S Paykel

This chapter deals with effects of recent psychosocial stress on the onset, maintenance and relapse of depression. Three aspects will be discussed: life events, persisting stress, and social support. They have not always been defined.

The term *life event* usually means a change in the external environment that occurs fairly rapidly. This involves several elements. There should be a change, it should be rapid rather than slow (for instance it should be datable, to within about a month), and it should involve the environment, usually the social environment, rather than just representing an internal change in perception. A change that is solely subjective, such as the realisation that one's job is boring, is not a life event, although it may have important consequences. Neither is adolescence, as it is both internal and slow, although it is very important in any life. There is one exception: the development of a personal physical illness is usually regarded as a life event since, although it is an internal change, it is externally verifiable, datable and similar in effects on life to many major external events.

Persistent stressful situations in the absence of change have received less attention. They figure particularly in the work of Brown and colleagues (Brown and Harris 1978), who use the term *difficulties* to describe them.

Social support also refers to a particular kind of situation, usually persistent, conceived of as protective although its absence is really a specific kind of chronic stress. Social support involves provision of help to a person. It is a multidimensional concept, involving emotional concern, love, caring, attention, practical (instrumental) aid, information, and other aspects. This may come from a person's close or wider social network (Brugha 1995).

Since the 1960s, there has been a large volume of literature on effects of recent life events on psychiatric disorder. The basic findings are well established. There is also a large body of literature on social support, although less of it is specifically psychiatric: rather it comes mainly from the social science literature. Space does not permit reference here to the large number of individual studies of these aspects, which will be found in the reviews cited.

RESEARCH METHODS

Most studies of life stress involve retrospective reporting. It is particularly difficult to study life events before they occur. Some precautions are necessary to obtain reliable and valid information.

First, there is a need to obtain accurate reporting. This may be distorted because of ordinary forgetfulness and because of mistaken perceptions due to psychiatric illness (for example, the guilt of depression). In addition, anyone who has had an illness will look for an explanation, the so-called *effort after meaning*, and this explanation may include an event. Furthermore, timing of life events is important in reporting. It is difficult to remember exactly when an event occurred, and subjects may volunteer events well outside the period under consideration.

A second problem is that psychiatric illness may itself produce new life events, which are consequences, not causes of the disorder (for example, job loss due to depression). Two methods can assist in eliminating such events. First, one can date symptom onset and consider only occurrences preceding it. Second, the judgment of independence introduced by Brown and Harris (1978) can be used. Detailed circumstances of an occurrence are examined to infer the likelihood of external origin.

A third issue is quantifying the stress. A count of the number of events is too simple and assumes all events are equal. Asking the subject if an event was stressful is risky as events preceding illness will inevitably be rated high. Various alternative methods have been used, including adding scores for events derived from separate scaling studies, or grouping events by their qualities. Probably the best are methods based on rater judgments using surrounding circumstances to make a rating as to how stressful the event would be to an average person in these circumstances – the rating of contextual threat first introduced by Brown and colleagues (Brown and Harris 1978).

The earliest studies of life events and psychiatric disorder collected data by pencil-and-paper checklists. It is now clear that these are not sufficiently reliable or valid (Paykel 1983). It is hard to define the event adequately and to date its occurrence without the prompts of a detailed interview. An interview method also permits further rating judgments regarding the nature and quality of events, to allow quantification. A variety of interviews have been devised and found useful in research. The two that have been used most commonly are the Bedford College Interview (Brown and Harris 1978) and the Interview for Recent Life Events (Paykel 1996).

The most common research design has been the controlled comparison between life stress occurring before onset in depressed patients and in a control group of normal subjects or of subjects with another disorder. Effects on outcome of depression have also been studied in follow-up studies. Epidemiological community studies identifying subjects with depression have also been used similarly. This is a good way of ruling out selection factors that lead some subjects to treatment. However, depressions treated in the community may be milder, more understandable, and potentially more related to stress than those treated by psychiatrists or in hospital. Another method of study is the prospective study, in which all subjects experiencing a specific effect are followed up. This is an excellent way of studying modifying factors. However, outside the realm of major catastrophes and post-traumatic stress disorder, only small proportions of individuals undergoing the common life stresses develop overt clinical disorder, although milder distress may be more common.

STUDIES OF LIFE EVENTS AT ONSET OF UNIPOLAR DEPRESSION

There have been many studies of life events and depression. The full literature is reviewed in detail elsewhere (Paykel and Cooper 1992; Paykel 1994, 2001; Tennant 2002). Studies have compared life events at onset of depression in samples of depressed patients with general population controls.

The earliest study examining a full range of events this way compared 185 depressed patients with 185 matched subjects from the general population and found the depressed people experienced more events in the 6 months before onset (Paykel et al. 1969). The events spanned a range of stressful experiences, but did not include an excess of events classified as desirable or entrances to the immediate social field of the respondent, while differences were marked for desirable events and exits from the social field. Since then, virtually all such studies have found an excess of events prior to depression onset.

This effect might not be limited to depression; other studies have used comparison groups with other psychiatric disorders. Studies comparing depressives with schizophrenics have tended to find higher rates for preceding life events in depressives, indicating a stronger effect on depression, although not all studies are consistent. Where suicide attempters (parasuicides) have been compared, consistently the suicide attempters, often young and not satisfying diagnostic criteria for depression, have a higher rate of preceding life events than depressives. Studies of comorbidity have found that patients with other primary diagnoses, such as heroin addiction, alcoholism and schizophrenia, who are also depressed have higher rates of preceding life events than those with the primary diagnosis only (Paykel and Cooper 1992).

Life events seem to be important at all ages. Goodyer and colleagues (1987) found that children attending child psychiatry clinics had experienced more severe negative events than community child controls. This effect was not specific to children with depression, but exit events were particularly important in those with severe mood disorder. Studies of elderly patients have also found higher rates of life events in depressed people than in general population controls.

A specific hypothesis would suggest that depression, and not other disorders, is induced by certain types of events. In depression research, loss has received particular attention. This concept is somewhat diffuse and has included interpersonal separations, bereavements, loss of self-esteem and other losses. The most specific meaning is the interpersonal loss by death or by separation. Many studies have found more such events in depressed people than in the general population. Studies comparing depressed people with other psychiatric patients have generally found increased separations in the depressed sample, which suggests more specificity. Events that involve the threat of separation, such as arguments and discord with important interpersonal figures, are also common in depression studies.

Blows to the self-esteem and failures have not usually been explicitly reported, but are probably also common. However, many different kinds of events precede depression. In general, studies suggest only weak specificity. There is some relationship between depression and interpersonal losses, but these also occur before other disorders and many depressions are not preceded by them. The strongest relationship appears when events are categorised in rather broad terms such as threatening or undesirable. Studies of other disorders, such as anxiety disorder, show a similar range of events to be involved, but with some differences.

STUDIES BY BROWN AND COLLEAGUES

The studies by George Brown and colleagues have mainly been based on community samples rather than depressed patients, and almost all have been in women only. The most influential studies were summarised in a seminal book (Brown and Harris 1978). A semi-structured, probing schedule was devised, incorporating the new concepts of independence and threat. In women in Camberwell, independent events and difficulties with long-term threat were found to precede depression.

Subsequent work extended beyond life events and difficulties to background factors modifying consequences of events. A distinction was made between *provoking agents* (life events and difficulties), and *vulnerability factors*, capable of influencing development of depression only when provoking agents were present. The model also involved *symptom-formation factors*, which influenced only the form and severity of depression, but these have received less attention.

In Camberwell, four vulnerability factors were found – lack of a confiding relationship, early loss of mother, presence at home of three or more children, and not working outside the home. In a study in the Hebrides, these factors were modified. Work outside the home was not significant, but absence of churchgoing (a marker of being outside the predominant social group in this community) was.

Subsequent work has involved effects on outcome of depression, effects on other psychiatric and psychosomatic disorders, refinement of different kinds of events, magnitude of effect, and effects of earlier adversity in adulthood and childhood, studied in the retrospective frame. Among follow-up studies, occurrence of fresh start events have been shown to predict better outcome at 1 year (Brown et al. 1988). Experience of humiliation and entrapment in events has been found to predict depression (Brown et al. 1995).

OUTCOME OF DEPRESSION

There is a considerable literature on life stress and the outcome of depression. There is some evidence that depressed people who have an adverse life event before the onset of the episode have a better outcome on follow-up, but some studies have been negative.

More studies have examined events after onset, usually those concurrent with the follow-up period. Short-term remission has been found to be less likely if negative events occur and more likely if a positive event occurs that neutralises an earlier event, or if there is a fresh start event.

Further findings have emerged in the past few years from studies of severe depressions that are recurrent. Two prospective studies of severe recurrent depressions (Andrew et al. 1993; Paykel et al. 1996) found that life events had little effect on relapse or recurrence in these patients. This is in keeping with studies that have compared life stress in earlier or first episodes of depression with later episodes and which have found less life stress preceding the later episodes, suggesting less causative effect (Kendler et al. 2000). Evidently, the course of severe recurrent depression becomes more autonomous or dependent on factors other than life stress.

MELANCHOLIA AND BIPOLAR DISORDER

Two classifications of depression are particularly relevant to life stress. The first is melancholia. Much of the earlier literature on stress and depression was bound up with the concept of endogenous depression and its distinction from reactive depression. This concept as it evolved was complex, in that endogenous depression was considered to show not only absence of life stress at onset but also a specific symptom pattern characterised by what now would be termed *melancholia*, or ICD-10 somatic syndrome. In addition, endogenous depressives were regarded as distinguished from reactive or neurotic depressives by absence of a vulnerable or neurotic personality.

It is now clear that, although some depressions are relatively unrelated to life stress and some depressions do show the melancholic pattern, the pictures in both cases are more often mixed. Furthermore, most studies have found either no relationship or a very weak one between absence of life stress and presence of melancholia.

Two recent studies have found some relationship, in both cases only in depressions that were already recurrent. Using a melancholic–psychotic score based on presence and severity of biological and psychotic symptoms, Brown et al. (1994), studying depressed women, found that severe life events were significantly less frequent in the melancholic–psychotic group. This did not apply to subjects undergoing their first depressive episode, and the difference emerged only when later episodes were examined separately. Frank et al. (1994), in a sample of people with highly recurrent depression, found fewer life events in endogenous than non-endogenous Research Diagnostic Criteria subtypes.

The second subclassification is bipolar disorder. There have been fewer life stress studies than in unipolar depression, but reports have been accumulating. Three studies have found more events before the onset of manic–depressive episodes than in general population control groups, but one study failed to find any difference (see Paykel and Cooper 1992). Recently Malkoff-Schwartz et al. (2000) reported more social rhythm disruption events prior to manic episodes than in control periods in the same subjects, and in those subjects compared with subjects with bipolar depressed episodes or unipolar depressed episodes. There was also a parallel elevation of severe events. This is the only study to make comparisons between bipolar and unipolar subjects. Mania is a disorder that produces increased activity and disinhibition, which readily lead to new events. Particular care therefore needs to be taken to define independent events in studies of mania, and this precaution has not always been observed. Clinically, international travel, which involves disruption of both biological and social rhythms, often leads to manic episodes, although travel may also sometimes be initiated by mania or hypomania.

Other studies have suggested elevations of life events in bipolar subjects experiencing depressive relapses, but these studies are not fully consistent. A sudden peak of relapses was found in bipolar depression in a lithium clinic after a hurricane – clearly an independent event, although one in which impaired medication-taking could have been the causative factor (this is also a possible mediating factor in other studies). Overall, the findings tend to suggest weaker effects on onset and relapse of illness in bipolar than in unipolar disorder.

A further depressive variant is post-partum depression. There is good evidence from both retrospective and prospective studies that recent life events, poor marital relationships and absence of social support are important antecedents of milder post-partum depressions. This is in contrast to the findings in more severe post-partum psychoses, which may be linked to bipolar disorder, and in which three studies have failed to find any relationship with life stress.

MAGNITUDE OF EFFECT

Is the effect of recent life stress on genesis of depression important or trivial? Case–control studies of the kind examined in this review can give a misleading picture. Although differences in life stress occurrence between the two groups may be substantial, if the causative factor is common and the consequential disorder not very common, many occurrences of life stress will not be followed by disorder. Prospective studies of specific events show that, although subsequent distress is common, major clinical disorder is uncommon. Most life events experienced by depressed people before onset are in the moderate range: unpleasant and undesirable, but common in a society where people die, relationships break up, and jobs may be lost.

There have been attempts to quantify the causative effect. Brown and Harris (1978) used the concept of *brought-forward time*: an estimate of the average time from an onset brought about by an event to the time a spontaneous onset would have occurred if no event were present. They concluded that the effect was large in magnitude and formative for depression, but smaller and only triggering for schizophrenia.

Paykel (1978) used an epidemiological measure, the *relative risk*, or ratio of the rate of disease among those exposed to a causative factor to the rate among those not exposed. This can be applied to the control studies using an approximation, *relative odds*. The risk of developing depression in the 6 months after the most stressful classes of events was increased about sixfold, falling off rapidly with time after the event. The relative risks for schizophrenia were much lower, at only two to three over 6 months, but for suicide attempts they were higher.

An alternative epidemiological measure is the population *attributable risk*, expressed as a percentage. This is an estimate of the proportion of disorder caused by life events, and is most easily applied to epidemiological general population studies. Applying this to published studies of depression has produced values ranging from 29 to 69 per cent, but mainly around 40 per cent.

Relative and attributable risks of this magnitude indicate effects that are important, but not exclusive. They suggest disorders with multifactorial causation, in which any single factor may account for only a relatively small proportion of the variance. Although events are important, a large part in determining whether an event is followed by disorder must be attributed to other modifying factors. There may be a whole host of these, both genetic and environmental, ranging from the biochemical, through personality and coping mechanisms, to social experiences, early or recent.

CHRONIC STRESSES

Relatively little work has focused specifically on chronic stresses, separately from change events or social support. Included in the work of Brown and colleagues have been *difficulties*, defined as problems which last at least 4 weeks. In most studies using Brown's methods, difficulties have been amalgamated with life events rather than analysed separately. In the original study by Brown and Harris (1978), difficulties (other than those involving health) that were rated high on threat and had lasted more than 2 years were associated with increased depression. The effect was manifested in the absence of severe events, but presence of both events and difficulties resulted in little increase of depression over that for either one singly.

Another form of chronic stress, not usually discussed in the life stress context, is high family expressed emotion. In studies of depressed patients, this is most commonly in the form of high criticism from the marital partner, rather than over-involvement. There is some evidence that high expressed emotion and high criticism predict relapse, but studies are not consistent, with at least one study suggesting that this does not occur in severe recurrent depression (Hayhurst et al. 1997).

SOCIAL SUPPORT

Social support and other aspects of psychosocial stress are not clearly separated. For instance, an exit event involving a key support person may lead to a subsequent absence of social support. The overlap with difficulties is more marked: social support is defined in the positive direction, but its absence is a chronic stress. High family criticism may readily be associated with poor family support.

The concept of independence has received little attention in the social support literature. It is clear that social support available to an individual will to some extent depend on that individual's own capacity for generating it, by selecting supportive social environments, and generating and fostering friendships and intimate personal relationships.

The social support literature makes distinctions between perceived and objective support, between wider social networks and close networks, between emotional support and instrumental (practical) support. Another distinction, resulting in much empirical research, is whether the effects of absence of social support are directly stressful, or whether the effect of social support is a stress-buffering one, acting only to mitigate effects where adversity (principally as stressful life events) is present.

Studies of social support and depression are summarised elsewhere (Paykel and Cooper 1992; Paykel 1994). A detailed review volume dealing with a wide range of psychiatric aspects is provided by Brugha (1995). Most studies have been on depressed subjects in the community, rather than psychiatric patient samples. Many have been cross-sectional, and far fewer longitudinal. Only longitudinal studies can distinguish well between poor social support that is a consequence of depression or of life events, and that which is pre-existing and prior to onset. The studies suggest that there is both a direct stressful effect on disorder of absence of social support and a stress-buffering effect of social support in moderating effects of life events. Close support appears to have greater influence than wider aspects of network support, but studies are not fully consistent.

Brown and colleagues have investigated social support in working-class women in the community in a longitudinal study (1986). They found poor self-esteem and poor social support correlated. The combination of both, particularly when it involved absence of expected social support from a core tie, was associated with a greatly increased risk of depression after a severe event or major difficulty.

In an influential study of British civil servants in which work status and conditions were found to be important determinants of health, poor social support from work colleagues and supervisors was associated with more frequent and longer spells of sickness absence (Stansfeld et al. 1997).

Several studies have used interventions based on aspects of social support in groups at high risk of disorder, such as women in the postnatal period, women with poor social networks, and psychiatric patients receiving long-term case management in the community (reviewed in Brugha 1995). Results show some initial promise, but well-designed randomised trials have rarely been undertaken. Social skills training may also enhance social support.

ANTECEDENTS OF LIFE EVENTS

In recent years, pathways to disorder have become acknowledged to be complex. As an aspect of this, there have been studies of the origins of life events themselves. These are reviewed in Paykel (2001). Dependent events in the Brown sense are more common in unipolar depressions than in normal controls, and more common in recurrent depressions than in first episodes. These studies confirm that depression can generate events.

There is a growing research examining genetic elements contributing to events. Raised event rates have been found in family members of depressed people, although this familial evidence does not necessarily indicate factors that are genetic rather than environmental, including shared social environment. More conclusively, higher correlations for life events have been found between monozygotic than dizygotic twins.

Kendler and colleagues have used the large Virginia twin registry to explore genetic and environmental elements in more detail. They found that correlations for events in the previous year were a little higher between monozygotic twins than between dizygotic twins. Genetic and environmental elements each accounted for about 20 per cent of the variance. Genetic elements were predominant in *network* events (affecting individuals in the respondent's social networks), whereas environmental elements were predominant in *personal* events (directly affecting the respondent). In later studies, genetic influences affected liability to develop depression after life events. Genetic liability to major depression increased the risk of being exposed to life events, mainly personal ones, outside the depressive episode. About a third of the association between life events and depression appeared to be due to self-selection into high-risk environments. In a further paper in the series (Kendler et al. 1999) (which also contains references to the earlier work), no evidence was found for genetic effects on independent events of personal or network classes, but network events showed considerable effects of family environment. Dependent events of both classes showed genetic effects. Recently, this group has also found genetic elements in social support (Agrawal et al. 2002).

In a different kind of genetic study, Farmer et al. (2001) used a sib-pair analysis to examine interrelationships between sensation-seeking measured on a questionnaire, life events and depression. Sensation-seeking scores showed a familial element and were associated with higher numbers of events of low threat, but were not associated with the more threatening events related to depression, and showed a negative association with depression itself.

Longitudinal cohort studies can examine childhood antecedents of adult events. A very long-term follow-up found that children who had shown emotional or behavioural disturbance when aged 10 years had markedly higher rates of highly threatening events and difficulties, both dependent and independent, when studied in their late 20s. A study using a British longitudinal 1946 birth cohort similarly found that stressful life events in midlife were predicted by high neuroticism in childhood. Absence of social support for people aged 50–70 years has been found to be strongly predicted by alcohol abuse, smoking and depression at age 50 (see Paykel 2001).

IMPLICATIONS FOR PREVENTION

Findings on life stress may have potential implication for prevention. In societies and times in which severe and catastrophic stresses are common, changing social conditions may be very helpful, although difficult. However, in developed Western societies, most of the life stresses involved in depression are not catastrophic but are common consequences of the human condition, including disrupted interpersonal relationships and mortality. In these circumstances, primary prevention by preventing life stresses is unlikely to be feasible. At best, there may be some limited opportunities for people with maladaptive life patterns to acquire new social and problem-solving skills and thus to avoid some life events and to increase social support.

What may be more feasible is a crisis intervention approach, in which occurrence of a stressful event is used as a signal that intervention is indicated in someone known to be vulnerable by previous history. Such intervention would aim to enhance social support and to foster solutions to prevent personal crisis and distress escalating into disorder. Although there are clear possibilities, the amount of research into application is limited, and currently the evidence does not exist for widespread application of these techniques in practice. It may be a fruitful avenue for future research.

REFERENCES

Agrawal A, Jacobson KC, Prescott CA, Kendler KS (2002) A twin study of sex differences in social support. *Psychological Medicine* 32:1155-64.

Andrew B, Hawton K, Fagg J, Westbrook D (1993) Do psychosocial factors influence outcome in severely depressed female psychiatric in-patients? *British Journal of Psychiatry* 163:747-54.

Brown GW, Harris TO (1978) *Social Origins of Depression: A study of psychiatric disorder.* London: Tavistock.

Brown GW, Adler Z, Bifulco A (1988) Life events, difficulties and recovery from chronic depression. *British Journal of Psychiatry* 152:487-98.

Brown GW, Harris TO, Hepworth C (1994) Life events and endogenous depression. A puzzle reexamined. *Archives of General Psychiatry* 51:525-34.

—— (1995) Loss, humiliation and entrapment among women developing depression: A patient and non-patient comparison. *Psychological Medicine* 25:7-21.

Brown GW, Andrews B, Harris TO, Adler Z, Bridge L (1986) Social support, self-esteem and depression. *Psychological Medicine* 16:813-31.

Brugha TS (1995) *Social Support and Psychiatric Disorder: Research findings and guidelines for clinical practice.* Cambridge: Cambridge University Press.

Farmer A, Redman K, Harris T, Mahmood A, Sadler S, McGuffin P (2001) Sensation-seeking, life events and depression: The Cardiff Depression Study. *British Journal of Psychiatry* 178:549-52.

Frank E, Anderson B, Reynolds CF, Ritenour A, Kupfer DJ (1994) Life events and the research diagnostic criteria endogenous subtype. A confirmation of the distinction using the Bedford College methods. *Archives of General Psychiatry* 51:519-24.

Goodyer IM, Kolvin I, Gatzanis S (1987) The impact of recent undesirable life events on psychiatric disorders in childhood and adolescence. *British Journal of Psychiatry* 151:179-84.

Hayhurst H, Cooper Z, Paykel ES, Vearnals S, Ramana R (1997) Expressed emotion and depression. A longitudinal study. *British Journal of Psychiatry* 171:439-43.

Kendler KS, Karkowski LM, Prescott CA (1999) The assessment of dependence in the

study of stressful life events: Validation using a twin design. *Psychological Medicine* 29:1455-60.
Kendler KS, Thornton LM, Gardner CO (2000) Stressful life events and previous episodes in the etiology of major depression in women: An evaluation of the 'kindling' hypothesis. *American Journal of Psychiatry* 157:1243-51.
Malkoff-Schwartz S, Frank E, Anderson BP, Hlastala SA, Luther JF, Sherrill JT, et al. (2000) Social rhythm disruption and stressful life events in the onset of bipolar and unipolar episodes. *Psychological Medicine* 30:1005-16.
Paykel ES (1978) Contribution of life events to causation of psychiatric illness. *Psychological Medicine* 8:245-53.
—— (1983) Methodological aspects of life events research. *Journal of Psychosomatic Research* 27:341-52.
—— (1994) Life events, social support and depression. *Acta Psychiatrica Scandinavica. Supplementum* 377:50-8.
—— (1996) The interview for recent life events. *Psychological Medicine* 27:301-10.
—— (2001) The evolution of life events research in psychiatry. *Journal of Affective Disorders* 62:141-9.
Paykel ES, Cooper Z (1992) Life events and social stress. In Paykel ES (ed), *Handbook of Affective Disorders*, 2nd edn. Edinburgh: Churchill Livingstone.
Paykel ES, Myers JK, Dienelt MN, Klerman GL, Lindenthal JJ, Pepper MP (1969) Life events and depression. A controlled study. *Archives of General Psychiatry* 21:753-60.
Paykel ES, Cooper Z, Ramana R, Hayhurst H (1996) Life events, social support and merital relationships in the outcome of severe depression. *Psychological Medicine* 26:121-33.
Stansfeld SA, Rael EG, Head J, Shipley M, Marmot M (1997) Social support and psychiatric sickness absence: A prospective study of British civil servants. *Psychological Medicine* 27:35-48.
Tennant C (2002) Life events, stress and depression: A review of recent findings. *Australian and New Zealand Journal of Psychiatry* 36:173-82.

CHAPTER 10

THE NEUROBIOLOGY OF DEPRESSION

Isaac Schweitzer
and Virginia Tuckwell

Our knowledge of the neurobiology of depression is expanding exponentially, but is far from being fully defined. The research focus has shifted from neurotransmitters and their receptors and neurohormones – the emphasis is now on gene expression and neuroprotection. The various neurochemical changes that are associated with depression ultimately affect gene expression.

There is considerable evidence supporting the involvement of central nervous system (CNS) serotonergic and noradrenergic neuronal dysregulation and their interrelationships in the pathophysiology of depression. It is also likely that alterations of other neurotransmitters are involved. Concurrent with the studies of neurotransmitters and their receptors has been extensive work in neuroendocrinology, which implicates dysregulation of the hypothalamic–pituitary–adrenal (HPA) axis and other endocrine axes, including the hypothalamic–pituitary–thyroid axis and the hypothalamic–growth hormone axis, in depression. Structural neuroimaging is identifying associated brain regions, and functional neuroimaging is now revealing more specific information regarding brain metabolism and neurotransmitter and receptor activity.

Researchers are using increasingly sophisticated techniques to investigate corticotrophin-releasing factor (CRF), other neuropeptides such as substance P, and intracellular pathways such as G proteins, second and third messenger systems, cyclic AMP response element binding protein (CREB) and brain-derived neurotrophic factor (BDNF), further expanding the number of associated abnormalities that putatively underlie depression. Recent advances in genetics and the completion of the Human Genome Project provide the potential to identify the genes that confer vulnerability to depression.

In this chapter, we describe research findings in depression over the past four decades that contribute to our understanding of the neurobiology of depression and the theories they have generated. We have focused on unipolar major depression; however, in some early studies, diagnosis was described simply as *depression*. Much of the evidence is indirect and is extrapolated from work on the mechanism of action of antidepressants. The abnormalities described herein are not found in all depressed patients and in many cases have also been found in other psychiatric disorders, confusing the significance of the findings. The issue of cause and effect must be considered and the heterogeneity of depression underlies the interpretation of all data.

GENETIC FACTORS

Depression is known to run in families, although this is more common in bipolar disorder than unipolar depression. (The genetic epidemiology of depression is the subject of Chapter 7.)

Current data indicate a significant genetic role in depression. It is postulated that genes confer a vulnerability to depression, or provide protection for the individual. To date, no specific genes have been identified, although research via linkage and association studies has been extensive. It is likely that various genes may contribute to a predisposition to depression and that each gene may bestow only a small effect. Environmental stressors may precipitate biochemical changes in genetically predisposed people that lead to depression. The psychosocial origins of depression are discussed in Chapter 9.

Genetic factors also may underlie a susceptibility to environmental stressors in depressed patients. It is proposed that *genes for depression* may be partly expressed by making individuals more prone to experiencing stressful life events, that is, by causing them to expose themselves to high-risk environments. It has also been proposed that social support is determined to a degree by genetic mechanisms underlying mood disorders (Kendler and Karkowski-Shuman 1997).

BIOGENIC AMINES

The biogenic amine models of depression were proposed during the 1960s. Musselman et al. (1998) provide a good history of these models. The catecholamine hypothesis was formulated in 1964 by Schildkraut and expanded by Bunney and Davis in 1965, who suggested a depletion of the concentration or receptor function of noradrenaline. Coppen in 1967 and Lapin and Oxenkrug in 1969 presented the indoleamine hypothesis, which attributed increased vulnerability to depression due to decreased serotonergic activity. Prange and his colleagues posited that a depletion of synaptic serotonin promoted a fall in noradrenaline, the so-called *permissive biogenic amine* hypothesis. A further variation was the proposal by Janowsky et al. in 1972 of an association between depression and a relative increase in the ratio of cholinergic to noradrenergic activity. Later research proved these hypotheses to be oversimplifications; however, there are many data supporting the involvement of noradrenaline and serotonin dysregulation in depression.

The biogenic amine hypotheses originated from pharmacological observations. Reserpine, which depletes CNS neurons of monoamines, was observed to precipitate depression in some patients. A drug for tuberculosis that inhibited the breakdown of monoamines caused an elevation in mood. Antidepressants increase the functional levels of biogenic amines in the brain: tricyclic antidepressants block the reuptake of noradrenaline and serotonin, serotonin precursors (such as L-tryptophan and 5-hydroxytryptophan) increase serotonin, and monoamine oxidase inhibitors increase synaptic serotonin and noradrenaline. In their turn, these models of depression have led to the development of new classes of antidepressants. The newer antidepressants, the selective serotonin reuptake inhibitors and the serotonin noradrenaline reuptake inhibitors, such as venlafaxine, duloxetine, mirtazapine, reboxetine, nefazodone and trazodone, all work by increasing serotonin and/or noradrenaline availability at the synaptic cleft.

There is an interrelationship between the serotonergic and noradrenergic systems, with reciprocal modulation. An intact serotonin system is required for optimal functioning of noradrenergic neurons. Several brain regions are thought to be involved in depression, and these are served by serotonin- and noradrenaline-containing neurons. The monoaminergic systems are distributed extensively in the limbic, striatal and prefrontal cortex regions. The hypothalamus is associated with appetite, libido and sleep, the amygdala with emotions, and the cortical areas with cognition. Serotonin has been linked to aggression, sleep and appetite, and noradrenaline-containing neurons are involved in many functions that are disturbed in depression, including mood, appetite and drives. Dopamine is important for pleasure, sex and psychomotor activity.

The biogenic amine hypotheses have generated extensive research. The measurement of concentrations of neurotransmitters and their metabolites and receptors in blood, urine and cerebrospinal fluid (CSF) and in the post mortem brain provide direct evidence of dysfunction. Studies show inconsistent alterations in neurotransmitter concentrations, suggesting neurotransmitter dysregulation. Abnormalities have been identified in concentrations of the catecholamines noradrenaline and dopamine, and the indoleamine serotonin and their metabolites, 3-methoxy-4-hydroxyphenylglycol, homovanillic acid and 5-hydroxyindoleacetic acid (5-HIAA), respectively, in blood, urine and CSF of depressed patients. Overall, although there are many data, the evidence is equivocal, as these abnormalities have not been demonstrated consistently in depressed patients.

Post mortem studies of neurotransmitter change are influenced by a variety of factors that make interpretation of post mortem data problematic, not the least being a definitive ante mortem diagnosis. Studies measuring the concentrations of serotonin and noradrenaline are inconclusive. Those investigating neurotransmitter receptors were thought to be more robust, as there is evidence that receptors are less affected by post mortem factors; however, results are still inconsistent. Brain imaging of neurotransmitters, a relatively new technique, may provide more meaningful data, as there are not the problems inherent in post mortem studies. (The contribution of post mortem studies to the understanding of mood disorders is the subject of Chapter 13.)

?-Adrenergic and serotonin receptor binding sites were found to be decreased after long-term, but not short-term, treatment with a range of antidepressants, putatively by down-regulation of noradrenaline and serotonin receptor density. Receptor sensitivity and dysregulation hypotheses were generated from these findings; however, they too have subsequently been modified.

Neuroendocrine studies of neurotransmitter function provide a means of assessing brain function indirectly. Changes in central serotonergic and noradrenergic function may be reflected by challenge tests and measurement of various hormonal responses, such as prolactin, adrenocorticotrophic hormone (ACTH) and growth hormone. The prolactin response to L-tryptophan, a serotonin precursor, is blunted in depressed patients, but produces a robust increase in plasma prolactin concentrations in non-depressed subjects. Prolactin responses to fenfluramine, a serotonin releasing agent and reuptake blocker, have been inconsistent. Some studies report a blunted response in depressed patients compared with healthy subjects, but other studies have found no difference. Ipsapirone, a selective serotonin 1A agonist, produces a decrease in temperature in healthy subjects and a blunted hypothermic response in depressed patients.

Clonidine is an β_2-adrenergic receptor agonist. In response to a clonidine challenge, depressed patients have consistently shown a reduced growth hormone response compared with normal volunteers, supporting a noradrenergic abnormality. Desipramine, a tricyclic antidepressant that is predominantly a noradrenaline reuptake inhibitor, causes an increase in growth hormone that appears to be mediated by stimulation of postsynaptic α_2-adrenergic receptors. Yohimbine, an α_2-adrenergic receptor antagonist, produces increased cortisol and blood pressure response in depressed patients compared with healthy controls.

During the past decade, the biogenic amine transporters have been cloned and selective radioligands developed. Frazer et al. (1999) provided evidence supporting the key role of these transporters in regulating synaptic levels of neurotransmitters. Second messenger systems such as cyclic adenosine 3′,5′-monophosphate (cAMP) dependent protein kinase and protein kinase C are likely to regulate acute transporter function. Post-transcriptional events are implicated in long-term regulation of transporter function.

Cumulative data clearly support a link between dysfunction of both the serotonergic and noradrenergic systems and depression. Presynaptic serotonin dysfunction in depression is supported by lower plasma tryptophan concentration, reduced CSF 5-HIAA level, decreased platelet serotonin uptake (platelets are used as a model of neuronal tissue as they share many properties with brain receptors), and blunted prolactin response to tryptophan and fenfluramine. Postsynaptic, but not presynaptic, dysregulation of the noradrenergic system has been demonstrated. Data supporting this include increased α_2-adrenergic receptor binding in platelets, increased β-adrenergic receptors in the brains of suicide victims, and decreased growth hormone response to clonidine and desipramine.

The neurotransmitters dopamine, acetylcholine, opiates and γ-aminobutyric acid (GABA) have not been studied as intensively as serotonin and noradrenaline, but are also likely to be implicated in depression. Dopamine dysfunction has been observed in some forms of depression, but may have a more important role in bipolar disorder than in unipolar depression. The concentration of muscarinic receptors is increased in depression, implicating the cholinergic system. Concentrations of GABA have been reported to be reduced in the CSF, plasma and brains of depressed subjects. Glutamate is a major excitatory neurotransmitter in the brain and can be neurotoxic in excess. There are high concentrations of the glutamate *N*-methyl-D-aspartate (NMDA) receptor in the hippocampus in depressed subjects. Recent publications have speculated on a possible role for glutamate in depression (Belsham 2001).

NEUROENDOCRINE ABNORMALITIES

As neurotransmitters influence secretion of hormones from the hypothalamus and pituitary, alterations in endocrine abnormalities may be predicted when they are dysregulated. Neuroendocrine measures have been regarded as a window to the brain. Disturbances of the limbic–hypothalamic–pituitary–adrenal axis, which mediates the endocrine stress response, have been one of most extensively researched areas in depression. Patients suffering from endocrine disorders such as Cushing's syndrome frequently experience a mood disturbance. Neurons in the paraventricular nucleus of the hypothalamus secrete CRF, which, with arginine-vasopressin, stimulates the synthesis and release of ACTH from the pituitary gland. ACTH acts on the adrenal cortex to produce glucocorticoids (primarily cortisol), which exert a wide range of effects on metabolism and behaviour. Inhibitory feedback mechanisms operate at the level of the hypothalamus, pituitary and hippocampus. Cortisol inhibits ACTH and CRF synthesis and release, and thus its own production, to maintain homeostasis. Negative feedback is mediated by glucocorticoid receptors, of which there are at least two types in the brain: glucocorticoid receptors are found throughout the brain with high concentrations in the hippocampus and hypothalamus, whereas the mineralocorticoid receptors are more restricted to the hippocampus.

Chronic HPA axis overactivity has been consistently found in at least 50 per cent of depressed patients. Evidence points to an impairment at the hypothalamic level and higher centres. Indices of HPA axis hyperactivity in depression include increased basal concentrations of cortisol and ACTH, as measured in plasma, saliva and CSF; increased urinary 'free' cortisol levels and increased CRF concentrations in the CSF, which return to normal after treatment; and enlargement of the adrenal and pituitary glands (Nemeroff 1998). Neuroendocrine challenge tests have supported these data. The dexamethasone suppression test demonstrated a lack of normal suppression of cortisol following an oral dose of 1 mg dexamethasone, a synthetic corticosteroid, in depressed patients. CRF has been used as a neuroendocrine probe of pituitary function – the ACTH response to CRF is blunted in depression compared with non-depressed controls, whereas the cortisol response is not different. In the dexamethasone–CRF test, depressed patients show a significantly increased ACTH and cortisol response compared with normal controls. A dexamethasone–CRF test using increasing doses of dexamethasone supports the theory of impairment of central glucocorticoid receptor function. It has also been found that depressed patients who do not show a normalisation of HPA axis changes in response to effective treatment are at risk of relapse (Schweitzer et al. 1987; Holsboer 2001).

Several brain pathways control HPA axis activity. The hippocampus exerts an inhibitory effect on CRF neurons in the hypothalamus, and the amygdala exerts an excitatory effect (Nestler et al. 2002). Amygdala hyperactivity correlates with severity of depression, a reflection of the effect of the amygdala on CRF or cortisol on the amygdala. These return to normal levels on effective antidepressant treatment (Manji et al. 2001). GABA-containing neurons are located in the amygdala, hippocampus and paraventricular nucleus, and exert an inhibitory effect on central CRF neurons. There is significant serotonergic and noradrenergic innervation of the hypothalamus, hippocampus, amygdala and cortical areas. Serotonin and noradrenaline are both involved in the regulation of a variety of hormones and neuropeptides, including cortisol, ACTH and growth hormone. Cortisol in its turn interacts with these brain pathways and with neurotransmitters and neuropeptides.

The HPA axis feedback mechanism regulates hippocampal and paraventricular nucleus neurons, and it has been proposed that sustained elevated levels of cortisol may be associated with damage to hippocampal neurons by a failure of the negative feedback inhibition. This is the *glucocorticoid cascade* hypothesis proposed by Sapolsky et al. (1986), whereby hypersecretion of cortisol down-regulates hippocampal glucocorticoid receptors, reducing the inhibitory feedback of the hippocampus on the HPA axis and thus perpetuating hypercortisolaemia and, putatively, loss of hippocampal neurons. This region is high in glucocorticoid receptors, and chronic exposure to glucocorticoids may be neurotoxic.

Overall, evidence points to central CRF overactivity, together with hypercortisolaemia, as the main driver of alterations in HPA axis regulation contributing to depression. The role of CRF is discussed further in the following section on neuropeptides.

The pituitary also secretes growth hormone and thyroid-stimulating hormone (TSH), and abnormalities have been reported in depression. Some depressed patients are found to be hypothyroid (0.7 per cent); however, subclinical abnormalities are more common. Elevated concentrations of TSH are found in about 4 per cent of depressed patients; the TSH response to thyrotrophin-releasing hormone is blunted in 25 per cent of patients and exaggerated in 15 per cent. The effectiveness of augmentation of antidepressant treatment by thyroid hormone supports dysfunction of the hypothalamic–pituitary–thyroid axis in depression. Decreased nocturnal and increased daytime growth hormone secretion and a decreased growth hormone response to clonidine and apomorphine challenge are also reported in depressed patients (Musselman et al. 1998).

The incidence of major depression in women is twice that in men. Oestrogen has been implicated in the regulation of mood and in the neurobiology of mood disorders. Depression has been associated with times of hormonal change such as puberty, post partum, premenstrually and in the perimenopause. It has been suggested that there may be a subtype of depression associated with hormonal factors. Clinical trials of oestrogen treatment of depression in perimenopausal women have demonstrated some positive results (Halbreich and Kahn 2001). The paucity of well-designed studies outside this group is disappointing.

NEUROPEPTIDES

Neuropeptides that have been investigated in depression include CRF, somatostatin, β-endorphin, ACTH, thyrotrophin-releasing hormone, vasopressin, substance P, cholecystokinin, neuropeptide Y and melatonin-stimulating hormone. They are short-chain amino acids that are located in the CNS. They may act as neurotransmitters or neuromodulators; many are colocalised and co-released with the classical neurotransmitters such as serotonin, noradrenaline, dopamine and acetylcholine.

CRF is a hypothalamic hormone and a neurotransmitter within the CNS, mediating autonomic and behavioural responses to stress. CRF neurons are distributed throughout the brain. The release of CRF is mediated by several neurotransmitters; noradrenaline input from the medulla may be primary. CRF secretion is enhanced by serotonergic, noradrenergic and cholinergic inputs, and inhibited by GABA and glucocorticoids. Two CRF receptor subtypes, CRF_1 and CRF_2, have been cloned and sequenced; each has a distinct localisation and pharmacology. Antagonists at the CRF_1 receptor show promise as novel antidepressants. Glucocorticoid antagonists have been investigated as potential antidepressants, but they have significant side effects and, as these drugs affect central HPA activation, they appear to have limited long-term utility (Arborelius et al. 1999; Holsboer 2001).

Increased concentrations of CRF in the CSF have been reported in depressed patients in many studies, but not all. This elevation was described in other disorders as well, but all subjects had comorbid depression. It appears to be state-dependent, as it is reversed by antidepressant treatment (Arborelius et al. 1999; Nemeroff 2002). Post mortem studies report findings of increased CRF-producing neurons in the hypothalamus and increased expression of CRF genes in depressed patients when compared with controls (Nemeroff 1998). There is evidence of reduced CRF binding sites in the frontal cortex of depressed suicide victims, possibly as a compensatory response to increased CRF (Arborelius et al. 1999). Direct intracerebroventricular administration of CRF in laboratory animals induces behaviours reflecting depressive symptomatology. These data, together with the blunted response of ACTH to CRF in depressed patients compared with controls, indicate a hypersecretion of CRH in depression. Nemeroff (2002) has postulated that this hypersecretion leads to a down-regulation of CRF receptors in the frontal cortex and hypothalamus and resultant decreased pituitary response to CRF.

Somatostatin is a hypothalamic neuropeptide and is also found in significant amounts in other brain regions, including the amygdala, hippocampus and prefrontal cortex. Somatostatin inhibits growth hormone, CRF, GABA, TSH and ACTH secretion. Decreased concentrations of somatostatin have been found in the CSF of depressed patients when compared with controls. This finding is reported in other disorders.

Substance P belongs to the neurokinin family of neuropeptides. It is widely distributed in the CNS and interacts with noradrenergic, serotonergic, dopaminergic and GABAergic pathways. Although there is little direct evidence to date that overactivity of substance P pathways is involved in the pathophysiology of depression, several lines of indirect evidence support this. Substance P binds preferentially to neurokinin 1 (NK1) receptors, which are highly expressed in neuroanatomical regions associated with depression (such as amygdala, hippocampus and hypothalamus), is co-localised with biogenic amine neurotransmitters, and plays a role in mediating the stress response. In animals, central injection of substance P provokes anxiety-like behaviours, which are blocked by substance P antagonists. These properties led to inhibition of the substance P–NK1 pathway as a potential treatment for depression. Substance P antagonists are one of the new types of antidepressant currently being trialled in international clinical studies (Kramer et al. 1998).

Arginine-vasopressin is a hypothalamic neuropeptide, which, like CRF, activates the HPA axis and is thought to have a role in the pathophysiology of depression. Elevated levels of arginine-vasopressin have been described in the brain and plasma of depressed patients in some studies, and a correlation with hypercortisolaemia and an association with depressive symptomatology have been described, although there is currently insufficient evidence (Scott and Dinan 2002).

SLEEP CHANGES

Sleep abnormalities are common in depression, and sleep electroencephalography (polysomnography) changes are well documented. Disturbances of sleep continuity, sleep architecture and rapid eye movement (REM) sleep are characteristic of depression. Decreased slow-wave sleep and reduced REM latency (time from sleep onset to first REM period) with increased REM density occurs. Reduced REM latency is probably reversed by antidepressants.

Sleep deprivation and selective REM sleep suppression have antidepressant effects. Neurobiological research of sleep deprivation has implicated serotonin, dopamine, GABA, growth hormone-releasing hormone (GHRH) and CRF, but the role of each is still inconclusive. The effect of sleep deprivation on gene expression is a current area of study.

IMMUNOLOGY

Activation of the inflammatory response system, involving an increase in pro-inflammatory cytokines, and its interaction with the serotonergic system and HPA axis contribute to the pathobiology of depression. Maes and colleagues published the monocyte and T lymphocyte hypothesis of major depression in 1993, and it is now posited that dysregulation of the immune–endocrine system may underlie depression (Leonard 2001).

Immunological measures that provide evidence supporting this theory include leukocyte functioning, leukocyte trafficking (numbers of different types of circulating leukocytes) and markers of immune function. Although there are methodological and technical issues in this area, in depression there appears to be impairment in lymphocyte function, a decrease in natural killer cell activity and a higher frequency of immune activation (Kronfol 2002). These immune abnormalities normalise with effective antidepressant treatment.

Several pro-inflammatory cytokines, such as interleukins (IL) 1 and 6, and tumour necrosis factor α, have potent effects on central serotonergic and noradrenergic systems and the activity of the HPA axis. For example, IL-1 is a potent inducer of CRF synthesis. HPA axis dysfunction may be a consequence of these increased cytokines. Various neurotransmitters, including serotonin, noradrenaline, dopamine and acetylcholine, together with glucocorticoids, CRF, thyroid hormones, growth hormone, prolactin, neuropeptide Y and oestrogens and androgens also affect the immune system. The interrelationships are complex and bidirectional.

The field of psychoneuroimmunology may conceivably be a candidate area in the development of novel treatments for depression.

NEUROIMAGING

Neuroimaging technology has evolved rapidly, allowing examination of structural, metabolic and physiological changes in the brains of living depressed patients. Ever-increasing resolution enables more precise imaging of brain regions. Evidence implicates various brain areas, all interconnected, in the mediation of depressive symptoms. The neocortex and hippocampus may mediate memory impairment, feelings of worthlessness and guilt, suicidality; the striatum and amygdala, emotional memory and possibly anhedonia, anxiety and decreased motivation; the hypothalamus, neurovegetative symptoms such as sleep, appetite and energy (Nestler et al. 2002).

Structural

Generalised and localised structural changes in the brains of depressed patients have been reported in many studies using computed tomography and magnetic resonance imaging (MRI). Among these are enlarged ventricles, sulcal widening and a reduction in grey matter volume in the prefrontal cortex and ventral striatum. In addition, increases in deep white matter hyperintensities, periventricular hyperintensities and subcortical grey matter hyperintensities, common in normal controls, are more extensive in depressed patients. The lesions are more severe in depressions that have a later age of first episode onset, less family history, and are associated with some evidence of cognitive impairment (Schweitzer et al. 2001). The finding of more severe white matter lesions in late onset depression led Alexopoulos and colleagues (1997) and Krishnan and colleagues (1997) to propose the concept of *vascular depression*, with a cerebrovascular aetiology, a poor prognosis and increased likelihood for the development of dementia. The link of a *vascular depression* that progresses to a *vascular dementia* is supported by recent neuropathological findings.

Late life depression has tended to be studied as a separate entity; however, the depressions that begin for the first time in late middle age or later (late onset depression), although less common than early onset depression, have been the subject of considerable research interest over the past decade or so. Clinical and biological differences between late onset and early onset depression have been reported. There is evidence that cerebral cortical atrophy and ventricular enlargement are greater in late onset than early onset depression, although that regarding temporal lobe structures, in particular the hippocampus, is conflicting (reviewed by Schweitzer et al. 2001).

MRI volumetric studies have found reduced volumes in the hippocampus, frontal cortex, caudate nucleus, putamen and amygdala during depression, but not all studies are in agreement (Sheline 2000). Inconsistencies in data may be explained by sex, age and chronicity of depression, and changing imaging technologies. Over the past decade, resolution, sensitivity and acquisition and post-acquisition analysis techniques have continued to improve.

Hippocampal volume loss has been demonstrated in recent studies that have used high resolution MRI of depressed patients in remission and with chronic treatment resistance but not in remission. An association with memory impairment has been described. The hippocampus is part of the limbic system and the serotonergic pathway and is involved in memory and learning. Reduced hippocampal volume may be caused by neuronal cell loss from glucocorticoid neurotoxicity or glial cell loss, or be due to impaired neurogenesis. It is also possible that elevated CRF and decreased BDNF may be responsible for hippocampal loss. Significant changes in hippocampal volume may be measurable only after repeated episodes of depression, and it is not known if it is reversible. Longitudinal studies are required to determine this (Sheline 2000; Manji et al. 2001).

Neuropathology studies support many of these MRI findings, with reductions in cortical thickness, neuronal size and neuronal and glial cell densities in the left prefrontal cortex, but also in the amygdala and hippocampus being reported (Sheline 2000; Davidson et al. 2002).

Functional

Positron emission tomography (PET) studies have demonstrated different patterns of activity, as measured by regional cerebral blood flow and glucose metabolism, in a range of prefrontal cortical and limbic areas in depressed patients when compared with normal controls.

The prefrontal cortex, particularly the subgenual prefrontal cortex, has been implicated relatively consistently in depression. Effective treatment subsequently causes a return to normal (Drevets 2000). Decreased activation of the anterior cingulate cortex in depressed people compared with controls has been reported in PET, single photon emission computed tomography (SPECT) and functional magnetic resonance imaging (fMRI) studies, with an increase on remission. An association with this hypoactivation and impaired executive function and blunted affect has been posited (Davidson et al. 2002).

Resting cerebral blood flow and glucose metabolism are elevated in the amygdala in depression, and there is a positive correlation with severity of depression. These indices return to normal on response to antidepressant treatment (Drevets 2000). Abnormalities in glucose metabolism have been reported in the hippocampus (Davidson et al. 2002).

The abnormalities detected by these functional imaging techniques tend to be subtle. Differences between studies in image acquisition, analysis and other parameters remain unresolved issues and contribute to inconsistencies in the data. What does this information on functional and structural abnormalities mean? We know there are reciprocal connections between the regions of the brain and that affective and cognitive symptomatologies are related to these regions, but the meaning of the specific abnormalities, the specific brain regions and their relationship to causality are yet to be determined. This will be a key area for future work.

MOLECULAR BIOLOGY

The focus of biological research in depression has shifted to the intracellular pathways linked to the monoamine neurotransmitters and regulation of gene expression. The tools of molecular biology now allow investigation of neurotransmitter and receptor action, the role of G proteins, signal transduction pathways, DNA transcription and mRNA translation.

New hypotheses emphasise the role for intracellular signal transduction pathways and neuronal plasticity. They are based on the effects of acute and chronic antidepressant treatment, particularly the delay of therapeutic response to antidepressant treatment and the effects of stress (Duman et al. 2000; Vaidya and Duman 2001).

Duman et al. (1997) have proposed a molecular and cellular hypothesis of depression. They suggest that monoamines ultimately act to control neuron functioning via mediation of post-receptor intracellular signal transduction pathways and specific target genes. Although the immediate effects of antidepressant treatment are to increase availability of monoamines at the synapse and cause subsequent down-regulation of receptors, this does not provide a complete explanation for antidepressant action. The long-term effects of antidepressants are adaptation at a cellular level.

There are multiple intracellular signal transduction pathways. They interact at various levels and it is likely they are involved in psychological, cognitive and vegetative functions (Manji et al. 2001). There are two main categories of transduction pathways: the first is regulated by G-protein-receptor-coupled second messengers, such as cAMP and Ca^{2+}, and the second is regulated by receptors coupled to protein tyrosine kinase and controlled by neurotrophins and cytokines. Receptors in the latter category activate intracellular cascades such as the mitogen-activated protein (MAP) kinase pathway.

G-protein-linked receptors include almost all monoamine and neuropeptide receptors. Binding of a neurotransmitter to these G-protein-linked receptors activates intracellular proteins that in turn set off a cascade of biochemical events within the neuron. One effect of G proteins is to regulate enzymes that produce a large number of second messengers, including cAMP. Second messengers exert their effect by regulating protein kinases (for example, cAMP-dependent protein kinases) and protein phosphatases, which act by phosphorylation of specific substrate proteins that regulate cellular function and can enter the nucleus and alter the expression of genes (for example, the transcription factor CREB). Transcription factors control gene expression by binding to particular sections of DNA. One such sequence of DNA responds as a binding site for proteins that can be phosphorylated by cAMP-dependent protein kinases (Duman et al. 1997).

An intracellular second messenger cascade of interest in the mechanism of action of antidepressant treatment response is the cAMP signal transduction pathway regulated by serotonin and noradrenaline. Research in this area shows activation of the cAMP system increases function and expression of CREB in several brain areas, including the hippocampus, during long-term treatment with most classes of antidepressants. In a post mortem study of depressed patients, levels of CREB were found to be reduced in the temporal cortex. CREB may be an intracellular target for different classes of antidepressants (Duman et al. 1997; Nestler et al. 2002). There are several potential target genes in the cAMP system; one is the BDNF gene.

Neuronal plasticity includes adaptations of neuronal cells and intracellular signal transduction pathways and gene expression. There is plasticity at the neurotransmitter level as well as at the neuron level. Depression may arise when the adaptations of neuronal systems are dysfunctional. The adaptive response is mediated by alterations in gene expression, reflected in neurotransmitter and receptor density and function, activity at multiple levels of intracellular pathways and neuron morphology (Vaidya and Duman 2001). Hence the relevance of transcription factors such as CREB and one of the target genes, the BDNF gene. Dysfunction of the function or expression of CREB and subsequent gene expression may underlie depression.

BDNF is involved in the growth and maintenance of neurons in the brain, that is, in neuronal plasticity, function and survival. Increased expression of BDNF has been found in neurons in the hippocampus after long-term antidepressant treatment. An extrapolation of this is the possible contribution of BDNF down-regulation to hippocampal atrophy. BDNF mediates the receptors coupled to protein tyrosine kinase via MAP kinase cascades.

Studies in this area are only beginning, and no conclusions can be reached regarding the precise role of CREB, BDNF and the cAMP pathway in the pathophysiology of depression. There are other genes regulated by this pathway and other signalling pathways that may be involved (Duman et al. 1997). Much of the current evidence comes from animal studies, and the findings need to be replicated in vivo.

CONCLUSION

Considerable progress has been made in our knowledge of factors implicated in the neurobiology of depression, and hypotheses of pathophysiology of depression have been modified with this increase in knowledge. Evidence points to a pathophysiological heterogeneity and, as depression is a diverse disorder, this confers a further degree of complexity. The consensus view is that depression arises from a complex interaction of multiple genes conferring both vulnerability and protection from environmental factors.

Brain neurotransmitter systems are intricate and specialised; they interact with each other and affect each other's functions. Neuropeptides are co-localised and co-released with neurotransmitters and modulate their activity. Disturbances in one system produce a series of changes that affect multiple other systems. Changes in signalling pathways may underlie the various abnormalities demonstrated to occur in depression. The HPA axis and the immune system are posited to affect central serotonergic and noradrenergic systems. These changes are believed to culminate in alterations in neuronal plasticity.

The hippocampus is involved in regulation of the HPA axis. It is involved in memory, learning and emotions. Changes have been demonstrated on structural and functional neuroimaging. However, abnormalities have been described in other brain regions that have been associated with regulation of the symptoms of depression, such as the amygdala. Researchers have speculated on how the multiple structural and functional abnormalities that have been published and their reciprocal connections might be integrated in a model of the pathophysiology of depression. We are unable to determine if these abnormalities are a cause or consequence of depression.

Data from studies of neurotransmitters and their metabolites, receptors, hormones and neuropeptides and from neuroimaging studies provide a basis for the theory of the pathophysiology of depression. Many of the abnormalities are not detected in all depressed patients. Neither can they be allocated to any specific subgroup of depressed patients, nor do they have predictive value. It has been suggested that some abnormalities may in fact be a reflection of the dysfunction of another system; on the other hand, they may represent a biological subtype. The cascade of changes produced by the interaction of the neurotransmitter systems can mask whether a change or abnormality is causal or a consequence of the disorder being expressed, that is, primary pathophysiology that causes depression or a secondary response to alterations or adaptations in gene expression.

Some of the abnormalities found in depression have also been reported in other psychiatric disorders. Van Praag postulated a dimensional neurochemical disturbance common to certain psychiatric disorders. Selective serotonin reuptake inhibitors, which have broad effectiveness in a variety of mood-related conditions, indirectly support this notion.

The prevalence of depression in women may be due to sex differences in brain structure or function, or in hormonal factors. We are no closer to understanding these differences and this field needs to be further embraced.

Much of our knowledge of the neurobiology of depression has been derived from the development of new antidepressants. Promising areas of antidepressant research are the CRF and glucocorticoid antagonists, substance P antagonists and, possibly, specific oestrogen receptor modulators.

The future promises further elucidation of the precise neurobiological changes underlying depression. Identification of genes involved in depression and advances in neuroimaging will allow us to map the neural circuits and molecular processes and further unravel the complex neurobiology of depression.

REFERENCES

Alexopoulos GS, Meyers BS, Young RC, Kakuma T, Silbersweig D, Charlson M (1997) Clinically defined vascular depression. *American Journal of Psychiatry* 154:562-5.

Arborelius L, Owens MJ, Plotsky PM, Nemeroff CB (1999) The role of corticotropin-releasing factor in depression and anxiety disorders. *Journal of Endocrinology* 160:1-12.

Belsham B (2001) Glutamate and its role in psychiatric illness. *Human Psychopharmacology* 16:139-46.

Davidson RJ, Pizzagalli D, Nitschke JB, Putnam K (2002) Depression: Perspectives from affective neuroscience. *Annual Review of Psychology* 53:545-74.

Drevets WC (2000) Neuroimaging studies of mood disorders. *Biological Psychiatry* 48:813-29.

Duman RS, Heninger GR, Nestler EJ (1997) A molecular and cellular theory of depression. *Archives of General Psychiatry* 54:597-606.

Duman RS, Malberg J, Nakagawa S, D'Sa C (2000) Neuronal plasticity and survival in mood disorders. *Biological Psychiatry* 48:732-9.

Frazer A, Gerhardt GA, Daws LC (1999) New views of biogenic amine transporter function: Implications for neuropsychopharmacology. *International Journal of Neuropsychopharmcology* 2:305-20.

Halbreich U, Kahn LS (2001) Role of estrogen in the aetiology and treatment of mood disorders. *CNS Drugs* 15:797-817.

Holsboer F (2001) Stress, hypercortisolism and corticosteroid receptors in depression: Implications for therapy. *Journal of Affective Disorders* 62:77-91.

Kendler KS, Karkowski-Shuman L (1997) Stressful life events and genetic liability to major depression: Genetic control of exposure to the environment? *Psychological Medicine* 27:539-47.

Kramer MS, Cutler N, Feighner J, Shrivastava R, Carman J, Sramek JJ, et al. (1998) Distinct mechanism for antidepressant activity by blockade of central substance P receptors. *Science* 281:1640-5.

Krishnan KR, Hays JC, Blazer DG (1997) MRI-defined vascular depression. *American Journal of Psychiatry* 154:497-501.

Kronfol Z (2002) Immune dysregulation in major depression: A critical review of existing evidence. *International Journal of Neuropsychopharmacology* 5:333-43.

Leonard BE (2001) The immune system, depression and the action of antidepressants. *Progress in Neuropsychopharmacology and Biological Psychiatry* 25:767-80.

Manji HK, Drevets WC, Charney DS (2001) The cellular neurobiology of depression. *Nature Medicine* 7:541-7.

Musselman DL, DeBattista C, Nathan KI, Kilts CD, Schatzberg AF, Nemeroff CB (1998) Biology of mood disorders. In Schatzberg AF, Nemeroff CB (eds), *Textbook of Psychopharmacology*. Washington, DC: American Psychiatric Press, pp. 549-88.

Nemeroff CB (1998) The neurobiology of depression. *Scientific American* 278:42-9.

—— (2002) New directions in the development of antidepressants: The interface of neurobiology and psychiatry. *Human Psychopharmacology* 17 Suppl 1:S13-16.

Nestler EJ, Barrot M, DiLeone RJ, Eisch AJ, Gold SJ, Monteggia LM (2002) Neurobiology of depression. *Neuron* 34:13-25.

Sapolsky RM, Krey LC, McEwen BS (1986) The neuroendocrinology of stress and aging: The glucocorticoid cascade hypothesis. *Endocrine Reviews* 7:284-301.

Schweitzer I, Tuckwell V, Ames D, O'Brien J (2001) Structural neuroimaging studies in late-life depression: A review. *World Journal of Biological Psychiatry* 2:83-8.

Schweitzer I, Maguire KP, Gee AH, Tiller JW, Biddle N, Davies B (1987) Prediction of outcome in depressed patients by weekly monitoring with the dexamethasone suppression test. *British Journal of Psychiatry* 151:780-4.

Scott LV, Dinan TG (2002) Vasopressin as a target for antidepressant development: An assessment of the available evidence. *Journal of Affective Disorders* 72:113-24.

Sheline YI (2000) 3D MRI studies of neuroanatomic changes in unipolar major depression: The role of stress and medical comorbidity. *Biological Psychiatry* 48:791-800.

Vaidya VA, Duman RS (2001) Depression – emerging insights from neurobiology. *British Medical Bulletin* 57:61-79.

CHAPTER 11

BRAIN IMAGING OF MOOD DISORDERS

FUNCTIONAL UNDERSTANDING OF NEUROANATOMY AND NEURAL CIRCUITS

Gin S Malhi,
Jim Lagopoulos,
Jair C Soares
and Eduard Vieta

Thomas Willis and his forerunner Sylvius (Franciscus de le Boë) successfully diverted the attention of seventeenth-century neuroanatomists from the ventricles of the brain to its substance, namely the cortex. Willis localised brain function to three regions – the corpus striatum, corpus callosum, and cerebral cortex – which mediated sensus communis, imagination, and memory, respectively. This fundamental shift marked a step towards cerebral localisation; however, progress was slow and often thwarted by religious and political concerns. By the beginning of the nineteenth century, Gall (the originator of phrenology) had named twenty-seven mental qualities or faculties and localised them to specific gyri termed *centres* or *organs*. It is interesting to note that all but eight of these were thought to be common to both humans and animals and that emotions such as friendship, love of offspring and pride were not exclusive to mankind. Pierre Flourens opposed the concept of localisation, and contributed to the abnegation of phrenology. However, he proposed an equally flawed theory of cerebral equipotentiality, in which the cerebrum was thought to lack excitability, and intellectual and perceptual functions were diffusely represented throughout the brain. This prompted scientists from a variety of disciplines to combine their expertise and distil their knowledge in an attempt to correlate structure and function. This endeavour continues more than a century later.

In this brief chapter we cannot do justice to the enormous range of studies and literature that has been amassed with respect to functional localisation even with respect to a single domain such as emotion. We have therefore chosen to provide a select perspective of our growing appreciation of emotional processing and its disorders, in the hope that it provides some interesting insights.

Brain imaging is an attractive research tool as it sheds light on the workings of the mind. Rapid technological advancement has made neuroimaging increasingly sophisticated and widely accessible and enhanced its clinical relevance. However, despite its mind-boggling complexity, findings from neuroimaging studies of the brain are best interpreted against a neuroanatomical background.

THE NEUROANATOMY OF EMOTION

The limbic system

The *limbic system* embraces a variable number of subcortical nuclei and the allocortex. It is phylogenetically older than the neocortex and is sometimes described as the *emotional brain*. However, it is difficult to definitively state which groups of cells make up the limbic system because different authors have failed to agree on its composition. Delineation is further compounded because functionally the limbic system is not a true system per se. It is therefore more useful to consider the individual structures that make up the limbic system and examine their connectivity, circuits and functions.

In this regard, midline cerebral structures deep within the brain are particularly important, as they have long been implicated in the mediation of emotion. In the second half of the nineteenth century, Broca outlined the great limbic lobe, a midline cortical region that forms a border around the brainstem. More than half a century later, Papez (1937) described what he considered to be a closed circuit comprising neuronal interconnections beginning and ending in the hippocampus, and he hypothesised the anatomical basis of emotional experiences. It was on the basis of this and other such ideas that the concept of a limbic system eventually took form, and the term was first used definitively by MacLean (1958) to describe the cortex of the limbic lobe and associated brainstem structures. Interestingly, Papez pre-empted our current views. He considered the cingulate to be the final destination for affective impulses and suggested that, via cortical projections, it could influence other brain regions in matters of emotional valence. He also proposed that parallel emotional, cognitive and motor corticothalamic circuits subserve differential brain functions, a concept that receives support in modern neuropsychiatry, albeit in more sophisticated form.

Neural circuits

Many limbic structures have extensive neuronal connections with anterior thalamic nuclei, resulting in the latter sometimes being referred to as the *limbic thalamus*. The latter receives inputs via the mammillothalamic tract and fornix, and projects topographically to the cingulate cortex. Based on the connections of these projections, the limbic system can be separated either into medial parahippocampal and lateral orbitoinsular portions or into anterior and posterior sections, with corresponding partitioning of the cingulate.

Limbic structures such as the cingulate have also been incorporated into a basal ganglia–thalamocortical circuit described by Alexander and colleagues (1990), called the *limbic circuit*. This consists of projections from the anterior cingulate and medial orbitofrontal cortices to the nucleus accumbens, and from the olfactory tubercle to the ventral pallidum and the medial dorsal nucleus of the thalamus, with returning fibres completing the circuit. This particular circuit is thought to be a positive feedback loop, and a subsidiary circuit involving the subthalamic nucleus provides negative feedback. The limbic circuit also receives significant amygdala input and stretches still further the concept of a limbic system by incorporating the basal ganglia. Broadly, it is thought to be involved in the experience of emotions, with dysfunction resulting in affective disturbances and perhaps contributing to mood disorders.

Another circuit implicated in mood disorders is the *dorsolateral prefrontal circuit*, which, like the lateral orbitofrontal circuit, arises from a cortical region of the same name and connects the caudate, globus pallidus, substantia nigra and medial dorsal nucleus of the thalamus. However, in contrast to the limbic circuit, dysfunction of the orbitofrontal circuit has been implicated in obsessive–compulsive disorder.

Anterior and posterior limbic systems

Based on cytoarchitectural, connectivity and functional differences, the limbic system can also be divided into anterior and posterior components. In this division, the anterior limbic system (which consists of the orbitofrontal, anterior cingulate and insular cortices, the amygdala, septum and ventral striatum) deals predominantly with affective functions, whereas the posterior limbic system (which consists of the dorsal striatum, posterior parietal, parahippocampal and cingulate cortices and hippocampus) is more concerned with learning and memory. In keeping with this, the cingulate is also divided into anterior and posterior components, with the latter mediating sensory and motor functions while the former is involved in executive functioning.

Summary

The anatomical basis of emotional processing has been of scientific interest for a considerable time, with successive refinements of putative models producing increasingly sophisticated concepts for theorising and testing. Testing has hitherto only been possible in humans by observing natural experiments involving brain trauma and illness or somewhat indirectly by applying neuropsychological and neurophysiological techniques. However, in the past two decades, neuroimaging has allowed unprecedented in vivo access to cognitive, affective and behavioural aspects of brain functioning using techniques and technologies that determine structure, neurochemistry, blood flow and metabolism, making it possible to map and in some cases tap the neural circuits of the brain.

BRAIN IMAGING IN MOOD DISORDERS

Structural imaging

GENERALISED BRAIN ABNORMALITIES In patients with mood disorders, a range of generalised brain abnormalities have been reported. These include cerebral atrophy, hyperintensities, cerebral and ventricular volume changes and changes in sulcal width and grey and white matter brain volume.

BRAIN SIZE Most studies that have compared the size of the lateral and third ventricles in unipolar depressed patients with healthy controls have reported no significant differences. However, in patients with bipolar disorder, several studies have found a significant increase in the size of these structures, or at least a similar trend, with one study associating ventricular enlargement with illness severity and another with subtype (bipolar I). Studies that have examined sulcal change in unipolar depressed patients have, on the whole, failed to identify significant differences, and although some have reported increased sulcal atrophy – more pronounced in the elderly – the findings across studies are inconsistent. Therefore, it appears that patients with mood disorders have significant ventricular enlargement and possible sulcal prominence when compared with healthy controls, but that this is much less than that found in schizophrenia. What remains unclear is the pathogenesis and clinical significance of these putative changes, and whether they occur as a consequence of mood disturbance or are in themselves aetiological factors.

Most neuroimaging studies that have compared total brain volume in patients with unipolar or bipolar disorder with healthy controls have found no significant differences, even with grey and white matter differentiation. However, studies that have examined patients with respect to age and onset of illness suggest that neurodegenerative mechanisms may contribute, particularly to the pathophysiology of bipolar disorder. It is therefore interesting to note that recent longitudinal and cross-sectional studies have identified increased total grey matter volumes in lithium-treated bipolar patients, suggesting that this underpins its neuroprotective effects.

HYPERINTENSITIES The most consistent neuroimaging finding regarding mood disorders is that of T2 signal hyperintensities, indicating a change of water content in the brain. A meta-analysis of studies (Videbech 1997) in unipolar patients reported an increased risk of hyperintensities, implicating them aetiologically, and suggested that this occurs perhaps by disrupting mood-regulating networks (Soares and Mann 1997a).

A similar association is noted in patients with bipolar disorder, especially in subcortical grey, periventricular and deep white matter. The likelihood of various *types* of hyperintensities, for example periventricular or deep white matter, is reportedly associated with subtype (bipolar I), poor outcome, and possibly age. However, most of these findings await robust replication and as yet there is little consensus. Furthermore, the pathophysiological significance of signal hyperintensities remains unresolved as they lack anatomical and diagnostic specificity – occurring commonly with ageing and in a variety of clinical disorders, including dementia and schizophrenia.

REGIONAL BRAIN ABNORMALITIES

Cortical regions

Idiopathic and acquired mood disorders are thought to involve dorsolateral and orbitofrontal circuit dysfunction within the prefrontal cortex (Cummings 1993; Soares and Mann 1997b). Most studies examining prefrontal cortical volume report reductions in unipolar depressed patients compared with healthy subjects and in patients with bipolar disorder have correlated these changes with neuropsychological deficits. However, studies that have defined prefrontal regions in patients with bipolar disorder report variable changes, ranging for instance from no significant differences in dorsolateral prefrontal cortex grey matter volume (Schlaepfer et al. 1994) to smaller prefrontal grey matter volumes (Lopez-Larson et al. 2002) and smaller subgenual prefrontal cortex volume accompanied by an abnormal decrease in metabolic activity (Drevets et al. 1997). These findings are consistent with those from post mortem histological studies that report reduced subgenual dorsolateral prefrontal cortical glial cell density in patients with bipolar disorder (Ongur et al. 1998; Rajkowska et al. 2001). However, these findings are confounded by the effects of medication.

Many of the studies that have examined temporal lobe volumes in unipolar depressed patients have found no difference from healthy controls; however, structural MRI voxel-based morphometric analysis has identified reduced temporal cortex grey matter density affecting in particular the anterior hippocampus in patients with chronic treatment-resistant depression. It is possible, however, that these changes are a consequence of chronicity or treatment as opposed to causing the disorder. In contrast, temporal lobe changes in bipolar disorder are far less consistent, with reports of decreases and increases, and some studies finding no significant differences. Furthermore, many of the findings have not been successfully replicated, with the exception of amygdala enlargement (Altshuler et al. 2000; Hirayasu et al. 2000), which supports its role in emotional processing. In patients with unipolar disorder, amygdala changes include asymmetry (Mervaala et al. 2000) and reduced core nuclei volume (Sheline et al. 1998). Taken together, temporal lobe changes seem to distinguish unipolar and bipolar disorder, in that the hippocampus is reduced in size in unipolar depressed patients but largely unaltered in patients with bipolar disorder, whereas the amygdala is enlarged in patients with bipolar disorder but generally unaltered in those with unipolar depression. Hippocampal structural changes in patients with unipolar depression are of particular interest, as several studies have linked hippocampal shrinking with illness duration, its severity and age at onset, positing that neuronal loss occurs secondary to glucocorticoid neurotoxicity.

Subcortical regions

Anatomically, the thalamus is pivotal to various mood-related cortical–subcortical circuits and is therefore strongly implicated in the pathophysiology of mood disorders. However, the evidence from structural MRI studies is unconvincing, with no consistent changes reported in unipolar depressed patients, and the number of studies that found an increase in size in bipolar patients was the same as the number that did not find an increase. It is important to note, however, that thalamic nuclei are difficult to delineate, making reliable measurement unfeasible.

In patients with unipolar depression, decreased caudate and putamen volumes have been reported in several studies and replicated by some, but not others. In contrast, basal ganglia enlargement has been reported in patients with bipolar disorder, although inconsistently. These varying findings strongly implicate striatal pathology in the pathophysiology of mood disorders, especially in unipolar depression and elderly patients.

Many other regions, including the cerebellum, corpus callosum, pituitary and brainstem, have been studied with interesting volumetric changes noted. However, there are many inconsistencies across these studies and the majority of tentative findings await robust replication. These have therefore not been considered in this chapter.

SUMMARY Computed tomography and magnetic resonance imaging studies have identified structural differences between patients with mood disorders and healthy controls (for review see Monkul et al. In press). Phenotypic changes have also been reported; however, diagnostic heterogeneity and the fact that early studies were technically less advanced limit interpretation. Nevertheless, these studies clearly suggest that detectable structural changes occur in patients with mood disorders within relevant neural circuits, and support the need for further investigation.

Functional imaging

Functional imaging techniques have allowed the assessment of cerebral change. In vivo examination has naturally provided much greater functional insight and will continue to do so as novel technologies emerge and existing techniques are refined.

POSITRON EMISSION TOMOGRAPHY AND SINGLE PHOTON EMISSION COMPUTED TOMOGRAPHY Positron emission tomography (PET) and single photon emission computed tomography (SPECT) rely on the emission of positrons and photons, respectively. PET is considerably more expensive than SPECT, but has greater spatial resolution and yields quantitative data. Both techniques, using radiotracers such as 18FDG and 99mT-HMPAO, can measure absolute (PET) and relative (SPECT) cerebral blood flow, and can track receptors using specific receptor-binding ligands.

Studies in healthy subjects involving the transient induction of different types of emotion have revealed regional changes indicative of functional localisation (George et al. 1995). Studies that have examined cerebral blood flow and metabolism in patients with primary depression and bipolar disorder have consistently identified decreased anterior paralimbic and cortical activity. In depressed patients, this prefrontal cortical deficit, which is signalled by diminished blood flow, attenuates with successful treatment of the illness – except when using electroconvulsive therapy, in which case there is a further decrease in anterior cerebral activity. In depressed bipolar patients, there is additional increased metabolism in subcortical paralimbic structures (Ketter et al. 2001), supporting a limbic–cortical dysregulation model of depression (Mayberg et al. 1997). This model proposes that dorsal neocortical hypofunction can produce ventral paralimbic overactivity and that this inverse relationship is reciprocal (Mayberg 1997).

Despite significant heterogeneity across mood disorder studies (which can be partly attributed to symptom variation), successful treatment irrespective of modality (pharmacological and psychological) is able to normalise baseline cerebral blood flow and metabolic abnormalities. However, the specific components of emotion-related circuits that therapeutic interventions engage are yet to be elucidated. Early indications suggest that differing treatments possess selectivity for different components.

Evidence for the above model also emanates from disorders that involve components of the basal ganglia thalamocortical circuits. Assuming that these circuits do mediate emotion, then disruption of the networks involved should result in psychopathology and neuroimaging findings similar to those found in mood disorders. Indeed this is so, with a wide variety of diseases such as epilepsy, Parkinson's disease, stroke and Alzheimer's disease, which are often associated with affective changes (that is, secondary depression), also showing anterior cerebral hypoactivity that is proportional to the severity of the depression.

With the development of biochemically specific radiotracers, PET and SPECT can be used to examine the levels of neurotransmitters, receptors and second messenger signalling pathways pertinent to mood-related neuronal circuits in patients with mood disorders (Yatham and Malhi In press). The process of neurotransmission is complex and involves several steps, including the uptake or reuptake of neurotransmitters into nerve terminals, their storage and timely release into the synaptic cleft upon receipt of a suitable signal, and the subsequent engagement of neurotransmitters, with both pre- and postsynaptic receptors triggering second messenger pathways, which culminate in biological responses.

Most radiotracer studies in patients with mood disorders have focused on aspects of serotonergic and dopaminergic neurotransmission. Serotonin studies have examined the serotonin transporter and both 5-HT_{1A} and 5-HT_{2A} receptors. PET studies that have examined serotonin transporter binding (Dahlstrom et al. 2000; Ichimiya et al. 2002) have found that, compared with controls, there are significant increases in the thalamus but not in the midbrain. Subanalysis by phenotype suggests that the increase in binding potential is similar across both major depression and bipolar disorder; however, SPECT studies in depressed patients report both increased and decreased availability in the midbrain and increased availability in the hypothalamus (Malison et al. 1998; Dahlstrom et al. 2000). Therefore, in both major depression and bipolar disorder, thalamic serotonin transporter is elevated. However, with respect to other regions such as the midbrain, findings are as yet inconclusive.

PET studies that have examined 5-HT_{1A} receptors in patients with bipolar depression and major depression have identified significant reductions in receptor binding in frontal, temporal and limbic cortical regions. PET studies in patients with major depression that have examined 5-HT_{2A} receptors similarly report either decreases or no change when compared with controls.

Dopamine studies, like those investigating serotonin, have examined transporters and receptors. However, some studies have also examined amphetamine-induced dopamine release. These SPECT studies are interesting, as they have found no difference in amphetamine-induced presynaptic dopamine release in bipolar patients, instead placing dopaminergic abnormalities postsynaptically at receptor sites or within second messenger signalling pathways (Anand et al. 2000). This is borne out to some extent by the finding that the transport of dopamine from cytoplasm to storage vesicles is intact in bipolar disorder (Zubieta et al. 2000). Another study in bipolar patients found a modest reduction in cerebral dopamine D1 receptor density, suggesting that this may be a trait marker for bipolar disorder (Suhara et al. 1992). In contrast, studies that have examined dopamine D2 receptor binding in patients with bipolar disorder suggest that increased D2 receptor density occurs only in those with psychotic mania. Indeed, D2 receptor density is unchanged in people with non-psychotic bipolar disorder, indicating that it is unrelated to bipolar disorder per se and that it is perhaps a putative marker of psychosis.

In summary, radiotracer studies that have examined patients with mood disorders have produced a variety of interesting findings, many of which are difficult to interpret and await replication. PET and SPECT studies that have examined healthy subjects and patients in resting conditions and varying mood states, natural and induced, have identified regions of interest with respect to emotion processing and provided a good basis for more sophisticated neurochemical and functional investigation.

SPECTROSCOPY In general, the application of spectroscopy to research in mood disorders has been relatively limited. Spectroscopy permits the chemical biopsy of brain tissue in vivo and, although this is a tremendous development, the chemicals (metabolites) that can be accurately visualised are very limited, with many having little relevance to clinical disorders and the processing of emotion. However, both unipolar and bipolar patients have been investigated for neurochemical markers and the changes brought about by pharmacotherapy.

Proton spectroscopy studies of depressed adults with either major depression or bipolar disorder have shown moderate increases in the concentration of choline in the basal ganglia (Hamakawa et al. 1998; Kato et al. 1998) and anterior cingulate. These alterations are more pronounced in patients that are responsive to selective serotonin reuptake inhibitors, such as fluoxetine, and tend to normalise with suitable antidepressant treatment. These tentative pharmacotherapeutic findings that associate basal ganglia choline concentration changes with clinical status (Stoll et al. 1996) await replication using fluorinated metabolite studies. However, it is clear that the concentration of choline in the basal ganglia varies with depression severity and that this is possibly state-dependent. Choline concentration changes have also been observed in the frontal lobes of depressed adolescents, further supporting a pathophysiological role in depression for choline-containing compounds.

Similar increases, attributed to membrane phospholipid metabolism changes, are observed in depressed patients with bipolar disorder, both medicated and unmedicated (Deicken et al. 1995). Magnetic resonance spectroscopy studies using 31P have demonstrated elevations of phosphomonoesters in the frontal lobes of symptomatic unipolar and bipolar patients along with changes of phosphocreatine. These increased choline and phosphomonoester measurements may in fact denote changes in phosphocholine or be due to lithium treatment, which inhibits choline transport and increases intracellular choline-containing compounds.

Proton spectroscopy studies of patients with bipolar disorder reveal diminished dorsolateral prefrontal *N*-acetyl-aspartate (NAA) (Winsberg et al. 2000) and creatine (Hamakawa et al. 1999) concentrations, imputing decreased neuronal density or neuronal dysfunction and state-dependent changes in metabolism. Decreased NAA ratios have also been found in the basal ganglia of patients with bipolar disorder, especially in older patients with later onset of illness. However, it is noteworthy that no such differences have been found in adolescents and children with bipolar disorder, which suggests that disease processes may differ with age. Perhaps equally important is the partitioning of grey and white matter shown in a recent study (Cecil et al. 2002), which found reduced NAA within the orbitofrontal grey matter of patients with bipolar disorder. This study also reported reduced levels of choline; however, some patients had mania, highlighting the importance of mood-state as a variable in interpreting metabolite changes.

Phosphorus spectroscopy has demonstrated changes in high-energy phosphate metabolism that have been less consistent, but warrant further investigation because of the important role of second messenger systems in the pathophysiology of bipolar disorders. A handful of studies have used lithium (^{7}Li) spectroscopy to determine the relationship between brain lithium concentrations and therapeutic response – with initial indications that the two are closely coupled. However, further investigation is necessary to elucidate the precise effects of lithium on brains of people with bipolar disorder, especially during the various phases of the illness.

Recent studies of patients with mood disorders have shown significant reductions in the concentrations of cortical GABA and anterior cingulate glutamate. Treatment studies, examining the metabolite changes before and after the administration of antidepressants or ECT, correlate biochemical and clinical parameters (for review see Malhi et al. 2002).

In summary, spectroscopy allows determination of cerebral metabolites such as choline and *N*-acetyl-aspartate. There is a pressing need to extend its application to more clinically relevant metabolites, such as serotonin and dopamine. One finding reported with some consistency is increased choline in basal ganglia of depressed patients and those with bipolar disorder. However, even this has to be treated as being tentative given the enormous number of confounding factors that can alter the neurochemical composition of the brain. Future studies should continue to examine the neurochemistry of depression and bipolar disorder and perhaps conduct longitudinal studies so as to differentiate state and trait changes.

FUNCTIONAL MAGNETIC RESONANCE IMAGING The neuronal mechanisms that subserve emotion have been investigated in healthy subjects and patients with major depression and bipolar disorder using positron emission tomography (PET) and functional magnetic resonance imaging (fMRI).

This body of research has helped develop useful functional models of major depression (Mayberg 1997, 2003; Phillips et al. 2003), in which emotion-related interconnected brain regions are partitioned into functional compartments: ventral–limbic and dorsal–cortical. The rostral anterior cingulate is not included in either, and is ascribed a separate role by virtue of its reciprocal connections with both regions, its cytoarchitectural characteristics, and its imputed role in treatment responsiveness (Mayberg et al. 1997).

A similar model for bipolar disorder is yet to be formulated. However, studies that have examined patients with bipolar disorder (Blumberg et al. 1999; Berns et al. 2002) suggest abnormal affective responsiveness, specifically a difficulty with emotional discrimination (Yurgelun-Todd et al. 2000), suggesting that examining emotions in the context of their interplay with cognitive and executive functions may help in understanding and delineating their neural substratum (Malhi 2004).

To this end, functional neuroimaging studies using a wide variety of affective stimuli have begun to identify brain regions that contribute to complex functions such as emotional experiences. It is important to note that many of the findings from functional studies are inconclusive and based on many assumptions. However, a relatively consistent finding across functional neuroimaging studies of unipolar depressed patients is diminished blood flow to the dorsal prefrontal cortex (BA9), which improves with effective treatment (Mayberg 1997; Mayberg et al. 1999). Responses in this region have also been reported in healthy subjects during memory-driven sadness and happiness (George et al. 1995), supporting the notion that the right prefrontal cortex (BA9) is an important destination for limbic projections and may play a role in modulating attention in affective states. Specifically, BA9 responses may indicate emotional awareness that involves attention to internal emotional state and entails greater cognitive emotional processing. Thus the medial prefrontal cortex is thought to have a general role in emotional processing that involves the modulation and evaluation of emotion and emotion-dependent decision-making.

Another region that contributes to emotional decisions and is functionally important to the experience of emotion, by virtue of its reciprocal connections to the orbitofrontal cortex, insula, amygdala, septal nuclei and hypothalamus, is the anterior cingulate. Functional activation and resting-state treatment studies (George et al. 1995; Drevets et al. 1997; Mayberg et al. 1999) strongly implicate the subgenual cingulate (BA25) in the pathogenesis of clinical depression, a region that is thought to play a central role in sadness such as autobiographical script-induced sadness. However, it has been suggested that it may simply process the cognitive aspects of internally generated emotion (Reiman et al. 1997), as opposed to sadness itself.

Furthermore, recall-induced sadness activates the orbitofrontal, temporal and insular cortices (Pardo et al. 1993; George et al. 1995; Lane et al. 1997; Blair et al. 1999), and the latter is also involved in autonomic responses and visceral sensations via its extensive connections to the temporopolar and orbital cortex and amygdala.

The amygdala is particularly interesting, and is activated in many functional imaging studies as it is thought to be involved in the detection of environmental threat and the experience of fear (Morris et al. 1998); however, its function may be more general – determining for instance the dangerousness of affective stimuli or simply their salience irrespective of valence. Hence, in addition to aversive and fearful stimuli, sad and happy affect has been shown to produce amygdala activation in functional neuroimaging (Blair et al. 1999).

SUMMARY Functional neuroimaging, particularly fMRI, has provided us with truly exciting possibilities. For the first time, there is a genuine confluence of technology and cognitive neuroscience. For instance, the ability to present sophisticated neuropsychological stimuli within the scanner environment to generate specific emotions has allowed investigators to 'see' the brain regions involved in emotional appreciation. Functional imaging studies have successfully validated findings from other lines of investigation and significantly enhanced our capabilitiy to test ideas. With respect to mood, emotions and mood disorders, functional imaging studies implicate in particular the anterior cingulate – perhaps as a decision-making modulator impinging upon brain regions that generate emotions cognitively, such as the orbitofrontal and medial prefrontal cortices. Via iterative connections with limbic brain regions and subcortical centres such as the thalamus, these cortices regulate emotional processing accommodating contextual and environmental information. Dysfunction in different regions could explain the many subtypes of mood disorders and the fact that patients with bipolar disorder not only swing from one extreme to the other but also have mixed states in which they experience composites of emotions.

CONCLUSION

An understanding of the neuroanatomy of the brain is essential for identifying neural circuits. These in turn provide a basis for imputing functional connectivity and the potential communication that may take place when processing specific simple and complex functions. However, it is the ability with the aid of neuroimaging techniques to invoke these changes and examine them while doing so that has opened up a new window to the brain. The structural, chemical and functional changes that take place can now be corroborated, and most promising of all is the fact that differential patterns of activation are emerging that may eventually separate subtypes of mood disorders or identify specific symptoms. These findings may in the very near future force a re-evaluation of our current phenomenology-based classifications of mood disorders and enable us to generate diagnoses that have greater relevance to pharmacological and psychological management and clinical outcome.

REFERENCES

Alexander GE, Crutcher MD, DeLong MR (1990) Basal ganglia-thalamocortical circuits: Parallel substrates for motor, oculomotor, 'prefrontal' and 'limbic' functions. *Progress in Brain Research* 85:119-46.

Altshuler LL, Bartzokis G, Grieder T, Curran J, Jimenez T, Leight K, et al. (2000) An MRI study of temporal lobe structures in men with bipolar disorder or schizophrenia. *Biological Psychiatry* 48:147-62.

Anand A, Verhoeff P, Seneca N, Zoghbi SS, Seibyl JP, Charney DS, et al. (2000) Brain SPECT imaging of amphetamine-induced dopamine release in euthymic bipolar disorder patients. *American Journal of Psychiatry* 157:1108-14.

Berns GS, Martin M, Proper SM (2002) Limbic hyperreactivity in bipolar II disorder. *American Journal of Psychiatry* 159:304-6.

Blair RJ, Morris JS, Frith CD, Perrett DI, Dolan RJ (1999) Dissociable neural responses to facial expressions of sadness and anger. *Brain* 122:883-93.

Blumberg HP, Stern E, Ricketts S, Martinez D, de Asis J, White T, et al. (1999) Rostral and orbital prefrontal cortex dysfunction in the manic state of bipolar disorder. *American Journal of Psychiatry* 156:1986-8.

Cecil KM, DelBello MP, Morey R, Strakowski SM (2002) Frontal lobe differences in bipolar disorder as determined by proton MR spectroscopy. *Bipolar Disorders* 4:357-65.

Cummings JL (1993) Frontal-subcortical circuits and human behavior. *Archives of Neurology* 50:873-80.

Dahlstrom M, Ahonen A, Ebeling H, Torniainen P, Heikkila J, Moilanen I (2000) Elevated hypothalamic/midbrain serotonin (monoamine) transporter availability in depressive drug-naive children and adolescents. *Molecular Psychiatry* 5:514-22.

Deicken RF, Weiner MW, Fein G (1995) Decreased temporal lobe phosphomonoesters in bipolar disorder. *Journal of Affective Disorders* 33:195-9.

Drevets WC, Price JL, Simpson JR, Jr., Todd RD, Reich T, Vannier M, et al. (1997) Subgenual prefrontal cortex abnormalities in mood disorders. *Nature* 386:824-7.

George MS, Ketter TA, Parekh PI, Horwitz B, Herscovitch P, Post RM (1995) Brain activity during transient sadness and happiness in healthy women. *American Journal of Psychiatry* 152:341-51.

Hamakawa H, Kato T, Murashita J, Kato N (1998) Quantitative proton magnetic resonance spectroscopy of the basal ganglia in patients with affective disorders. *European Archives of Psychiatry and Clinical Neuroscience* 248:53-8.

Hamakawa H, Kato T, Shioiri T, Inubushi T, Kato N (1999) Quantitative proton magnetic resonance spectroscopy of the bilateral frontal lobes in patients with bipolar disorder. *Psychological Medicine* 29:639-44.

Hirayasu Y, McCarley RW, Salisbury DF, Tanaka S, Kwon JS, Frumin M, et al. (2000) Planum temporale and Heschl gyrus volume reduction in schizophrenia: A magnetic resonance imaging study of first-episode patients. *Archives of General Psychiatry* 57:692-9.

Ichimiya T, Suhara T, Sudo Y, Okubo Y, Nakayama K, Nankai M, et al. (2002) Serotonin transporter binding in patients with mood disorders: A PET study with [11C](+)McN5652. *Biological Psychiatry* 51:715-22.

Kato T, Murashita J, Kamiya A, Shioiri T, Kato N, Inubushi T (1998) Decreased brain intracellular pH measured by 31P-MRS in bipolar disorder: A confirmation in drug-free patients and correlation with white matter hyperintensity. *European Archives of Psychiatry and Clinical Neuroscience* 248:301-6.

Ketter TA, Kimbrell TA, George MS, Dunn RT, Speer AM, Benson BE, et al. (2001) Effects of mood and subtype on cerebral glucose metabolism in treatment-resistant bipolar disorder. *Biological Psychiatry* 49:97-109.

Lane RD, Reiman EM, Ahern GL, Schwartz GE, Davidson RJ (1997) Neuroanatomical correlates of happiness, sadness, and disgust. *American Journal of Psychiatry* 154:926-33.

Lopez-Larson MP, DelBello MP, Zimmerman ME, Schwiers ML, Strakowski SM (2002)

Regional prefrontal gray and white matter abnormalities in bipolar disorder. *Biological Psychiatry* 52:93-100.

MacLean PD (1958) The limbic system with respect to self-preservation and preservation of the species. *Journal of Nervous and Mental Disease* 127:1-11.

Malhi GS, Lagopoulos J, Ward PB, Kumari V, Mitchell PB, Parker GB, Ivanovski B, Sachdev P (2004) Cognitive generation of affect in bipolar depression: An fMRI study. *European Journal of Neuroscience* 19:742-54.

Malhi GS, Valenzuela M, Wen W, Sachdev P (2002) Magnetic resonance spectroscopy and its applications in psychiatry. *Australian and New Zealand Journal of Psychiatry* 36:31-43.

Malison RT, Price LH, Berman R, van Dyck CH, Pelton GH, Carpenter L, et al. (1998) Reduced brain serotonin transporter availability in major depression as measured by $[^{123}I]$-2 beta-carbomethoxy-3 beta-(4-iodophenyl)tropane and single photon emission computed tomography. *Biological Psychiatry* 44:1090-8.

Mayberg HS (1997) Limbic-cortical dysregulation: A proposed model of depression. *Journal of Neuropsychiatry and Clinical Neurosciences* 9:471-81.

—— (2003) Modulating dysfunctional limbic-cortical circuits in depression: Towards development of brain-based algorithms for diagnosis and optimised treatment. *British Medical Bulletin* 65:193-207.

Mayberg HS, Brannan SK, Mahurin RK, Jerabek PA, Brickman JS, Tekell JL, et al. (1997) Cingulate function in depression: A potential predictor of treatment response. *Neuroreport* 8:1057-61.

Mayberg HS, Liotti M, Brannan SK, McGinnis S, Mahurin RK, Jerabek PA, et al. (1999) Reciprocal limbic-cortical function and negative mood: Converging PET findings in depression and normal sadness. *American Journal of Psychiatry* 156:675-82.

Mervaala E, Fohr J, Kononen M, Valkonen-Korhonen M, Vainio P, Partanen K, et al. (2000) Quantitative MRI of the hippocampus and amygdala in severe depression. *Psychological Medicine* 30:117-25.

Monkul ES, Malhi GS, Soares JC (2003) Mood Disorders – Review of structural MRI studies. *Acta Neuropsychiatrica* 15:368-80.

Morris JS, Friston KJ, Buchel C, Frith CD, Young AW, Calder AJ, et al. (1998) A neuromodulatory role for the human amygdala in processing emotional facial expressions. *Brain* 121:47-57.

Ongur D, Drevets WC, Price JL (1998) Glial reduction in the subgenual prefrontal cortex in mood disorders. *Proceedings of the National Academy of Sciences of the United States of America* 95:13290-5.

Papez JW (1937) A proposed mechanism of emotion. *Archives of Neurology and Psychiatry* 38:725-43.

Pardo JV, Pardo PJ, Raichle ME (1993) Neural correlates of self-induced dysphoria. *American Journal of Psychiatry* 150:713-19.

Phillips ML, Drevets WC, Rauch SL, Lane RD (2003) Neurobiology of emotion perception II: Implications for major psychiatric disorders. *Biological Psychiatry* 54:515-28.

Rajkowska G, Halaris A, Selemon LD (2001) Reductions in neuronal and glial density characterize the dorsolateral prefrontal cortex in bipolar disorder. *Biological Psychiatry* 49:741-52.

Reiman EM, Lane RD, Ahern GL, Schwartz GE, Davidson RJ, Friston KJ, et al. (1997) Neuroanatomical correlates of externally and internally generated human emotion. *American Journal of Psychiatry* 154:918-25.

Schlaepfer TE, Harris GJ, Tien AY, Peng LW, Lee S, Federman EB, et al. (1994) Decreased regional cortical gray matter volume in schizophrenia. *American Journal of Psychiatry* 151:842-8.

Sheline YI, Gado MH, Price JL (1998) Amygdala core nuclei volumes are decreased in recurrent major depression. *Neuroreport* 9:2023-8.

Soares JC, Mann JJ (1997a) The anatomy of mood disorders – Review of structural neuroimaging studies. *Biological Psychiatry* 41:86-106.

—— (1997b) The functional neuroanatomy of mood disorders. *Journal of Psychiatric Research* 31:393-432.

Stoll AL, Sachs GS, Cohen BM, Lafer B, Christensen JD, Renshaw PF (1996) Choline in the treatment of rapid-cycling bipolar disorder: Clinical and neurochemical findings in lithium-treated patients. *Biological Psychiatry* 40:382-8.

Suhara T, Nakayama K, Inoue O, Fukuda H, Shimizu M, Mori A, et al. (1992) D1 dopamine receptor binding in mood disorders measured by positron emission tomography. *Psychopharmacology* 106:14-18.

Videbech P (1997) MRI findings in patients with affective disorder: A meta-analysis. *Acta Psychiatrica Scandinavica* 96:157-68.

Winsberg ME, Sachs N, Tate DL, Adalsteinsson E, Spielman D, Ketter TA (2000) Decreased dorsolateral prefrontal *N*-acetyl aspartate in bipolar disorder. *Biological Psychiatry* 47:475-81.

Yatham LN, Malhi GS (2003) Neurochemical brain imaging studies in bipolar disorder. *Acta Neuropsychiatrica 15:381-7.*

Yurgelun-Todd DA, Gruber SA, Kanayama G, Killgore WD, Baird AA, Young AD (2000) fMRI during affect discrimination in bipolar affective disorder. *Bipolar Disorders* 2:237-48.

Zubieta JK, Huguelet P, Ohl LE, Koeppe RA, Kilbourn MR, Carr JM, et al. (2000) High vesicular monoamine transporter binding in asymptomatic bipolar I disorder: Sex differences and cognitive correlates. *American Journal of Psychiatry* 157:1619-28.

CHAPTER 12

THE NEUROPSYCHOLOGY OF MOOD DISORDERS

Peter Gallagher
and Richard J Porter

It is widely accepted that cognitive impairment is one of the core features of episodes of affective disturbance (depression, mania, hypomania and mixed affective states) in major depressive disorder and bipolar disorder. This has a marked effect on psychological wellbeing and on social and occupational functioning. Studies have investigated the degree of impairment during and between episodes, the specific neuropsychological functions affected, and the origin of these abnormalities. In this chapter we give a brief overview of the assessment of neuropsychological functioning and examine the profile, magnitude and factors contributing to the impairment found in mood disorders.

PRINCIPLES OF NEUROPSYCHOLOGICAL ASSESSMENT

Neuropsychology is an applied science concerned with the behavioural expression of brain function (Lezak 1995). Traditionally, neuropsychological testing has been used to investigate abnormalities in individual subjects. This approach has been developed to permit the systematic investigation of neuropsychological function in groups of subjects with particular clinical diagnoses. Increasingly, more sensitive measures, particularly computer-based test batteries, are being developed, allowing identification of more subtle impairment. Such assessments not only allow the profiling of functional performance but may also provide an objective marker of underlying neuroanatomical or neurochemical disturbance.

COGNITIVE ARCHITECTURE OF HUMAN MEMORY

The many conflicting theories, classifications and ways of testing human cognitive function have, in the past, led to considerable confusion. Below, we present a simple model for understanding the literature on neuropsychological dysfunction in mood disorder.

Memory

One of the oldest distinctions is between *working memory* (sometimes referred to as *short-term memory*) and *long-term memory*. Working memory is involved in the temporary maintenance of information. It is sometimes divided into visuospatial and auditory–verbal modalities. Long-term memories, on the other hand, are maintained from hours to years, and are usually separated into two distinct systems: *declarative* (effortful, or cognitive, learning) and *non-declarative* (habit-like learning, such as skills or procedures). Declarative memory is sometimes further subdivided into *semantic* memory (memory for facts) and *episodic* memory (memory for events and personal experiences).

Numerous different *forms* of memory have also been postulated, such as verbal memory or recognition memory. Similarly, specific impairments are often discussed in terms of memory *processes*, such as acquisition or encoding, rehearsal, consolidation, and retrieval. These contribute to memory formation, but are not memory systems in themselves. It is also important to remember that, although particular tasks can be relatively specific to a particular memory system, several memory systems and processes may contribute to performance on any given test.

Attention and executive function

Executive functions are sometimes referred to as *higher-order* cognitive processes, and are responsible for aspects of planning, judgment, decision-making, anticipation or reasoning, control of attention, and task management. The neuroanatomical locus of these processes has historically been considered the frontal lobes, in particular the prefrontal cortex. However, it is now understood that such processes activate diverse neural frontal–subcortical circuitry (Alexander et al. 1986). The control of working memory processes and attentional resources are also thought to be functions of the executive system ('central executive': Baddeley 1990). Impairments in these domains appear to be one of the few consistent findings across neuropsychological studies of major affective illness.

Functional imaging has allowed investigators to study, in humans, the areas of the brain activated by particular neuropsychological tests. This technique has added to previous studies of the effects of brain lesions on neuropsychological function in animals and humans. Many of the neuropsychological tests described below have been investigated to determine which parts of the brain are activated during their performance.

TESTS OF NEUROPSYCHOLOGICAL FUNCTION

A vast array of tasks has been used to test neuropsychological function in patients with mood disorders. Here we will highlight a few of the most commonly used (for a more detailed discussion, see Lezak 1995).

Memory span

It is thought that verbal–auditory and spatial information are dealt with in separate subcomponents of working memory. Consequently, separate tasks are typically used to assess memory span. The most commonly used are digit span, in which subjects must remember and repeat back a series of random numbers which increase in length over successive presentations; and spatial span (usually based on the Corsi Block task), in which random spatial locations are used as the stimuli. Some of these tasks have now been computerised, increasing the methodological rigour of testing.

Verbal learning and memory

Typically, verbal declarative memory is assessed using tasks such as the California Verbal Learning Test or Rey-Auditory Verbal Learning Test. These tests involve the presentation of a list of words or items in the form of an imaginary 'shopping list', which subjects are required to learn over successive presentations. The benefits of such tasks lie in the number of different outcome measures that can be derived, such as immediate memory span, learning indices, and long-term recall and recognition measures.

Non-verbal learning and memory

The development of computerised test batteries has increased the possibility of more accurate examination of non-verbal abilities. These range from simple pattern and spatial recognition tests to more complex tasks. Examples of these include delayed-match-to-sample (in which subjects must remember an abstract pattern and select this stimulus from several very similar stimuli, across varying retention intervals), and paired associative learning (in which a series of abstract patterns must be paired with the spatial location at which they were first seen). The advantage of these tasks is that most are derived from – or in some cases are exactly the same as – tests used in the animal literature and therefore have a good theoretical underpinning.

Executive function

Owing to the diverse number of processes subserved by the central executive, many different tasks are used to assess different facets of executive function. Some of the most common include:

- tests of verbal/category fluency, which require subjects to generate words according to a prescribed set of rules, such as beginning with a particular letter or from a given semantic category
- tests of planning, such as the Tower of London, which require subjects to plan and execute a series of sorting manoeuvres in a minimum number of moves
- tests of concept or attentional set-shifting, such as the Wisconsin Card Sorting Test or Trail Making Test, which require subjects to deduce a set

of rules and then 'shift' to an alternative, previously irrelevant sorting principle or shift attention between sets

- tests of inhibitory control, such as the Stroop Colour and Word Test, in which subjects are presented with a list containing the names of colours, printed in an incongruous colour (for example, the word red is printed in blue ink, and subjects must state the colour of the ink).

Many of these tasks allow the function of particular neuroanatomical structures or systems to be assessed (however, note the caveat discussed earlier, that several memory systems may contribute to performance on any given test). For example, tasks such as the Tower of London depend upon the integrity of the dorsolateral prefrontal cortex (Rowe et al. 2001), whereas tasks such as the Stroop rely heavily on the anterior cingulate (MacLeod and MacDonald 2000) – the function of both structures is believed to be significantly compromised in mood disorders.

NEUROPSYCHOLOGY OF MAJOR DEPRESSION

Historically, psychometric or neuropsychological tests were used to differentiate organic from functional disorders, as it was generally believed that there was an absence of objective impairment in the latter. However, cases of *endogenous* depression, in which the impairment was so severe it was said to be functionally indistinguishable from organic dementia (pseudodementia), were increasingly recognised. Since then, many studies have investigated the pattern of impairment in major depression, partly to help differentiate severe cases from dementias and partly to add to knowledge about the pathophysiology of the condition.

Pattern and magnitude of impairment

Thousands of studies have investigated the neuropsychological phenotype of major depression and have yielded highly variable results, demonstrating impairment of virtually every conceivable neuropsychological function. Two main factors account for this variability. First, few studies are sufficiently methodologically rigorous, with adequate selection criteria and matching of control subjects. For instance, both Veiel (1997) and Zakzanis et al. (1998) identified fewer than twenty-five studies deemed to possess sufficient methodological rigour. Second, the clinical heterogeneity of major depression means that multiple demographic and illness-related factors interact to affect the profile observed. Some of the more important factors in determining the neuropsychological profile are discussed below.

Effects of depressive subtype

A continuing issue is whether melancholia is a distinct entity with a greater genetic component, particular biological abnormalities, better response to biological treatment, fewer psychosocial stressors and less evidence of personality dysfunction, or whether it is simply a more severe depression (see Chapters 3 and 4).

Studies investigating the relationship between melancholia and neuropsychological impairment have not shown a definitively different pattern unrelated to measures of severity. Austin et al. (1999) found that predominantly mnemonic tasks were impaired in a large sample of depressed patients, compared with controls. When a narrow definition of melancholia was used (CORE or Newcastle scales), executive dysfunction was found in melancholic patents compared with controls. However, there were no significant differences when the subtypes of depression were compared and severity used as a statistical covariate.

A further problem in comparing melancholic and non-melancholic patients is that psychomotor slowing is an essential part of most definitions of melancholia. This may bias melancholic patients towards exhibiting impairments on neuropsychological tests that use latency as an outcome measure.

Studies comparing the performance of psychotic unipolar depressed patients with non-psychotic patients have consistently shown that the neurocognitive impairment in psychotic depression is significantly more widespread and severe. Studies that have failed to find such differences have generally used smaller sample sizes with a post-hoc division into subjects with and without psychotic features, rather than recruiting such groups from the outset. Jeste et al. (1996) studied a cohort of 218 patients aged over 45 years: thirty had unipolar major depression with psychotic features, twenty-eight had non-psychotic unipolar major depression, and 160 had schizophrenia. The performance of patients with psychotic depression was similar to that of patients with schizophrenia. Both groups were more impaired than the patients with non-psychotic depression on measures of psychomotor speed, motor function, verbal learning, attention and aspects of executive functioning. In contrast, memory retention was similar across the groups.

Severity of depression

Evidence regarding the effects of current severity is inconsistent. Some studies show an association with selected aspects of neuropsychological performance, while others fail to. Several possibilities may explain this, including general methodological differences between studies, differences in other underlying clinical and demographic factors, and the possibility that the relationship is not linear or monotonic, as is assumed when using a correlational approach. Interestingly, some depression rating scales may be better suited than others for use in this respect. Elliott et al. (1996) found significant correlations between severity of depression and several tests of visuospatial learning and memory when using the Montgomery–Asberg Depression Rating Scale, but not the Hamilton Depression Rating Scale.

Studies that have examined the effects of hospitalisation on neuropsychological performance have consistently demonstrated more severe impairment in inpatients than outpatients. Using the intradimensional/extradimensional set-shifting task (a test said to be analogous to the Wisconsin Card Sorting Test) in young depressed patients, Purcell et al. (1997) classified the 50 per cent who completed the task as an *unimpaired group* and the 50 per cent who failed as an *impaired group*. The groups did not differ according to severity of depression, age of onset or length of illness, age, years of education, IQ or medication status. However, patients in the impaired group were more likely to have reported a history of inpatient hospitalisation compared with the unimpaired group. Similarly, Elliott et al. (1996) examined a cohort of middle-aged depressed patients, after separating them by current hospitalisation. The two groups did not differ in terms of age, IQ or severity; however, the eleven inpatients were significantly more impaired on tests of delayed matching to sample, spatial span and response to failure (see 'Catastrophic response to failure' below) than the seventeen outpatients. It is especially interesting that this is found both in currently hospitalised patients and in those with a past history of hospitalisation (Elliott et al. 1996; Purcell et al. 1997).

As with many of the factors discussed in this section, it is often difficult to isolate the major contributory factor when, for most factors, a significant degree of overlap exists between subgroups. Inpatients are more likely to be melancholic, suicidal, and probably have episodes which are more severe, longer, recurrent or more treatment-resistant. All these factors may affect neuropsychological performance.

Effects of age

Age is associated with a progressive decline in neurocognitive functioning. It has been suggested that the specific domains that are affected are the same as those that are impaired in more severe (and melancholic-type) depression, and therefore that age must always be viewed as a significant confound (Austin et al. 2001). In their meta-analysis, Christensen et al. (1997) reported a larger magnitude of effect in patients over 60 years of age than in those under 60 years. Individually, many studies have used age as a covariate in their statistical analyses or have examined the correlation between age and neurocognitive performance, although relatively few have directly compared the performance of older and younger depressed subjects against groups of matched healthy controls.

Tarbuck and Paykel (1995) and Lockwood et al. (2002) both examined neuropsychological profile in groups of depressed patients older and younger than 60 years. The groups were otherwise well matched and were assessed on a comprehensive battery of tests. Overall, significant effects of age were observed on most tests, particularly of psychomotor speed. Selected complex or executive tasks were disproportionately impaired in the older depressed group.

Recent studies have divided elderly patients into those with early onset (younger than 60 years) and late onset (older than 60 years) depression. This distinction appears to have important implications for the neurobiological findings, in addition to neuropsychological abnormalities. This may be because of a significantly greater contribution of vascular pathology in the late onset cases of depression (Baldwin and O'Brien 2002).

Effects of medication

The effects of antidepressant and other psychotropic medication, and their withdrawal may be of particular importance in studies of neuropsychological function in less severely depressed or non-melancholic people, whose impairment may be more subtle. It appears that antidepressants with anticholinergic properties impair aspects of neuropsychological function, while there may be less effect of selective serotonin reuptake inhibitors or monoamine oxidase inhibitors. Many studies have attempted to control for antidepressant effects by using a washout period. Unfortunately, in some cases this has not been long enough, because although onset of antidepressant discontinuation symptoms is usually within several days of stopping an antidepressant, symptoms may last several weeks. Very few studies have examined patients who are drug-naïve, or even following a drug-free period of more than a few weeks. Studies that have attempted to recruit such patients are often negative because of the very mild illness severity of subjects that are able to participate.

In a recent study, we examined a group of forty-four patients with major depression who had been medication-free for at least 6 weeks (including twenty-six who were entirely drug-naïve) and forty-four matched healthy control subjects (Porter et al. 2003). The patients were predominantly first-episode, non-melancholic outpatients with a moderate to severe depressive illness, but displayed significant neuropsychological impairment compared with control subjects. Impairment was found on tests of sustained attention and executive function, including verbal fluency and strategy formation, as well as visuospatial recognition and working memory, and delayed matching to sample. However, verbal declarative learning and memory, motor speed, and psychomotor functions were unimpaired. Importantly, severity of depression was correlated with almost all tests of learning and memory but no tests of executive function. This may suggest that executive functions are more sensitive, being adversely affected regardless of the severity of depression, while learning and memory functions are impaired only with increased severity of depression. An alternative is that executive deficits may represent a relatively stable trait marker, while mnemonic impairment is related to clinical state. This is in line with studies that have shown a complete absence of residual memory impairment after clinical recovery, while executive dysfunction persists.

NEUROPSYCHOLOGY OF BIPOLAR DISORDER

There are far fewer studies on the neuropsychology of bipolar disorder than on major depressive disorder. Early studies often grouped the two together, making any interpretation of results with respect to distinct profiles impossible (Bearden et al. 2001).

Comparison between unipolar and bipolar depression

Comparisons of unipolar and bipolar depression have generally been small and report no differences between the groups in general intellectual functioning (Mojtabai et al. 2000). In that study, the researchers also administered a range of tests of attention, memory and executive function and found no differences on any measure. In contrast, Borkowska and Rybakowski (2001) found significantly greater impairment in bipolar disorder than in major depression across a range of executive functions, as well as in general intellectual functioning. The discrepancy may be due to the confounding effect of depressive subtype, as all subjects in the study by Mojtabai et al.

were psychotic. This highlights the importance of illness variables on performance and raises the question of whether the two disorders can ever be compared satisfactorily. For example, even if the groups could be matched for demographic profile and the severity of current episode, it would be impossible to equate overall illness characteristics such as medication, hospitalisations and previous affective episodes (of depression or mania).

Mania

Very few studies have examined patients in the manic state, because of the inherent difficulty of testing patients when manic. Those that have been carried out suggest that the degree of impairment is greater in the manic state than in either bipolar or unipolar depression.

Clark et al. (2001) used discriminant function analysis to classify manic patients and controls on the basis of their neuropsychological test performance. Performances on tests of verbal learning (the California Verbal Learning Test) and sustained attention (the rapid visual information processing task), when combined, could be used to classify correctly 87 per cent of manic subjects and 91 per cent of subjects overall. This is a particularly important finding in light of the report by Swann et al. (2003), who found increased commission errors in manic patients compared with both euthymic patients and controls on the Immediate Memory–Remote Memory Task (which reflects risk of impulsivity). Interestingly, both patient groups (manic and euthymic) scored higher than controls on a questionnaire measuring impulsivity, suggesting not only that attentional processing may be impaired in mania but that aspects such as impulsiveness may also pervade in clinical remission.

State versus trait?

Specific impairments, present during euthymia, may represent trait markers that indicate specific neurobiological impairment in bipolar disorder. In a review of the literature, Chowdhury et al. (2003) highlighted the issues surrounding this topic, including methodological problems such as the way in which euthymia is defined. Even minor residual affective symptoms appear to affect the degree of impairment observed and must therefore be controlled, either in the design of the study or in the subsequent statistical analysis.

These issues aside, two distinct profiles of trait abnormality have been suggested, with some degree of overlap but with differing views regarding the contribution of working memory. One profile suggests that deficits such as impaired attention, planning, verbal fluency and response inhibition in euthymia can be conceptualised as an impairment in the executive control of working memory. Others have rejected a working memory interpretation. This is largely because there is some evidence that sustained attention tasks with no working memory load are impaired while those with working memory load are performed at normal levels. However, as discussed previously, attempting to equate task performance to specific memory systems is complex, and a task engaging the working memory system need not involve memory per se.

Although there is debate on the precise nature of the deficit, the identification of a trait abnormality in executive function is further strengthened by studies in high-risk groups, such as first-degree relatives of bipolar patients. It has been shown that these subjects exhibit subtle impairment in neuropsychological functioning, despite having no personal history of bipolar disorder (Chowdhury et al. 2003).

ORIGIN OF NEUROPSYCHOLOGICAL IMPAIRMENT

Many authors have examined mechanisms that may explain the neuropsychological impairment of depression. Theories have generally been either entirely psychological, based on the symptomatology of depression (for example, reduced motivation, altered cognitive style) or entirely biological, based on neurobiological findings (for example, altered hypothalamic–pituitary–adrenal (HPA) axis function, regional changes in brain activity). The true explanation may lie in a combination of several of these factors.

Psychological

EFFORTFUL VERSUS AUTOMATIC PROCESSING Some authors have suggested that effort is the principal factor mediating neuropsychological changes in depression. It is hypothesised that performance on tasks requiring effortful processing is more impaired than performance on more automatic tasks. Support for this comes from a recent meta-analysis which reported minimal effect sizes on tests of primary, semantic and working memory (relatively automatic processes), with the most prominent effects being in memory processes, such as the effortful encoding of information and inefficiency of retrieving poorly encoded information from declarative memory (Zakzanis et al. 1998). It also appears that some of the greatest comparative impairment seen in mood disorders is on tests of attention and executive function, both domains typically requiring effortful processing. However, as already discussed, impairment in these domains may also represent a relatively stable trait deficit, present in even mild affective episodes or persisting in euthymia. Furthermore, this hypothesis does not explain why deficits are often reported on non-effortful tasks. Our own work has found not only high-effort tasks to be impaired in major depression but also relatively automatic processes, such as recognition memory in both visual and verbal domains, despite intact verbal declarative memory (Porter et al. 2003).

A related theory is that all deficits are related to a general reduction in motivation (Schmand et al. 1994). This is closely related to the effortful processing hypothesis; however, it is difficult to explain the lack of impairment in certain cognitive domains and the specificity of the profile seen in others if reduced motivation is the major factor in mediating neuropsychological dysfunction.

CATASTROPHIC RESPONSE TO FAILURE In elderly patients, Beats et al. (1996) described a catastrophic response to perceived failure on the Tower of London task. They found that once patients made an error, subsequent performance deteriorated markedly. Subsequently, Elliott et al. (1996) reported a different response to failure on the delayed matching to sample task and the new Tower of London task in depressed patients compared with control subjects. In normal subjects, receiving feedback that the wrong response has been given tends to increase the likelihood of succeeding on subsequent trials. This was not seen in depressed patients. A similar phenomenon has been reported in dysphoric subjects using the Wisconsin Card Sorting Test. However, some subsequent studies have failed to replicate these findings. This may be related to the statistical procedures used, or to the exact nature of the task or feedback (for a discussion, see Murphy et al. 2003).

MOOD-RELATED BIAS IN INFORMATION PROCESSING Various studies have shown altered neuropsychological performance, depending on the emotional valence of the stimuli used (usually words) in testing. For instance, in a task of set shifting (a commonly tested executive function), depressed patients showed abnormalities that could be interpreted as a bias towards verbal stimuli with negative emotional valence, whereas manic patients exhibited an opposite bias, towards words with a positive emotional valence (Murphy et al. 1999). Given the findings of impairment on tasks with no discernible emotional content, this mechanism is probably part of, but not an explanation for, the neuropsychological profile of depression.

Biological

HYPERCORTISOLISM Abnormal HPA axis function is frequently described in mood disorders. High levels of cortisol have been shown to impair learning and memory in humans, both in Cushing's disease, a condition characterised by a chronic elevation of cortisol secretion, and following administration of exogenous corticosteroids to healthy volunteers. It has therefore been proposed that abnormal cortisol secretion is one of the principal causes of neuropsychological impairment.

Several studies have proposed a relationship between cortisol secretion or measures of HPA axis feedback (the dexamethasone suppression test) and neuropsychological impairment (McAllister-Williams et al. 1998). However, recent work (including a large study in the elderly) has not always confirmed this, and it may be that other factors such as vascular pathology are so variable, particularly in the elderly, that a direct relationship is unlikely.

Levels of the adrenal steroid dehydroepiandrosterone (DHEA), a functional antagonist to cortisol, may be important in modifying the effects of cortisol on the brain. The ratio of cortisol to DHEA may therefore be important, and has been found to be elevated even in younger, non-melancholic outpatients (Young et al. 2002), although in that study the ratio did not correlate with measures of neuropsychological function (Porter et al. 2003). Therefore, evidence is still inconclusive, probably complicated by other factors mediating cognitive impairment and by the complexity of the HPA axis. Also, corticosteroids have very specific effects on different stages of information processing and as yet this has not been fully explored in mood disorders.

FRONTOSTRIATAL DYSFUNCTION As discussed earlier, the neuroanatomical locus of executive functions has long been believed to be the frontal lobes, but it is now understood that that such processes activate frontal–subcortical loops. Dysfunction of this circuitry is believed to be central to many of the observed neuropsychological impairments in mood disorders, although the precise manner in which the deficits manifest is still somewhat unclear. Rogers et al. (1998) have speculated that the executive deficits in non-melancholic depression may be purely frontal, whereas those in melancholic depression are frontostriatal with accompanying motor disturbance. Alternatively, frontostriatal deficits may be present in all major depression, with dysfunction of the motor circuit restricted to melancholic depression. Continuing development in neuroimaging techniques which allow the assessment of activated neural circuitry will be used in studies of drug-free patients to resolve these issues.

CONCLUSION

An increasing body of literature is describing neuropsychological deficits in mood disorders. This confirms the subjective reports of many patients who describe problems in everyday memory and concentration, leading to considerable distress and impairment of social and occupational functioning. The pattern and magnitude of neuropsychological impairment is varied, ranging from individuals who exhibit no discernible dysfunction at all, to those with severe motor and cognitive impairments. This variability can, in part, be explained by the clinical heterogeneity of these disorders, with factors such as subtype, severity and age affecting the profile of deficits. One aim for the future is to identify those individuals who are particularly susceptible, and the underlying biological substrates causing the deficits. This would then provide a potential therapeutic target to ameliorate such deficits.

REFERENCES

Alexander GE, DeLong MR, Strick PL (1986) Parallel organization of functionally segregated circuits linking basal ganglia and cortex. *Annual Review of Neuroscience* 9:357-81.

Austin MP, Mitchell P, Goodwin GM (2001) Cognitive deficits in depression: Possible implications for functional neuropathology. *British Journal of Psychiatry* 178:200-6.

Austin MP, Mitchell P, Wilhelm K, Parker G, Hickie I, Brodaty H, et al. (1999) Cognitive function in depression: A distinct pattern of frontal impairment in melancholia? *Psychological Medicine* 29:73-85.

Baddeley AD (1990) *Human Memory: Theory and practice*. Hillsdale, NJ: Lawrence Erlbaum.

Baldwin RC, O'Brien J (2002) Vascular basis of late-onset depressive disorder. *British Journal of Psychiatry* 180:157-60.

Bearden CE, Hoffman KM, Cannon TD (2001) The neuropsychology and neuroanatomy of bipolar affective disorder: A critical review. *Bipolar Disorders* 3:106-50.

Beats BC, Sahakian BJ, Levy R (1996) Cognitive performance in tests sensitive to frontal lobe dysfunction in the elderly depressed. *Psychological Medicine* 26:591-603.

Borkowska A, Rybakowski JK (2001) Neuropsychological frontal lobe tests indicate that bipolar depressed patients are more impaired than unipolar. *Bipolar Disorders* 3:88-94.

Chowdhury R, Ferrier IN, Thompson JM (2003) Cognitive dysfunction in bipolar disorder. *Current Opinion in Psychiatry* 16:7-12.

Christensen H, Griffiths K, Mackinnon A, Jacomb P (1997) A quantitative review of cognitive deficits in depression and Alzheimer-type dementia. *Journal of the International Neuropsychological Society* 3:631-51.

Clark L, Iversen SD, Goodwin GM (2001) A neurophysiological investigation of prefrontal cortex involvement in acute mania. *American Journal of Psychiatry* 158:1605-11.

Elliott R, Sahakian BJ, McKay AP, Herrod JJ, Robbins TW, Paykel ES (1996) Neuropsychological impairments in unipolar depression: The influence of perceived failure on subsequent performance. *Psychological Medicine* 26:975-89.

Jeste DV, Heaton SC, Paulsen JS, Ercoli L, Harris J, Heaton RK (1996) Clinical and neuropsychological comparison of psychotic depression with nonpsychotic depression and schizophrenia. *American Journal of Psychiatry* 153:490-6.

Lezak MD (1995) *Neurophysiological Assessment*, 3rd edn. New York: Oxford University Press.

Lockwood KA, Alexopoulos GS, Van Gorp WG (2002) Executive dysfunction in geriatric depression. *American Journal of Psychiatry* 159:1119-26.

MacLeod CM, MacDonald PA (2000) Interdimensional interference in the Stroop effect: Uncovering the cognitive and neural anatomy of attention. *Trends in Cognitive Sciences* 4:383-91.

McAllister-Williams RH, Ferrier IN, Young AH (1998) Mood and neuropsychological function in depression: The role of corticosteroids and serotonin. *Psychological Medicine* 28:573-84.

Mojtabai R, Bromet EJ, Harvey PD, Carlson GA, Craig TJ, Fennig S (2000) Neuropsychological differences between first-admission schizophrenia and psychotic affective disorders. *American Journal of Psychiatry* 157:1453-60.

Murphy FC, Robbins MTW, Sahakian BJ (2003) Neurophysiological impairment in patients with major depressive disorder: The effects of feedback on task performance. *Psychological Medicine* 33:455-67.

Murphy FC, Sahakian BJ, Rubinsztein JS, Michael A, Rogers RD, Robbins TW, et al. (1999) Emotional bias and inhibitory control processes in mania and depression. *Psychological Medicine* 29:1307-21.

Porter RJ, Gallagher P, Thompson JM, Young AH (2003) Neurocognitive impairment in drug-free patients with major depressive disorder. *British Journal of Psychiatry* 182:214-20.

Purcell R, Maruff P, Kyrios M, Pantelis C (1997) Neuropsychological function in young patients with unipolar major depression. *Psychological Medicine* 27:1277-85.

Rogers MA, Bradshaw JL, Pantelis C, Phillips JG (1998) Frontostriatal deficits in unipolar major depression. *Brain Research Bulletin* 47:297-310.

Rowe JB, Owen AM, Johnsrude IS, Passingham RE (2001) Imaging the mental components of a planning task. *Neuropsychologia* 39:315-27.

Schmand B, Kuipers T, Van der Gaag M, Bosveld J, Bulthuis F, Jellema M (1994) Cognitive disorders and negative symptoms as correlates of motivational deficits in psychotic patients. *Psychological Medicine* 24:869-84.

Swann AC, Pazzaglia P, Nicholls A, Dougherty DM, Moeller FG (2003) Impulsivity and phase of illness in bipolar disorder. *Journal of Affective Disorders* 73:105-11.

Tarbuck AF, Paykel ES (1995) Effects of major depression on the cognitive function of younger and older subjects. *Psychological Medicine* 25:285-95.

Veiel HO (1997) A preliminary profile of neuropsychological deficits associated with major depression. *Journal of Clinical and Experimental Neuropsychology* 19:587-603.

Young AH, Gallagher P, Porter RJ (2002) Elevation of the cortisol-dehydroepiandrosterone ratio in drug-free depressed patients. *American Journal of Psychiatry* 159:1237-9.

Zakzanis KK, Leach L, Kaplan E (1998) On the nature and pattern of neurocognitive function in major depressive disorder. *Neuropsychiatry, Neuropsychology, and Behavioral Neurology* 11:111-19.

CHAPTER 13

POST MORTEM BRAIN STUDIES

Understanding the pathology of mood disorders

Brian Dean and
Elizabeth Scarr

In opening any review on the use of post mortem tissue, it is important to highlight that such research is always dependent on the decision by relatives to allow the brain of a recently deceased person to be removed for research. Such remarkable gestures have underpinned ongoing research into the causes of psychiatric illness. Thus, it could be argued that post mortem studies represent the ultimate partnership between psychiatric research and society.

As science moves into the twenty-first century, it is perhaps reasonable to consider why studies involving the use of post mortem brain tissue still play an important role in the quest to understand the pathology of mood disorders. The reasons post mortem tissue is still used in such studies are, like the disorders themselves, varied and complex. Many predicted the demise of post mortem studies with the availability of neuroimaging techniques permitting the study of the living human brain. However, neuroimaging techniques have limitations that place boundaries on the studies using these technologies. Thus, in the case of the functional neuroimaging techniques such as single photon emission computer tomography and positron emission tomography, the relatively slow development of radioactive compounds suitable for imaging studies, constraints on the amount of radioactivity that can be injected into a subject, and the limits of resolution of the technologies have prevented these techniques from superseding post mortem brain tissue studies. Also, limitations in resolution and tracing technologies have meant that structural neuroimaging techniques, such as magnetic resonance imaging, have not been able to completely substitute for the intensive study of changes in the cellular make-up of post mortem brain tissue from subjects with mood disorders. Studies using post mortem brain tissue or neuroimaging techniques form complementary approaches to the study of the brain from subjects with mood disorders, and people interested in the area need to keep abreast of both approaches. However, this chapter will focus on the contribution of the study of post mortem brain tissue to our understanding of the two major mood disorders, major depression and bipolar disorder.

CONFOUNDING ISSUES

The major confounding issue faced by researchers using post mortem brain tissue from subjects with mood disorders is that it is now most unusual for brain tissue to be collected from subjects who have not received drug treatments before death. Thus, it is necessary to consider the potential mix of pathological and pharmacological changes that may be present in brain tissue from subjects with mood disorders that may be detected when post mortem tissue is used.

There are various strategies that have been developed to control for this problem. First, results from subjects with mood disorders can be compared with those from another disease cohort that have received the same drugs before death. If differences do not transcend diagnosis, this is a strong indicator that the differences observed are not a simple drug effect. Added to this approach is to compare results between individuals who were 'off' drugs for a considerable period before death and those who were 'on' drugs at death. Changes that are present only in subjects on drug at death could be an effect of the drug treatment. In addition, determining if changes in human tissue from subjects who have received specific drugs are present in the brains of animals treated with same drugs is a common approach to determining if changes are simply due to drug treatment. By carefully combining these controlling factors, it is possible to predict which changes are associated with the pathology of diseases such as the mood disorders.

One issue that is of particular relevance to the study of mood disorders is that the increased incidence of suicide means that studies using post mortem brain tissue will usually include tissue from a number of donors who died in this fashion. Therefore, the possible confounding effects of a pathology of suicide must also be considered when examining results in studies on mood disorders. This confounding factor is relatively easily controlled by comparing results within suicide but across diagnosis on the premise that a pathology of suicide would not be diagnostically specific.

A CONVERGENCE OF SCIENTIFIC DISCIPLINES

To completely understand the outcomes of the full gamut of research using post mortem brain tissue requires knowledge of human neuroanatomy and molecular brain functioning that cannot be presented in this chapter but can be obtained from classic texts on these subjects (Kandel et al. 1991). Combined with this information, there is a need for an understanding of the basic concepts of diagnosing psychiatric illnesses according to standardised protocols and an understanding of the actions of drugs used to treat psychiatric illnesses.

NAVIGATING THE HUMAN BRAIN

What is becoming increasingly apparent is that changes in the brains of subjects with mood disorders show discrete regional localisation. Unfortunately, descriptions of brain regions are not uniform across publications; in this chapter, discussion on the regions of the brain is restricted and unified to descriptions of broad areas, definitions of which can be found in most human brain atlases (England and Wakely 1991). However, many publications use Brodmann's concepts of cortical regionalisation, which are based on his studies of the topographic analysis of the human cerebral cortex founded on variation in cellular structure. These concepts are clearly outlined in the translation of Brodmann's text from German to English by Garey (1994).

From structural to cellular organisation

With whole books being devoted to the different approaches to using post mortem brain tissue in psychiatric research (Dean et al. 1999), it should be appreciated that experiments using such tissue can range from global measurements, such as measuring brain weight at autopsy, to examining changes in the molecular architecture of the brain. It is important to note that processing the brain varies depending on the methodology for which it is to be used. Thus, careful fixation is required to maintain cellular integrity for cell counting studies, whereas rapid freezing is necessary to preserve the integrity of proteins and mRNAs. This often means that researchers cannot extend their studies from, for example, counting neurons to measuring specific proteins in the same tissue sample. This remains an unavoidable limitation to identifying changes in the human brain that underlie psychiatric illnesses.

Macro and cellular changes

It has been suggested recently that there are significant reductions in the volume of some brain regions and a complex series of changes in the cellular make-up of certain regions of the brain from subjects with bipolar disorder (Rajkowska 2002). It is perhaps not surprising, given some of the similarities of the mood disorders, that there have been similar findings in the brains of subjects with major depression (Drevets 2000). Although the changes in specific structures in the brain are suggested by neuroimaging studies, it is recent post mortem studies that are providing data to suggest that the volume changes observed are due to complex changes in the cellular make-up of the brain.

At the structural level, post mortem studies have shown changes in the lamina formations of the entorhinal cortex of subjects with bipolar disorder and major depression (Baumann and Bogerts 2001). Cortical laminae are discrete and well-defined cytoarchitectural layers that make up the human cortex. The entorhinal cortex forms part of the temporal lobe, and further studies of the temporal lobe have revealed other abnormalities in this important brain region. For example, unlike in schizophrenia, the decrease in cortical thickness does not appear to be accompanied by an overall change in neuronal density in subjects with bipolar disorder and major depression. Thus, there appear to be significant differences in the underlying cause of the reduction in cortical thickness between schizophrenia and the mood disorders. Importantly, such gross changes in cortical structure would have to occur early in development, supporting the concept that psychiatric illnesses are due, at least in part, to deficits in neurodevelopment.

As in the entorhinal cortex, a reduction in cortical thickness also been reported for the dorsolateral prefrontal cortex in bipolar disorder, major depression and schizophrenia (Baumann and Bogerts 2001). The importance of this finding is that the dorsolateral prefrontal cortex forms part of the neocortex, which controls the higher and cognitive functions of the human brain (Monuki and Walsh 2001). As these functions seem to alter markedly in mood disorders, a better understanding of the changes in the neocortex will be important in elucidating the pathology of these illnesses.

It is also clear that changes in the brain associated with mood disorders are not limited to the neocortex. Reduced numbers of non-pyramidal neurons have been reported in the CA2 region of the hippocampus in bipolar disorder (Baumann and Bogerts 2001). Importantly, these reductions were also found in brain tissue from subjects with schizophrenia. What is the significance of findings that are apparently not disease-specific? Clearly, in psychiatric disorders such findings may be related to the genesis of symptoms, such as psychoses, that are present in both bipolar disorder and schizophrenia.

The temporal cortex represents one of the oldest phylogenic regions of the mammalian brain and therefore it seems that the search for the cause of psychiatric illness cannot be limited to the neocortex. This argument is further supported by the finding in the cingulate cortex that there is a decrease in glial cells in laminae VI from subjects with major depression or schizophrenia, but not bipolar disorder.

With regard to findings in the cortex, one important question relates to how subjects with bipolar disorder and depression have a decrease in cortical thickness with no loss of neurons. This question seems to be answered by the finding that there is a decrease in the density of glial cells in the dorsolateral prefrontal and orbital cortex from subjects with major depression and bipolar disorder (Davidson et al. 2002). Glial cells were long thought simply to provide a passive structural support for neurons in the brain. However, more recently it has been shown that glia and neurons are extremely interactive. Thus, psychiatric illness may be caused by changes in the *neuropil*, that is, the total cellular population of the brain, rather than just the neurons. Clearly, current data question the long-held belief that abnormalities of neuronal function must be the cause of psychiatric illnesses and make the growing understanding of glial–neuronal interaction (Derouiche et al. 2002) an important aspect of understanding the pathology of mood disorders.

In considering the complexity of the pathology of psychiatric disorders, it is important to examine the regional specificity of changes in post mortem brain tissue. Adjacent to the dorsolateral prefrontal cortex is the foremost part of the brain, the frontal pole. In contrast to the dorsolateral prefrontal cortex, findings in the frontal pole have shown that the decrease in glial density is limited to laminae VI, the deepest laminae of the cortex, in tissue from subjects with bipolar disorder and schizophrenia (Davidson et al. 2002). Interestingly, this finding was limited to brains from subjects with major depression where there was a strong family history of mental illness. Hence, in depression, the susceptibility to develop that disorder may be a genetic predisposition to abnormal brain development. This hypothesis is supported by the finding that there is a decrease in the number of glial cells in a region of the cingulate cortex in subjects with bipolar disorder and major depression, and this decrease is most pronounced in subjects with a family history of mood disorder.

Significantly, unlike in neurological disorders such as Parkinson's disease, Huntington's chorea and Alzheimer's disease, no gross neuroanatomical lesion has been found in the brains of subjects with psychiatric disorders. The failure to find such lesions in the brains of subjects with mood disorders has led to the postulate that macroscopic changes in brain structure are not the cause of these illnesses. Extending this hypothesis, it then seems likely that the cause of psychiatric illnesses is change in the molecular architecture of the brain.

Changes in molecular architecture

Studies trying to determine the molecular changes that underlie mood disorders were initially based on the hypothesis that the molecules targeted by proven clinical agents could be involved in the pathology of the disorders. In the case of antidepressants, this suggested that components of the serotonergic and noradrenergic systems could be affected by the disorder. The picture in bipolar disorder is obviously more complex, with the use of mood stabilisers, antipsychotics and antidepressants.

Early research to identify the causes of bipolar disorder focused on the G proteins, because they are modulated by both lithium and antidepressants (Dean 2002). G proteins are the components of the cell that allow a signal to pass from the receptor to the intracellular milieu (Marinissen and Gutkind 2001). To date, various studies have shown changes in the levels of different members of the G-protein family in post mortem brain tissue from subjects with bipolar disorder (Dean 2002) and in depression (Stockmeier 1997). This suggests that the communication between receptors and their signal transduction pathways through the G proteins is disrupted in both disorders. A careful comparison of changes in the different G proteins in different regions of the brain will be required to determine if different members of this family of proteins are affected in the two different mood disorders.

At present, it is not clear how changes in G proteins may precipitate the symptoms of mood disorders. However, it has been shown that there is a disruption in the interaction between the serotonin 1A receptor and its associated G proteins in the brains of subjects with bipolar disorder (Dean 2002). Moreover, it has been suggested that changes in the serotonin 1A (Stockmeier et al. 1998) and serotonin 2A (Yates et al. 1990) receptors are present in the brains of people with depression. Given the findings of changes in these important components of the serotonergic system in mood disorders, it is significant that a recent study, using a high-throughput screening technique to examine the levels of expression of multiple genes, found that the gene encoding the serotonin transporter is over-expressed in the frontal lobe from subjects with bipolar disorder (Sun et al. 2001). Thus, data from post mortem studies seem to support the long-held hypotheses that changes in the serotonergic systems of the brain are core deficits in depression (Arango et al. 2002) and bipolar disorder (Vawter et al. 2000). It is now necessary to determine exactly how changes in the serotonergic system can precipitate at least some of the symptoms of either depression or bipolar disorder. However, at present, it seems likely that changes in serotonergic systems of the brain are central to generating the symptoms of depression that are common to many psychiatric disorders.

The major body of data in bipolar disorder and depression at the molecular level has focused on the serotonergic system, its receptors, and the G proteins. However, there are now some findings (which remain to be replicated) that are potentially of great interest as they may shed light on the pathological processes associated with bipolar disorder and depression. One intriguing finding suggests that there may be a change in the subunit composition of the γ-aminobutyric$_A$ (GABA$_A$) receptor in the dorsolateral prefrontal cortex from subjects with bipolar disorder. The GABA$_A$ receptor has a variety of functional binding sites, one of which binds the benzodiazepines. In the dorsolateral prefrontal cortex from subjects with bipolar disorder, the number of benzodiazepine binding sites on the GABA$_A$ receptors is increased (Dean 2002). The endogenous ligand for the benzodiazepine binding site on the GABA$_A$ receptor has yet to be identified. However, given that benzodiazepines are potent modulators of mood, it seems likely this site is involved in the physiological modulation of mood. Hence, it could be that changes in the subunit composition of the GABA$_A$ receptor may be involved in the mood swings prominent in bipolar disorder. Other studies have reported decreases in synaptophysin, growth-associated protein 43 and complexin I and II in anterior cingulate cortex from subjects with bipolar disorder. These proteins are all associated with the functioning of the *presynaptic* neuron (Graham et al. 2002), the neuron that releases neurotransmitters into the synaptic cleft. Of particular interest is the possible consequence of changes in synaptophysin, which forms part of the vesicular docking mechanism of the presynaptic neuron. If this process is aberrant in the brains of people with bipolar disorder, it is possible that there are widespread abnormalities in neurotransmitter release involved in the pathology of the illness.

In the case of depression, it has been suggested that there is a decreased number of noradrenaline transporters in the locus coeruleus of subjects with the disorder (Klimek et al. 1997). This finding, in conjunction with the presence of a decrease in the number of serotonin transporters in the prefrontal cortex from subjects with depression (Arango et al. 2002), seems to support the argument developed from clinical neuropsychopharmacology that abnormalities in the serotonergic and noradrenergic systems of the brain are involved in depression.

From the limited review of post mortem brain research focusing on the changes in the molecular architecture of the brain in mood disorders, it is becoming clear that the causes of these illnesses are complex. To date, attempts to identify the pathology of the mood disorders have depended upon hypothesis-driven research that has progressed on a gene-by-gene basis. Technologies have been developed recently that can measure the levels of thousands of proteins or their mRNAs at one time. These technologies are likely to have a substantial impact on our understanding of the changes in the brain that cause mood disorders. It is the combination of these technologies with post mortem brain research that is leading the search for genes that might be involved in bipolar disorder and depression.

COMPARISON OF PATHOLOGIES OF PSYCHIATRIC ILLNESSES

It has been questioned whether the mood disorders may share some common genetic susceptibility and therefore are a spectrum of mental illness rather than discrete diseases (Gershon 2000). To address this issue, it is necessary to compare the underlying abnormalities in both disorders in a controlled fashion using brains from carefully selected donors with either bipolar disorder or depression. This is now occurring under an initiative known as the Stanley Foundation Neuropathology Consortium (Knable et al. 2001). This consortium is supplying tissue from subjects with schizophrenia, bipolar disorder and depression to laboratories for specific investigations as to the changes that may be involved in the differing pathologies of these disorders.

In a meta-analysis of the data currently available to the consortium, it was concluded that the changes in the brains from subjects with bipolar disorder are more similar to those in subjects with schizophrenia than to those with depression. This was suggested because most changes in the brains of subjects with the three psychiatric illnesses have not proven to be disease-specific. Only two changes, decreased dynorphin mRNA and increased levels of cytochrome oxidase 4, are specific to bipolar disorder. Only one change, increased immunoreactive nitric oxide synthase, is specific to depression. Superficially, it appears that the pathologies of bipolar disorder and depression are similar in nature.

THE RIVER OF PSYCHIATRIC ILLNESS

From current studies of human post mortem brain tissue, there appear to be common factors that underlie mood disorders and there seem to be few disease-specific differences in the brains of subjects with schizophrenia, bipolar disorder or depression. Moreover, these abnormalities do not appear to be restricted to the neurons but may also involve the much more abundant glial cells. However, different mood disorders can be clearly delineated, so it must be asked how illnesses with such apparent commonalities present with such different aetiologies.

In considering the aetiologies of psychiatric illness, it must be acknowledged that an increasing body of data suggests that there are some common neural abnormalities that must occur to produce the symptoms of psychiatric illness such as depression or psychoses. These abnormalities may stem from mutations that make an individual susceptible to mental illness (Gershon 2000). Moreover, there are ever-increasing findings that implicate specific neurotransmitter systems as being common to the generation of symptoms across disease. Thus, overactive dopaminergic pathways are required for the genesis of psychoses, and changes in serotonergic activity are central to the onset of depression across all diseases that display these symptoms.

However, it seems very likely that the symptoms common between diseases, such as psychoses and depression, result from changes to central pathways that may be induced by changes in different pathways in the brain. The focus on these common systems has come about because they are the targets for therapeutic agents that are known to be beneficial in treating symptoms, independent of the overarching disease that has generated the symptom. Extending this argument, it seems logical that it is the *upstream* changes that differ between psychiatric disorders. To make an analogy, the processes involved in inducing psychiatric symptoms could be modelled using a river system. At present, following clues from the neuropsychopharmacology of symptom treatment, it is probable that we have searched for the sources of the disorders in the main body of the river, where the level of the river is a result of a series of different inputs from many tributaries. From this model, the goal must be to move from the main body of the river into the tributaries, the levels of which are affected only by limited local factors. This approach would identify factors that cause specific symptomatology, but in disease-specific processes. Given that existing therapies can effectively treat specific symptoms, why is this journey necessary? First, in better targeting the epicentre of a disease or symptom pathology, it is likely that therapeutic benefits could be obtained with fewer unwanted side effects, a problem of all existing therapies. In addition, it would be expected that the pathologies in subjects who are treatment-resistant will be identified, and drugs developed that will be useful in treating these subjects.

As suggested previously, technologies are now available to study the molecular make-up of the brain, providing the opportunity to take the journey up river to its source. These technologies are known as *high-throughput screening techniques*, and can measure the levels of thousands of proteins and their messenger RNA at one time (Colantuoni et al. 2000). As the genes identified as being affected by the pathology of the illness are discovered on an a priori basis, the potential outcomes of such studies are to identify genes that would not be considered by hypothesis-driven research based on earlier findings. One such study has used such an approach based on microarray technology to identify genes that are differentially expressed in the frontal cortex from subjects with bipolar disorder (Bezchlibnyk et al. 2001). The expression level of 1200 genes was examined, and twenty-four of these genes were differentially expressed in the tissue from subjects with bipolar disorder. The authors of the study suggested that three differentially expressed genes that might be important in the pathology of bipolar disorder are transforming growth factor β1, caspase-8 precursor, and transducer of erbB2. These three genes are involved in neuroprotection, cell death and the regulation of mitogenesis, respectively. This list of genes shows that high-throughput screening techniques can change the perception of potential key pathways affected by the pathology of a disorder. It is also clear that there will be considerable further research required to understand the role of such genes in precipitating the pathology of psychiatric illnesses such as the mood disorders.

CONCLUSION

The likely outcome that must be expected from post mortem brain research into mood disorders is to identify potential drug target sites. When a drug is developed to target such a site and is proven effective in the treatment of a mood disorder, then the debt owed to those who have allowed tissue to be used in such research will be partly repaid.

REFERENCES

Arango V, Underwood MD, Mann JJ (2002) Serotonin brain circuits involved in major depression and suicide. *Progress in Brain Research* 136:443-53.

Baumann B, Bogerts B (2001) Neuroanatomical studies on bipolar disorder. *British Journal of Psychiatry. Supplement* 41:s142-7.

Bezchlibnyk YB, Wang J-F, McQueen GM, Young LT (2001) Gene expression differences in bipolar disorder revealed by cDNA array analysis of post-mortem frontal cortex. *Journal of Neurochemistry* 79:826-34.

Colantuoni C, Purcell AE, Bouton CM, Pevsner J (2000) High throughput analysis of gene expression in the human brain. *Journal of Neuroscience Research* 59:1-10.

Davidson RJ, Lewis DA, Alloy LB, Amaral DG, Bush G, Cohen JD, et al. (2002) Neural and behavioral substrates of mood and mood regulation. *Biological Psychiatry* 52:478-502.

Dean B (2002) Changes in the molecular structure of the brain in bipolar disorder: Findings using human postmortem brain tissue. *World Journal of Biological Psychiatry* 3:125-32.

Dean B, Kleinman JE, Hyde TM (1999) *Using CNS Tissue in Psychiatric Research.* Sydney: Harwood Academic Press.

Derouiche A, Anlauf E, Aumann G, Muhlstadt B, Lavialle M (2002) Anatomical aspects of glia-synapse interaction: The perisynaptic glial sheath consists of a specialized astrocyte compartment. *Journal de Physiologie (Paris)* 96:177-82.

Drevets WC (2000) Neuroimaging studies of mood disorders. *Biological Psychiatry* 48:813-29.

England MA, Wakely J (1991) *A Colour Atlas of the Brain and Spinal Cord.* London: Wolfe Publishing.

Garey LJ (1994) *Brodmann's Localisation in the Cerebral Cortex.* London: Smith-Gordon.

Gershon ES (2000) Bipolar illness and schizophrenia as oligogenic diseases: Implications for the future. *Biological Psychiatry* 47:240-4.

Graham ME, Washbourne P, Wilson MC, Burgoyne RD (2002) Molecular analysis of SNAP-25 function in exocytosis. *Annals of the New York Academy of Sciences* 971:210-21.

Kandel ER, Schwartz JH, Jessell TM (1991) *Principles of Neural Science*, 3rd edn. Norwalk: Appleton Lange.

Klimek V, Stockmeier C, Overholser J, Meltzer HY, Kalka S, Dilley G, et al. (1997) Reduced levels of norepinephrine transporters in the locus coeruleus in major depression. *Journal of Neuroscience* 17:8451-8.

Knable MB, Torrey EF, Webster MJ, Bartko JJ (2001) Multivariate analysis of prefrontal cortical data from the Stanley Foundation Neuropathology Consortium. *Brain Research Bulletin* 55:651-9.

Marinissen MJ, Gutkind JS (2001) G-protein-coupled receptors and signaling networks: Emerging paradigms. *Trends in Pharmacological Sciences* 22:368-76.
Monuki ES, Walsh CA (2001) Mechanisms of cerebral cortical patterning in mice and humans. *Nature Neuroscience* 4 Suppl:1199-206.
Rajkowska G (2002) Cell pathology in bipolar disorder. *Bipolar Disorders* 4:105-16.
Stockmeier CA (1997) Neurobiology of serotonin in depression and suicide. *Annals of the New York Academy of Sciences* 836:220-32.
Stockmeier CA, Shapiro LA, Dilley GE, Kolli TN, Friedman L, Rajkowska G (1998) Increase in serotonin-1A autoreceptors in the midbrain of suicide victims with major depression – postmortem evidence for decreased serotonin activity. *Journal of Neuroscience* 18:7394-401.
Sun Y, Zhang L, Johnston N, Torrey E, Yolken R (2001) Serial analysis of gene expression in the frontal cortex of patients with bipolar disorder. *British Journal of Psychiatry. Supplement* 41:s137-41.
Vawter MP, Freed WJ, Kleinman JE (2000) Neuropathology of bipolar disorder. *Biological Psychiatry* 48:486-504.
Yates M, Leake A, Candy JM, Fairbairn AF, McKeith IG, Ferrier IN (1990) 5HT2 receptor changes in major depression. *Biological Psychiatry* 27:489-96.

SECTION

IV

Management

CHAPTER 14

THE CLINICAL MANAGEMENT OF DEPRESSION

Peter R Joyce

The clinical management of patients with depression involves:

- performing a diagnostic assessment
- evaluating and ensuring safety
- providing education to the patient and, when relevant, to his/her family
- establishing a therapeutic alliance
- providing support and care
- providing advice, and recommendations for specific treatments (for example, evidence-based psychotherapies or antidepressants)
- monitoring treatment response
- enhancing treatment compliance
- evaluating and managing associated impairments
- preventing relapse.

Clinical management, compared with specific psychotherapies or antidepressant drugs, has been under researched and undervalued. When clinical management has been formally evaluated in clinical trials, it has sometimes been surprisingly effective, and this may be part of the reason for high placebo response rates in some clinical trials of depression. The best study to date, which demonstrated the comparative efficacy of good clinical management, was the National Institute of Mental Health Collaborative Treatment Study of Depression. In this large multicentre study, patients with major depression were randomly allocated to one of four treatment groups: clinical management plus placebo, clinical management plus imipramine, cognitive therapy, or interpersonal psychotherapy. Clinical management included evaluation, education, encouragement and support, but specific psychotherapeutic methods were not allowed (Fawcett et al. 1987). In patients with mild to moderate depression (Hamilton depression rating scale [HDRS] <20), there were no differences in treatment efficacy across the four treatment groups. In patients with a moderate to severe depression (HDRS ≥ 20), imipramine plus clinical management had the best results. The two psychotherapies were not as good as imipramine, but were better than clinical management plus placebo (Elkin et al. 1989). In an accompanying editorial commenting on the results from this study, a key issue highlighted was the effectiveness of clinical management.

INITIAL EVALUATION AND MANAGEMENT

Making and sharing the diagnosis

When patients present on the first occasion, they suspect that there is something wrong with them, but they may have little idea as to what is wrong. They will also bring to the first session some opinion, knowledge, fear and prejudice about the nature of mental illness in general and of depression in particular. Even patients who consider that they may have some general medical disorder (for example, cancer) will have their own knowledge and opinions about depression. Indeed, dealing with the opinions and fears about depression in patients who present with somatic symptoms or who are convinced of a general medical explanation of their symptoms can be a major management challenge.

In primary care and general medical settings, the skills involved in a successful referral to mental health services can be considerable, especially in patients who tend to deny the possible existence of a mental disorder within themselves. Understanding the basis of this denial (for example, fear, prejudice or stigma) may be a necessary first step to providing care and treatment. Sometimes, presenting depression as a biological (rather than psychological) disorder associated with chemical changes in the brain can assist in obtaining agreement to treatment in those who wish not to have a 'mental' disorder. However, there are dangers in excessive use of this approach, and the prescribing of antidepressant drugs to assist 'sleep' is fraught with its own difficulties.

Once a sufficient history of depressive symptomatology has been obtained from patients, it is important to the provision of care and treatment that both healthcare professional and patient understand the viewpoints of each other. Thus, sharing the diagnosis of major depression involves considerably more than the doctor saying, 'You have depression; now, take these tablets'. It is usually important that patients have some understanding of the concept of clinical depression, and that it is not synonymous with depressed mood. Some explanation of current knowledge about the symptomatology, aetiology, outcome and treatment of depression is important. In other words, there should be discussion about what it is (symptoms and diagnosis), what caused it (aetiology), what will happen (outcome), and what can be done about it (treatment). As this should be a two-way discussion, it is not just the doctor's view of symptomatology, aetiology, outcome and treatment but also the patient's view of these issues that should be covered. The patient might have views about diagnosis, aetiology or treatment that are at odds with the professional viewpoint to an extent that may hinder treatment. It is also relevant that fear about depression could hinder care and treatment. Many patients have had some experience of depression or its treatment in family, friends or through the media, and negative experiences or perceptions of hospitalisation, medications or psychotherapy may hinder their acceptance of care and treatment for themselves. Alternatively, knowing someone who has received good care and made an excellent recovery may lead patients to expect similarly good results for themselves. Finally, patients may fear the power of psychiatrists to commit them under the Mental Health Act and have a fear of being locked away in a psychiatric hospital.

Providing initial clinical management

After the making and sharing of a depressive diagnosis, the ingredients of good clinical management are to ensure safety, and provide education, support and encouragement. In people with depression, the evaluation of safety is of paramount importance, as around half of all depressed patients will have some degree of suicidal ideation, and perhaps up to a quarter of all people with depression will make a suicide attempt at some time. Although 2–10 per cent of people with depression ultimately die by suicide, and the suicide risk is real, it is very unusual for people with depression to make a suicide attempt early in their care if they perceive that they are receiving good clinical management. The danger times are before presentation or diagnosis, when patients perceive they are not receiving adequate care, or when treatments have failed to provide relief from depression. Therefore, if newly diagnosed depressed patients are engaged in a plan for clinical care, most can be treated on an outpatient basis and only a small minority should ever require inpatient care.

In the evaluation of suicide risk, it is important to enquire about the frequency and intensity of suicidal ideation, any suicide plans (such as timing or methods), circumstances that could provoke action (for example, loss of a partner) and factors that may prevent patients acting on their thoughts (such as religious beliefs that suicide is a sin). It is also important to know a patient's family history and past history of suicidal behaviour, and to have some idea of personality traits (especially impulsivity).

Suicide is not the only safety issue that needs to be considered in the management of people with depression. In severely depressed people, a belief that the world or person is 'bad' may lead to the ideation that a patient's family would also be better off dead. Therefore, some murder–suicides involve a depressed patient and, in depressed women with young children, the depressed patient may be thinking about killing her children as well as herself.

Once safety issues have been considered, the key ingredients of clinical management include education, care, encouragement and a plan for evaluating symptomatology and response to intervention. Education can be enhanced by providing written material on depression (such as a pamphlet), and it is sometimes surprising what patients learn from the written material that was discussed during an appointment but not retained. Written material can also be a helpful way for patients to share the diagnosis and management of their depression with a family member or a friend. This eliciting of helpful support and education can be very useful in their ongoing management. Conversely, a spouse who has no understanding or sympathy about the nature of depression can undermine successful treatment.

As depression is not cured by a single appointment or the provision of a single prescription, an essential part of any management plan is to review the symptomatology over time. If a depressive episode is mild to moderate in severity, then specific treatments may not be required at the first appointment, although treatment options could be discussed. At a second arranged appointment (for example, a week later) to review symptomatology, discuss treatment options, and to provide further education, support and encouragement, the doctor should not be misled by an improvement in symptoms following the first interview and assume that no further evaluation is necessary. Often, there will be deterioration in symptomatology from the second to the third appointment and the transient improvement following initial diagnosis, education and support will have passed. Specific treatments may be clearly indicated at that later time.

It is also important to note that, following a suicide attempt, a transient improvement in symptomatology, from a few days to several weeks, is common. Too often, no review of symptomatology is arranged 2–4 weeks after the initial assessment and, without an explicit arrangement to return for review, many patients fall through the gaps in service provision and are not seen again for treatment to be more clearly offered.

Treatment options

For depressive episodes that are of mild severity, short duration and that lack melancholic or psychotic features, there is no real evidence that specific treatments are better than good clinical management. For instance, in trials using antidepressant drugs, it is relatively clear that placebo will not be worse than antidepressant drugs in mild, short duration, non-melancholic major depressive episodes (Fairchild et al. 1986; Peselow et al. 1992; Rush 2000; Schatzberg and Kraemer 2000; Kupfer and Frank 2002). To prescribe drugs that have side effects and that can be dangerous in overdose must, therefore, be considered dubious practice. Anti-anxiety drugs, even if they produce early symptom relief, may be problematic and worse than placebo in the longer term.

In considering treatment options, and in discussing them with depressed patients, it is important to keep in mind that depression tends to be chronic or recurrent. A person who has a single uncomplicated episode in a lifetime is the exception, and both management and treatment should be planned with this understanding. Similarly, treatment options are not mutually exclusive, and both pharmacological and psychotherapeutic approaches may be tried over time. Discussing both general modalities early in management may be helpful in preventing the development of unhelpful either/or dichotomies.

If patients are voluntarily seeking assistance, then there is probably an implied consent for diagnosis, monitoring, education, support and encouragement. However, when management moves beyond diagnosis and clinical care, information about specific treatment modalities (whether psychotherapy, cognitive therapy, antidepressant drugs, or electroconvulsive therapy) should be provided to patients so that they are informed about efficacy, side effects, adverse effects and monitoring of treatment response before specific treatments begin.

There is no evidence that antidepressant drugs interfere with psychotherapy or that psychotherapy adversely affects response to antidepressant drugs (Rounsaville et al. 1981). In many clinical situations it is not feasible, nor are there advantages to combining antidepressant drugs with psychotherapy. However, in patients with severe or chronic depression (Thase et al. 1997; Keller et al. 2000) and in the elderly (Reynolds et al. 1992), there may be real therapeutic advantages to combining antidepressant drugs with psychotherapy. Sequential treatment may often be successful (Frank et al. 2000), and this may be more feasible in many clinical situations and more cost-effective.

In general, it is useful for patients to be made aware of potential treatment options early, even when patients are stating a strong preference for either a psychotherapeutic or pharmacological approach. Indeed, as no treatment for depression exists that is uniformly beneficial for all patients, extra effort should be made to discuss all treatment options for patients who have strong views about one treatment approach.

The sick role

For most new patients presenting with depression, it can be useful to discuss depression as a disorder or as an illness. This can often alleviate fears that it is a general medical disorder or belief that it is due to personal inadequacy, and that if only they 'pulled themselves together' they would recover. In explicitly using an illness model, it becomes legitimate for patients to have the usual rights and expectations of someone who is sick. For some, it may be appropriate to consider whether the patient should be relieved of normal roles (whether at work, school or home). Too often, depressed patients struggle on with all sorts of expectations (both externally and internally imposed), and explicit discussion of time off or time out may be helpful.

Similarly, while individuals are acutely unwell it is generally desirable for them to defer any major personal decisions (such as to separate, change partner, change job or change house). Although deferment of major personal decisions is probably advisable with all illnesses, it is especially important in depression, as patients' views about their partner, job or house may change dramatically upon recovery from their depressive disorder. Too often, patients make major decisions they later regret.

During the acute phase of treatment of depression, it is also useful to discuss with the patients and the family what their expectations of the patient should be, and what expectations the patients should have of their family. Although being 'sick' may excuse the patient from some normal duties at home and at work, this does not give the patient the right to be angry at, or rude to, family or friends. Discussion about the extent of the patient's involvement in family activities may help decrease unnecessary friction. For example, while it may be reasonable for the depressed patient to be excused social functions and meeting new people, it seldom seems justified for patients to avoid family meal times, even if the patient is quieter and eats less than usual.

Recovery from depression may also be assisted by patients trying to keep to regular daily activities and schedules (for example, regular meal times, bed time and getting-up time), and avoiding excessive alcohol or other drugs. For patients who do shift work, consideration of avoiding these disruptions to daily rhythms may be of value.

MONITORING SYMPTOMATOLOGY

If the initial management plan involves clinical management only, then if there are no marked improvements in symptomatology over about 4 weeks, specific treatments may need to be added. Even if there has been improvement, there should be an arrangement for a review of symptomatology (even by telephone) after 2–3 months. Too often, the mood deteriorates after discharge and, for a variety of reasons, the patient fails to seek help again.

When the initial management plan involves prescribing antidepressant medication, part of the explanation about the drugs involves the likely time course of response. It is unsatisfactory just to say that they take 6 weeks to work – some patients may show some improvement by 1 week, and many will experience improvement during the second and third weeks. Improvement requires that they be taking the drug and at an adequate dosage, so dosage adjustments may be required if there is no improvement by 3 weeks. If there is no response after 4–6 weeks on an adequate dose, then it is unlikely that the current antidepressant will work, although antidepressant response may take longer than 6 weeks in the elderly. Even though the patient-may show some improvement by 1–3 weeks, this is not to say they will have recovered and be symptom-free by this time.

Indeed, it is vital in management for clinicians to distinguish between *better* (improved) and *better* (recovered). Patients often respond affirmatively when asked if they are better, but they mean they are better than they were, not that they are recovered. The clinician may misinterpret the patient in this way. This misunderstanding often leads to a collusion between patient and clinician, especially when the patient is grateful for small gains, does not want to worry the clinician, and perhaps believes that small gains are all that should be expected.

When the initial management involves a short-term psychotherapy, such as cognitive behaviour therapy or interpersonal psychotherapy, which normally involve ten to fifteen sessions, improvement should be monitored and be apparent over 6–12 weeks. If a patient is severely depressed or has melancholic feature, no symptom improvement by 6–8 weeks may suggest the need for the addition of antidepressant medication. For a patient with mild to moderate depression, a detailed review after the ten to fifteen sessions will indicate whether other treatment modalities may be indicated.

Thus, regardless of treatment modality offered, if a patient's depression is moderate to severe, no symptom change by 6–8 weeks necessitates review of treatment options, and for a depression which is mild to moderate, a review of treatment options should be mandatory after 3 months. Too often, patients are left on antidepressant drugs that are not providing symptom relief for months and longer without review, or receive psychotherapy over months or longer without review. Neither situation is appropriate management, and patients need to be made aware of the need for review over time.

PREVENTING RELAPSE AND RECURRENCE

Preventing relapse

Relapse is now generally defined as a return of depressive symptoms after only a short period of improvement (for example, less than 2–3 months) (Frank et al. 1991). It is important for treating clinicians to be aware of the high likelihood of relapse, and if the specific treatment offered was antidepressant medication, it is important to educate and advise patients about the need to continue with a full dosage of medication during the months following recovery. For a first episode of depression, the antidepressant medication should be continued for 6–12 months. The duration of continuation with medication should be longer with chronic depressions (including major depression superimposed on dysthymia), with very severe depressions, and when past history or family history suggest the probability of recurrence is higher.

The possibility of relapse may be reduced by the patient experiencing or creating his or her own *fresh start* life events. Thus, new relationships, new jobs and changed circumstances may assist in a sustained recovery. Certainly, the epidemiological data support the association between such fresh start life events and recovery. It is intriguing to note how often patients initiate their own life changes, not only in treatments such as interpersonal psychotherapy but also during antidepressant drug treatment. Conversely, patients who remain trapped in situations with ongoing adverse life stressors or chronic interpersonal difficulties may have much greater difficulty sustaining improvements.

Preventing and managing recurrence

In providing care for patients with depression, recurrence or chronicity is the rule rather than the exception. For a patient experiencing a first episode of depression, there is a greater than 50 per cent chance of suffering a recurrence. For patients in their second episode, the probability of yet another episode is probably greater than 80 per cent, and for those suffering their third or subsequent episode, the probability of yet another is certainly over 90 per cent. All patients need to be educated about the probabilities of recurrence, if only to facilitate early and appropriate help-seeking behaviour if or when the next episode happens.

The data from the Pittsburgh maintenance treatment study of recurrent depression provide overwhelming evidence for the efficacy of maintaining full-dose antidepressants (imipramine with blood level monitoring at a mean dose of over 200 mg daily) in recurrent depression. However, the Pittsburgh study also provided some evidence that maintenance interpersonal psychotherapy (once a month over 3 years) reduced the likelihood of recurrence compared with clinical management and placebo, but it was not as effective as full-dose imipramine (Frank et al. 1990; Kupfer et al. 1992). Even after 3 years of sustained recovery on imipramine, reducing the dose usually led to recurrence (Frank et al. 1993).

TREATMENT-RESISTANT DEPRESSION

Review of diagnosis and treatment

Treatment-resistant depression is not a unitary phenomenon, and involves people who remain severely depressed despite adequate treatment trials. Although this may be a common view of what treatment resistance means, people whose depression is completely unchanged by treatment are relatively few. A much larger group of patients with treatment-resistant depression are those who have a partial response (that is, better but not right) or have brief responses (for example, much better for a few days to a few weeks) but then slip back to either the initial level of severity or to the level of a partial response. In some respects, these patients with partial or brief responses are more problematic for management than those who remain severely and unremittingly depressed (Kornstein and Schneider 2001; Thase et al. 2001; Fava 2003; Nelson 2003).

The first step in reviewing the management of a patient who has been thought of as treatment-resistant is to review the diagnosis. A diagnosis of a major depressive disorder implies that the depressive symptoms are not due to a general medical disorder (such as hypothyroidism), are not substance-induced (for example, by alcohol, cannabis or prescribed drugs) and are not part of a schizophrenic or other psychotic disorder. However, the presence of an axis II personality disorder or a history of sexual abuse does not alter a diagnosis of major depression. These may also be present in a patient with a major depressive disorder, and may also need to be addressed, but they do not explain the depressive syndrome. The re-labelling of a patient with treatment-resistant depression as now having 'just a personality disorder' or as being 'just a victim' of sexual abuse is inappropriate management and says more about the clinician than the patient.

The second step in reviewing the management of a patient with treatment-resistant depression is to review what treatments the patient has actually received. That a patient has seen a psychotherapist for thirty sessions over 6 months does not mean that the patient received adequate psychotherapy. That a patient was prescribed a tricyclic antidepressant for 6 months does not ensure that the patient received an adequate antidepressant trial. For instance, did the patient comply with treatment, and was the dose (and blood levels when available) adequate? How many adequate antidepressant trials has a patient received, or did the treatment consist of multiple, short-duration, low-dose antidepressant prescriptions that were poorly complied with?

The third step in reviewing the management of a patient with treatment-resistant depression is to review comorbid conditions. Thus, if a patient had a primary diagnosis of panic disorder, obsessive–compulsive disorder, post-traumatic stress disorder, somatisation disorder or anorexia nervosa, and then developed a major depressive disorder, the probability of recovery from the major depression may be lower than for a depressed patient without such a comorbid disorder. In these circumstances, treatment may need to be directed at both the depression and the comorbid disorder. The second group of comorbid diagnoses that need to be considered are physical disorders, such as diabetes. Although diabetes is not causative of depression and thus it is inappropriate to diagnose a depression due to a general medical disorder, the outcome of treatment of depression in the context of diabetes is generally poorer than in a patient who is physically healthy. Third, it is important to consider comorbid axis II personality disorders. A personality disorder does not explain the depression, but when present may adversely affect the response to treatment of the depression (Mulder 2002). Thus, it may be necessary to address the personality disorder psychopathology as well as the depressive psychopathology.

The fourth step in reviewing the management of a patient with treatment-resistant depression is to consider the current social environment of the patient. Is the patient living in a situation with chronic marital conflict, caring for sick or dependent relatives, ongoing violence, or poverty? Although these current environmental factors may lower the probability of a good response to treatment of depression and may need to be addressed, the possibly surprising observation is how often patients make good recoveries from depression despite living in difficult circumstances. On recovery, patients may describe how they are now coping much better with their difficult, but possibly unchanged, circumstances.

Depression as a chronic disorder

About 10 per cent of patients treated for depression will still be depressed in 1 year's time, despite optimal management and treatment. In addition to the 10 per cent still meeting full criteria for major depression, a further 10–20 per cent may have had a partial rather than a full response. This lack of improvement in at least 10 per cent of depressed patients is not the patient's fault (that is, it is not that they are just personality-disordered), and it does not mean that the clinician has done something wrong or is incompetent. The lack of improvement reflects our current ignorance about the causes and treatments of depression, and in providing ongoing care it is important that 'blame' of the patient or by the patient is appropriately addressed. Similarly, clinicians must deal appropriately with their own sense of inadequacy or failure.

If the diagnosis of depression is correct and if the patient has really been resistant to various treatment trials, it becomes important to discuss the notion of treatment-resistant depression. It is useful to be realistic but optimistic: realistic in the sense that the probability of recovery over the next

3 months and with the next treatment option is low, optimistic in the sense that even after years of depression it is possible for depression to undergo a natural remission regardless of treatment. There are case histories of individuals with a 10–20-year history of depression who awake one day and the depression has lifted. However, in accepting that the probability of recovery in the short term is low, it is often appropriate to move from a *sick role* model of depression to a *rehabilitation* model. Thus, the issues are no longer excusing patients from some responsibilities because they are acutely ill, but helping them function optimally despite suffering from chronic depression. During the provision of ongoing care, careful attention to activities of daily living and their planning can produce small but useful gains. In depression, it is important to recognise the inertia that patients generally suffer; explicit planning of daily activities may overcome some of this inertia. Furthermore, if some activities are undertaken during a day, this decreases self-recrimination and guilt at the end of the day for doing nothing. Regular exercise may make a limited contribution. Note, however, that these management strategies are about coping with chronic depression, rather than cure.

During chronic depression, it is still appropriate to keep trying alternative treatment options. If the patient is severely depressed, then electroconvulsive therapy should be tried. Changes to antidepressant medication should be tried, looking for even small therapeutic benefits. In general, it is important not to expect too much of any specific treatment modality, and treatment trials should be for a longer duration (2 or 3 months) with any medication change.

Finally, in chronic depression it is necessary to keep in mind the possibility that demoralisation may be added to depression. Not only may the patient be demoralised, but treating clinicians may also feel demoralised and experience a sense of hopelessness and futility. When chronic depression is compounded by hopelessness and futility, the ever-present risk of suicide in depression may increase. However, ongoing care of patients with chronic depression can be satisfying, if demanding, and unexpected improvements and gains may often be observed over time.

REFERENCES

Elkin I, Shea MT, Watkins JT, Imber SD, Sotsky SM, Collins JF, et al. (1989) National Institute of Mental Health Treatment of Depression Collaborative Research Program. General effectiveness of treatments. *Archives of General Psychiatry* 46:971-82.

Fairchild CJ, Rush AJ, Vasavada N, Giles DE, Khatami M (1986) Which depressions respond to placebo? *Psychiatry Research* 18:217-26.

Fava M (2003) Diagnosis and definition of treatment-resistant depression. *Biological Psychiatry* 53:649-59.

Fawcett J, Epstein P, Fiester SJ, Elkin I, Autry JH (1987) Clinical management – imipramine/placebo administration manual. *Psychopharmacology Bulletin* 23:309-21.

Frank E, Prien RF, Jarrett RB, Keller MB, Kupfer DJ, Lavori PW, et al. (1991) Conceptualization and rationale for consensus definitions of terms in major depressive disorder. Remission, recovery, relapse, and recurrence. *Archives of General Psychiatry* 48:851-5.

Frank E, Kupfer DJ, Perel JM, Cornes C, Mallinger AG, Thase ME, et al. (1993) Comparison of full-dose versus half-dose pharmacotherapy in the maintenance treatment of recurrent depression. *Journal of Affective Disorders* 27:139-45.

Frank E, Grochocinski VJ, Spanier CA, Buysse DJ, Cherry CR, Houck PR, et al. (2000) Interpersonal psychotherapy and antidepressant medication: Evaluation of a sequential treatment strategy in women with recurrent major depression. *Journal of Clinical Psychiatry* 61:51-7.

Frank E, Kupfer DJ, Perel JM, Cornes C, Jarrett DB, Mallinger AG, et al. (1990) Three-year outcomes for maintenance therapies in recurrent depression. *Archives of General Psychiatry* 47:1093-9.

Keller MB, McCullough JP, Klein DN, Arnow B, Dunner DL, Gelenberg AJ, et al. (2000) A comparison of nefazodone, the cognitive behavioral-analysis system of psychotherapy, and their combination for the treatment of chronic depression. *New England Journal of Medicine* 342:1462-70.

Kornstein SG, Schneider RK (2001) Clinical features of treatment-resistant depression. *Journal of Clinical Psychiatry* 62 Suppl 16:18-25.

Kupfer DJ, Frank E (2002) Placebo in clinical trials for depression: Complexity and necessity. *JAMA* 287:1853-4.

Kupfer DJ, Frank E, Perel JM, Cornes C, Mallinger AG, Thase ME, et al. (1992) Five-year outcome for maintenance therapies in recurrent depression. *Archives of General Psychiatry* 49:769-73.

Mulder RT (2002) Personality pathology and treatment outcome in major depression: A review. *American Journal of Psychiatry* 159:359-71.

Nelson JC (2003) Managing treatment-resistant major depression. *Journal of Clinical Psychiatry* 64 Suppl 1:5-12.

Peselow ED, Sanfilipo MP, Difiglia C, Fieve RR (1992) Melancholic/endogenous depression and response to somatic treatment and placebo. *American Journal of Psychiatry* 149:1324-34.

Reynolds CF, Frank E, Perel JM, Imber SD, Cornes C, Morycz RK, et al. (1992) Combined pharmacotherapy and psychotherapy in the acute and continuation treatment of elderly patients with recurrent major depression: A preliminary report. *American Journal of Psychiatry* 149:1687-92.

Rounsaville BJ, Klerman GL, Weissman MM (1981) Do psychotherapy and pharmacotherapy for depression conflict? – Empirical evidence from a clinical trial. *Archives of General Psychiatry* 38:24-9.

Rush AJ (2000) The use of placebos in unipolar major depression: The current status. *Biological Psychiatry* 47:745-7.

Schatzberg AF, Kraemer HC (2000) Use of placebo control groups in evaluating efficacy of treatment of unipolar major depression. *Biological Psychiatry* 47:736-44.

Thase ME, Friedman ES, Howland RH (2001) Management of treatment-resistant depression: Psychotherapeutic perspectives. *Journal of Clinical Psychiatry* 62 Suppl 18:18-24.

Thase ME, Greenhouse JB, Frank E, Reynolds CF, 3rd, Pilkonis PA, Hurley K, et al. (1997) Treatment of major depression with psychotherapy or psychotherapy–pharmacotherapy combinations. *Archives of General Psychiatry* 54:1009-15.

CHAPTER 15

THE MANAGEMENT OF BIPOLAR DISORDER

Philip B Mitchell,
Gin S Malhi
and Jillian Ball

Over the past decade, there has been a resurgence of interest in the treatment of bipolar disorder. For the first time, there has been pharmaceutical industry interest in the development of new effective compounds for this condition. Parallel with this has been the establishment of well-studied psychological therapies. Particular therapeutic areas of unmet need such as bipolar depression, rapid-cycling illness and mixed episodes are also starting to be addressed.

In this chapter, we initially outline the principles of clinical assessment for each phase of the illness, then review the current status of the therapies of interest. The reader should be aware that there have been no controlled treatment studies of bipolar II disorder exclusively. Consequently, knowledge derived from studies of bipolar I samples is extrapolated to the bipolar II population – a less than satisfactory state of affairs.

ACUTE TREATMENT OF MANIA AND MIXED EPISODES

Principles of initial assessment

For acutely manic patients, referral to a specialist psychiatric service for community, outpatient or inpatient care is necessary because aggression, excessive spending and disinhibited behaviour (for example, sexual indiscretions) are likely to damage the person's reputation. Insight and judgment are usually impaired early, even in the absence of delusions. Although outpatient treatment is preferable, and admission with consent occasionally possible, involuntary hospitalisation is frequently required. The latter can protect the patient and family from the damage that could follow impaired judgment. The decision to admit is often traumatic for both patient and family, all of whom will need support. A useful rule to guide decisions about hospitalisation is that manic patients are generally worse than they appear. Corroborative information from family, friends or general practitioner is invaluable in assessment.

If treatment occurs in an outpatient setting, close monitoring of risky behaviour, particularly sexual, financial or that which leads to potential harm to others (such as hazardous driving), is crucial. A financial power-of-attorney may be necessary, particularly with a history of excess spending. Because mania produces chaotic behaviour, outpatient attendance is often erratic. Legally enforced community treatment may be an option, using options such as a *community treatment order.*

Once the urgency is contained, a full psychiatric history and mental state and physical examinations are necessary to confirm the diagnosis, rule out organic causes (including prescription medications or illicit drugs), identify physical complications (for example, dehydration), and ascertain level of risk to self or others. As noncompliance with ongoing mood-stabilising medications often causes relapse, this should always be considered. Any concurrent antidepressant should be ceased.

Acute pharmacological treatment

LITHIUM Despite recent controversy about lithium's efficacy, a series of meta-analyses (see below) confirm its value for both acute episodes and for prophylaxis. Indeed, lithium remains the benchmark for regulatory authorities such as the US Food and Drug Administration and the Australian Therapeutic Goods Administration when evaluating new mood stabilisers.

CARBAMAZEPINE With a few exceptions, the quality of the randomised controlled trials (RCTs) of carbamazepine in acute mania has been surprisingly poor. Only two double-blind, placebo-controlled monotherapy trials have been carried out (Ballenger and Post 1980); carbamazepine was effective in both. In another study (Post et al. 1987), responders tended to be dysphoric or rapid-cyclers. In trials comparing the efficacy of carbamazepine and lithium (for example, Lerer et al. 1987), no difference was found between the two, but samples were small and intention-to-treat analyses not undertaken.

VALPROATE Valproate (valproic acid) is usually administered as a sodium salt; other forms are valpromide (the amide) and divalproex sodium (sodium valproate and valproic acid in a 1:1 molar ratio). The term *valproate* will cover all forms unless otherwise specified. Three studies of valproate in treating mania have involved comparisons with placebo and/or lithium. Pope et al. (1991) found valproate significantly more effective than placebo, whereas Freeman et al. (1992) demonstrated no difference between valproate and lithium except in patients with mixed mania, where valproate was superior. Both studies were limited by small samples.

Bowden et al. (1994), in a large trial comparing valproate, lithium and placebo, found significantly greater (but equal) improvement with the active drugs compared with placebo. Lithium and valproate were also equally effective for people with rapid cycling. Swann et al. (1997) later reported that valproate was more effective than lithium for dysphoric mania in this sample. In the only comparison of valproate and carbamazepine in acute mania (albeit open label), Vasudev et al. (2000) found valproate more effective.

Oral loading (initial treatment with a high oral dosage) of valproate may lead to a more rapid antimanic response. In an open random-assignment comparison with blind evaluators, McElroy et al. (1996) found 20 mg/kg divalproex was as effective as haloperidol in patients with mania, with most improvement occurring within three days. Although a prompt response with oral loading is likely, a confirmatory comparison of standard and oral loading doses in an adequate sample has yet to be done.

LAMOTRIGINE No placebo-controlled RCTs using lamotrigine in patients with mania or mixed episodes have been reported.

CLOZAPINE No RCTs in bipolar disorder have been done, but in a small number of open case series clozapine has been found to be useful in the acute treatment of mania and in prophylaxis.

OLANZAPINE In two RCTs for mania (Tohen et al. 2000), olanzapine was more effective than placebo, and from the first week. Although olanzapine appears to be as effective as the typical antipsychotic haloperidol (Shi et al. 2002), there have been no published comparisons against lithium. There have been two RCTs comparing olanzapine and valproate in mania and mixed states, but with discrepant results. One found olanzapine to be superior to valproate (Tohen et al. 2002), but the other reported no difference between these two agents (Zajecka et al. 2002). A 12-month continuation study (Tohen et al. 2003) has demonstrated maintenance of the benefit of olanzapine.

RISPERIDONE No placebo-controlled studies of risperidone monotherapy in mania or mixed states have been reported. However, Sachs et al. (2002) compared risperidone with haloperidol and placebo – with each as an adjunct to a mood stabiliser (lithium or valproate). Risperidone and a mood stabiliser was more effective than placebo and a mood stabiliser, but not more so than haloperidol and a mood stabiliser.

Electroconvulsive therapy

In the single randomised (but small) comparison of electroconvulsive therapy (ECT) and lithium in acute mania (Small et al. 1988), ECT was more effective than lithium at 6–8 weeks. Patients who did not respond to unilateral ECT improved with bilateral ECT.

Meta-analyses of acute treatment

Two published meta-analyses of the acute drug treatment of mania have been done, but no Cochrane reviews have been reported. Poolsup et al. (2000) identified twelve RCTs of lithium (658 patients). The response rate compared with placebo was 1.95 (95% CI, 1.17–3.23). The mean number needed to treat (NNT) was 5 (95% CI, 3–20). Lithium was more likely to achieve remission than chlorpromazine, but was no more effective globally than haloperidol. Carbamazepine and valproate were not more effective than lithium. Emilien et al. (1996) compared lithium, valproate and carbamazepine. Although valproate was more effective than placebo, the three drugs did not differ in efficacy.

ACUTE TREATMENT OF BIPOLAR DEPRESSION

Clinical assessment

A full psychiatric history and mental state and physical examinations are necessary to confirm the diagnosis, exclude underlying organicity (such as hypothyroidism), identify physical complications and ascertain the risk of self-harm. As compliance is a frequent cause of relapse, this should therefore always be suspected.

Acute pharmacological treatment

LITHIUM In the nine RCTs of lithium, eight used a crossover design. Lithium was superior to placebo, with up to 80 per cent of patients achieving at least a partial response. However, abrupt cessation of lithium before the double-blind phase may have increased the likelihood of early relapse into mania or depression, and contributed to lithium's advantage. When stringent criteria are applied to evaluate response, only a modest antidepressant effect emerges. This contrasts with the efficacy of lithium in augmenting antidepressants, for which there is robust evidence in both unipolar and bipolar depressed patients. An additional limit of lithium in bipolar depression is the delay of 6–8 weeks before it exerts an antidepressant effect, much slower than its antimanic effect, which occurs within 6–10 days.

CARBAMAZEPINE With no specific placebo-controlled study of carbamazepine in acute bipolar depression, we have to look at trials with mixed groups of bipolar and unipolar depressed patients (for example, Ballenger and Post 1980). These suggest an antidepressant effect for carbamazepine, significant given that most open and controlled studies have examined it in depressed lithium non-responders.

VALPROATE No controlled studies of valproate for bipolar depression have been done, but of interest is a double-blind trial (Young et al. 2000) which found that adding a second mood stabiliser (lithium or valproate) was as effective, though less well-tolerated than adding paroxetine.

LAMOTRIGINE A study of lamotrigine 200 mg daily in 195 patients with bipolar depression found that it was superior to placebo (Calabrese et al. 1999). Lamotrigine is emerging as an effective agent with a distinct therapeutic profile in that it works for depression but not for mania.

Antidepressants

To treat bipolar depression, antidepressants have been borrowed from unipolar depression, akin to the overspill of anticonvulsants from antiepileptic use. There have been fear studies undertaken specifically in bipolar depressed samples..

RISK OF SWITCHING AND RAPID CYCLING In uncontrolled studies, antidepressant-induced switch rates of up to 70 per cent have been reported. These have been lower in controlled studies, for example, in a meta-analysis, Peet (1994) reported a switch rate of only 2–3 per cent for the selective serotonin reuptake inhibitors (SSRIs), which was no different from placebo. The highest switch rate (11 per cent) was associated with a tricyclic antidepressant (TCA), a pattern found by several other investigators. Concurrent use of a mood stabiliser, especially lithium, may protect from switching. Other antidepressants have been less well studied, but SSRIs and moclobemide, with their relatively low switch rates, may be useful in patients with a history of antidepressant-induced mood instability or rapid-cycling bipolar disorder.

SELECTIVE SEROTONIN REUPTAKE INHIBITORS Fluoxetine and paroxetine have been investigated in double-blind, placebo-controlled studies (for example, Nemeroff et al. 2001). SSRIs are effective in bipolar depression, offering advantages over TCAs in having lesser side effects, safety in overdose and low propensity for switching.

TRICYCLIC ANTIDEPRESSANTS A few studies have determined the efficacy of TCAs in the treatment of bipolar depression (Sachs et al. 1994). Controlled studies indicate that bipolar depression may be less responsive acutely to TCAs than unipolar depression is. The use of TCAs is often associated with troublesome side effects, and is further limited by incurring a significant risk of switching.

MONOAMINE OXIDASE INHIBITORS A small number of studies have examined the efficacy of monoamine oxidase inhibitors (MAOIs) in the treatment of bipolar depression. Tranylcypromine is at least as effective, if not more so, than some of the TCAs, especially in patients with anergia (Himmelhoch et al. 1991). The MAOI diet is very restrictive, as are the many potential drug interactions, so it is disappointing that moclobemide, which is better tolerated, appears to be less effective.

OTHER ANTIDEPRESSANTS The role of second-generation antidepressants, such as trazodone, has not been adequately investigated. Third-generation antidepressants, such as venlafaxine, mirtazapine, nefazodone and reboxetine have not been assessed in controlled studies.

Antipsychotics

Recently, an RCT has found olanzapine, as monotherapy and in combination with fluoxetine, to be more effective than placebo, with the combined therapy being apparently of greater value (Tohen et al. 2003). The long-term use of olanzapine is, however, limited by sedation and weight gain.

Electroconvulsive therapy

In a review of nine studies (more than 700 patients) on ECT's efficacy for depression (Zornberg and Pope 1993), seven compared it with antidepressants, and ECT was more effective in five of these studies. When unilateral and bilateral ECT in unipolar and bipolar depression are compared, the outcomes are similar; however, bipolar patients responded more rapidly regardless of electrode placement and stimulus dose (Daly et al. 2001). ECT is recommended for bipolar depression after an antidepressant trial has failed.

PROPHYLAXIS OF BIPOLAR DISORDER

Most patients who experience mania have further episodes of mania, as well as depression. The frequency is 0.37–0.66 episodes a year in people with established illness. The difficult issue of selecting patients for long-term treatment is debatable. Using actuarial techniques, Grof et al. (1979) concluded that at least two episodes of mania or depression in a 2-year period was the best criterion, as this correctly classified 61 per cent of patients who had a recurrence within 2 years. The National Institute of Mental Health (NIMH) Consensus Development Panel (1985) recommends that having a single manic episode, or both hypomanic and depressed episodes, are grounds for prophylaxis, but factors such as suicide attempts in the past, psychotic symptoms and functional incapacity associated with episodes need to be considered. Goodwin and Jamison (1990) recommended maintenance treatment after a second episode, regardless of frequency.

Clinical assessment

As noncompliance is the most common factor in relapse, clinicians try to improve compliance by strategies such as educating patients and families about the disorder and its treatment and possible side effects. Trying to minimise the side effects is obviously a crucial task. Patients fear the potentially abrupt loss of control and its embarrassing consequences. They may resist accepting the diagnosis and need for treatment despite experiencing several episodes. Active bipolar disorder support groups are widespread and contribute usefully to a treatment program. Written material about bipolar disorder and its treatment (provided by health authorities and non-government organisations such as SANE) is helpful to enhance patient knowledge.

An under acknowledged aspect of long-term care of bipolar disorder is its continuity, relevant to both patient and clinician. Contact with the same clinician enhances early identification of recurrence, and facilitates joint awareness of the continuing impact of the illness. Unfortunately, clinicians move about frequently (particularly in public systems). Bipolar disorder is also linked to a peripatetic lifestyle in a proportion of patients.

Pharmacological treatments

LITHIUM Lithium remains the mainstay of prophylaxis. Many placebo-controlled trials demonstrate that it reduces both frequency and severity of manic and depressive episodes: lesser recurrence in 50 per cent of patients, and no relapse at all in 20 per cent.

Unfortunately, noncompliance is common among patients with bipolar disorder (18–53 per cent) (Goodwin and Jamison 1990). In a major study, patients cited four main reasons for this: dislike of medication controlling mood; resisting the idea of having a chronic illness; feeling depressed; and side effects, particularly lethargy, incoordination and dulling of the senses. In the same study, clinicians attributed noncompliance to the patient seeing no need to continue medication when well, missing the highs of hypomania, and being bothered by the idea of having a chronic illness (Jamison et al. 1979). One consequence of noncompliance with lithium is that rapid discontinuation leads to a high rate of relapse, greater than the natural pattern (Suppes et al. 1991). Fifty per cent of patients experience a relapse within 5 months (with mostly mania).

CARBAMAZEPINE The single placebo-controlled prophylactic study of carbamazepine (Okuma et al. 1981), with twenty-two patients over 1 year, failed to demonstrate its superiority over placebo. Five methodologically acceptable randomised double-blind comparative prophylactic studies against lithium have been reported, and most found no difference between the two treatments. The study by Denicoff et al. (1997b) is worthy of comment: fifty-two outpatients with bipolar disorder were randomised in a double-blind fashion to 1 year of lithium or carbamazepine, with a crossover in the second year, and the combination in the third year. Lithium was more effective than carbamazepine in preventing mania, but not depression, and the combination better than monotherapy. Greil et al. (1997), in an open, randomised prospective study over 2.5 years, found lithium superior to carbamazepine in bipolar I but not bipolar II patients. No head-to-head prophylactic studies comparing lithium and carbamazepine have been done in rapid-cycling patients.

VALPROATE In the one double-blind trial of the prophylactic value of valproate for bipolar disorder (Bowden et al. 2000), 372 patients recently recovered from a manic episode were given valproate, lithium or placebo for 1 year. There was no difference in time to the recurrence of any mood episode, possibly because of the inclusion of milder cases of this illness. The largest open randomised study (Lambert and Vernaud 1992) compared valpromide and lithium in bipolar and recurrent unipolar patients over 18 months; patients experienced a reduction in depressed and manic episodes with both lithium and valpromide. No details were offered in the Bowden et al. maintenance trial for rapid-cycling illness; open studies indicate prophylactic antimanic and anti-mixed, but not antidepressant, activity.

LAMOTRIGINE A recently published trial by Bowden et al. (2003) has reported that lamotrigine is more effective in preventing bipolar depressed episodes than lithium or placebo, but appears to be less effective than lithium in preventing manic relapses. Frye et al. (2000) undertook a placebo-controlled randomised crossover trial of lamotrigine and gabapentin in patients, most of whom had refractory bipolar (mainly rapid-cycling) disorder. Lamotrigine was globally more effective than both gabapentin and placebo, but findings were not given for bipolar and unipolar groups.

COMBINATION DRUG THERAPIES In practice, combinations of mood stabilisers are used frequently, particularly in prophylaxis. There is now growing, albeit still minimal, evidence from RCTs that the combination of lithium and carbamazepine and/or valproate enhances efficacy. Kramlinger and Post have reported, in both acute mania and depression, that a substantial proportion of non-responders to carbamazepine respond to the addition of lithium. With regard to prophylaxis, Denicoff et al. (1997b) found a combination of lithium and carbamazepine more effective than either alone. Denicoff et al. (1997a) also compared the efficacy of valproate plus lithium in twenty-four patients who had completed a 3-year trial comparing lithium, carbamazepine, and their combination; the investigators found that a third of patients had moderate or marked responses to valproate plus lithium.

Suicide prevention

Consistent with prior reports, a recent study of suicide attempts and completed suicides of bipolar disorder patients in two large US integrated health plans by Goodwin et al. (2003) found that rates were less with lithium than divalproex (valproate). While not examined specifically in that paper, prior reports (Baldessarini et al. 1999) had suggested that this apparent anti-suicide effect may be independent of lithium's antidepressant activity. Lithium discontinuation can elevate the risk. Baldessarini et al. (1999) reported a 6.5-fold reduction in suicide risk with treatment and a 20-fold increase in the first year after discontinuation.

Psychological treatments

Although pharmacotherapy remains the primary treatment for bipolar disorder, associated psychological treatments are valuable. The limitations of medication in alleviating symptoms and functional impairment highlight the need for psychosocial interventions, which aim to reduce symptoms, prevent relapse and recurrence, restore psychosocial functioning and provide support to patient and family. Specific goals include a therapeutic alliance, medication adherence, promoting regular cycles of activity and sleep, identifying prodromes, improving symptoms and coping, and addressing varied psychosocial effects of the illness. The patient also faces significant psychological adjustments during the recovery process, including stigma associated with the illness, fears of recurrence, interpersonal difficulties, marital, family and parenting issues, educational or occupational disruption, and negative consequences arising from acute episodes.

A range of treatments is available, but the style, intensity and focus varies for each patient. Psychological treatments are presented separately below, but in clinical practice a range of different interventions may be applied.

PSYCHOEDUCATION Psychoeducation offers the patient and family a conceptual and practical approach for understanding and coping with the illness and its treatment. Psychoeducation increases satisfaction with treatment and adherence. Brief psychoeducation can enhance adherence and identify early warning signs. In one RCT, Perry et al. (1999) found that teaching patients to recognise early symptoms of mania and to seek treatment led to improvement in time to first relapse, social functioning and employment.

COGNITIVE THERAPY The roles of cognitive vulnerabilities and stressful life events in unipolar depression have been well researched; the little work that has been conducted on bipolar disorder suggests that negative coping styles combined with stressful life events can lead to episodes of depression and mania (Reilly-Harrington et al. 1999). Furthermore, people with bipolar disorder tend to have more dysfunctional attitudes (even when euthymic) compared with normal controls. Their self-esteem appears to be more unstable, they have a greater need for social approval, perfectionist tendencies are more marked, and they often show poorer problem-solving skills.

Cognitive therapy (CT) aims to identify and manage stress, prodromes and symptoms, and to prevent relapse or recurrence through monitoring and challenging negative assumptions and thoughts. The clinical advantages of this approach are its brevity, its coherent theoretical framework and the fostering of self-efficacy.

The adaptation of CT to the particular needs of patients with bipolar disorder has been described in case reports and open trials. Controlled trials of individual CT show varying efficacy. Treatment, adherence, recognition of prodromes and symptomatic management have been principal targets of therapy. Most studies show improved mood, coping and adherence, and reduced admissions; gains are greater for depressive than manic symptoms.

Schema-focused CT has also been recommended in treating bipolar disorder (Newman et al. 2002; Ball et al. 2003) on the premise that it may delay the onset of a new episode, reduce the duration and severity, and promote adaptation to the condition. Whereas CT uses measures to alter distorted beliefs, schema-focused CT involves emotive, interpersonal, cognitive and behavioural interventions. Schemas are changed most effectively at times of high arousal.

INTERPERSONAL AND SOCIAL RHYTHM THERAPY Interpersonal and social rhythm therapy (IPSRT) proposes that stressful life events influence the course of bipolar disorder by disrupting daily routines, social patterns, and sleep–wakefulness habits. Patients are guided to regulate their social rhythms when stressed and to address interpersonal problems linked to the onset and persistence of bipolar episodes. IPSRT is under evaluation at the University of Pittsburgh; preliminary results show that patients after a year of IPSRT are advantaged compared with those in intensive clinical management.

GROUP THERAPY Group therapy has been successfully applied as an adjunct to medication with an emphasis on adherence and 'here and now' interpersonal issues, lithium monitoring and problem-solving. Bauer and McBride (1997) have reported on an effective group therapy program for patients with bipolar disorder, comprising psychoeducation and realistic goal setting. Colom et al. (2003) recently reported on an RCT in which group psychoeducation was found to prevent recurrence of episodes in bipolar I and II patients.

FAMILY-FOCUSED TREATMENT Family-focused treatment covers such aspects as communication, problem-solving skills and psychoeducation. In the latter, multiple family stresses leading to high levels of expressed emotion are examined and dealt with. Family-focused treatment has been evaluated in two RCTs on patients who had experienced an acute bipolar episode. The comparison group in the first received two sessions of family education followed by crisis management as required: and, in the second, individual therapy concentrating on symptom management and problem-solving. Miklowitz and colleagues (2000) found that patients receiving family-focused treatment had fewer depressive (but not manic) symptoms than comparison group patients, especially in families with high expressed emotion. Goldstein and colleagues (1996) found effects favouring family-focused treatment only after 2 years of follow-up.

Family therapy can improve quality of life and decrease the relapse rate in dysfunctional families. Standard treatment (medication plus clinical management), standard treatment plus family therapy, and standard treatment plus multifamily group therapy have been compared (Miller et al. 2000); the two family treatments have proved superior, but in dysfunctional families only.

Meta-analyses of prophylaxis

Of two Cochrane meta-analyses of the prophylactic value of lithium, the first (Burgess et al. 2002) examined lithium as a maintenance treatment. Using relapse rate as the principal outcome measure, three studies included only bipolar disorder patients, or had separately randomised bipolar disorder groups. Lithium was more effective than placebo in preventing relapse (OR, 0.28; 95% CI, 0.09–0.93); the NNT ranged from 4 (95% CI, 3–6) to 14 (95% CI, 4–∞). When manic and depressive relapses were examined separately, results were similar but not significant. In the other analysis (Macritchie et al. 2002) – of the Bowden et al. (2000) study – lithium and valproate were not more effective than placebo in preventing relapse in bipolar disorder. Dardennes et al. (1995) undertook a meta-analysis of four studies of the role of carbamazepine and lithium in preventing relapse in bipolar disorder, and concluded that the question of the efficacy of carbamazepine was still open.

Focusing on the random-assignment, double-blind, placebo-controlled and case–control matched-subject studies of lithium in the prevention of recurrence in bipolar disorder patients (n = 514), Davis et al. (1999) found that the drug reduced the rate by half (82 per cent with placebo, 32 per cent with lithium). Carbamazepine was only a little less efficacious than lithium, the difference not significant (60 per cent with lithium and 55 per cent with carbamazepine).

CONCLUSION

Although there is now a wide range of effective therapies for bipolar disorder, there are two major limitations in contemporary treatment. First, although this is a highly genetic condition, the specific genes involved have yet to be elucidated, and the molecular mechanisms of this illness as yet remain elusive. This lack of knowledge of the disease mechanisms limits the development of therapies tailored to the specific pathophysiology of this condition.

Second, despite the availability of effective therapies, community studies have shown that treatment uptake is low. For example, Kessler et al. (1997) reported that although 93 per cent of bipolar I patients had received treatment at some point, only 45 per cent had been treated in the previous year.

Furthermore, only half of that 45 per cent were helped in the health care sector. Similarly, Mitchell et al. (2004) have shown low treatment rates in an analysis of the Australian National Survey of Mental Health and Wellbeing. Only 60 per cent of Australian bipolar disorder patients received any medications in the 12-month period, and only 33 per cent had any contact with a mental health professional.

Thus, there are two major challenges to the field: first, the need to understand mechanisms to enable the development of rational therapies; and second, efficient application and availability of the existing proven therapies.

ACKNOWLEDGMENTS

Some of the material included in this chapter has also appeared in the following publications: Mitchell PB, Malhi GS (2002) The expanding pharmacopoeia for bipolar disorder. *Annual Review of Medicine* 53:173–88; and Mitchell PB, Malhi GS, Redwood BL, Ball J (2004) Australian and New Zealand Clinical Practice Guideline for the treatment of bipolar disorder. *Australian and New Zealand Journal of Psychiatry*.

REFERENCES

Baldessarini RJ, Tondo L, Hennen J (1999) Effects of lithium treatment and its discontinuation on suicidal behavior in bipolar manic–depressive disorders. *Journal of Clinical Psychiatry* 60 Suppl 2:77-84.

Ball J, Mitchell P, Malhi G, Skillecorn A, Smith M (2003) Schema-focused cognitive therapy for bipolar disorder: Reducing vulnerability to relapse through attitudinal change. *Australian and New Zealand Journal of Psychiatry* 37:41-8.

Ballenger JC, Post RM (1980) Carbamazepine in manic–depressive illness: A new treatment. *American Journal of Psychiatry* 137:782-90.

Bauer M, McBride R (1997) *Structured Group Psychotherapy for Bipolar Disorder. The Life Goals Program*. New York: Springer.

Bowden CL, Brugger AM, Swann AC, Calabrese JR, Janicak PG, Petty F, et al. (1994) Efficacy of divalproex vs lithium and placebo in the treatment of mania. The Depakote Mania Study Group. *JAMA* 271:918-24.

Bowden CL, Calabrese JR, Sachs G, Yatham LN, Asghar SA, Hompland M, et al. (2003) A placebo-controlled 18-month trial of lamotrigine and lithium maintenance treatment in recently manic or hypomanic patients with bipolar I disorder. *Archives of General Psychiatry* 60:392-400.

Bowden CL, Calabrese JR, McElroy SL, Gyulai L, Wassef A, Petty F, et al. (2000) A randomized, placebo-controlled 12-month trial of divalproex and lithium in treatment of outpatients with bipolar I disorder. Divalproex Maintenance Study Group. *Archives of General Psychiatry* 57:481-9.

Burgess S, Geddes J, Hawton K, Townsend E, Jamison K, Goodwin G (2002) Lithium for maintenance treatment of mood disorders. *Cochrane Database of Systematic Reviews* 3.

Calabrese JR, Bowden CL, Sachs GS, Ascher JA, Monaghan E, Rudd GD (1999) A double-blind placebo-controlled study of lamotrigine monotherapy in outpatients with bipolar I depression. Lamictal 602 Study Group. *Journal of Clinical Psychiatry* 60:79-88.

Colom F, Vieta E, Martinez-Aran A, Reinares M, Goikolea JM, Benabarre A, et al. (2003) A randomized trial on the efficacy of group psychoeducation in the prophylaxis of recurrences in bipolar patients whose disease is in remission. *Archives of General Psychiatry* 60:402-7.

Daly JJ, Prudic J, Devanand DP, Nobler MS, Lisanby SH, Peyser S, et al. (2001) ECT in bipolar and unipolar depression: Differences in speed of response. *Bipolar Disorders* 3:95-104.

Dardennes R, Even C, Bange F, Heim A (1995) Comparison of carbamazepine and lithium in the prophylaxis of bipolar disorders. A meta-analysis. *British Journal of Psychiatry* 166:378-81.

Davis JM, Janicak PG, Hogan DM (1999) Mood stabilizers in the prevention of recurrent affective disorders: A meta-analysis. *Acta Psychiatrica Scandinavica* 100:406-17.

Denicoff KD, Smith-Jackson EE, Bryan AL, Ali SO, Post RM (1997a) Valproate prophylaxis in a prospective clinical trial of refractory bipolar disorder. *American Journal of Psychiatry* 154:1456-8.

Denicoff KD, Smith-Jackson EE, Disney ER, Ali SO, Leverich GS, Post RM (1997b) Comparative prophylactic efficacy of lithium, carbamazepine, and the combination in bipolar disorder. *Journal of Clinical Psychiatry* 58:470-8.

Emilien G, Maloteaux JM, Seghers A, Charles G (1996) Lithium compared to valproic acid and carbamazepine in the treatment of mania: A statistical meta-analysis. *European Neuropsychopharmacology* 6:245-52.

Freeman TW, Clothier JL, Pazzaglia P, Lesem MD, Swann AC (1992) A double-blind comparison of valproate and lithium in the treatment of acute mania. *American Journal of Psychiatry* 149:108-11.

Frye MA, Ketter TA, Kimbrell TA, Dunn RT, Speer AM, Osuch EA, et al. (2000) A placebo-controlled study of lamotrigine and gabapentin monotherapy in refractory mood disorders. *Journal of Clinical Psychopharmacology* 20:607-14.

Goldstein MJ, Rea MM, Miklowitz DJ (1996) Family factors related to the course and outcome of bipolar disorder. In Mundt C, Goldstein MJ, Hahlweg K, Fiedler P (eds), *Interpersonal Factors in the Origin and Course of Affective Disorders.* London: Gaskell.

Goodwin FK, Jamison KR (1990) *Manic–Depressive Illness.* New York: Oxford University Press.

Goodwin FK, Fireman B, Simon GE, Hunkeler EM, Lee J, Revicki D (2003) Suicide risk in bipolar disorder during treatment with lithium and divalproex. *JAMA* 290:1467-73.

Greil W, Ludwig-Mayerhofer W, Erazo N, Schochlin C, Schmidt S, Engel RR, et al. (1997) Lithium versus carbamazepine in the maintenance treatment of bipolar disorders – a randomised study. *Journal of Affective Disorders* 43:151-61.

Grof P, Angst J, Karasek M, Keitner G (1979) Patient selection for long-term lithium treatment in clinical practice. *Archives of General Psychiatry* 36:894-7.

Himmelhoch JM, Thase ME, Mallinger AG, Houck P (1991) Tranylcypromine versus imipramine in anergic bipolar depression. *American Journal of Psychiatry* 148:910-16.

Jamison KR, Gerner RH, Goodwin FK (1979) Patient and physician attitudes toward lithium: Relationship to compliance. *Archives of General Psychiatry* 36:866-9.

Kessler RC, Rubinow DR, Holmes C, Abelson JM, Zhao S (1997) The epidemiology of DSM-III-R bipolar I disorder in a general population survey. *Psychological Medicine* 27:1079-89.

Lambert PA, Vernaud G (1992) Comparative study of valpromide versus lithium as prophylactic treatment in affective disorders. *Nervure Journal Psychiatrie* 7:1-9.

Lerer B, Moore N, Meyendorff E, Cho SR, Gershon S (1987) Carbamazepine versus lithium in mania: A double-blind study. *Journal of Clinical Psychiatry* 48:89-93.

Macritchie KAN, Geddes JR, Scott J, Haslam DRS, Goodwin GM (2002) Valproic acid, valproate and divalproex in the maintenance treatment of bipolar disorder. *Cochrane Database of Systematic Reviews* 3.

McElroy SL, Keck PE, Stanton SP, Tugrul KC, Bennett JA, Strakowski SM (1996) A randomized comparison of divalproex oral loading versus haloperidol in the initial treatment of acute psychotic mania. *Journal of Clinical Psychiatry* 57:142-6.

Miklowitz DJ, Simoneau TL, George EL, Richards JA, Kalbag A, Sachs-Ericsson N, et al. (2000) Family-focused treatment of bipolar disorder: 1-year effects of a psychoeducational program in conjunction with pharmacotherapy. *Biological Psychiatry* 48:582-92.

Miller IW, Keitner GI, Ryan CE, Solomon D (2000) Family treatment of bipolar disorder. *Society for Psychotherapy Research*. Braaga, Portugal.

Mitchell PB, Slade T, Andrews T (2004) Twelve-month prevalence and disability of DSM-IV bipolar disorder in an Australian general population survey. *Psychological Medicine* (In press).

National Institute of Mental Health (NIMH/NIH) Consensus Development Conference Statement (1985) Mood disorders: Pharmacologic prevention of recurrences. Consensus Development Panel. *American Journal of Psychiatry* 142:469-76.

Nemeroff CB, Evans DL, Gyulai L, Sachs GS, Bowden CL, Gergel IP, et al. (2001) Double-blind, placebo-controlled comparison of imipramine and paroxetine in the treatment of bipolar depression. *American Journal of Psychiatry* 158:906-12.

Newman CF, Leahy RL, Beck AT, Reilly-Harrington NA, Gyulai L (2002) *Bipolar Disorder: A cognitive therapy*. Washington, DC: American Psychological Association.

Okuma T, Inanaga K, Otsuki S, Sarai K, Takahashi R, Hazama H, et al. (1981) A preliminary double-blind study on the efficacy of carbamazepine in prophylaxis of manic–depressive illness. *Psychopharmacology* 73:95-6.

Peet M (1994) Induction of mania with selective serotonin re-uptake inhibitors and tricyclic antidepressants. *British Journal of Psychiatry* 164:549-50.

Perry A, Tarrier N, Morriss R, McCarthy E, Limb K (1999) Randomised controlled trial of efficacy of teaching patients with bipolar disorder to identify early symptoms of relapse and obtain treatment. *BMJ* 318:149-53.

Poolsup N, Li Wan Po A, de Oliveira IR (2000) Systematic overview of lithium treatment in acute mania. *Journal of Clinical Pharmacy and Therapeutics* 25:139-56.

Pope HG, Jr, McElroy SL, Keck PE, Jr, Hudson JI (1991) Valproate in the treatment of acute mania. A placebo-controlled study. *Archives of General Psychiatry* 48:62-8.

Post RM, Uhde TW, Roy-Byrne PP, Joffe RT (1987) Correlates of antimanic response to carbamazepine. *Psychiatry Research* 21:71-83.

Reilly-Harrington NA, Alloy LB, Fresco DM, Whitehouse WG (1999) Cognitive styles and life events interact to predict bipolar and unipolar symptomatology. *Journal of Abnormal Psychology* 108:567-78.

Sachs GS, Grossman F, Ghaemi SN, Okamoto A, Bowden CL (2002) Combination of a mood stabilizer with risperidone or haloperidol for treatment of acute mania: A double-blind, placebo-controlled comparison of efficacy and safety. *American Journal of Psychiatry* 159:1146-54.

Sachs GS, Lafer B, Stoll AL, Banov M, Thibault AB, Tohen M, et al. (1994) A double-blind trial of bupropion versus desipramine for bipolar depression. *Journal of Clinical Psychiatry* 55:391-3.

Shi L, Namjoshi MA, Zhang F, Gandhi G, Edgell ET, Tohen M, et al. (2002) Olanzapine versus haloperidol in the treatment of acute mania: Clinical outcomes, health-related quality of life and work status. *International Clinical Psychopharmacology* 17:227-37.

Small JG, Klapper MH, Kellams JJ, Miller MJ, Milstein V, Sharpley PH, et al. (1988) Electroconvulsive treatment compared with lithium in the management of manic states. *Archives of General Psychiatry* 45:727-32.

Suppes T, Baldessarini RJ, Faedda GL, Tohen M (1991) Risk of recurrence following discontinuation of lithium treatment in bipolar disorder. *Archives of General Psychiatry* 48:1082-8.

Swann AC, Bowden CL, Morris D, Calabrese JR, Petty F, Small J, et al. (1997) Depression during mania. Treatment response to lithium or divalproex. *Archives of General Psychiatry* 54:37-42.

Tohen M, Baker RW, Altshuler LL, Zarate CA, Suppes T, Ketter TA, et al. (2002)

Olanzapine versus divalproex in the treatment of acute mania. *American Journal of Psychiatry* 159:1011-17.
Tohen M, Ketter TA, Zarate CA, Suppes T, Frye M, Altshuler L, et al. (2003) Olanzapine versus divalproex sodium for the treatment of acute mania and maintenance of remission: A 47-week study. *American Journal of Psychiatry* 160:1263-71.
Tohen M, Jacobs TG, Grundy SL, McElroy SL, Banov MC, Janicak PG, et al. (2000) Efficacy of olanzapine in acute bipolar mania: A double-blind, placebo-controlled study. *Archives of General Psychiatry* 57:841-9.
Vasudev K, Goswami U, Kohli K (2000) Carbamazepine and valproate monotherapy: Feasibility, relative safety and efficacy, and therapeutic drug monitoring in manic disorder. *Psychopharmacology (Berl)* 150:15-23.
Young LT, Joffe RT, Robb JC, MacQueen GM, Marriott M, Patelis-Siotis I (2000) Double-blind comparison of addition of a second mood stabilizer versus an antidepressant to an initial mood stabilizer for treatment of patients with bipolar depression. *American Journal of Psychiatry* 157:124-6.
Zajecka JM, Weisler R, Sachs G, Swann AC, Wozniak P, Sommerville KW (2002) A comparison of the efficacy, safety, and tolerability of divalproex sodium and olanzapine in the treatment of bipolar disorder. *Journal of Clinical Psychiatry* 63:1148-55.
Zornberg GL, Pope HG, Jr (1993) Treatment of depression in bipolar disorder: New directions for research. *Journal of Clinical Psychopharmacology* 13:397-408.

CHAPTER 16

ANTIDEPRESSANT DRUGS

Trevor R Norman,
James S Olver and
Graham D Burrows

It is nearly 50 years since the first report of the antidepressant activity of imipramine was published by Kuhn (1958). At about the same time, two studies confirmed the antidepressant activity of a monoamine oxidase inhibitor, iproniazid (Crane 1957; Kline 1958). These two drugs formed the prototype of classes of antidepressant agents known collectively as *tricyclic antidepressants* (TCAs), based on the similarity of chemical structure, and *monoamine oxidase inhibitors* (MAOIs), based on the similarity of biochemical actions. Although these drugs were rightly regarded at the time as breakthroughs in the treatment of major depression, it was apparent in clinical practice that they were not panaceas. Lack of clinical response in a substantial minority of patients, relatively slow onset of action, intolerable side effects, and the dangers of over-dosage made it clear that newer agents were necessary to alleviate the symptoms of depression in all patients. It was almost 20 years before the introduction of a class of agents with pharmacological actions different from either the TCAs or MAOIs. Agents relatively selective for their effects on the reuptake of serotonin into nerve terminals, or *selective serotonin reuptake inhibitors* (SSRIs), were first subject to broad clinical testing in the 1970s. The first of these agents was zimelidine (Ross and Renyi 1975), which was subsequently withdrawn from the market. The first commercially successful SSRI was fluvoxamine.

Although further new agents with putatively different mechanisms of action have been marketed in the past few years, perennial problems remain:

response rates and time before onset of action are little changed from the past. In part, the failure to substantially speed the onset of action may be explained by the continued focus on neuronal reuptake of monoamines as the putative mechanism of action of antidepressant medications. To some extent, it may result from an approach to the use of the drugs that fails to recognise important individual differences between patients. Diagnostic issues may also reduce apparent response rates by inappropriate prescription, on occasion, for patients suffering from the vicissitudes of life. Furthermore, the notion of depression as a unitary diagnosis is unhelpful in deciding treatment regimens. Despite this apparent gloomy outlook in respect of the pharmacotherapy of depression, there have been significant advances. In particular, newer medications tend to be better tolerated and tend to pose a reduced risk of death on overdose, partly because of a safer cardiovascular profile.

PHARMACOLOGICAL EFFECTS

Acute effects

A distinction is drawn between the acute and chronic pharmacological effects of antidepressants, as acute effects have generally been held responsible for the initial side effects experienced by patients receiving these drugs. Chronic effects, on the other hand, are regarded as responsible for the alleviation of the symptoms of depression and thus the mechanism of action of these agents. The distinction is based on the perceived time course of response to antidepressant drugs, with therapeutic response requiring several weeks. This is, of course, an arbitrary distinction, as there are late-occurring side effects of antidepressants, while therapeutic responses may be measurable in some patients at as early as 1 week (Davies et al. 1975; Davies et al. 1977; Parker 1996).

Soon after the introduction of TCAs, it was recognised that these drugs share the common property of inhibiting the neuronal reuptake of noradrenaline and serotonin. As reuptake into the nerve terminal represents one of the main mechanisms for terminating the action of these monoamines, the TCAs, by increasing the synaptic concentration of monoamine neurotransmitters, were suggested to correct a hypothesised deficiency. MAOIs were thought to act in an analogous manner, enhancing transmitter availability by preventing transmitter metabolism by monoamine oxidase. Both classes of antidepressant drugs enhanced functional activity of one or more brain monoamine transmitters by actions at the presynaptic neuron. Such a simplistic mechanism of action does not sit well with the complex effects that antidepressant drugs have in the central nervous system (CNS), in terms of both their acute effects and adaptations that occur on chronic administration. Furthermore, some drugs developed after the TCAs and MAOIs have no effect or only weak effects on noradrenaline and serotonin reuptake, yet are clinically effective antidepressants. On the other hand, some drugs that have potent effects on reuptake mechanisms (for example, cocaine) are not clinically effective antidepressants. Most antidepressants developed after this time also have effects on the reuptake of noradrenaline, serotonin or both, and others have effects on dopamine reuptake.

In addition to their common effects on reuptake mechanisms, antidepressants from all classes have potent effects on a range of receptors for various neurotransmitters (Table 16.1). The differential affinity of drugs for these receptors is generally regarded as the explanation of the side effects that most patients experience at the initiation of therapy. Effects on the α_1-adrenergic receptor by TCAs and MAOIs are responsible in part for postural hypotension and dizziness noted in some patients. Sedative effects are probably mediated through antagonism of histamine H_1 receptors, and anticholinergic effects such as dry mouth and blurred vision are mediated by actions at all five muscarinic cholinergic receptor subtypes. As noted in Table 16.1, there are significant effects at other receptors as well, and these can be used to explain differences in side effect profiles between antidepressants from different classes.

Table 16.1
Binding of antidepressant drugs at selected neurotransmitter receptors

	Catecholamine		Serotonin	Histamine	Cholinergic
Drug	α_1	α_2	5-HT_2	H_1	M
Paroxetine	0	0.006	0.005	0.005	0.9
Citalopram	0.05	0.007	0.04	0.2	0.05
Fluvoxamine	0.01	0.007	0.02	0.0009	0.0004
Fluoxetine	0.02	0.008	0.5	0.02	0.05
Amitriptyline	4	0.1	3	91	6
Imipramine	1	0.03	1.3	9	1
Clomipramine	3	0.03	4	3	3
Desipramine	0.8	0.01	0.4	0.9	0.5
Mirtazapine	0.2	0.7	6	700	0.15
Venlafaxine	0	0	0	0	0
Reboxetine	0.01	NA	0.02	0.3	0.02
Nefazodone	4	0.02	30	5	0.01

NOTE Affinity is expressed as $1/10^7 \times$ Kd where Kd is the equilibrium dissociation constant. Higher numbers indicate greater potency at the designated receptor.

SOURCE Leonard and Richelson (2000).

Chronic effects

RECEPTOR DOWN-REGULATION Conventional clinical wisdom suggests that antidepressant therapy is associated with a lag phase of 2–4 weeks before the onset of a beneficial effect. Effects on noradrenaline and serotonin reuptake in the brain occur acutely, even after single doses. Thus, the time frame for the two events does not coincide, and adaptive changes following continuous drug administration are likely to be more important in understanding how antidepressants work. Such adaptive changes following chronic drug administration may occur both pre- and postsynaptically.

Postsynaptic central β_1-adrenoceptor sensitivity

The chronic administration of antidepressants (TCAs, MAOIs, SSRIs and repeated electrically induced convulsions) is associated with a reduction in the number of β_1-adrenoceptor recognition sites in the frontal cortex of rodents. This phenomenon is known as *down-regulation of receptors.* Several drugs without antidepressant properties but with specific effects on noradrenaline reuptake (for example, cocaine and chlorpromazine) fail to bring about β_1-adrenoceptor down-regulation.

How such down-regulation occurs is not clear. A key finding was the observation that the responsiveness of noradrenaline-stimulated adenylate cyclase in rodent limbic forebrain is diminished by all forms of long-term antidepressant treatment. Acute treatment does not down-regulate the system. This is an indirect effect, since lesioning of locus coeruleus noradrenaline neurons prevents down-regulation. Similar down-regulation occurs in β_1-adrenoceptors located in the pineal gland. Possible explanations for drug-induced down-regulation include:

- increased noradrenaline in the synaptic cleft (so-called *agonist-induced down-regulation*, a general phenomenon)
- changes in receptor density, that is, the number of receptors
- alterations in the activity of phosphodiesterase
- changes in the coupling factors and modifications of the properties of the cell membrane.

Whatever the explanation, these observations have led to speculation that, in part, depression may arise because of a functional hyperactivity of certain noradrenergic neuronal systems. These hypersensitive receptors may serve to amplify incoming stimuli and cause hyperexcitability. A hyper-responsive noradrenergic system may be a cause of depression, and antidepressant drugs act to desensitise the system. Note that this view is radically different from the original hypothesis, which proposed a deficiency of noradrenaline at central synapses.

It is inappropriate to unequivocally view the super-sensitivity hypothesis as the sole mode of action of antidepressants, as a range of pharmacological observations do not accord with this notion.

Presynaptic central α_2-adrenoceptor sensitivity

Most physiological systems examined respond to α_2-adrenoceptor agonists with a decrease in noradrenaline release, whereas there is an increase in noradrenaline release following treatment with α_2-antagonists. α-Adrenoceptors are believed to occur in several different sites:

- An inhibitory postsynaptic receptor located on a cell body or dendrites (somatodendritic receptor), as might occur for example in the nucleus locus coeruleus (LC). Binding at this receptor exerts an inhibitory input to the LC neurons. Activation decreases the firing of these neurons and reduces noradrenaline release from axon terminals.
- Hypothetical inhibitory extrasynaptic receptor located on cell bodies or dendrites.

- Presynaptic inhibitory α_2-adrenoceptor (an autoreceptor) situated on an axon terminal. Activation of this receptor causes local inhibition of release of noradrenaline at the terminal on which it is situated without affecting release of noradrenaline from other axon branches of the neuron.
- Presynaptic α_2-adrenoceptor (a *heteroreceptor*) located on the terminal of a non-adrenergic neuron.

A role for α_2-adrenoceptors in the mechanism of action of antidepressants has been suggested. In particular, a drug-induced subsensitivity of central presynaptic α_2-autoreceptors would play a critical role. Desensitisation of presynaptic α_2-receptors following chronic antidepressant treatment has been demonstrated by electrophysiological studies and radio-receptor binding studies. This down-regulation is believed to occur on continued exposure to the agonist noradrenaline (due to reuptake blockade by the drug). The consequence of autoreceptor down-regulation is enhanced release of noradrenaline into the synaptic cleft. The antidepressant effect can be related to a correction of a pre-existing defect whereby presynaptic α_2-adrenoceptor number is increased in depression. The mechanism of action of antidepressants can be summarised as: chronic drug administration induces subsensitivity of presynaptic α_2-adrenoceptors, leading to increased noradrenaline availability in the synaptic cleft. Hyperinnervation by noradrenaline leads to a decreased receptor number of postsynaptic β_1-adrenoceptors.

Central serotonin receptor sensitivity

There is considerable evidence from clinical studies to suggest an involvement of serotonin in the aetiology of depression. Most of this evidence is indirect. The bulk of the evidence points to a deficiency of serotonin function in the CNS as a possible cause of depression. Antidepressant drugs are believed to act to reverse this defect by increasing serotonin function. Because of the heterogeneity of serotonin receptor subtypes and the imprecise definition of their function, it is not clear how this arises.

A key role for serotonin neurons is suggested by the observation that β_1-adrenoceptor down-regulation does not occur in the absence of an intact serotonin system. Second, chronically administered antidepressant drugs down-regulate the number of 5-HT_2 recognition sites in brain. This property is common to TCAs, MAOIs and other antidepressants. However, repeated electrically induced convulsions are associated with an increased number of 5-HT_2 recognition sites. Thus, the role of 5-HT_2 receptors in mediating antidepressant effects of pharmacological treatments is somewhat confusing.

Increasingly the 5-HT_{1A} receptor has been scrutinised as a major determinant of antidepressant drug action. Evidence for the involvement of 5-HT_{1A} receptors in the mechanism of action of antidepressant drugs is mostly derived from animal behavioural studies:

- reduction in 8-OH-DPAT-induced hypothermia by chronically administered drugs, a 5-HT_{1A}-mediated presynaptic effect
- diminished response of raphe nuclei cells to applied serotonin, indicating a subsensitivity of 5-HT_{1A} somatodendritic autoreceptors

- impaired serotonin-mediated adenylate cyclase response in hippocampal cells, a postsynaptic 5-HT_{1A} response.

This hypo-responsiveness occurs on chronic antidepressant administration in the absence of a reduction in 5-HT_{1A} receptor number either pre- or postsynaptically. Thus, the resistance to up- or down-regulation of the 5-HT_{1A} receptor on chronic agonist exposure suggests that drug effects occur beyond the receptor, possibly at the second messenger system, for example, G proteins, intracellular enzyme levels, or even at the gene.

Signal transduction

A recent focus of attention in attempting to understand the mechanism of action of antidepressants has been on changes induced in the intracellular signalling pathways linked to noradrenergic and serotonergic receptors. Two main areas of interest have been protein phosphorylation and gene expression. Such studies have led to a variety of findings, which suggest that these events are important for understanding the mechanism of action of antidepressants. Furthermore, they suggest that targets beyond the receptor may be fruitful in the development of new agents for the treatment of depressive disorders.

In these intracellular signalling pathways, antidepressants (because of their effects on synaptic monoamine concentrations) lead to perturbations in intracellular signal transduction pathways, which in turn lead to alterations in gene expression. A key change is in the activity of protein kinases. Phosphorylation by protein kinases may represent a major regulatory mechanism for intracellular events. A key event in the cascade appears to be the activation by chronic administration of antidepressants of the enzyme protein kinase A (PKA). In turn, PKA can phosphorylate the transcription factor CREB (cyclic AMP response element binding protein). This protein binds to specific promoter sites to produce changes in the expression of certain genes, including, of particular importance, the gene for brain-derived neurotrophic factor (BDNF) and its receptor trkB. Chronic but not acute administration of antidepressants increases mRNA for CREB as well as the level of CREB in the brain. Furthermore, associated with these changes are increases in the production of BDNF, particularly in the hippocampus.

Such findings suggest that a reassessment of the hypothetical basis of depression is needed. In particular, the new hypothesis posits that depression may arise as a consequence of a chronic stress-induced atrophy of neurons in the brain, particularly the hippocampus. As BDNF is involved in differentiation and growth of new neurons in the developing brain, and in maintenance and survival of neurons in the adult brain, it may oppose stress-induced changes. Antidepressants then exert their effects by facilitating increases in BDNF production.

INDICATIONS FOR ANTIDEPRESSANT USE

Antidepressants tend to be broad-spectrum agents finding therapeutic uses across several psychiatric disorders. In addition to depression, various anxiety disorders are responsive to antidepressant treatment. This may reflect symptom overlap between anxiety and depressive disorders or may indicate that the nosology of these disorders is in need of revision. On the other hand, it may suggest that anxiety and depression have a common biological substrate which is acted upon, albeit indirectly as noted above, by these agents.

Depression

Once a diagnosis of depression has been established, choice of treatment is usually based on the severity of the current episode. Illness severity can be assessed on the basis of a clinical impression or by using a formal rating scale. Both clinician-rated scales (for example, the Hamilton Depression Rating Scale or the Montgomery-Asberg Depression Rating scale) and patient self-rated scales (for example, the Beck Depression Inventory or the Carroll scale) can provide an anchor point against which progress of treatment can be judged. Mild depression (Hamilton Depression Rating score ≤12) usually requires psychotherapeutic treatments alone, whereas severe depression with serious suicidal intent may require electroconvulsive therapy (ECT). Moderate to severe depression will, for most patients, require a combination of psychotherapy and pharmacotherapy.

The mainstay of treatment for depressive disorders has been the antidepressant drugs. Medications have dramatically altered the course of depression and the costs to society of the disorder. When used in appropriate doses, controlled clinical trials suggest that between 70 and 80 per cent of patients will show a significant clinical improvement following a course of antidepressant medication. Such responses are observed irrespective of the apparent aetiology of the illness, that is, depression arising for no obvious reason (primary or endogenous depression), or in response to an adverse life experience (secondary or reactive depression). Antidepressants from each of the various classes are equally effective in controlled clinical trials. This does not preclude the possibility that, for an individual patient, one drug may be more useful than another. The first choice of drug for an individual is made on the basis of a past history of response to that agent either by the patient or by a first-degree relative. When this information is not available, the choice of drug may be made on the adverse event profile. Other considerations such as the toxicity of the drug on overdose, especially in suicidal patients, may also be relevant. Most clinicians would suggest that venlafaxine, mirtazapine and the SSRIs are first-line drugs in the treatment of major depression. They are generally better tolerated than TCAs and MAOIs and are more likely to be used at therapeutic doses. The MAOIs are unlikely to be first-line treatment owing to the risk of hypertensive crises as a result of the interaction with tyramine in foods (the *cheese effect*). The reversible inhibitor of MAO, moclobemide, is less likely to cause this effect than the older, irreversible inhibitors, particularly when the drug is consumed after meals.

Recommended doses for antidepressants are shown in Table 16.2. It should be noted that there is no fixed dosage for any antidepressant. Dose must be titrated to individual requirements. Some patients will require considerably more than average, while others may derive therapeutic benefits from low doses. At high doses, careful monitoring of adverse events and cardiovascular effects is necessary. Although such doses may be well tolerated in younger, physically healthy patients, the elderly often do not tolerate even low doses very well. Postural hypotension and the associated potential for falls and fractures are a problem with TCAs, MAOIs, and with some of the newer agents when used in the elderly.

Table 16.2
Some suggested dose ranges for antidepressants

Drug	Dose (mg/day)
Selective serotonin reuptake inhibitors (SSRIs)	
Fluoxetine	20–80
Paroxetine	20–60
Sertraline	50–200
Citalopram	20–40
Fluvoxamine	50–250
Serotonin noradrenaline reuptake inhibitor (SNRI)	
Venlafaxine	75–300
5-HT_2 antagonists	
Nefazodone	100–600
Noradrenaline reuptake inhibitor	
Reboxetine	4–12
Reversible inhibitor of monoamine oxidase	
Moclobemide	150–600
Tetracyclic antidepressants	
Mianserin	60–150
Mirtazapine	30–60
Tricyclic antidepressants (TCAs)	
Amitriptyline	50–300
Clomipramine	50–300
Desipramine	50–300
Dothiepin	50–300
Doxepin	50–300
Imipramine	50–300
Nortriptyline	50–300
Trimipramine	50–300
Monoamine oxidase inhibitors (MAOIs)	
Phenelzine	30–90
Tranylcypromine	10–50

When using tricyclic antidepressants, most of the starting dose can be administered at night to take advantage of the sedative effects of these drugs. Both the MAOIs and SSRIs are best administered in the morning or early afternoon, as their activating properties will cause sleep difficulties with nocturnal administration. Titration of the dose during the first 2–3 weeks to the maximum dose is generally advisable to minimise side effects.

DURATION OF TREATMENT Clear signs of improvement should be apparent within 2 weeks, once the maximum tolerated dose is achieved. Sleep disturbance and altered appetite are generally the first symptoms to be relieved, followed by agitation, anxiety, depressed mood and hopelessness. Low energy, poor concentration, decreased libido and helplessness are affected later. Full antidepressant effect may not be apparent for a further 2–6 weeks. In patients who respond, antidepressant medications should be continued at full doses for up to 12 months or the length of a previous episode, whichever is longer. In recurrent depression, prophylactic treatment has been shown to be effective in reducing the number and severity of such recurrences. Severe previous episodes, significant suicidal ideation and impaired psychosocial function are other indicators that may suggest prophylactic treatment. Full doses of drugs have been advocated by some people, whereas minimum effective doses have been recommended by others. In either case, regular monitoring is required and further treatment should be implemented at the first signs of the recurrence of symptoms. For patients who have experienced three or more discrete episodes of depression, lifelong maintenance therapy should be considered. Psychotherapy is a useful adjunct treatment throughout any maintenance or prophylactic phases, as well as the acute phase of treatment.

TREATMENT FAILURE Up to 30 per cent of patients may fail to respond to the first course of an antidepressant medication. For many, this is due either to problems with dosing, usually too low, or to noncompliance. If these factors can be eliminated as the cause of non-response, then a switch to a drug of another class should be considered. Empirical evidence suggests that changing between different TCAs is usually ineffective and an SSRI, tricyclic antidepressant (mirtazapine), venlafaxine or nefazodone should be used. Moclobemide, the reversible MAOI, may also be considered as an alternative treatment. When changing between drugs, adequate washout periods should be allowed to avoid potential drug–drug interactions. In true cases of treatment-resistant depression, augmentation therapy, such as adding lithium, may be necessary. These cases may require inpatient admission, at least in the initial stages of treatment.

Anxiety disorders

In addition to their use for the treatment of depression, several antidepressant drugs have been widely evaluated in the treatment of panic disorder and obsessive–compulsive disorder (OCD), and there is some evidence for efficacy in the treatment of generalised anxiety disorder and post-traumatic stress disorder. Klein and Fink (1962) demonstrated the differential effect of imipramine for the treatment of panic attacks, and the usefulness of MAOIs for the treatment of anxiety was demonstrated as early as 1959 (West and Dally 1959). Subsequent studies have confirmed the effect of imipramine in panic disorder (Judd et al. 1986). Other TCAs have not been as widely evaluated for the treatment of panic disorder. The best evidence for efficacy exists for clomipramine, a compound with relatively potent effects on serotonin reuptake. The effect of these agents on panic attacks is independent of their antidepressant effect, as the initial level of dysphoria in patients does not influence the ultimate outcome. Nevertheless, antidepressants have incidental beneficial effects in patients with comorbid depression. The disadvantages of the TCAs in panic disorder are the same as those in depression treatment: slow onset of action and their numerous associated side effects (anticholinergic effects, orthostatic hypotension, activation syndrome).

The MAOIs phenelzine and tranylcypromine are effective in the treatment of panic attacks (Rosenberg 1999). Response to medication is relatively slow, and dietary restrictions, side effects and drug interaction potential of these agents have limited their use, particularly in anxious patients. A recent review has provided a mixed picture for the efficacy of moclobemide in panic disorder (Bandelow et al. 2002). Generally, it seems that this drug has reduced efficacy compared with other agents.

The efficacy of fluvoxamine, paroxetine, sertraline and citalopram is well recognised in the treatment of panic disorder (Bandelow et al. 2002). For fluoxetine, the evidence is not so clear, owing to a comparative lack of studies, but there is no reason to believe it is less effective than the other SSRIs. No differences in efficacy are found between SSRIs and TCAs in the treatment of panic disorder, but the SSRIs are better tolerated. There is a risk of jitteriness, restlessness, insomnia and increased panic attacks at the start of treatment with SSRIs; this often leads to poor compliance. For newer antidepressants (reboxetine, nefazodone, mirtazapine), there are too few controlled trials on which to form a judgment. Effective pharmacotherapy in panic disorder is generally recommended for 6–12 months, as the disorder is chronic and recurrence is common when treatment is ceased. Cognitive behaviour therapy should also be commenced concomitantly with medication to provide patients with a strategy for coping once medication is ceased.

The efficacy of SSRIs in the treatment of OCD has been well demonstrated in many clinical trials (Bandelow et al. 2002). Initial effects are seen after 4–6 weeks, but maximum benefits from medications often require up to 16 weeks. The TCA clomipramine is also effective in doses of up to 250 mg/day. Until the advent of the SSRIs it was the standard treatment, but it is associated with side effects that limit its acceptability by patients. Other TCAs are not effective in the treatment of OCD. There is no convincing evidence for the efficacy of MAOIs in OCD, and newer antidepressants such as nefazodone, mirtazapine, venlafaxine and reboxetine have not been evaluated in controlled studies.

The effectiveness of antidepressants in post-traumatic stress disorder has not been extensively investigated, but recent trials suggest that the SSRIs sertraline and paroxetine are beneficial. Limited clinical data suggest that amitriptyline, imipramine and phenelzine may also be effective for post-traumatic stress disorder. Similarly, in social anxiety disorder (social phobia), the evidence suggests that SSRIs are effective. There is some evidence for the efficacy of the MAOI phenelzine in social phobia, but the data with moclobemide are equivocal. In all but the most severe cases of social phobia, the benefits of non-pharmacological treatments may outweigh those of pharmacological management.

Generalised anxiety disorder is responsive to treatment with the serotonin noradrenaline reuptake inhibitor venlafaxine.

Other disorders

In keeping with their broad spectrum of pharmacological effects, antidepressants have been variously used for the treatment of pain (for example, amitriptyline for trigeminal neuralgia; citalopram for diabetic neuropathy), nocturnal enuresis (imipramine), eating disorders (SSRIs) and Tourette's syndrome (fluvoxamine). Most of these indications are based on case reports, case series or small trials. In other instances, such as imipramine for nocturnal enuresis in children, antidepressant use has been replaced by safer, equally effective, non-pharmacological treatments.

ADVERSE EVENTS WITH ANTIDEPRESSANTS

Side effects of antidepressant drugs are an extension of their pharmacological actions and can generally be related to interactions with various receptors and their subtypes. Interaction of TCAs with the subtypes of the muscarinic cholinergic receptor, for example, leads to the well-known spectrum of side effects with these agents (blurred vision, urinary retention, dry mouth). Similarly, the indirect serotonin agonist actions of the SSRIs are in part responsible for their gastrointestinal effects and the instances of akathisia sometimes noted early in their use. Common side effects with the different classes of antidepressant drugs are noted in Table 16.3. More troublesome adverse events, which arise less frequently, are discussed here.

Table 16.3
Common side effects of antidepressants

System	Symptoms
Anticholinergic	Dry mouth; loss of visual accommodation; palpitations, tachycardia, dizziness; urinary hesitancy; constipation; paralytic ileus; oedema; memory impairment
Noradrenergic	Jitteriness; tachycardia; tremor
Central nervous system	Insomnia; seizure; twitching; dysarthria; ataxia
Cardiovascular	Orthostatic hypotension; conduction delays; arrhythmias; contractility impairment
Miscellaneous	Weight gain; sexual dysfunction; skin reactions; blood dyscrasias (agranulocytosis, leukopenia, leukocytosis, neutropenia, eosinophilia

Cardiovascular effects

Although the SSRIs and other newer antidepressants are relatively free of major adverse effects on the cardiovascular system, this is not so for the TCAs and MAOIs (Sloman et al. 1983). Postural hypotension, hypotension, hypertension, tachycardia, aggravation of congestive cardiac failure, cardiac arrhythmia, myocardial infarction, atrioventricular block and an increased incidence of sudden death among cardiac patients have all been attributed to TCAs. These effects occur infrequently, but electrocardiographic effects of TCAs are clinically important. Therapeutic doses of TCAs have been associated with ST-T wave flattening, QRS broadening, tachycardia and arrhythmias. Such effects suggest that TCAs should be used with caution in the elderly and in patients with pre-existing heart disease. Few studies have systematically examined the effects of TCA prescription on the electrocardiogram in such patient groups. Of greater concern is that overdoses of TCAs are associated with heart block, bundle branch block, dysrhythmias, and QRS interval prolongation. The effects of overdose are often unpredictable, and serious complications may result from relatively small doses in some patients. In children, doses of 350 mg imipramine have been reported to be fatal.

There is less systematic study of the effects of MAOIs. Generally, these drugs are regarded as safe in usual therapeutic doses, with two exceptions. There is a well-recognised postural hypotensive effect of these agents, which suggests a particular caution in elderly patients. The *cheese effect* is also important – this results in severe headache and hypertension from the co-ingestion of foodstuffs containing tyramine. An interaction with sympathomimetic amines also results in severe headache and hypertension. Both reactions can be fatal, with findings at autopsy often revealing subarachnoid haemorrhage.

Some third-generation antidepressants have been associated with cardiovascular effects (Olver et al. 2001). Venlafaxine has been reported to show a dose-dependent elevation in blood pressure in controlled clinical trials. In placebo-controlled studies, about 6 per cent of patients treated with doses in excess of 200 mg had increases of diastolic blood pressure ≥15 mmHg from baseline. In some instances, the diastolic blood pressure was ≥105 mmHg (Feighner 1995). Sinus tachycardia and atrioventricular ectopic beats have been associated with reboxetine use in controlled clinical trials. Increased blood pressure has been observed in patients taking doses of reboxetine in excess of 12 mg/day. For both drugs, the effects can probably be attributed to an increase in noradrenaline concentrations.

Haematological effects

Leukopenia and eosinophilia may occur with TCAs and are usually benign and transient. Agranulocytosis is rare with TCAs, but can be fatal. The effect is probably due to a hypersensitivity reaction, and routine monitoring of blood counts is generally not predictive. Sudden onset of fever and infection are often the first signs. Blood dyscrasias are more likely to occur in elderly women than in healthy younger adults. These effects are not frequently reported with other antidepressants, with the possible exception of mianserin where, although rare, blood dyscrasias may occur more frequently than with TCAs. Mirtazapine, a structural analogue of mianserin, has been associated with an incidence of neutropenia of around 1 in 1000 cases. Based on patient exposure years, this incidence is only slightly higher than amitriptyline. Blood dyscrasias with SSRIs and other antidepressants appear to occur less frequently than with TCAs. It should not be assumed that these effects do not occur at all; as these agents become much more frequently used, rare instances of the abnormalities may occur.

Discontinuation reactions

Discontinuation has been defined as a collection of signs and symptoms temporally related to either dose reduction or cessation of a drug. The syndrome is characterised by a predictable onset, duration and offset, with psychological and physical symptoms that were not present before the initiation of therapy (Lader 1983). Discontinuation reactions have been described following abrupt cessation of antidepressant drugs, and discontinuation symptoms, including dry mouth, sweating, dizziness and paraesthesias, were first noted in the original report on the antidepressant activity of imipramine (Kuhn 1958). Similar symptoms have been reported for MAOIs, SSRIs and venlafaxine (Olver et al. 1999). Generally, symptoms of the syndrome appear within 1–3 days of discontinuation of a drug, and may last for up to 2 weeks. For most patients, symptoms tend to be mild to moderate and are transient. Differences between classes of agents exist with respect to the symptoms of the syndrome. Flu-like symptoms as well as anxiety, agitation, muscle tension and nervousness are common during TCA and SSRI discontinuation. A phenomenon of electric shocks in the extremities has been described during SSRI withdrawal. Symptoms noted during antidepressant cessation are shown in Table 16.4. Discontinuation syndromes may occur with normal or high doses of the drugs. Among the SSRIs, there is some evidence to suggest that paroxetine is more likely and fluoxetine least likely to be associated with a discontinuation syndrome (Olver et al. 1999).

Table 16.4
Withdrawal symptoms with antidepressant drugs

Symptom group	Characteristic signs
General somatic symptoms	Fatigue, headache, sweating, myalgia, flu-like syndrome, anxiety, agitation, muscle tension, nervousness
Sleep	Insomnia, vivid dreams
Movement	Unsteady gait, abnormal involuntary movements, akathisia
Affect	Lowered mood, crying, irritability, lability
Miscellaneous	Dizziness, paraesthesias, electric shocks in arms and legs (most characteristic of SSRI withdrawal)

Weight gain

Antidepressants are sometimes associated with weight gain of up to 5 kg. This is more likely to occur with the TCAs and with mianserin and mirtazapine. It is notable that these drugs are associated with histamine H_1 blockade, which can induce considerable daytime sedation and consequent physical inactivity. In addition, carbohydrate craving has been reported with citalopram, mianserin and mirtazapine. A further mechanism for altering weight may be through the effects that these agents have on 5-HT_{2C} receptors. The SSRIs and venlafaxine do not usually cause significant weight gain.

Other adverse events

Individual agents and classes of drugs have been linked to rarer side effects. There may be an increased incidence of the syndrome of inappropriate secretion of antidiuretic hormone and resultant hyponatraemia with SSRIs, especially in the elderly. Extrapyramidal symptoms and akathisia occur to a small extent with the SSRIs, and delirium and a fine resting tremor have been noted rarely with TCAs. These rarer events are summarised in Table 16.5.

Table 16.5
Rarer adverse reactions with antidepressant drugs

Adverse event	Description	Agents involved
Sexual dysfunction	Erectile dysfunction, delayed ejaculation, anorgasmia	TCAs, SSRIs, MAOIs, venlafaxine
Galactorrheoa, amenorrheoa		TCAs
Extrapyramidal syndrome	Akathisia, acute dystonia, parkinsonism	SSRIs
Delirium	Anticholinergic effect	TCAs
Cholestatic jaundice		TCAs, MAOIs
Switch to hypomania		All antidepressants
Teratogenicity	Some evidence to suggest SSRIs may be safe	All antidepressants
Seizures		TCAs

DRUG INTERACTIONS

Drug interactions can occur whenever the presence of one chemical substance alters the pharmacological effects of an administered medication. The notion of chemical substance needs to be thought of in the broadest possible context, and could include tobacco, alcohol, illicit drugs, foods, and food additives, as well as other medications. Clearly, some populations of patients treated with antidepressants are at greater risk for drug–drug interactions than others. Vulnerable populations include medically ill people treated with several drugs, elderly and debilitated people, people with renal or hepatic disease, and people treated with single drugs that are potent isozyme inhibitors.

Drug interactions can be described as either *pharmacokinetic* or *phar-*

macodynamic. As their name suggests, pharmacokinetic interactions imply the alteration of the kinetics of one drug by the other. This may result in a pharmacodynamic effect as well. For example, the inhibition of the metabolism of triazolobenzodiazepines (triazolam, alprazolam) by nefazodone increases not only the plasma concentration of the drug but also the sedative effect. On the other hand, pharmacodynamic effects do not necessarily result from changes in kinetics. Rather, these effects may occur by interaction at receptor sites. For example, the serotonin syndrome (see below) results from excessive action of serotonin at its receptor sites due to the action of two serotonin agonists administered concomitantly. Pharmacokinetic interactions are often qualitatively, if not quantitatively, predictable based on the knowledge of the pharmacokinetic properties of the interacting agents. In practice, such interactions are most likely related to interactions at metabolic enzymes. By contrast, pharmacodynamic interactions are not always predictable.

Pharmacokinetic interactions

The main, but not exclusive, source of pharmacokinetic interactions is the inhibition or induction of hepatic P450 enzymes by co-prescribed medications. It is beyond the scope of this article to review all of these potential interactions in detail. Extensive lists of inducers, inhibitors and substrates of cytochrome P450 enzymes are available. Reviews of pharmacokinetic interactions based on inhibition or induction of the P450 system are widely available (for example, Nemeroff et al. 1996), and these detail interactions with various isozymes and their relevance to the metabolism and interaction potential of newer antidepressants. Much less work is extant on the older TCAs and MAOIs with respect to specific P450 isozymes involved in drug interactions. However, it is well recognised that the metabolism of TCAs is inhibited by phenothiazines, oestrogen and cimetidine, probably because of inhibition of CYP2D6. Similarly, some SSRIs elevate plasma concentrations of TCAs through inhibition of metabolism, raising the risk of cardiac arrhythmias. On the other hand, tobacco smoking, carbamazepine, barbiturates and phenytoin lower plasma concentrations of TCAs because of induction of liver enzymes.

SSRIs can potentially affect the metabolism of other drugs because they are metabolised in the liver. Generally, SSRIs are inhibitors of cytochrome P450 enzymes, but there are differences in potency between them (see Table 16.6). Clinically significant interactions have been reported because of inhibition of CYP3A4, causing elevations of terfenadine and cisapride plasma levels and leading to cardiac arrhythmias. Similarly, CYP1A2 inhibition increases plasma levels of clozapine, theophylline and some TCAs, giving rise to severe adverse effects.

Table 16.6
Effects of newer antidepressant drugs on cytochrome P450 enzymes

	Cytochrome P450 enzyme				
Drug	**1A2**	**2C9**	**2C19**	**2D6**	**3A4**
Fluoxetine	+	++	+/++	+++	+/++
Sertraline	+	+	+/++	+	+
Paroxetine	+	+	+	+++	+
Fluvoxamine	+++	++	+++	+	++
Citalopram	0/+	0	0	+	0
Nefazodone	0	0	0	0	+++
Venlafaxine	0	0	0	0	0
Mirtazapine	0	–	–	+	0
Reboxetine	0	0	?	0	0

SOURCE Greenblatt et al. (1998).

Pharmacodynamic interactions

Interactions between antidepressants and other agents leading to adverse pharmacodynamic effects have been long recognised. TCAs interfere with the antihypertensive effects of drugs that need to be taken up into the neuron (for example, guanethidine) to exert their effects. The sedative, psychomotor and cognitive impairments produced by benzodiazepines and alcohol are often potentiated by TCAs. The action of indirect-acting sympathomimetic amines and over-the-counter cold and flu remedies is potentiated by TCAs. The interaction of MAOIs with tyramine-containing foodstuffs is well recognised, and patients receiving these drugs should receive a card containing the foods to avoid.

Serotonin syndrome is a drug-induced condition usually resulting from the mixing of different classes of agents. The cause of the syndrome is increased serotonin within the central nervous system. The most frequent combination of therapeutic drugs able to induce the syndrome is the combination of MAOIs with drugs that inhibit serotonin reuptake. It should be noted that, in addition to SSRIs, other drugs (for example, tramadol, pethidine and sibutramine) are able to inhibit serotonin reuptake and cause a serotonin syndrome. The usual duration of an episode of serotonin toxicity is dependent on the drugs responsible. If the duration of action is less than 24 hours and the drugs are ceased, the effects will subside without specific treatment. Life-threatening or fatal cases of serotonin syndrome have resulted from combinations of an MAOI and an SSRI. In non-fatal cases, there is no firm evidence for permanent or long-term effects from the serotonin syndrome. Features that distinguish serotonin syndrome from other toxicities are hyperreflexia, myoclonus, fever, agitation and late-stage pyramidal rigidity and pyrexia (Sternbach 1991; Gillman 1999). Onset of the syndrome is rapid, with the patient exhibiting hypervigilance, tremor and hyperreflexia. Clonus and myoclonus start in the lower limbs and may become generalised.

Pyramidal rigidity is a late development and may impair respiration. Rigidity and a fever of >39.5°C indicate serious toxicity (Gillman 1999). The condition may deteriorate rapidly and is likely to require active medical intervention, including intensive care admission, cooling, 5-HT_{2A} antagonists and possible intubation. Cyproheptadine is effective for the milder cases, and chlorpromazine has been used for severe toxicity (Gillman 1999). The syndrome may be difficult to distinguishclinically from neuroleptic malignant syndrome.

Many other drug–drug interactions with new and old antidepressants have been reported, but a description is beyond the scope of this article. As newer agents become more widely used in clinical practice, there will no doubt be further reports of interactions. As noted above, many interactions are predictable on the basis of knowledge of the metabolic profiles, but pharmacodynamic effects are less predictable and can occur as an idiosyncratic reaction to drug combinations. The frail elderly, the very young, and patients with medical illness in addition to those already receiving medications for other disorders are most at risk.

CONCLUSION

Antidepressants are widely used and, despite their many potential drawbacks in terms of side effects and interaction potential, they remain relatively safe drugs. Advances in basic neuroscience research in the past decade have seen a greater understanding in their mechanism of action. An appreciation of the effects of antidepressants at the cellular level and the effects on second messenger systems offers the promise of agents acting outside of the monoamine paradigm. Recent findings (Santarelli et al. 2003) that antidepressant effects may be mediated by stimulation of neurogenesis in the hippocampus offer exciting prospects for the treatment of depression. Until agents developed from these insights are available, treatment will rely on the ever-increasing range of agents based on the monoamine hypothesis of the aetiology of depression. The search for the elusive goal of a fast-acting, highly effective antidepressant has heralded diminished use of TCAs and MAOIs, with SSRIs and serotonin noradrenaline reuptake inhibitors now the first choice of drug for most clinicians. Treatment of depression requires the development of a plan tailored to each individual and will combine elements of pharmacotherapy and psychotherapy as well as considerations of severity, sex, age and past response to medications.

USEFUL WEBSITES

General articles on antidepressants. <http://www.preskorn.com/column2.html>

Antidepressant mechanisms of action.
<http://www.psychiatrist.com/pcc/brainstorm/indexa.htm>

Drug interactions and lists of inducers and inhibitors.
<http://medicine.iupui.edu/flockhart/clinlist.htm>

Distinction of malignant neuroleptic syndrome and serotonin syndrome.
<http://www.vh.org/adult/provider/psychiatry/CPS/09.html>

Description and treatment of serotonin syndrome.
<http://www.currentpsychiatry.com/2003_05/0503_serotonin.asp>;
<http://www.psychotropical.com/ss.html>

REFERENCES

Bandelow B, Zohar J, Hollander E, Kasper S, Moller H-J (2002) Guidelines for the pharmacological management of anxiety, obsessive compulsive and post-traumatic stress disorders. *World Journal of Biological Psychiatry* 3:171-99.

Crane GE (1957) Iproniazid (Marsilid) phosphate, a therapeutic agent for mental disorders and debilitating disease. *Psychiatry Research Reports* 8:142-52.

Davies B, Burrows G, Poynton C (1975) A comparative study of four depression rating scales. *Australian and New Zealand Journal of Psychiatry* 9:21-24.

Davies B, Joshua S, Burrows G, Poynton C (1977) A sequential trial of viloxazine (Vivalan) and imipramine in moderately depressed patients. *Medical Journal of Australia* 1:521-2.

Feighner JP (1995) Cardiovascular safety in depressed patients: Focus on venlafaxine. *Journal of Clinical Psychiatry* 56:574-9.

Gillman PK (1999) The serotonin syndrome and its treatment. *Journal of Psychopharmacology* 13:100-9.

Greenblatt DJ, von Moltke LL, Harmatz JS, Shader RI (1998) Drug interactions with newer antidepressants: Role of human cytochromes P450. *Journal of Clinical Psychiatry* 59 Suppl 15:19-27.

Judd FK, Norman TR, Burrows GD (1986) Pharmacological treatment of panic disorder. *International Clinical Psychopharmacology* 1:3-16.

Klein DF, Fink M (1962) Psychiatric reaction patterns to imipramine. *American Journal of Psychiatry* 119:432-8.

Kline NS (1958) Clinical experience with iproniazid (Marsilid). *Journal of Clinical and Experimental Psychopathology* 19 (2 Suppl 1):72-8.

Kuhn R (1958) The treatment of depressive states with G22355 (imipramine hydrochloride). *American Journal of Psychiatry* 115:459-64.

Lader M (1983) Benzodiazepine withdrawal states. In Trimble MR (ed), *Benzodiazepines Divided*. New York: John Wiley & Sons.

Leonard BE, Richelson E (2000) Synaptic effects of antidepressants: Relationship to their therapeutic and adverse effects. In Buckley PF, Waddington JL (eds), *Schizophrenia and Mood Disorders: The New Drug Therapies in Clinical Practice*. Oxford: Butterworth-Heinemann.

Nemeroff CB, DeVane CL, Pollock BG (1996) Newer antidepressants and the cytochrome P450 system. *American Journal of Psychiatry* 153:311-20.

Olver JS, Burrows GD, Norman TR (1999) Discontinuation syndromes with selective serotonin reuptake inhibitors: Are there clinically relevant differences? *CNS Drugs* 12:171-7.

—— (2001) Third generation antidepressants: Do they offer advantages over the SSRIs? *CNS Drugs* 15:941-54.

Parker G (1996) On brightening up: Triggers and trajectories to recovery from depression. *British Journal of Psychiatry* 168:263-4.

Rosenberg R (1999) Treatment of panic disorder with tricyclics and MAOIs. In Nutt DJ, Ballenger JC, Lepine J-P (eds), *Panic Disorder: Clinical diagnosis, management and mechanisms*. London: Martin Dunitz, pp. 125-44.

Ross S, Renyi AL (1975) Tricyclic antidepressant agents. Comparison of the inhibition of the uptake of 3H-noradrenaline and 14C-5-hydroxytryptamine in slices and crude synaptosome preparations of the midbrain hypothalamus regions of the rat brain. *Neuropharmacology* 16:57-63.

Santarelli L, Saxe M, Gross C, Surget A, Battaglia F, Dulawa S, et al. (2003) Requirement of hippocampal neurogenesis for the behavioral effects of antidepressants. *Science* 301:805-8.

Sloman JG, Norman TR, Burrows GD (1983) Clinical studies of antidepressant cardiotoxicity. In Burrows GD, Norman TR, Davies BM (eds), *Drugs in Psychiatry*, Vol. 1: Antidepressants. Amsterdam: Elsevier Science Publishers, pp. 173-86.
Sternbach H (1991) The serotonin syndrome. *American Journal of Psychiatry* 148:705-13.
West ED, Dally PJ (1959) Effects of iproniazid in depressive syndrome. *BMJ* 1:1491.

CHAPTER 17

MOOD STABILISERS

Gordon F Johnson

The mood stabilisers comprise a group of drugs used in the treatment of bipolar disorder. The term was initially used to describe the actions of lithium. The demonstration of mood-stabilising properties of some anticonvulsants, such as carbamazepine, valproate and lamotrigine, has led to their inclusion in this group. The spectrum of action of mood-stabilising drugs in bipolar disorder includes treatment of acute mania, treatment of bipolar depression and long-term prevention of recurrences of mania and depression. Individual drugs show different profiles of action. Only lithium has an established efficacy across all phases of the illness, and is the benchmark for comparison with newer agents. Some properties of the mood stabilisers are summarised in Table 17.1.

LITHIUM

Lithium is an alkaline metal which is found in abundant quantities in the earth's crust and is an ingredient of spa waters. It possesses no known physiological function. Its therapeutic effects in bipolar disorder were first reported in 1949 by John Cade in the *Medical Journal of Australia*. Cade's report made little impact on psychiatry despite his conclusion, 'the effect is so specific that it inevitably leads to speculation as to the possible aetiological significance', which he initially speculated to be a lithium deficiency. There was a lag of 20 years between Cade's initial observations and the approval of lithium for the treatment of mania by the US Food and Drug Administration in 1970. The history of lithium was recounted at a meeting in 1999 celebrating the fiftieth anniversary of Cade's discovery (Mitchell et al. 1999).

Table 17.1
Some properties of mood stabilisers

	Lithium	Valproate	Carbamazepine	Lamotrigine
Dose range (mg/day)	500–2500	400–3000	200–1600	100–400
Oral loading dose	No	20–30 mg/kg per day	No	Contraindicated
Plasma concentration therapeutic range				
Mania	0.8–1.4 mEq/L	>315 mmol/L	17–50 mmol/L	Not useful
Maintenance	0.6–0.8 mEq/L	300–700 mmol/L	17–50 mmol/L	Not useful
Metabolism	None	Hepatic	Hepatic	Hepatic
CYP 450 drug metabolising enzymes	No effect	Inhibitor of lamotrigine and carbamazepine metabolism	Significant induction of its own metabolism and concomitantly administered drugs	Weak auto induction
Pregnancy classification	D	D	D	B3

Mode of action

Lithium has a wide variety of biological effects in animals and humans, but its mode of action remains unknown. Putative sites of action focused initially on ion transport and presynaptic neurotransmitter release. More recently, the focus has shifted to postsynaptic events, particularly the ability to alter patterns of intracellular signalling in critical regions of the brain, with downstream effects on gene regulation and neuroplastic changes underlying long-term mood stabilisation. Lithium-induced alteration in gene expression may also explain the recent findings of a neuroprotective effect of lithium in inhibiting apoptosis and cell death (Lenox and Frazer 2002).

Efficacy

MANIA Placebo-controlled crossover design studies carried out between 1954 and 1971 reported significant differences in response and remission rates between lithium and placebo. The early studies have been criticised because of the likelihood of carryover effects and the small sample sizes. The strongest evidence for efficacy is provided by a recent double-blind, controlled parallel design study comparing the efficacy of divalproex with placebo and lithium in patients with acute mania. It found lithium and valproate were significantly superior to placebo. Using a 50 per cent improvement, 49 per cent of the lithium group met criteria, compared with 25 per cent of the placebo group. The mean number needed to treat was 5. As 50 per cent of the patients in the lithium treatment group were prior lithium nonresponders, these results may underestimate lithium response rates (Bowden et al. 1994).

Studies comparing lithium with typical antipsychotics, which were the treatment of choice before the introduction of lithium, reported lithium to be superior to chlorpromazine and similar to haloperidol. Comparative studies of lithium monotherapy versus new atypical antipsychotics, risperidone or olanzapine monotherapy, have reported similar outcomes. However, low plasma lithium levels and small sample sizes may have been insufficient to establish differences between active drugs.

A meta-analysis of twelve randomised controlled trials of lithium in acute mania in 655 patients confirmed that lithium is more likely than chlorpromazine to induce remission, but no more effective than haloperidol. Neither carbamazepine nor valproate is more effective than haloperidol (Poolsup et al. 2000).

Combining an antipsychotic and a mood stabiliser is common clinical practice. The addition of olanzapine or placebo to patients partially responsive to lithium or valproate showed superior efficacy of the combination in treating manic or mixed bipolar episodes (Tohen et al. 2002). Similar findings have shown risperidone plus a mood stabiliser is more efficacious than mood stabiliser alone (Yatham et al. 2003). Given the lag of onset of lithium action of 5–10 days, and the more rapid action of antipsychotics, particularly on manic behaviour, the combined therapy could be more advantageous than either drug alone in severe mania.

BIPOLAR DEPRESSION There are no double-blind, prospective, placebo-controlled studies of lithium in bipolar depression. The evidence base for efficacy consists of placebo-control crossover design studies. In seven of the eight studies, lithium showed superior antidepressant efficacy, with up to 80 per cent of subjects showing partial response. However, only 36 per cent of lithium-treated patients achieved full remission (Keck and McElroy 1996). In one negative study, alternating 7–10-day periods of lithium and placebo may have been too short to assess efficacy. Controlled trials versus tricyclic antidepressants (TCAs) report similar efficacy, but lack sufficient numbers to distinguish differences between the active drugs. The antidepressant efficacy of lithium monotherapy in bipolar depression is less predictable than in mania, and clinically is often used in combination with short-term antidepressant therapy. This is consistent with established efficacy as an augmentation therapy in patients with major depression who are partially responsive to other antidepressants (Schweitzer et al. 1997).

Prophylaxis of mania and depression

Long-term prophylactic effects of lithium against recurrences of mania and depression were first systematically studied using patients as their own control during periods of 1–5 years. Comparisons in relapse frequency prior to and following lithium therapy showed a significant reduction during lithium administration (Angst et al. 1970). Double-blind, randomised studies of placebo substitution in matched patients maintained on lithium reported significantly higher recurrence rates among patients receiving placebo.

A recent Cochrane review of lithium prophylaxis in mood disorder included nine prospective studies in 825 patients randomly allocated to lithium or placebo (Burgess et al. 2001). Lithium was more effective than placebo in preventing relapse in mood disorder overall. The most consistent effect was found in bipolar disorder. In unipolar disorder, the direction of effect was in favour of lithium, but the result did not reach statistical significance. The direction of effect was the same in all studies. No study found a negative effect for lithium. The report concluded that lithium is an efficacious treatment for bipolar disorder. Evidence of effect size varied between individual studies. The number needed to treat to prevent one relapse during the first year of follow-up varied from 4 to 14.

A meta-analysis of nineteen double-blind, randomised controlled trials of lithium prophylaxis found this agent far superior to placebo in preventing recurrences: 74 per cent recurrence on placebo versus 29 per cent on lithium. This meta-analysis included discontinuation studies of patients on lithium maintenance with placebo substitution, which were not included in the Cochrane analysis. They concluded that in these mirror-image studies there was no evidence to support recurrence due to lithium withdrawal as an explanation for this difference (Davis et al. 1999).

A recent placebo-controlled 18-month trial of lithium and lamotrigine in bipolar I disorder found lithium to be significantly superior to placebo for the prevention of recurrence of a mood episode, particularly mania (see Lamotrigine below).

Comparative studies of lithium versus TCAs consistently show lithium to be more effective. The combination of lithium plus an antidepressant, a common treatment practice, showed no advantage of the combination over lithium alone in preventing recurrences of depression or mania. There are no published studies comparing lithium and antipsychotic drugs in the prophylaxis of bipolar disorder.

Side effects

Many of the side effects of lithium are dose-related and can be eliminated or reduced by dosage adjustment and fine-tuning of serum levels.

GASTROINTESTINAL Nausea, vomiting and diarrhoea may occur. This may be related to the formulation, associated with a rapid rise in plasma levels seen in the initial treatment of mania, or a sign of toxicity during maintenance.

NEUROMUSCULAR The most frequent adverse effect is tremor, which may occur in up to 30–50 per cent of patients. Tremor can be managed by adjustment of plasma level, change of dosage regimen, or use of a β-blocker.

RENAL Lithium blocks the action of antidiuretic hormone on the renal tubule, increasing obligatory water loss. Patients may notice increased thirst and urine output. This may persist with long-term lithium treatment, to a varying degree in up to 20 per cent of patients, leading to diabetes insipidus. Increased obligatory water loss carries a potential risk in circumstances of sodium depletion, excessive fluid loss or reduced intake. The impairment of urinary concentrating ability may be irreversible or only partly reversible upon lithium discontinuation.

An associated nonspecific interstitial nephropathy on renal biopsy has been reported. However, similar findings have been found in psychiatric patients who have never received lithium.

There is a negative correlation between maintenance serum lithium levels and urinary concentrating ability. In contrast, glomerular function remains relatively unscathed. Progressive impairment of renal function during lithium maintenance is the exception rather than the rule, and appears related more to age, episodes of lithium intoxication, concurrent drug administration and comorbid cardiovascular disease. Where there is progressive renal impairment with falling creatinine clearance, alternative medication should be considered. Management of diabetes insipidus includes reducing the lithium dose, ensuring adequate fluid intake, and administering a diuretic. Diuretics decrease obligatory water loss but increase lithium reabsorption, requiring lowering of lithium dosage to avoid toxicity. Amiloride is potassium-sparing (Boton et al. 1987).

THYROID FUNCTION Thyroid dysfunction is common with lithium therapy, and subclinical or overt hypothyroidism has been found in 4 per cent of patients (mostly women) with 1–5 years' treatment, rising to 21 per cent with 10 years' treatment. Based on ultrasonic evaluation, goitre was present in forty of 100 bipolar patients (Perrild et al. 1990). Presence of hypothyroidism or autoimmune disease was low. Both respond well to supplementary treatment with thyroxine, where clinically indicated, while lithium treatment is maintained.

OTHER EFFECTS Lithium may affect glucose and insulin regulation and is associated with weight gain. Less frequent side effects include dermatological reactions such as psoriasis and acneiform eruptions. Subjective memory impairment and concentration may be troublesome in some patients.

NEUROTOXICITY Symptoms may appear during the treatment of acute mania or emerge during long-term maintenance treatment. Intercurrent illness or administration of drugs that decrease lithium elimination, such as diuretics, non-steroidal anti-inflammatory drugs or angiotensin-converting enzyme inhibitors, raise plasma lithium levels and may precipitate neurotoxicity. The combination of neurological signs (tremor, hyperreflexia, dysarthria and ataxia) and delirium with alteration in level of consciousness, impaired mentation and disorientation are the hallmarks of lithium intoxication. Early prodromal symptoms that should alert the clinician to impending intoxication during lithium maintenance treatment are progressive tiredness, sluggishness, weakness, difficulty in thinking and concentration, increased tremor and shakiness, unsteadiness, increased thirst, and nausea and diarrhoea. The patient may look ill, with marked facial pallor.

Neurotoxicity may occur with plasma lithium levels in the therapeutic range, particularly in the elderly; however, levels in excess of 1.5 mmol/L are more likely to be associated with symptoms of neurotoxicity. In mild to moderate cases, symptoms remit depending on the rate of elimination after lithium withdrawal. Toxicity with impaired level of consciousness may require fluid and electrolyte replacement or haemodialysis. The latter is the most effective method available for the removal of lithium, particularly in the presence of renal impairment, and in severe lithium intoxication with serum levels >3.0 mEq/L it is the treatment of choice. Prolonged or severe intoxication may result in irreversible neurological sequelae (Johnson 1984).

Lithium use

PREPARATIONS AND DOSAGE Formulations contain lithium carbonate with dosage strengths of 250 mg (an immediate release) and 450 mg (a delayed release). Lithium is absorbed rapidly with peak serum concentrations achieved within 1–3 hours. The half-life of lithium is about 24 hours, and steady-state serum concentrations are reached in 5–7 days in patients with normal renal function. Lithium clearance is by the kidney. Total daily dosage ranges from 1 g to 2.5 g in mania and from 500 mg to 1.5 g in long-term maintenance treatment. It is adjusted according to the plasma level and clinical response. Recommended serum concentrations are based on a divided dosage regimen and need to be adjusted for a once-daily regimen. There is no established evidence that once-daily dosing leads to differences in efficacy or effects on renal function, compared with a divided dose.

PLASMA LEVEL MONITORING Monitoring of serum concentrations of lithium is mandatory, as it has a narrow therapeutic index and plasma levels are more accurate than dosage for indicating efficacy and side effects. Recommended therapeutic lithium concentrations are based on trough measurements 12 hours following the last dose and assuming that the patient is in steady state. Twelve-hour serum concentrations are 10–25 per cent higher after a single night-time dose. Serum concentrations of 0.8–1.4 mmol/L are required for control of acute mania.

For long-term maintenance, serum lithium concentrations between 0.6 and 0.8 mmol/L are recommended in most patients. Serum lithium concentrations of 1 mmol/L or above should be reviewed. Serum lithium concentrations should be monitored regularly every 1–3 months, depending on clinical response, side effects and patient compliance. Routine laboratory tests, carried out prior to lithium therapy and every 3 months, should include plasma electrolytes and serum creatinine, and thyroid function, which should be monitored at 6–12-month intervals.

CONTRAINDICATIONS AND PRECAUTIONS Recent myocardial infarction is a contraindication to lithium treatment. Lithium should be used with caution in patients at risk of cardiac arrhythmias such as the presence of cardiac disease, electrolyte abnormalities – particularly hypokalaemia – or in conjunction with drugs that can affect QT prolongation, and in patients with renal impairment.

Women taking lithium should avoid becoming pregnant. Initial reports of lithium use during pregnancy indicated a 10 per cent risk of teratogenicity. In more recent studies, the degree of risk has been revised downwards (Cohen et al. 1994).

The decision to maintain patients on lithium during pregnancy must take into account the risks of the exacerbation of bipolar disorder to both mother and fetus as against the risks of lithium to the fetus. During pregnancy, serum lithium levels should be carefully monitored as changes may occur, particularly in the third trimester. Transitory effects related to lithium reported in the newborn infant include thyroid dysfunction. No long-term developmental anomalies have been reported in studies of up to 5 years in infants exposed to lithium during pregnancy. Lithium is present in breast milk and may rarely have adverse effects on the infant. Mothers are advised not to breastfeed if receiving lithium. The puerperium is a time of high risk of recurrence for bipolar patients. For patients who have been well controlled on lithium prior to pregnancy, recommencement immediately following delivery is recommended (Schou 1990).

Lithium and suicidal behaviour

Several studies have reported a reduced risk of mortality in bipolar patients maintained on lithium. This is largely achieved by reduction in suicide rates. A meta-analysis of twenty-two studies comparing suicide rates on and off lithium in patients with major affective illness found suicide was 82 per cent less frequent during lithium treatment (Tondo et al. 2001). It remains unclear whether lithium has a direct anti-suicidal action or whether the reduced rates of suicide and suicidal behaviour reflect the mood-stabilising effects of lithium treatment. The 2001 Cochrane review on lithium's long-term effectiveness found no definitive evidence as to whether lithium has an anti-suicidal effect. No similar data been have reported with other mood stabilisers.

VALPROATE

Valproate is a carboxylic acid derivative initially marketed for the treatment of epilepsy. Studies of valpromide (a prodrug) in the 1960s in Europe reported benefit in the management of mood disorders, particularly mood stabilisation in patients followed up over many years.

Mode of action

Valproate potentiates γ-aminobutyric acid (GABA) in the brain and blocks voltage-dependent sodium channels. It is these properties that underlie its anticonvulsant action. Whether the GABA agonist properties contribute to its actions in bipolar disorder is unclear.

Recent research on intracellular signalling mechanisms and drug action has discovered that valproate shares with lithium a specific effect on protein regulation, a property that may underlie its mood-stabilising actions (Lenox and Frazer 2002).

Efficacy

MANIA Evidence of efficacy is provided by a double-blind, prospective study in 179 patients hospitalised with acute mania and randomly allocated to divalproex, placebo or lithium as an internal control. Treatment was terminated prematurely in 31 per cent of patients on valproate, 33 per cent on lithium and 51 per cent on placebo, because of lack of efficacy. The proportions of patients improving at least 50 per cent were significantly higher for divalproex (48 per cent) and lithium (49 per cent) than for placebo (25 per cent). The efficacy of divalproex appeared to be independent of prior responsiveness to lithium. A post-trial analysis suggested that even a modest level of pre-treatment depression-related symptoms was associated with a better response to divalproex than to lithium (Bowden et al. 1994).

Additional placebo-controlled comparisons have shown efficacy for valproate in lithium-refractory or -intolerant patients and in patients with mixed mania where response to valproate was superior to lithium. Two multicentre randomised trials of valproate versus olanzapine in mania have been reported. Olanzapine was superior to valproate in one study and similar in efficacy in the other. The difference in trial outcomes may reflect differences in dosage regimens of olanzapine and valproate in the trial designs.

PROPHYLAXIS OF RECURRENT BIPOLAR DISORDER A randomised, double-blind, parallel group, multicentre study compared the efficacy of divalproex, lithium and placebo over a 52-week maintenance period in 372 patients with bipolar disorder recently recovered from a manic episode. The primary outcome measure was time to recurrence of any mood episode. No significant differences were found on survival analysis between divalproex, lithium or placebo in time to any mood episode. Divalproex was superior to placebo in terms of lower rates of discontinuation and superior to lithium in longer duration of successful prophylaxis and less deterioration in depressive symptoms. Failure to distinguish lithium and valproate from placebo may have been due to inclusion of milder or less recurrent forms of bipolar disorder (Bowden et al. 2000).

An open randomised study comparing valpromide and lithium over an 18-month period reported a similar reduction in the number of both depressed and manic episodes with both lithium and valpromide.

BIPOLAR DEPRESSION There are no published placebo-controlled studies of valproate monotherapy for the treatment of bipolar depression. While open-label studies report partial remission rates of 30 per cent on valproate, a potential role in bipolar depression is yet to be defined.

Side effects

Valproate has a wide therapeutic index.

Nausea, appetite loss and vomiting may occur, are less common with the enteric-coated formulations, are dose-related, and may resolve with continuing treatment. Sedation is common and may be managed by adjustment of dose or dosage regimen and may diminish with continuing treatment. Tremor may occur at therapeutic doses. Weight gain occurs in a significant proportion of patients. This may be associated with increased appetite. Alopecia (hair loss) has been reported in up to 4 per cent of patients. This is usually self-limiting.

Minor abnormalities in hepatic transaminases are common and not usually progressive. Serious hepatotoxicity, which usually occurs during the first 6 months of therapy, is rare, with a reported incidence of 1 in 20 000.

Mild asymptomatic leukopenia and thrombocytopenia may occur; this is reversible upon drug discontinuation. Rare cases of pancreatitis have been reported. Polycystic ovary disease has been reported in women with seizure disorder receiving valproate.

It is recommended that haematological, renal, electrolyte and hepatic functions be assessed before valproate treatment. Haematological and hepatic function should be monitored at least each 3–6 months after treatment has been initiated.

Clinical use

Preparations for oral use contain both sodium valproate and valproic acid. They are available in enteric-coated formulations, which minimise gastrointestinal effects. Valproate is fully bioavailable and is metabolised in the liver. Half-life at steady state is 8–15 hours. It is highly protein-bound in plasma and may be displaced from binding sites by other highly protein-bound drugs, such as aspirin. It is an inhibitor of hepatic CYP450 enzymes and may increase serum level of concurrently administered drugs, such as lamotrigine.

Dose

Recommended initial dose is 400–800 mg/day orally in two divided doses, to be increased every 2–3 days by increments of 200–500 mg/day, depending on clinical response. Maximum recommended dose is 3 g. An acute loading dose strategy may be used in hospitalised patients, with an initial dose of 20–30 mg/kg.

A comparison of valproate oral loading 20 mg/kg versus haloperidol 0.2 mg/kg in acute mania showed equal effectiveness in reducing acute manic and psychotic symptoms over 3 days of treatment. Side effects were infrequent. Extrapyramidal effects were significantly more common with haloperidol. A valproate loading dose was found to be better tolerated than similar loading strategies with lithium in acute mania (Keck et al. 2000).

Plasma level monitoring

Plasma level monitoring is recommended as a guide to treatment response. In mania, minimum plasma valproate levels of 315 mmol/L are recommended. In long-term maintenance treatment, the relation between plasma concentrations and prophylactic mood-stabilising effects is less precise. The recommended range is similar for anticonvulsant effects (350–700 mmol/L). Plasma concentrations in excess of 700 mmol/L are associated with a greater likelihood of toxicity. The appropriate level for a particular patient is the level that controls symptoms satisfactorily.

Pregnancy and breastfeeding

Valproate has been associated with a 1–2 per cent incidence of spina bifida in women taking the drug during pregnancy. If a decision is made to continue anticonvulsants, the risk of neural tube defects may be reduced if folic acid is taken before and throughout the pregnancy. Use of valproate during breastfeeding is considered low-risk, as concentrations in breast milk are low because of high plasma protein binding.

CARBAMAZEPINE

Carbamazepine is a tricyclic compound that resembles imipramine in structure.

Mode of action

The ability of carbamazepine to block repetitive firing of action potentials in depolarised neurons through blockade of sodium channels is believed to mediate its anticonvulsant action. The ability of carbamazepine to attenuate or block electrically induced *kindling* in limbic areas of the brain has been hypothesised as the basis for its mood-stabilising effects (Post and Weiss 1989).

Efficacy

ACUTE MANIA Most double-blind trials of efficacy of carbamazepine in acute mania have been confounded by the co-administration of other drugs such as lithium and antipsychotics. A placebo-controlled, crossover study in lithium-resistant patients reported carbamazepine to be superior to placebo.

Two monotherapy controlled trials of lithium and carbamazepine have been published. In one, lithium was associated with the more favourable outcome. In the second study, the improvement rate was similar, but the numbers were small and there was a high dropout rate of 70 per cent in both lithium and carbamazepine groups because of lack of efficacy. Comparisons of carbamazepine and chlorpromazine have reported similar results in acute mania.

A meta-analysis of lithium compared with valproic acid and carbamazepine in mania reported no significant differences between the treatment effect of the three drugs compared in five studies (three lithium/carbamazepine and two lithium/valproic acid comparisons (Emilien et al. 1996).

BIPOLAR DEPRESSION There are no placebo-controlled, parallel design studies of carbamazepine in bipolar depression. A randomised controlled placebo crossover trial of carbamazepine in the treatment of acute bipolar depression reported marked improvement in 34 per cent of bipolar and unipolar depressed patients on carbamazepine compared with placebo. In the absence of further controlled studies, the antidepressant efficacy of carbamazepine remains uncertain.

MAINTENANCE TREATMENT A placebo-controlled study undertaken to assess the prophylactic action of carbamazepine in twenty-two bipolar manic–depressive patients over 1 year reported a significant difference in outcome, with 60 per cent of patients on carbamazepine showing marked to moderate clinical response while only 22 per cent of patients on placebo achieved a similar outcome. The use of adjunctive medication, however, limits the extent to which relapse rates can be directly compared.

A randomised comparative study of prophylactic effectiveness of lithium and carbamazepine in 144 patients with bipolar disorder over 2.5 years showed no statistically significant differences regarding hospitalisations and recurrences. Applying broader outcome criteria, including psychotropic co-medication and severe side effects, showed that the results were distinctly in favour of lithium. In patients who completed the study, recurrence occurred in 28 per cent of patients on lithium versus 47 per cent on carbamazepine

(Greil et al. 1997). Other controlled trials of carbamazepine versus lithium over periods of 1–3 years report similar efficacy.

A review of controlled or partly controlled studies in 191 patients showed a carbamazepine response rate of 63 per cent (Post and Weiss 1989). However, a meta-analysis of four studies of the comparative efficacy of lithium and carbamazepine reported that the prophylactic efficacy of carbamazepine was questionable (Dardennes et al. 1995).

Side effects

Common adverse effects of carbamazepine are dizziness, drowsiness, nausea, ataxia and diplopia. Central nervous system effects and sedation are usually dose-related, may be transient, and are often reversible with dosage reduction.

A wide variety of skin reactions of varying severity and seriousness can occur, including exfoliative dermatitis (Stevens-Johnson syndrome), which is potentially fatal. Discontinuation of carbamazepine was reported as necessary in approximately 15 per cent of patients because of skin reactions.

Leukopenia is the most frequent adverse haematological disturbance, transient changes in white cell count being relatively common. Rarely, agranulocytosis or aplastic anaemia may occur, and some patients have died. Monitoring of white cell count would appear desirable, and the drug should be discontinued if the white cell count falls below $2000/mm^3$.

Mild elevation of hepatic liver enzymes may occur. This is usually benign and non-progressive. A progressive rise should, however, lead to discontinuation of carbamazepine, as significant hepatic toxicity may occur.

Hyponatraemia may occur in 6–30 per cent of patients. This may be related to its antidiuretic hormone agonist-like activity at the renal level.

Haematological, renal, electrolyte and hepatic function should be assessed before commencing carbamazepine, and should be monitored throughout treatment. Most adverse effects occur in the first 3–6 months of treatment, but they can occur after more extended periods of treatment.

Carbamazepine is metabolised through the cytochrome P450 system. It induces its own metabolism as well as that of some concomitantly administered drugs, such as oral contraceptives, warfarin, antipsychotics and valproate, leading to reduced serum levels. Drugs that inhibit cytochrome P450 enzymes, such as fluoxetine and fluvoxamine, may increase carbamazepine levels and risk of toxicity. (For full list see *Psychotropic Drug Guidelines* 2000.)

Preparations and dosage

Carbamazepine is available in two oral formulations: an immediate release and a controlled release. The initial plasma half-life is 20–30 hours; however, as it induces its own metabolism, plasma half-life 2–4 weeks after initiation shortens to 10–15 hours.

Recommended initial doses are 200–400 mg orally, increased weekly by increments of 100–200 mg/day, depending on clinical response. A dose range of 800–1600 mg per day is associated with adequate therapeutic plasma levels for most patients. The controlled-release preparation may minimise intermittent central nervous system effects occurring around the time of peak plasma level.

Therapeutic drug monitoring

Evidence determining the therapeutic plasma concentration range for the use of carbamazepine as a mood stabiliser is lacking. In epilepsy, a concentration range of 17–50 µmol/L is recommended. This provides a guide for clinical use to establish compliance, to assess changes in plasma level associated with increase or decrease of carbamazepine metabolism due to auto-induction or concomitantly administered drugs, and to minimise the risk of toxicity at levels above the maximum range. Therapeutic ranges are based on the trough of plasma concentrations.

Contraindications and precautions

Carbamazepine is contraindicated where there is a history of drug-induced haematological reactions, bone marrow suppression, hypersensitivity to carbamazepine or other TCAs, or hepatic dysfunction. It should not be used in combination with clozapine. Use of carbamazepine in pregnancy has been associated with a 1 per cent incidence of spina bifida. In addition, craniofacial defects and developmental delay have been reported. The risk of neural tube defects may be reduced if folic acid is taken prior to and throughout the pregnancy. Carbamazepine is compatible with breastfeeding. Carbamazepine does occur in breast milk, but the clinical importance of this remains uncertain. The infant should be monitored for side effects, such as jaundice, drowsiness, poor suckling, vomiting and poor weight gain.

LAMOTRIGINE

Lamotrigine is a triazine derivative, structurally and pharmacologically unrelated to other anticonvulsant drugs.

Mode of action

Lamotrigine inhibits voltage-gated sodium channels, reducing the release of glutamate, an excitatory amino acid.

Efficacy

ACUTE MANIA Three published controlled studies have evaluated lamotrigine in the treatment of mania. Two placebo-controlled studies, one comparing lamotrigine, gabapentin and placebo and one as adjunctive or monotherapy compared with lithium, found no significant differences between active drugs and placebo. A direct comparison of lithium versus lamotrigine found similar efficacy. All three studies had methodological limitations, small patient numbers, high placebo response rates and low lithium levels.

BIPOLAR DEPRESSION Lamotrigine was compared with placebo in a 7-week, multicentre, double-blind trial in 195 bipolar I patients. Lamotrigine 50 mg and 200 mg was significantly superior to placebo, evident at 4–5 weeks (Calabrese et al. 1999).

This is the largest double-blind, placebo-controlled study of bipolar depression, and establishes efficacy of lamotrigine in the treatment of bipolar depression. Treatment-emergent hypomanic, manic or mixed episodes were significantly higher in the placebo group compared with the lamotrigine group.

PROPHYLAXIS OF MANIA AND DEPRESSION Evidence for prophylactic efficacy in bipolar I disorder was provided in a placebo-controlled 18-month trial of lamotrigine and lithium maintenance treatment. The subjects were 349 patients with bipolar I disorder who entered an open-label phase during a manic or hypomanic episode, and of whom 175 met stabilisation criteria on lamotrigine and were randomised to lamotrigine, lithium or placebo.

Both lamotrigine and lithium were superior to placebo at prolonging the time to intervention for any mood episode. Lamotrigine was superior to placebo at prolonging the time to a depressive episode and lithium was superior to placebo at prolonging the time to a manic, hypomanic or mixed episode (Bowden et al. 2003). A similar unpublished study using a similar study design in bipolar I patients with a recent depressive episode found lamotrigine and lithium were superior to placebo in delaying relapse or recurrence of mood episodes. Lamotrigine and lithium appear to have complementary actions, with lamotrigine preventing recurrence of depression and lithium primarily preventing recurrence of mania.

In a 6-month, blinded, randomised, parallel group study, lamotrigine was superior to placebo in time to intervention or early discontinuation for any reason in patients with rapid-cycling bipolar illness. After 6 months of monotherapy, 41 per cent of patients treated with lamotrigine were stable without relapse, compared with 26 per cent of placebo-treated patients.

Use

Lamotrigine is rapidly absorbed, with peak plasma concentrations occurring 2.5 hours after administration. Lamotrigine has a half-life of about 24 hours. This is considerably shortened with co-administration of drugs that are enzyme inducers, such as carbamazepine, and increased two-fold with valproate, which inhibits metabolism. Risk of interaction with other drugs metabolised by cytochrome P450 enzymes is low.

It is recommended that a careful lamotrigine dosing schedule be adhered to, to reduce the risk of skin reaction. Initial recommended dose is 25–50 mg/day for the first 2 weeks, followed by 50–100 mg/day given in two divided doses per day for the following 2 weeks. Thereafter, the dose should be increased until an optimum response is achieved. Dosage range is 200–400 mg/day. In patients taking sodium valproate, the dosage schedule should be halved. There are no data to support plasma level monitoring of lamotrigine.

Contraindications and precautions

Severe, potentially life-threatening rashes have been reported in association with the use of lamotrigine. It should be discontinued at the first sign of a rash unless it is clearly not drug-related. The risk of rash is strongly associated with high initial doses of lamotrigine and concomitant use of valproate. Rash may also occur as part of a hypersensitivity syndrome with fever and lymphadenopathy.

There are insufficient data available on the use of lamotrigine during pregnancy to evaluate its safety. Women taking lamotrigine during pregnancy should take a folate supplement. There is limited information on the use of lamotrigine during lactation. It passes into breast milk in concentrations of the order of 40–60 per cent of those in plasma levels at which pharmacological effects may occur.

Side effects

Side effects associated with lamotrigine are primarily related to the central nervous system, such as headache, dizziness, somnolence and tremor.

Skin rashes have been reported in 10 per cent of patients. The rash, usually maculopapular, generally appears within 8 weeks of starting treatment and resolves on withdrawal of lamotrigine. Serious, potentially life-threatening rashes, including Stevens-Johnson syndrome and toxic epidermal necrolysis, have been reported. The risk is considerably reduced by adhering to slow dosage titration.

OTHER ANTICONVULSANTS

Gabapentin

Gabapentin is a GABA analogue and increases GABAergic activity in the brain. In two placebo-controlled studies of the efficacy of gabapentin, either as monotherapy or added to lithium or valproate or the combination in the treatment of mania, gabapentin was similar to or significantly less effective than placebo. A study comparing gabapentin, lamotrigine or placebo in bipolar depression showed gabapentin to be no more effective than placebo.

Oxcarbazepine

Oxcarbazepine is a carbamazepine derivative. It has a different metabolic profile, fewer drug interactions and a reportedly more favourable side-effect profile.

Initial observations and treatment trials report good tolerability despite rapid dose titration. There are no placebo-controlled trials of efficacy.

Topiramate

The anticonvulsant topiramate is a sulfamate derivative of fructose. It inhibits sodium channels, enhances GABA action, and is a carbonic anhydrase inhibitor. A 3-week placebo-controlled, double-blind trial in mania comparing two doses of topiramate (256 mg and 512 mg) reported no significant difference among the three treatment arms (Chengappa et al. 2001). Common side effects are sedation, attention, concentration and memory problems, paraesthesia, nausea and anorexia. Renal calculi have been reported in 1.5 per cent of patients receiving topiramate for epilepsy. Its use is associated with weight loss.

REFERENCES

Angst J, Weis P, Grof P, Schou M (1970) Lithium prophylaxis in recurrent affective disorders. *British Journal of Psychiatry* 116:604-14.

Boton R, Gaviria M, Batlle DC (1987) Prevalence, pathogenesis, and treatment of renal dysfunction associated with chronic lithium therapy. *American Journal of Kidney Diseases* 10:329-45.

Bowden CL, Brugger AM, Swann AC, Calabrese JR, Janicak PG, Petty F, et al. (1994) Efficacy of divalproex vs lithium and placebo in the treatment of mania. The Depakote Mania Study Group. *JAMA* 271:918-24.

Bowden CL, Calabrese JR, Sachs G, Yatham LN, Asghar SA, Hompland M, et al. (2003) A placebo-controlled 18-month trial of lamotrigine and lithium maintenance treatment in recently manic or hypomanic patients with bipolar I disorder. *Archives of General Psychiatry* 60:392-400.

Bowden CL, Calabrese JR, McElroy SL, Gyulai L, Wassef A, Petty F, et al. (2000) A randomized, placebo-controlled 12-month trial of divalproex and lithium in treatment of outpatients with bipolar I disorder. Divalproex Maintenance Study Group. *Archives of General Psychiatry* 57:481-9.

Burgess S, Geddes J, Hawton K, Townsend E, Jamison K, Goodwin G (2001) Lithium for maintenance treatment of mood disorders. *Cochrane Database of Systematic Reviews* (2):CD003-13.

Calabrese JR, Bowden CL, Sachs GS, Ascher JA, Monaghan E, Rudd GD (1999) A double-blind placebo-controlled study of lamotrigine monotherapy in outpatients with bipolar I depression. Lamictal 602 Study Group. *Journal of Clinical Psychiatry* 60:79-88.

Chengappa KN, Gershon S, Levine J (2001) The evolving role of topiramate among other mood stabilizers in the management of bipolar disorder. *Bipolar Disorder* 3:215-32.

Cohen LS, Friedman JM, Jefferson JW, Johnson EM, Weiner ML (1994) A reevaluation of risk of in utero exposure to lithium. *JAMA* 271:146-50.

Dardennes R, Even C, Bange F, Heim A (1995) Comparison of carbamazepine and lithium in the prophylaxis of bipolar disorders. A meta-analysis. *British Journal of Psychiatry* 166:378-81.

Davis JM, Janicak PG, Hogan DM (1999) Mood stabilizers in the prevention of recurrent affective disorders: A meta-analysis. *Acta Psychiatrica Scandinavica* 100:406-17.

Emilien G, Maloteaux JM, Seghers A, Charles G (1996) Lithium compared to valproic acid and carbamazepine in the treatment of mania: A statistical meta-analysis. *European Neuropsychopharmacology* 6:245-52.

Greil W, Ludwig-Mayerhofer W, Erazo N, Schochlin C, Schmidt S, Engel RR, et al. (1997) Lithium versus carbamazepine in the maintenance treatment of bipolar disorders – a randomised study. *Journal of Affective Disorders* 43:151-61.

Johnson G (1984) Lithium. *Medical Journal of Australia* 141:595-601.

Keck PE, Jr, McElroy S (1996) Outcomes in the pharmacological treatment of bipolar disorder. *Clinical Psychopharmacology* 16:155-235.

Keck PE, Jr, McElroy SL, Bennett JA (2000) Pharmacologic loading in the treatment of acute mania. *Bipolar Disorder* 2:42-6.

Lenox RJ, Frazer A (2002) Mechanism of action of antidepressants and mood stabilisers. In Davis KL, Charney DS, Nemeroff CB (eds), *Neuropsychopharmacology: The fifth generation of progress*. Philadelphia: Lippincott, Williams & Wilkins, pp. 1139-63.

Mitchell P, Hadzi-Pavlovic D, Manji H (1999) Fifty years of treatments for bipolar disorder celebration of John Cade's discovery. *Australian and New Zealand Journal of Psychiatry* 33 Suppl:s1-122.

Perrild H, Hegedus L, Baastrup PC, Kayser L, Kastberg S (1990) Thyroid function and ultrasonically determined thyroid size in patients receiving long-term lithium treatment. *American Journal of Psychiatry* 147:1518-21.

Poolsup N, Li Wan Po A, de Oliveira IR (2000) Systematic overview of lithium treatment in acute mania. *Journal of Clinical Pharmacologyy and Therapeutics* 25:139-56.
Post RM, Weiss SRB (1989) Sensitization, kindling, and anticonvulsants in mania. *Journal of Clinical Psychiatry* 50 Suppl:23-30.
Schou M (1990) Lithium treatment during pregnancy, delivery, and lactation: An update. *Journal of Clinical Psychiatry* 51:410-13.
Schweitzer I, Tuckwell V, Johnson G (1997) A review of the use of augmentation therapy for the treatment of resistant depression: Implications for the clinician. *Australian and New Zealand Journal of Psychiatry* 31:340-52.
Tohen M, Chengappa KN, Suppes T, Zarate CA, Jr., Calabrese JR, Bowden CL, et al. (2002) Efficacy of olanzapine in combination with valproate or lithium in the treatment of mania in patients partially nonresponsive to valproate or lithium monotherapy. *Archives of General Psychiatry* 59:62-9.
Tondo L, Hennen J, Baldessarini RJ (2001) Lower suicide risk with long-term lithium treatment in major affective illness: A meta-analysis. *Acta Psychiatrica Scandinavica* 104:163-72.
Yatham L, Grossman F, Augustyns I, Vieta E, Ravindran A (2003) Mood stabilisers plus risperidone or placebo in the treatment of acute mania: International, double-blind, randomised controlled trial. *British Journal of Psychiatry* 182:141-7.

CHAPTER 18

PHARMACOGENETICS OF ANTI DEPRESSANTS AND MOOD STABILISERS

Martin A Kennedy,
Geraldine R Rogers
and Peter R Joyce

The term *pharmacogenetics* was coined more than 50 years ago. The dual goals of this field of research are to attempt to understand genetic susceptibility to adverse effects, and to better predict positive responses to drug treatment. In short, pharmacogenetics promises to make prescribing safer and more effective.

Among the first documented examples of the dramatic effects of inter-individual variability in response to drugs were hypersensitivity to the anti-hypertensive agent debrisoquine, malignant hyperthermia caused by administration of certain anaesthetics and muscle relaxants, and haemolysis in African-American males after administration of antimalarial drugs. Each of these effects was subsequently traced back to mutations or polymorphisms in the genes for specific enzymes. However, although we are now well aware of the genetic basis for several severe adverse drug reactions, and we have access to the complete human genome sequence, we are still a long way from understanding the interactions of environment (including other drugs) and genetics that lead to poor outcomes of drug treatment.

Our knowledge of inter-individual variability in metabolism of mood drugs, and the genetic variability of the targets of these drugs, supports the view that pharmacogenetics may be of value in guiding treatment of the mood disorders. In addition, there is some evidence that closely related individuals tend to show similarity in their responses to specific mood drugs, suggesting heritable components of these responses.

Antidepressants and mood stabilisers cause a wide range of side effects that are a major cause of treatment discontinuation. Minimising such effects would significantly improve the success of drug therapy, and this is one goal of pharmacogenetics. A parallel goal is to improve our ability to predict the most efficacious treatment for each patient with a mood disorder. Currently, optimising the treatment for each patient can be a difficult and lengthy process as drug therapy is initiated, doses adjusted and, if no benefit is observed, a washout period and trial with a new drug commenced. For the seriously ill patient, this may be occurring against a background of high morbidity and a considerably elevated risk of suicide. Treatment with any given antidepressant seems to be successful for about 50 per cent of patients; some patients will respond to the second or third antidepressant they try, and some will prove resistant to all forms of drug treatment. A similar pattern of response is seen with the mood stabilisers lithium and valproate. It is not possible to predict which drug will succeed or fail in a given patient for any of the drugs used to treat mood disorders.

As our understanding of human genome structure has increased, many of the genes and their variant forms implicated in pharmacogenetic phenomena have been identified (Evans and McLeod 2003). In parallel with human genome knowledge has come the ability to study the structure and expression of many genes, opening new possibilities for understanding the molecular basis of responses to drug treatment, and for improving the development and testing of new drugs. The application of human genome knowledge and technology in these ways is known as pharmacogenomics, which is really an extension of pharmacogenetic principles to the genome scale (Evans and Relling 1999). Pharmacogenomics relies on new tools that allow high-throughput analysis of gene expression or structure. Expression methods, such as microarrays, or gene chips, can be applied to explore the biological effects of drugs, either in human tissues or in laboratory models. This is becoming an important tool during preclinical phases of drug development. The other application of pharmacogenomics is to explore, on a genome scale, the nature of genetic variants in groups of patients displaying different responses to drugs (Roses 2000).

NATURE OF GENETIC VARIATION

All human beings have essentially the same genetic architecture. Although we share the same basic complement of genes, the precise sequence of those genes and the non-coding regions of our genomes show considerable diversity at the population level. Current estimates for the degree of such variability are that, on average, there is one difference every 1300 base pairs (bp) (Sachidanandam et al. 2001). Given that the human genome is about 3×10^9 bp in size, there are two to three million genetic differences between individuals. However, because only about 5 per cent of the genome encodes genes, most of these differences will not affect protein structure or expression.

Genetic variants arise by mutation of DNA through the course of evolution, and can display a wide variety of forms. The most common type of genetic variant is the alteration of a single base pair, but insertions and deletions of DNA are quite common. For practical purposes, it is usual to refer to a genetic variant that is maintained in a population at a frequency of greater than 1 per cent as a *polymorphism*, whereas variants that occur in less than 1 per cent of the population are *mutations* – although this is an operational rather than rigid distinction. The rationale for this definition is that a genetic variant that is common in a population is unlikely to be overtly deleterious, as it would be lost from the population through natural selection.

Polymorphisms are responsible for natural variation in the expression and function of genes, thus contributing to human diversity. However, in combination with certain environmental conditions, some polymorphisms will operate as the genetic alleles that underlie susceptibility to complex diseases such as the mood disorders. In addition, polymorphisms (as well as rarer mutations) can influence individual responses to drugs. Therefore, the focus of pharmacogenomics is on understanding genetic diversity of those genes that are likely to influence drug responses.

A great variety of polymorphisms and mutations has been documented, ranging from single base changes to deletions of entire genes or even chromosomal rearrangements. Repetitive sequence polymorphisms are common, including *microsatellites* (such as the dinucleotide and tetranucleotide repeats) and repeats of longer-sequence elements known as *variable number tandem repeats* (VNTRs). However, the most common type of polymorphism in the human genome is the single base change or *single nucleotide polymorphism* (SNP; pronounced 'snip') (Sachidanandam et al. 2001). Because they are so common, often leading to alterations in gene structure and expression, and simple automated assays to detect their occurrence can be developed, SNPs have become a major focus for pharmacogenomic studies (Roses 2000).

DETECTING PHARMACOGENETIC VARIATION

It is worth emphasising here that phenotyping of a patient, if it can be done by means of an enzyme assay, measurement of plasma drug levels, or treatment with a probe drug, can give valuable information that may not always be apparent through genetic analysis of specific genes (genotyping). In many instances, phenotyping may be the only means available for assessing in ter-individual variability in pharmacokinetics. However, once clear genotype–phenotype relationships are established, genotyping has the advantages that it can be performed on DNA extracted from buccal cells or a peripheral blood sample, the data it yields are not influenced by concurrent medication or disease states, and probe drugs do not have to be administered. In a research setting, it is most useful to explore pharmacogenetics with the benefit of phenotype measures if they are available. Once pharmacogenetic influences on a drug are well understood, it may be possible to simply apply genotyping.

High-quality DNA is easily extracted from a sample of peripheral blood, drawn in an EDTA tube (not heparin, as this can interfere with downstream analyses). Alternatively, a mouthwash sample or buccal scrapings will provide sufficient cells to yield enough DNA for genetic analyses. Because of the unique, detailed, and very personal information that can be determined by genetic analysis, collection of samples for DNA analysis must be carried out with informed consent under appropriate ethical and regulatory approvals (Rothstein and Epps 2001).

Analysis of genes can be carried out at two levels. Gene structure is surveyed broadly for deletions, insertions or duplications of material with the technique of *Southern blotting*. A sample of genomic DNA (typically 10 µg) is digested with a specific restriction enzyme that fragments the DNA in a predictable fashion. The digested DNA is then size-separated by electrophoresis on an agarose gel. This method is simple in principle: the agarose acts as a molecular sieve, and when an electric current is applied the negatively charged DNA fragments move through the gel at a rate that reflects their size. Smaller fragments move rapidly, while larger ones move more slowly. After several hours of electrophoresis (often overnight), the DNA is transferred out of the fragile agarose gel onto a robust nylon membrane. This procedure, called Southern blotting (after Edwin Southern, its inventor), is accomplished by simple capillary transfer, using tissues to draw buffer through the gel and onto the membrane, where the DNA becomes covalently attached. Once this copy of the gel has been created, the DNA regions of interest are visualised by annealing of radioactively or chemically labelled probe molecules that are complementary to part of the gene of interest. The blot is washed to remove nonspecifically bound probe, and either chemically treated or exposed to X-ray film (depending on the probe labelling method used) to visualise the DNA fragments of interest.

The Southern blot allows visual inspection of DNA regions of a few hundred base pairs in size to regions of up to 40 kilobase pairs (kb). With modifications to the DNA preparation method and separation system (pulsed field gel electrophoresis), much greater resolution (hundreds of kilobase pairs or millions of base pairs) can be obtained. These methods are useful for identifying complete gene deletions, such as those that occur in the cytochrome P450 2D6 (*CYP2D6*) gene (which encodes an important drug-metabolising enzyme), as well as intragenic deletions or other gross structural alterations of genes.

The second level of gene analysis, which is now much more commonly used in a wide variety of configurations, is the polymerase chain reaction (PCR) (Saiki et al. 1988). PCR is an in vitro DNA amplification procedure, involving sequential thermal cycling of a reaction mixture usually containing two oligonucleotide primers (short, single-stranded DNA molecules) that demarcate the fragment of interest, a thermally stable enzyme (Taq DNA polymerase), the four deoxyribonucleoside triphosphates (dATP, dCTP, dGTP and dTTP), and a small sample of genomic DNA (typically a few nanograms) from which the researcher aims to amplify a specific region. PCR amplification from minimal amounts of starting material yields sufficient DNA within a few hours for most genotyping analyses. If the polymorphism is a VNTR, the PCR product may be visualised directly on an agarose gel. If the polymorphism creates or removes a restriction site, the PCR product may be digested with a restriction enzyme before electrophoresis to detect whether the restriction site is present. Alternatively, the assay may be configured to carry out allele-specific amplification, in which case separate PCR products indicate the presence of one or both alleles of a SNP. Methods of polymorphism detection are evolving rapidly, and many automated PCR genotyping assays now involve fluorescent dyes or mass spectrometric detection rather than gel electrophoresis. Fluorescent and mass spectrometric genotyping methods generally depend on highly specialised, expensive items of equipment.

Pharmacogenetic research aimed at assessing the clinical relevance of polymorphism in a given candidate gene usually takes the form of an association study. Association between a polymorphism in a candidate gene and a phenotype, such as occurrence of adverse drug reactions or response to a drug, is sought. The distribution of the polymorphic variant between different groups of the study sample (for example, those with or without an adverse drug reaction) is statistically evaluated, and if there is a significant skewing of the distribution between the groups, the polymorphism is said to be associated with the phenotype. Association is a statistical measure: it says little about causality. If association is observed, the polymorphism may be a causative factor in the phenotype under study. Alternatively, the polymorphism may have no direct effect but be located close (in *linkage disequilibrium*) to some other genetic variant that is causative. Not uncommonly, as shown by the large numbers of non-replicated and contradictory association studies in the literature, the observed association may simply be by chance and of no biological consequence. Therefore, any observed association should be considered provisional, at least until confirmed in an independent sample and preferably until the underlying molecular biology is teased out and understood (Malhotra and Goldman 1999; Risch 2000).

Although it is not yet clear whether it will prove feasible, whole genome association studies are perceived as a potentially powerful method of identifying genes involved in complex disease and pharmacogenetic phenotypes (Kruglyak 1999). Conceptually, the approach is to carry out an association study using a large panel of polymorphisms spread throughout the genome. Rather than selecting one or a few candidate genes for testing (as in a conventional approach), the whole genome association study does not presuppose any knowledge of the biology underlying a phenotype, and simply asks, 'What regions of the genome are implicated in a given phenotype?'. Identifying regions of the genome that contribute to a phenotype would then allow identification and closer inspection of candidate genes in each region. At present, such studies would be prohibitive because of the large number of SNPs required, the cost of genotyping, and the sample size required to gain statistical power. However, as the haplotype structure of the human genome is clarified, it appears likely that a relatively manageable set of markers will be identified that effectively scans the genome. With continuing reductions in costs of genotyping, and improvements in the biostatistics required to evaluate such complex datasets, whole genome association studies may prove feasible and could eventually begin to yield insight into the pharmacogenetics and aetiology of complex diseases such as the mood disorders.

GENETIC EFFECTS ON PHARMACOKINETICS

Pharmacogenetics

When a drug is administered, it enters the bloodstream and travels to the target tissue, where it interacts with its molecular targets. Elimination of the drug from the body occurs by a variety of routes, usually involving enzymatic modification before excretion. The processes of absorption, distribution through the body, metabolism and elimination are collectively referred to as the *pharmacokinetics* of a drug. Genetic variability can affect any aspect of pharmacokinetics. Such variation may be of little consequence for drugs that are effective and non-toxic over a broad concentration. However, genetic differences may have a significant effect for many drugs that have relatively narrow therapeutic windows and can be quite toxic (such as tricyclic antidepressants). Rigorous examination of the role of genetic variability in all aspects of mood drug pharmacokinetics is not yet possible, particularly as we do not fully understand the enzymes and transporter molecules that mediate these processes. Although it is still far from complete, our understanding of the pharmacogenetics of drug metabolism is more advanced than for other aspects of pharmacokinetics.

Metabolic enzymes

It has long been known that steady-state plasma levels of nortriptyline in individuals receiving the same dose can vary by thirty- to forty-fold, largely because of genetic influences (Alexanderson et al. 1969). This inter-individual variability is due to differences in drug metabolism mediated by cytochrome P450 enzymes predominantly, but not exclusively, in the liver. We now understand such differences are due to genetic variability in genes encoding this family of enzymes. Individuals able to metabolise drugs effectively are known as *extensive metabolisers*, and those with low or absent enzyme activity are referred to as *poor metabolisers*. The term *intermediate metaboliser* refers to an individual with reduced enzyme function, although the distinction from extensive metabolisers is not absolute.

The cytochrome P450 enzymes of greatest importance to mood disorders are CYP2D6, CYP2C9, CYP2C19, CYP1A2 and CYP3A4/3A5 (Table 18.1). Bimodal distributions of activities for CYP2D6 and CYP2C19 are observed in populations. This indicates a high degree of functional polymorphism in these enzymes, and this has been confirmed by extensive genetic studies. However, genetic analysis has also revealed a range of variants for most other cytochrome P450 genes that have been explored, including *CYP2C9* and *CYP3A4/3A5*. The biological and clinical relevance of all of these genetic variants is an unfolding story, but it is quite clear that considerable diversity exists in metabolic enzymes that may affect metabolism of agents used to treat mood disorders.

Perhaps the best-studied example of this type is CYP2D6, which is relevant to psychiatry as many psychotropic drugs either inhibit or induce this enzyme, or are substrates of it. *CYP2D6* is highly polymorphic, even to the extent that about 7 per cent of Caucasians lack any functional copy of the

Table 18.1
Common antidepressants and cytochrome P450 enzymes involved in their metabolism[a]

Drug	CYP2D6	CYP2C9	CYP2C19	CYP3A4/5[b]	CYP1A2
Amitriptyline	+	+	+	+	+
Citalopram	+		+	+	
Clomipramine	+		+	+	+
Desipramine	+				+
Doxepin	+				
Fluoxetine	+	+	+	+	
Fluvoxamine	+		+		+
Imipramine	+	+	+	+	+
Mirtazapine	+	+		+	+
Nortriptyline	+				+
Paroxetine	+		+	+	+
Sertraline	+		+	+	
Venlafaxine	+			+	

NOTES a This is an indicative guide only, and as more experimental data are generated the metabolic profile for each drug may alter.
b The pharmacological action of CYP3A4 and CYP3A5 is virtually indistinguishable.

gene. In addition to various inactivating mutations, entire deletions of the gene are not uncommon in the population, and many other variants that modify or reduce the function of the gene exist. On the other hand, some individuals show an *ultra-rapid metaboliser* phenotype, at least a proportion of which appear to result from duplication of the gene. Individuals of this phenotype may suffer therapeutic failure or be wrongly suspected of non-compliance.

Plasma and brain levels of drugs will differ between patients because of genetic variability in metabolic enzymes. This was first described for nortriptyline in CYP2D6 poor metabolisers, where much greater plasma levels occur because removal by CYP2D6 action in the liver is impaired. Dosage adjustment during treatment with nortriptyline and other tricyclic antidepressants appears to reduce the occurrence of side effects, and recommendations have been made for CYP2D6 and CYP2C19 genotype-based dosages of antidepressants (Kirchheiner et al. 2001). However, these guidelines have yet to be widely adopted because appropriate genetic tests are not readily available and the value of this approach is still unclear.

Several case reports describe CYP2D6 poor metaboliser individuals who were prescribed antidepressants and suffered severe or fatal events. These cases represent extreme examples that come to light among many routine cases, and the precise frequency of such events is unclear. Some of these cases may result from other environmental or genetic factors, and it is yet to be established whether pharmacogenetic variation is the sole or major

Table 18.2
Selected genetic variants of potential pharmacogenetic importance to mood disorders

Gene name	Name of polymorphism(s)	Type of polymorphism(s)
CYP1A2 [a]	*CYP1A2*1C*	–3858G>A
	*CYP1A2*1F*	–164C>A
CYP2C9 [a]	*CYP2C9*2*	430C>T (R144C)
	*CYP2C9*3*	1075A>C (I359L)
CYP2C19 [a]	*CYP2C19*2A*	99C>T; 681G>A; 990C>T; 991A>G
	*CYP2C19*2B*	99C>T; 276G>C; 681G>A; 990C>T; 991A>G
	*CYP2C19*3*	636G>A; 991A>G; 1251A>C
CYP2D6 [a]	Multiple polymorphisms	
CYP3A4 [a]	Several polymorphisms	
CYP3A5 [a]	*CYP3A5*3A*	6986A>G; 31611C>T
	*CYP3A5*6*	14690G>A
GNB3 (G protein ß3 subunit gene)	825C>T	Intronic SNP
IMPA1 and *IMPA2* (inositol monophosphatase)	Several polymorphisms	
INPP1 (inositol poly-phosphate 1-phosphatase)	Several polymorphisms	
MAOA (monoamine oxidase)	MAOA-uVNTR	VNTR of 30bp repeat element in promoter
	MAOA-CAn	Dinucleotide repeat in intron 2
SLC6A2 (noradrenaline transporter)	A457P	237 G>C
SLC6A4 (serotonin transporter)	5HTTLPR	VNTR of 44bp repeat element in promoter region
	STin2	VNTR of 17bp repeat element in intron 3 (formerly intron 2)
SLC18A2 (VMAT2, vesicular monoamine transporter)	Several polymorphisms	
TPH [b] (tryptophan hydroxylase)	A218C	Coding SNP

NOTES a An up-to-date list of all alleles and their correct nomenclature is located at <http://www.imm.ki.se/cypalleles/>.
b The recent discovery of a second tryptophan hydroxylase gene (*TPH2*) and the suggestion that *TPH* is not expressed in the brain makes the relevance of this polymorphism uncertain.

Functional effect
Decreased enzyme activity
Higher inducibility
Amino acid change (Arg144Cys): decreased enzyme activity
Amino acid change (Ile359Leu): decreased enzyme activity
Splicing defect. No enzyme activity
Splicing defect and missense change. No enzyme activity
Stop codon. No enzyme activity
A wide range of effects, ranging from complete loss of function to varying effects on activity of the enzyme
Unknown function
Splicing defect. No expression
Splicing defect. No expression
Altered splicing leads to variant protein associated with an increased signal transduction and ion transport
Unknown effect. Lithium sensitive enzyme
Unknown effect. Lithium sensitive enzyme
Affects gene expression
Unknown function
Rare amino acid variant (Gly359Cys) with markedly reduced affinity for noradrenaline
Long alleles show higher gene expression
Regulates transcription of *SLC6A4*
Unknown function
Unknown function

contributing factor in such instances. Phenocopying (induction of a poor metaboliser state by drug–enzyme interaction) is an important cause of adverse effects, and fluoxetine is well known to have this effect on CYP2D6. Pharmacogenetics of metabolic enzymes may be of particular importance in situations where more than one drug is being used and the potential for inhibition of a metabolic enzyme occurs. Such interactions could conceivably be exacerbated in patients with reduced function of the relevant enzyme system due to otherwise benign polymorphisms.

Variants of other cytochrome P450 genes are likely to be of pharmacogenetic importance in treatment of mood disorders. For example, mutations of CYP2C19 appear to affect sertraline disposition, and patients who are poor metabolisers for this enzyme can show adverse reactions such as nausea and dizziness, presumably because toxic concentrations of the drug accumulate.

Of the mood stabilisers, valproate has three principal metabolic pathways (including CYP2C19), and because of this it is less susceptible to pharmacokinetic drug interactions. This may also mean that metabolism of valproate is not greatly influenced by pharmacogenetic variation in one or other of these pathways. Lithium is not metabolised, and is excreted in an unmodified form.

It is now established that several cytochrome P450 enzymes, including CYP2D6, are expressed in the brain, where they may operate in the metabolism of endogenous substrates such as neurotransmitters. This suggests that polymorphisms affecting such enzymes may have broader pharmacogenetic or behavioural effects in the central nervous system, in addition to influences on plasma and tissue levels of drugs.

The cytochrome P450 enzymes are part of the phase I metabolic system, responsible for oxidising drugs and other exogenous substances that are usually lipophilic, to produce more polar products that can be further modified by a second large group of enzymes, the phase II system. During phase II reactions, conjugation of endogenous substrates (such as glucuronic acid or sulfate) occurs, resulting in formation of very hydrophilic molecules that can be readily eliminated from the body. Although much of the focus in metabolism of drugs used for mood disorders has been on the phase I enzymes, variability in activity of phase II enzymes also may affect response to such drugs. For example, carbamazepine is metabolised primarily by CYP3A4/5, but it has an active epoxide metabolite that is generated in a phase II conjugation reaction.

Other pharmacokinetic activities

Our knowledge of genetic influences on the absorption, distribution and elimination of mood drugs within the body is poor. Studies in mice with a targeted mutation in the P-glycoprotein gene (*Mdr1a* or *Abcb1*) demonstrated that this molecule is important for removal of some antidepressant drugs, such as nortriptyline, from the brain via the blood–brain barrier (Uhr et al. 2000). We have described an association between a variant of the P-glycoprotein gene that appears to have reduced transporter function and postural hypotension in nortriptyline-treated patients (Roberts et al. 2002). Although this association remains to be confirmed, it illustrates the potential value of examining variability in relevant drug transporters.

Lithium is rapidly absorbed and circulates as a free ion in the blood, accumulating to different levels in different tissues. It is almost entirely excreted unmodified in the urine. An early study suggested the existence of at least one gene affecting uptake of lithium into red blood cells (Dorus et al. 1983). Uptake of valproate into rat brain is mediated by a medium-chain fatty acid transporter, and this may be a worthwhile target for pharmacogenetic analysis. Little further work has explored the molecular biology of transport and other pharmacokinetic processes of the mood-stabilising agents. The recent comprehensive description of polymorphic variants of many membrane-bound drug transporter proteins (Hoffmeyer et al. 2000; Leabman et al. 2003) may enhance our understanding of drug absorption and elimination processes for drugs used to treat mood disorders.

GENETIC EFFECTS ON PHARMACODYNAMICS

Genetic variability in drug targets

Interaction of a drug with its target and the pharmacological consequences of that interaction are referred to as *pharmacodynamics*. Genetic variability in drug targets may modify the drug–target interaction or its consequences, and this is an additional source of potential pharmacogenetic effect. The pharmacogenetics of drug targets is becoming quite well studied in the mood disorders, and attempts have been made to extend this work to biochemical pathways downstream of the primary drug targets. Some examples are considered below.

The serotonin transporter is the initial target of selective serotonin reuptake inhibitors (SSRIs). The gene for this protein (*SLC6A4*) has several polymorphisms, but of particular interest is a VNTR element in the promoter of the gene, called 5HTTLPR, which appears to influence basal levels of transcription (Lesch et al. 1996). Several studies have evaluated the effect of the 5HTTLPR polymorphism on antidepressant response, and although most authors conclude there is an effect on response to SSRIs, the findings are not consistent. Variant forms of 5HTTLPR and another VNTR present in intron 2 of the gene have been associated with response to fluoxetine, paroxetine, fluvoxamine, and pindolol augmentation of fluvoxamine treatment. However, few of these studies have been replicated, and there is little consistency in outcome for specific alleles. This confusing pattern most likely reflects mainly false-positive results, although the lack of consistency also suggests that if variability of the serotonin transporter gene has an effect on SSRI response it is not strong.

The noradrenaline transporter is the target for several antidepressants (including desipramine, nortriptyline, venlafaxine and doxepin) and a large number of SNPs have been identified in the gene, many of which lead to altered amino acid variants. The pharmacogenetic significance of these variants, if any, is unknown. Monoamine oxidase A (MAO-A) is a key enzyme in the metabolism of serotonin and is the target of monoamine oxidase inhibitors such as moclobemide. Although this class of antidepressants is not widely used, pharmacogenetic analysis of MAO-A may be of wider relevance to treatment with SSRIs and other drugs that act on the serotonergic system. A VNTR in the promoter of MAO-A appears to affect expression of the gene, although it is not yet clear whether this has any pharmacogenetic consequences.

The mechanisms by which lithium acts to modify mood are not fully understood, limiting our ability to approach the pharmacogenetics of targets for this drug. However, a great deal of evidence supports the notion that lithium responsiveness is a familial trait (Lerer and Macciardi 2002). Lithium has a broad range of complex effects in the brain, acting on several neurotransmitter systems, intracellular signalling pathways (particularly metabolism of inositol phosphate), gene transcription, and cell growth and survival (Detera-Wadleigh 2001). This complexity of action has, until fairly recently, inhibited the identification of clear drug targets that might provide a focus for lithium pharmacogenetics.

Two lithium-sensitive enzymes involved in inositol phosphate metabolism (inositol monophosphatase and inositol polyphosphate 1-polyphosphatase) have been examined for genetic variability, although no clear evidence for their involvement in lithium response has emerged. Candidate gene association studies in lithium-responsive patients have explored involvement of MAO-A, various GABAergic, serotonergic and dopaminergic genes, and the corticotrophin and pro-encephalin genes. From these studies, the only positive finding to emerge was an association of response with 5HTTL-PR. Numerous other candidate genes are coming to light, and these will be examined progressively. One example is the gene for glycogen synthase kinase 3ß, an enzyme inhibited by both lithium and valproate, and on which the signalling pathways modified by lithium converge.

Genetic variability in pathways associated with drug targets

Just as we expect that variability of drug targets may influence responses to drugs, it is also possible that inter-individual variability in key molecules that operate upstream or downstream of drug targets might influence responses. The range of such candidates is large, and includes molecules involved in synthesis or processing of neurotransmitters, or in transduction of signals received by neurotransmitter receptors. These candidates can be loosely categorised in function as presynaptic or postsynaptic. Examples of presynaptic candidates are enzymes involved in neurotransmitter generation, such as tryptophan hydroxylase, or in transport and storage of neurotransmitters, such as vesicular monoamine transporter, which pumps cytosolic monoamines into synaptic vesicles. Postsynaptic candidates include many G proteins and other molecules that transduce signals from neurotransmitter receptors, and the receptors themselves. Serotonin binds to a range of receptors and, although these are not necessarily drug targets, genetic variability influencing function of these receptors may indirectly affect response to antidepressants. Attention has recently focused on one G protein component, encoded by the G protein ß3 subunit gene (*GNB3*). A common SNP occurs in *GNB3*, the T allele of which is associated with an alternative RNA splicing event that generates an altered protein. This variant protein appears to mediate increased signal transduction, and the 825C>T SNP has been associated with antidepressant response in several studies.

Although single gene candidate studies can yield interesting data, new approaches are needed to identify candidates in biochemical pathways associated with mood disorders and their treatment. Given the complexity of effects caused by antidepressants and mood stabilisers, pharmacogenomics approaches that assess the expression patterns of many genes in model systems may provide useful targets for further analysis, and preliminary examples of such work have appeared (Choy and Thomas 1999; Cordeiro et al. 2000; Landgrebe et al. 2002; Yamada et al. 2002). There is evidence from simple model systems that valproate, lithium and carbamazepine all share a common mechanism of operation (Williams et al. 2002). It is also possible that antidepressants of various classes, despite their different targets and modes of action, may share common pathways of action. If such common targets or effectors of drug action can be identified, it may be possible, based on this knowledge, to develop a small set of clinically useful pharmacogenetic tests that predict response to these drugs.

CHALLENGES AND PROSPECTS

The most significant challenge ahead is the identification of polymorphisms that are of clinical utility in psychiatry. How an individual responds to an antidepressant or mood stabiliser is likely to be influenced by a complex interaction of environmental and genetic factors. Each gene may contribute only a small component of the effect, and it is not yet clear whether we can identify new genes that confer sufficient effect to be of clinical value.

Even the best-known pharmacogenetic polymorphisms, such as those that inactivate CYP2D6, are not currently part of the repertoire of routine testing laboratories as they are of unclear value to the practising psychiatrist. Recommendations to routinely screen cytochrome P450 mutations in psychiatric practice have been made (Kirchheiner et al. 2001), but these have not been widely adopted and it is not yet clear whether doing so will lead to safer prescribing and improved outcomes. Further research is required to clarify where pharmacogenetics tests should be applied, how these might improve treatment of mood disorders, and whether such approaches are cost-effective. Most studies to date have involved small numbers of patients with a particular polymorphism, and much larger and longer-term studies must be carried out to get definitive answers.

Assuming genetic tests that usefully guide prescribing can be developed, two further problems will remain. The first is how best to effectively communicate this pharmacogenetic information to the practitioner. This will require sound evidence of clinical utility and thorough dissemination of the information. The second problem is to ensure the accessibility of genetic tests for relevant polymorphisms, and this will most likely be solved by market forces. An additional challenge will be developing pharmacogenetic practices that are applicable or specific to different ethnic groups, as the frequency of specific polymorphisms can differ markedly with ethnicity (Nebert and Menon 2001).

Future developments likely to profoundly influence our understanding of pharmacogenetics include the application of increasingly sophisticated pharmacogenomics and *proteomics* (protein genome) methods to identify the genes and gene products that show altered behaviour during treatment with drugs. These analyses in cell culture and animal models, and in human tissues, will identify sets of genes that are most likely to influence occurrence of side effects and responses to treatments. Confirmation of a role for these genes can then be sought in clinical studies of treatment outcome and laboratory studies that determine the functional consequences of each polymorphism. Whether such gene sets can be usefully applied to guide prescribing and improve outcomes remains to be seen.

The combination of imaging techniques that allow real-time investigation of brain function, with pharmacogenetics and pharmacogenomics, also promises to accelerate our understanding of how genetic variability affects responses to drugs (Soares 2002). Observed differences in function between patient groups of different genotype, particularly during treatment with an antidepressant or mood stabiliser, may provide evidence of altered function due to variant genes. These types of studies will provide new information and considerably augment existing candidate gene association studies, which often lack biochemical evidence of altered function for polymorphic candidate genes.

Finally, as susceptibility genes for the mood disorders are identified over the next few years, it will be of interest to test variants of these genes for pharmacogenetic effects. Biochemical relationships between the underlying pathophysiology of such illnesses and the mechanism of action of drugs used in their treatment are likely to be intimate, and one of the immediate applications of knowledge about genes that increase individual risk of suffering a mood disorder may be as a guide to improved treatment.

REFERENCES

Alexanderson B, Evans DA, Sjoqvist F (1969) Steady-state plasma levels of nortriptyline in twins: Influence of genetic factors and drug therapy. *BMJ* 4:764-8.

Choy RK, Thomas JH (1999) Fluoxetine-resistant mutants in *C. elegans* define a novel family of transmembrane proteins. *Molecular Cell* 4:143-52.

Cordeiro ML, Umbach JA, Gundersen CB (2000) Lithium ions up-regulate mRNAs encoding dense-core vesicle proteins in nerve growth factor-differentiated PC12 cells. *Journal of Neurochemistry* 75:2622-5.

Detera-Wadleigh SD (2001) Lithium-related genetics of bipolar disorder. *Annals of Medicine* 33:272-85.

Dorus E, Cox NJ, Gibbons RD, Shaughnessy R, Pandey GN, Cloninger CR (1983) Lithium ion transport and affective disorders within families of bipolar patients. Identification of a major gene locus. *Archives of General Psychiatry* 40:545-52.

Evans WE, Relling MV (1999) Pharmacogenomics: Translating functional genomics into rational therapeutics. *Science* 286:487-91.

Evans WE, McLeod HL (2003) Pharmacogenomics – Drug disposition, drug targets, and side effects. *New England Journal of Medicine* 348:538-49.

Hoffmeyer S, Burk O, von Richter O, Arnold HP, Brockmoller J, Johne A, et al. (2000) Functional polymorphisms of the human multidrug-resistance gene: Multiple sequence variations and correlation of one allele with P-glycoprotein expression and activity in vivo. *Proceedings of the National Academy of Sciences of the United States of America* 97:3473-8.

Kirchheiner J, Brosen K, Dahl ML, Gram LF, Kasper S, Roots I, et al. (2001) CYP2D6 and CYP2C19 genotype-based dose recommendations for antidepressants: A first step towards subpopulation-specific dosages. *Acta Psychiatrica Scandinavica* 104:173-92.

Kruglyak L (1999) Prospects for whole-genome linkage disequilibrium mapping of common disease genes. *Nature Genetics* 22:139-44.

Landgrebe J, Welzl G, Metz T, van Gaalen MM, Ropers H, Wurst W, et al. (2002) Molecular characterisation of antidepressant effects in the mouse brain using gene expression profiling. *Journal of Psychiatric Research* 36:119-29.

Leabman MK, Huang CC, DeYoung J, Carlson EJ, Taylor TR, de la Cruz M, et al. (2003) Natural variation in human membrane transporter genes reveals evolutionary and functional constraints. *Proceedings of the National Academy of Sciences of the United States of America* 100:5896-901.

Lerer B, Macciardi F (2002) Pharmacogenetics of antidepressant and mood-stabilizing drugs: A review of candidate-gene studies and future research directions. *International Journal of Neuropsychopharmacology* 5:255-75.

Lesch K-P, Bengel D, Heils A, Sabol SZ, Greenberg BD, Petri S, et al. (1996) Association of anxiety-related traits with a polymorphism in the serotonin transporter gene regulatory region. *Science* 274:1527-31.

Malhotra AK, Goldman D (1999) Benefits and pitfalls encountered in psychiatric genetic association studies. *Biological Psychiatry* 45:544-50.

Nebert DW, Menon AG (2001) Pharmacogenomics, ethnicity, and susceptibility genes. *Pharmacogenomics Journal* 1:19-22.

Risch NJ (2000) Searching for genetic determinants in the new millennium. *Nature* 405:847-56.

Roberts RL, Joyce PR, Mulder RT, Begg EJ, Kennedy MA (2002) A common P-glycoprotein polymorphism is associated with nortriptyline-induced postural hypotension in patients treated for major depression. *Pharmacogenomics Journal* 2:191-6.

Roses AD (2000) Pharmacogenetics and the practice of medicine. *Nature* 405:857-65.

Rothstein MA, Epps PG (2001) Ethical and legal implications of pharmacogenomics. *Nature Reviews. Genetics* 2:228-31.

Sachidanandam R, Weissman D, Schmidt SC, Kakol JM, Stein LD, Marth G, et al. (2001) A map of human genome sequence variation containing 1.42 million single nucleotide polymorphisms. *Nature* 409:928-33.

Saiki RK, Gelfand DH, Stoffel S, Scharf SJ, Higuchi R, Horn GT, et al. (1988) Primer-directed enzymatic amplification of DNA with a thermostable DNA polymerase. *Science* 239:487-91.

Soares JC (2002) Can brain-imaging studies provide a 'mood stabilizer signature'? *Molecular Psychiatry* 7 Suppl 1:S64-70.

Uhr M, Steckler T, Yassouridis A, Holsboer F (2000) Penetration of amitriptyline, but not of fluoxetine, into brain is enhanced in mice with blood-brain barrier deficiency due to mdr1a P-glycoprotein gene disruption. *Neuropsychopharmacology* 22:380-7.

Williams RS, Cheng L, Mudge AW, Harwood AJ (2002) A common mechanism of action for three mood-stabilizing drugs. *Nature* 417:292-5.

Yamada M, Takahashi K, Tsunoda M, Nishioka G, Kudo K, Ohata H, et al. (2002) Differential expression of VAMP2/synaptobrevin-2 after antidepressant and electroconvulsive treatment in rat frontal cortex. *Pharmacogenomics Journal* 2:377-82.

CHAPTER 19

ELECTROCONVULSIVE THERAPY

John W G Tiller

Electroconvulsive therapy (ECT) was introduced in the late 1930s and was initially used to treat schizophrenia, for which it was the first effective treatment. Despite clinical use, it was decades before adequate research showed its acute efficacy. It proved more effective for severe depression and mania. It seems to remain the most effective treatment for severe acute affective episodes despite the introduction of antidepressants, antipsychotics, and mood stabilisers. Although most patients can be managed on continuation pharmacotherapy (most commonly an antidepressant, a mood stabiliser or a combination) after a course of ECT, some patients do not remain well on medication yet appear to remain well with maintenance ECT.

WHAT IS ECT?

Convulsive therapy has a long history in psychiatry, with references in Western medicine at least back to the sixteenth century (Mowbray 1959). In the early part of the twentieth century, chemicals, particularly camphor derivatives, were used to induce fitting. This was an unpredictable and potentially toxic way of inducing a fit. Furthermore, patients reported a most distressing sense of overwhelming apprehension after injection of the induction agent and immediately before the onset of the fit. The introduction by Cerleti and Bini (1938) of electrical stimulation provided the opportunity for the safer, more reliable and predictable induction of fits. The application of electrodes to the scalp avoided the problems seen in some early animal experimentation, in which the passage of electricity across the heart (when endeavouring to induce a fit) resulted in cardiac arrhythmias, and some deaths.

Electroconvulsive therapy is the name given to a number of treatment techniques which have as a common element the induction of a fit by an electric charge delivered to the scalp, resulting in electroencephalographic changes and a motor fit. ECT has evolved substantially over the past 60 years, although reports and reviews of studies tend to treat it as if it is only one treatment modality that has never been developed. ECT now refers to a range of treatment approaches and techniques, with differing outcomes. Research on ECT has tended to combine the outcomes of disparate studies using disparate therapeutic techniques. There is a paucity of studies on the safety and effectiveness of ECT as it is currently administered.

Major changes in ECT treatment include changes in electrode location (particularly right unilateral compared with bilateral treatment), the stimulation waveform (the introduction of square wave rather than sine wave stimuli), mode of treatment (the introduction of brief pulse rather than continuous waveform stimuli), electroencephalographic monitoring (observing changes in the post-stimulus electroencephalogram), and improved anaesthetics, including better anaesthetic agents, the use of muscle relaxants and pre-oxygenation. Better patient preparation, the management of concomitant medications and the elimination of anticonvulsants, where possible, have helped improve outcomes and minimise adverse events. A key element has been the introduction of specific ECT training for psychiatrists and nurses who are involved in administering the treatment. In addition, anaesthetics are now often administered by consultant anaesthetists rather than the psychiatrist, a general practitioner, or anaesthetist trainee, and this has improved safety, especially for frail and elderly patients who need ECT. Many ECT services now have anaesthetics administered only by consultant anaesthetists. The development of specialist treatment teams seems to reduce the risk of adverse outcomes.

CONTEMPORANEOUS ECT

Various developments have resulted in present recommendations for the administration of ECT. These are exemplified in Australasia by the Clinical Memorandum of the Royal Australian and New Zealand College of Psychiatrists (1999) and the book *ECT: An Australasian Guide* (Tiller and Lyndon 2003). These should not be seen as defining ECT treatment for all time, but rather as living documents that will change and evolve as new research and improved techniques provide the opportunity for better outcomes.

Two principal techniques are currently used in Australasia. These are high-dose right unilateral ECT after stimulus dosing and with dose adjustments over treatment, and low-dose bilateral ECT after stimulus dosing and with dose adjustments over treatment (Sackeim et al. 1987; Sackeim et al. 1993; Sackeim et al. 2000). With stimulus titration, the stimulus that just induces an electrical and motor response is called the threshold dose. With high-dose right unilateral treatment, effective treatments are associated with initial doses around three to six times the threshold. These doses need adjustment over the course of treatment as threshold rises. With bilateral treatment, the initial dose is normally about one and a half times the threshold. Bifrontal treatment has been proposed as a way of getting an effective result with fewer cognitive adverse events (Letemendia et al. 1993). It can be difficult to judge the appropriate dose, in part because people vary in the size and extent of frontal sinuses. That may also result in high flux densities in some adjacent tissues. This has the effect of varying (from patient to patient) the surface stimulus required to produce an effective response and the possibility, in theory at least, of tissue complications.

ECT ANAESTHETICS

ECT used to be administered without any anaesthetic. Patients could be quite apprehensive before ECT. There have been considerable advances in ECT anaesthetics, as detailed by the Australian and New Zealand College of Anaesthetists (1994; 1995; 2002).

With no pre-oxygenation, there was the potential for some hypoxia during treatment and a risk of cerebral ischaemia with consequent adverse events, including increased problems with disorientation and memory after treatment.

Pre-oxygenation reduces the risk of hypoxia during ECT, and the hyperventilation associated with pre-oxygenation reduces carbon dioxide levels and lowers the threshold for fitting (lowers the electrical dose required to induce the fit) (Holmberg 1953; McAndrew and Hauser 1967). The lower the stimulus dose, the fewer the cognitive adverse events, as long as the doses are adequate to result in an effective treatment with the particular technique used.

The absence of any muscle relaxant when ECT was introduced led to the potential for injury during the motor fit from excessive muscle activity, including crush fractures of the spine, with these especially occurring in the tonic phase. The introduction of muscle relaxants dramatically reduced the risk of injury from excessive muscle contractions during ECT. The most commonly used is suxamethonium, a depolarising muscle relaxant. This drug is mostly well tolerated, but some patients experience considerable muscle aches and pains, especially following the first treatment, when there is prolonged muscle relaxation associated with electrical dose titration. This post-muscle-relaxant pain is mostly well managed with a non-steroidal analgesic such as diclofenac or paracetamol. Rarely, a patient has a pseudo-cholinesterase deficiency with prolonged muscle relaxation. Such patients need to be ventilated until muscle activity and spontaneous respiration is restored. Recovery of adequate muscle activity may take hours, and facilities must be available to support the patient for that period. Curare-like agents are alternative muscle-relaxing agents, but are slower-acting, longer-lasting and not as predictable as depolarising agents.

The traditional anaesthetic agent was the barbiturate sodium thiopentone. In many centres this agent was replaced by methohexitone, which was regarded as a less potent anticonvulsant (less likely to interfere with the induction of a fit) and with more predictable action. The withdrawal of the latter agent from the market in Australia resulted in many centres moving to the use of propofol. Even though propofol may cause problems with an increased stimulus threshold because of its potent anticonvulsant activity, this is not insurmountable in practice and the reliability of the agent and the ease of recovery seems of benefit to patients.

It is essential that the same anaesthetic be used for each treatment, as different agents given in different doses can result in varying electrical thresholds and may impair treatment, or be associated with excessive dosage with particular treatments.

ECT anaesthetics were administered by the treating psychiatrist in many centres until about the 1970s, but modern techniques and safety considerations result in most ECT anaesthetics being administered by a consultant anaesthetist. The administration of ECT now normally occurs in a specialist ECT facility with adequate oxygen supplies, suction facilities and resuscitation equipment, or in a hospital operating theatre or recovery area with similar facilities.

ECT STIMULUS

The introduction of brief pulse square-wave stimulation has resulted in the capacity to induce a fit with therapeutic effectiveness at a lower energy than was required with continuous sine-wave stimulation. Dosing is now usually determined by electrical charge rather than energy, as the latter may vary depending on the electrical resistance with the electrodes on the scalp. Present-day machines are typically *constant current* machines. Most of these can deliver up to about 1000 mC, with most patients being treated at doses between 50 and 500 mC.

Any fit, no matter how induced, results in a potent anticonvulsant response in the brain to stop that fitting. This is seen in response to ECT with a progressive increase in threshold over a course of treatment. The threshold typically doubles from the beginning to the end of an acute course of about nine treatments. One theory of how ECT works relates to this anticonvulsant response, which is generated in response to ECT treatment and persists for some time after each treatment.

ELECTROENCEPHALOGRAM RESPONSE

Before the stimulus, there is a typical low-voltage, desynchronised, fast-wave beta activity when patients are resting with their eyes open, or alpha activity when patients have their eyes lightly closed. This is usually regarded as a baseline status. Following the stimulus and the stimulus artefact, there is a brief period of recruitment on the electroencephalogram associated with the tonic motor phase followed by a high-amplitude *spike-and-wave* phase associated with clonic motor activity. Motor activity typically ceases about 10 seconds before the high-amplitude phase on the electroencephalogram, which settles to a low-voltage trace called the *phase of post-ictal suppression* (Tiller and Lyndon 2003). One indirect measure of the efficacy of a particular treatment is called the *post-ictal suppression index*, which reflects how quickly and to what degree the EEG amplitude falls just after the end of the seizure. It compares the mean amplitude over a 3-second epoch at the phase of peak amplitude with the mean amplitude over 3 seconds in the post-ictal phase. Effective treatment is usually associated with more than 80 per cent suppression, while the common recommendation is that the patient should have a re-stimulation at a higher dose if the index is below about 75 per cent.

When treatment is marginally supra-threshold, the motor response is typically short (less than 10 seconds), the amplitude of the electroencephalogram is low, there is asymmetry between the traces from the right and left side of the brain, and the EEG duration of the fit is brief (commonly under 20 seconds), although occasionally can be very prolonged (greater than 120 seconds). Sometimes, with marginally supra-threshold doses there is normal post-ictal suppression followed by a recurrence of fitting. The latter may or may not be associated with motor movements. Such fitting is normally associated with profound post-ictal confusion and disorientation and increased rates of memory difficulties compared with a satisfactory treatment.

LOW-DOSE BILATERAL ECT

Bilateral electrode placement with bitemporal electrodes was used when ECT was first introduced. Bitemporal placement, or any placement across the head, avoided the risk of passing electrical stimuli through the heart and risking the induction of potentially fatal cardiac arrhythmias. There was no monitoring of the electroencephalogram when ECT was first introduced. EEG monitoring was not widely introduced until the 1990s. Before then, the adequacy of any one treatment was estimated by duration of the motor fit, using that as a surrogate measure for efficacy.

The initial bilateral technique used a sinusoidal current, which provided a high-energy stimulus. A particular problem with the initial use of a sinusoidal current is that the higher the energy, the greater the likelihood of eliciting an adequate therapeutic response. In addition, the risk of cognitive adverse events is higher with greater energy.

An advantage of bilateral ECT is that any dose that elicits an electrical and motor fit is likely to be efficacious. On average, it seems that a dose of about one and a half times threshold is more appropriate for bilateral treatment. In addition, bilateral ECT seems to result in more adverse cognitive events than high-dose unilateral ECT, although brief pulse, square-wave, constant current techniques are now used, needing less charge than continuous sinusoidal stimuli.

HIGH-DOSE RIGHT UNILATERAL ECT

This technique was introduced in an attempt to reduce the nature and frequency of adverse events with bilateral treatment. Bitemporal electrode placement is associated with a higher rate of cognitive adverse events. In practice, everyone has immediate post-ECT confusion, and most have some impairment to memory, which is cumulative over the course of treatment.

This memory impairment particularly relates to autobiographical memory (memory of personal events). In addition, bitemporal electrode placement means that there is stimulation near the speech areas of the brain. Some patients can have quite a marked speech dysfunction with ECT, especially with difficulties in word finding and expression. Although this may be a transient effect immediately after treatment, it can be quite distressing.

Treatment with electrodes placed over the non-dominant hemisphere avoids stimulation near the speech areas, and appears to reduce speech difficulties after ECT. Even left-handed patients predominantly have left-sided cortical dominance, so it is the rare patient where speech problems arise, and the decision may then be taken to use left unilateral treatment.

Unfortunately, low-dose right unilateral treatment is ineffective, and can result in prolonged fitting after stimulation and high levels of cognitive adverse events. Increasing the dose to about three times threshold appears to be optimal in terms of therapeutic effectiveness while minimising very high doses that can result in increased cognitive adverse events. The fact that right unilateral treatment needs to be administered in a dose which falls in a therapeutic window (neither too low nor too high) means that the team administering ECT, and particularly the treating psychiatrist, needs to be able to change and modify the stimulus dose so that it remains in that window throughout treatment. At locations where training is limited and skills not developed adequately for such adjustments, bilateral treatment is likely to be more reliable in effectiveness, though at the expense of more adverse events involving memory.

Some authors advocate six times threshold as the optimal dose for high-dose right unilateral ECT. In practice, this may not differ from those who advocate three times threshold as the dose. If the initial dose is three times threshold, and the dose is modified over an acute course of ECT, the final dose is likely to be about six times the initial threshold. This process provides the opportunity for effectiveness while minimising cognitive adverse events. An initial dose of six times threshold which is maintained through treatment may result in more early cognitive adverse events than a three times threshold dose, but is more likely to be efficacious and with fewer cognitive adverse events than circumstances when the treatment dose is lower and not adequately increased as treatment progresses.

The skills to effectively assess, judge and modify the treatment dose over a course of ECT are a central part of ECT training.

A common system is to commence with high-dose right unilateral treatment and move to bilateral treatment if unilateral treatment is not efficacious. Alternatively, one moves to unilateral treatment if cognitive adverse events are unacceptable with bilateral treatment.

BIFRONTAL ECT

A bifrontal electrode placement has been advocated as a technique that can be as efficacious as bitemporal treatment, with less confusion and a lower risk of speech problems (Letemendia et al. 1993). This technique is vulnerable to inter-individual differences in the size and location of the frontal sinuses. For some patients this is not an issue; for others, there is the potential for the electrodes to be kept quite some distance from the brain surface by large frontal sinuses. In such circumstances, there is the possibility of a high flux density around the sinus margins, including in the immediate supra-orbital area, and this can affect the eye. It has not been properly defined whether this technique may be useful once the location of frontal sinuses has been determined by X-ray. Electrodes can then be placed away from the sinus, but in the frontal area. At present, this electrode placement is mostly regarded as experimental, rather than in widespread routine clinical use.

TREATMENT FREQUENCY IN AN ACUTE COURSE

In Australasia, for an acute course of ECT, three times a week treatment is commonly used. This has been found empirically to provide a reasonable balance between achieving rapid treatment response and minimising cognitive effects. If confusion, disorientation or memory problems are a substantial problem, then treatment is normally spread out to twice a week, or even once a week.

With weekly treatment, there is the possibility that mood may be maintained but not further improved, so two or three times a week treatment is usually advocated for acute therapy.

More frequent ECT administration, as exemplified by approaches in the 1970s with multiple ECT treatments in a single session or attempting an entire treatment course in a single session, resulted in profound confusion and seemingly no more therapeutic benefit than from a normal single treatment. In the United Kingdom, twice a week treatment is recommended. This may partly relate to the UK preference for bilateral treatment, which has a higher rate of cognitive adverse events (National Institute for Clinical Excellence 2003).

CONTINUATION ECT

At the end of a course of ECT, there may be concern that post-ECT pharmacotherapy is not fully established. There may be a slight relapse in the patient's clinical status if the post-treatment pharmacotherapy is not effective and before alternative pharmacotherapy has an opportunity to work. The administration of one or two ECT treatments at weekly intervals can help maintain mood over this transitional period. Continuation ECT is the term applied to such treatments given in the first 6 months after an acute course of treatment.

MAINTENANCE ECT

Although most patients remain well with pharmacotherapy after an acute course of ECT, some patients do not respond to pharmacotherapy even though they have responded well to ECT. In such instances, maintenance ECT may be considered. Maintenance ECT is a continuation of ECT for periods up to 12 months or longer.

There is no consensus on the frequency of maintenance ECT treatments. This may vary from as frequently as weekly, to intervals up to 6 weeks or more. The essence of maintenance ECT is that the patient's mood should remain satisfactory and without relapse between treatments. If there is a relapse after 1 or 2 weeks, or any other interval, the frequency of maintenance ECT treatments should be increased so there is no relapse between treatments. The normal process is to start with weekly intervals and then progressively increase the interval between treatments, observing that the patient remains well over this time.

The duration of maintenance ECT is not known. Mostly it has commenced when patients have failed multiple pharmacotherapy treatments. A period of at least a year of good health could be considered before withholding such treatment. The patient's history might indicate that maintenance treatment over 2 or more years could be warranted for some.

Because of the paucity of data on maintenance ECT, some authorities recommend it should never be used (National Institute for Clinical Excellence 2003). That is to avoid a possible error of commission, but not an error of omission. The comparison between the prolonged and severe disability of the patient with, for example, unresponsive depressive illness and response to maintenance ECT can be dramatic. For this reason, even though research data are at present inadequate, maintenance ECT should be considered for those who are unresponsive or inadequately responsive to pharmacotherapy, or where ECT appears especially effective.

ECT FOR DEPRESSION

Many studies over the past 50 years support the effectiveness of ECT for depressive illness. A useful recent systematic review and meta-analysis of this area considering both efficacy and safety of ECT is that of Carney et al. (2003). There was a consistent finding that real ECT is significantly more effective than simulated ECT (six trials). ECT was significantly more effective than antidepressant pharmacotherapy in eighteen trials. Bilateral ECT was moderately more effective than unilateral ECT. High-dose ECT was more effective than low-dose ECT.

The Northwick Park trial (Johnstone et al. 1980), which addressed cognitive functioning with ECT for depression, indicated that the fourteen patients treated with real ECT were better able to retrieve recent memories than patients treated with simulated ECT, who had more word recognition errors immediately after treatment. At 6 months, no significant difference was noted between patients treated with real ECT or simulated ECT on subjective memory impairment, new learning, and remote memory. Recovery of orientation was longer for patients treated with bilateral compared with unilateral ECT, and testing of retrograde memory a week after the end of a course of ECT showed greater impairment among patients treated with bilateral ECT. A deficiency in our understanding of cognitive adverse events with different ECT treatments is the small size of studies.

Regarding frequency of treatment, there was no difference in efficacy between twice a week and three times a week, or between once a week and three times a week treatments.

This review highlighted the lower overall mortality in patients treated with ECT compared with those not treated in three out of four studies.

ECT FOR THE DEPRESSED ELDERLY

A Cochrane review in 2003 identified only three trials that could be included (Van der Wurff et al. 2003). It emphasised the major methodological shortcomings with these studies. The reviewers regarded the conclusion of one study that real ECT was superior to simulated ECT as needing to be interpreted cautiously. A second trial showed efficacy of unilateral over bilateral ECT, but the reviewers felt this was not a convincing result. Importantly, there are no adequate data on the efficacy and safety of ECT in the depressed elderly with concomitant dementia, cerebrovascular disorders or Parkinson's disease. The review concluded that none of the objectives of the review to assess the efficacy and safety of ECT (compared with simulated ECT or antidepressants) in the depressed elderly could be adequately tested because of the lack of firm randomised evidence.

Clinically, ECT appears to be an effective treatment for the depressed elderly, although patients who have evidence of dementia may be troubled with greater cognitive adverse events than non-demented patients. This can be addressed by preferentially using high-dose right unilateral treatment, and treating patients twice a week rather than three times a week. This is different from patients with depressive pseudo-dementia, who may respond successfully to three times a week treatment.

BIPOLAR DEPRESSION

Most studies on the effectiveness of ECT do not identify whether patients have bipolar depression. The presence of vegetative and melancholic symptoms was believed to have useful predictive value, but is now largely regarded as of historical interest. One study showed that the bipolar–unipolar distinction has no predictive value in determining ECT outcome (Daly et al. 2001). In three double-blind treatment protocols of 228 patients, the trend was for bipolar patients to show more rapid clinical improvement and to need fewer treatments than patients with unipolar depression. Given the hundreds of references to ECT for bipolar depression in a simple search of the topic, it is surprising that there are so few controlled data to guide clinical decision-making.

MANIA

ECT for mania has been extensively reviewed (Mukherjee et al. 1994), with the assessment that ECT has equivalent or superior antimanic properties compared with lithium and chlorpromazine. ECT has also been suggested as the primary treatment for manic delirium because it is rapidly effective and said to have a high safety margin.

MIXED AFFECTIVE STATES

There are limited data suggesting that ECT is effective for patients with mixed manic–depressive states, even in medication-refractory patients (Devanand et al. 2000; Ciapparelli et al. 2001).

There is ongoing discussion whether ECT for depression induces mania, and if it does then what to do about it. One argument is to continue ECT even if a depressed patient does become manic during a course of treatment, as ECT is also effective antimanic therapy (Kellner 1999).

ECT IN PREGNANCY

Reports of the use of ECT in pregnancy have been favourable. It can be considered when pharmacotherapy is contraindicated or ineffective. It is also a therapeutic option for women who need treatment for depression, mania or mixed states in the puerperium when they wish to breastfeed (Moreno et al. 1998; Bhatia et al. 1999).

PATIENT CONCERNS

Surprisingly for a treatment that is arguably the most effective for severe psychiatric disorders, ECT is subject to marked community fear, ignorance, and often an inappropriate desire to avoid the treatment. There are various reasons for this, discussed by Tiller and Lyndon (2003). A lot of public information comes from the cinema or drama, where ECT may be depicted as it was believed to have occurred in the 1940s and 1950s, but rarely as it is contemporaneously practised. There are beliefs about ECT destroying the brain or causing brain damage, notwithstanding the absence of demonstrated structural brain changes after ECT with lifetime or previous ECT treatments.

There may be excessive and inappropriate concern about memory loss, with beliefs that patients will lose all memories of their past. Although some concerns may have been appropriate with treatments given decades ago (in the absence of any effective alternative treatments), these are inappropriate concerns in respect of properly conducted contemporaneous ECT. It is inevitable that the patient will suffer some memory loss relating to the period of treatment, particularly autobiographical memories. There may also be some awareness of memory loss for the interval when the patient was very depressed before ECT commenced. Although memory loss has been reported after the end of a course of ECT, this is usually mild and lessens with the passage of time.

The provision of effective contemporaneous information for patients and their families about ECT is essential to demystify the treatment. This will help people be aware of the benefits and potential adverse effects of treatment on a rational basis, rather than having their decision-making coloured by inappropriate and inaccurate supposition, conjecture or gossip. The patient is then empowered to make an informed decision about having or not having the treatment.

OTHER ELECTRICAL TREATMENTS

Transcranial magnetic stimulation (Burt et al. 2002) and vagal nerve stimulation techniques (George et al. 2000) to treat depression are sometimes proposed as alternatives to ECT. These treatments are linked ECT because they involve magnetic or electrical stimulation in the therapeutic process. They are quite different treatments and unrelated to ECT. Neither treatment has been shown to be either equal or superior to ECT.

Electroconvulsive therapy has also been confused at times with electrical stimuli for aversive therapy, a behavioural psychological treatment technique. Aversive therapy has fallen out of favour for a variety of reasons, including perceptions of patient abuse and abuse of a power relationship in the therapeutic setting.

CONCLUSION

ECT has undergone major advances since it was first introduced. It is being recognised as a valuable treatment for mood disorders, and may be uniquely effective for patients with medication resistance or those who are very severely ill. There is an urgent need for large-scale effective studies of contemporaneous ECT, compared with modern alternatives. Despite the limited data, more than half a century of clinical experience shows the continued value of this treatment and its life-saving potential.

REFERENCES

Australian and New Zealand College of Anaesthetists (1994) Recommended Mininum Facilities for Safe Anaesthetic Practice in ECT. Review T4. Melbourne: ANZCA.

—— (1995) Guidelines for the Care of Patients Recovering from Anaesthesia. Review P4. Melbourne: ANZCA.

—— (2002) T2 Recommendations on Minimum Facilities for Safe Anaesthesia Practice Outside Operating Suites. Melbourne: ANZCA.

Bhatia SC, Baldwin SA, Bhatia SK (1999) Electroconvulsive therapy during the third trimester of pregnancy. *Journal of ECT* 15:270-4.

Burt T, Lisanby SH, Sackeim HA (2002) Neuropsychiatric applications of transcranial magnetic stimulation: A meta analysis. *International Journal of Neuropsychopharmacology* 5:73-103.

Carney S, Caowen P, Dearness K, Eastaugh J (2003) Efficacy and safety of electroconvulsive therapy in depressive disorders: A systematic review and meta-analysis. *Lancet* 361:799-808.

Cerletti U, Bini L (1938) Un neuvo motodo di shockterapie 'L'elettroshock'. *Bollettino Accademia Medica Roma* 64:136-8.

Ciapparelli A, Dell'Osso L, Tundo A, Pini S, Chiavacci MC, Di Sacco I, et al. (2001) Electroconvulsive therapy in medication-nonresponsive patients with mixed mania and bipolar depression. *Journal of Clinical Psychiatry* 62:552-5.

Daly JJ, Prudic J, Devanand DP, Nobler MS, Lisanby SH, Peyser S, et al. (2001) ECT in bipolar and unipolar depression: Differences in speed of response. *Bipolar Disorders* 3:95-104.

Devanand DP, Polanco P, Cruz R, Shah S, Paykina N, Singh K, et al. (2000) The efficacy of ECT in mixed affectives states. *Journal of ECT* 16:32-7.

George MS, Sackeim HA, Marangell LB, Husain MM, Nahas Z, Lisanby SH, et al. (2000) Vagus nerve stimulation. A potential therapy for resistant depression? *Psychiatric Clinics of North America* 23:757-83.

Holmberg G (1953) The factor of hypoxemia in electroshock therapy. *American Journal of Psychiatry* 110:115-18.
Johnstone EC, Deakin JF, Lawler P, Frith CD, Stevens M, McPherson K, et al. (1980) The Northwick Park electroconvulsive therapy trial. *Lancet* 2:1317-20.
Kellner CH (1999) ECT and manic switching: Bipolar IV disorder. *Journal of ECT* 15:243-4.
Letemendia FJ, Delva NJ, Rodenburg M, Lawson JS, Inglis J, Waldron JJ, et al. (1993) Therapeutic advantage of bifrontal electrode placement in ECT. *Psychological Medicine* 23:349-60.
McAndrew J, Hauser G (1967) Preventilation of oxygen in electroconvulsive treatment: A suggested modification of technique. *American Journal of Psychiatry* 124:251-2.
Moreno ME, Munoz JM, Valderrabanos JS, Gutierrez TV (1998) Electroconvulsive therapy in the first trimester of pregnancy. *Journal of ECT* 14:251-4.
Mowbray RM (1959) Historical aspects of electric convulsant therapy. *Scottish Medical Journal* 4:373-8.
Mukherjee S, Sackeim HA, Schnur DB (1994) Electroconvulsive therapy of acute manic episodes: A review of 50 years' experience. *American Journal of Psychiatry* 151:169-76.
National Institute for Clinical Excellence (2003) Guidance on the Use of Electroconvulsive Therapy – Technology Appraisal 59. London: National Institute for Clinical Excellence.
Royal Australian and New Zealand College of Psychiatrists (1999) RANZCP Clinical Memorandum #12: Electroconvulsive therapy. Melbourne: RANZCP.
Sackeim HA, Decina P, Kanzler M, Kerr B, Malitz S (1987) Effects of electrode placement on the efficacy of titrated, low-dose ECT. *American Journal of Psychiatry* 144:1449-55.
Sackeim HA, Prudic J, Devanand DP, Kiersky JE, Fitzsimons L, Moody BJ, et al. (1993) Effects of stimulus intensity and electrode placement on the efficacy and cognitive effects of electroconvulsive therapy. *New England Journal of Medicine* 328:839-46.
Sackeim HA, Prudic J, Devanand DP, Nobler MS, Lisanby SH, Peyser S, et al. (2000) A prospective, randomized, double-blind comparison of bilateral and right unilateral electroconvulsive therapy at different stimulus intensities. *Archives of General Psychiatry* 57:425-34.
Tiller J, Lyndon R (eds) (2003) *Electroconvulsive Therapy: An Australasian guide.* Melbourne: Australian Postgraduate Medicine.
Van der Wurff FB, Stek ML, Hoogendijk WL, Beekman ATF (2003) *Electroconvulsive Therapy for the Depressed Elderly*, The Cochrane Library, Issue 2. Oxford: Update Software.

CHAPTER 20

PSYCHOLOGICAL THERAPIES FOR DEPRESSION

Janice M McKenzie,
Janet D Carter and
Suzanne E Luty

Major depression causes a great deal of suffering both for the patients and for people close to them. Despite this, there is overwhelming evidence that depression remains seriously undertreated, with one of the main reasons being the failure of providers to consider psychotherapeutic approaches (Hirschfeld et al. 1997).

An understanding of psychotherapeutic principles greatly assists in the assessment of a depressed patient and aids in treatment planning. Psychotherapy may be used alone or in combination with medication. Although psychodynamic therapy has been used in the treatment of depression for many years, the past 30 years have seen significant advances in the research of short-term psychotherapies specifically developed for depression.

This chapter describes some of the key theoretical concepts underpinning the three short-term psychotherapies used in treatment for depression: interpersonal psychotherapy, cognitive behaviour therapy, and short-term psychodynamic therapy. The evidence for the efficacy of these psychotherapies is reviewed, followed by an outline of practical treatment strategies and therapeutic considerations.

THEORETICAL CONSIDERATIONS

Psychodynamic psychotherapy

Freud's work provides an important foundation for today's psychodynamic theory. Within this large body of theory, various writers have considered the origins of depression. In one of Freud's major works, *Mourning and Melancholia* (1917), he related the development of depression to the experience of loss. Although grief is specifically attached to actual loss of a loved one, depression may result from an actual or perceived loss. Furthermore, the intense self-criticism often seen in depression is explained as 'anger turned upon oneself', rather than the anger attaching to whoever had triggered the perceived loss. Freud also linked the later development of depression to difficulties experienced in the oral stage of development. However, he also cautioned that not all depression will necessarily have a psychodynamic origin.

Klein (1934) suggested that depression in later life may result from the individual failing to successfully negotiate a specific phase of childhood – she called this phase the *depressive position*. Klein suggested that, during this time, the infant begins to experience guilt because of destructive fantasies for the loved object, particularly the mother. The resulting experience is a feeling of having lost the loved object and with this the part of themselves that is loveable (Karasu 1990a, b).

Bibring (1953) and Jacobson (1971) have both described depression as being related to a loss of self-esteem. They also considered that depression could result from difficulties occurring in any stage of development.

Arieti (1977) postulated that a depressed person is often in an intense relationship with a *dominant other*. The depressed person is trying to please or live through the other person. The dominant other may also be an ideal or institution. The person thus feels helpless and unable to make any changes for him- or herself.

Many writers have emphasised the need in early development to have good relationships that initiate and maintain a sense of wellbeing and self-esteem. If the early relationships are unsatisfactory, the person may develop maladaptive ways of seeking praise or approbation to make up for deficiencies in their sense of self. Overall, key themes contributing to the future development of depression relate to difficulties with or separations from early attachment figures, resulting in problems maintaining a positive sense of self (Gabbard 1994).

Interpersonal psychotherapy

Interpersonal psychotherapy (IPT) is derived from a range of theoretical, empirical and clinical sources. These include the ideas of Adolph Meyer, whose psychobiological approach to understanding psychiatric disorders placed an emphasis on the patients' relationship to their environment. The interpersonal theory developed by Harry Stack Sullivan, linking psychiatric disorders and interpersonal relations, has also played a significant role in the development of IPT, mainly through the interpersonal school, which emerged in the Washington–Baltimore area of the United States during the 1930s and 1940s.

The empirical basis from which the understanding and treatment of depression with IPT is derived has several sources. These include studies that demonstrate the role of social supports and intimacy as protection against depression, as well as studies that explore the effect of chronic social and interpersonal stress on the onset of depression. The works of Bowlby, which emphasise the importance of attachment and loss, and data that suggest a strong association between marital disputes and depression are also important sources (Weissman et al. 1979).

Cognitive behaviour therapy

Several theorists have contributed to the development of cognitive-behavioural approaches over the years. It was in the 1960s and 1970s, however, that the application of cognitive-behavioural approaches to depression came to the fore. This was due to a variety of coinciding factors (see Dobson and Block 1988 for review). For example, there was growing dissatisfaction with the extent to which the strict behaviourist model could account for all of human behaviour. It was becoming increasingly apparent that this approach was not always appropriate for problems in which the behavioural targets were not readily apparent (for example, obsessive thinking in obsessive–compulsive disorder). Clinicians and researchers were placing increasing importance on mediational processes in the development and maintenance of psychopathology. There was also growing dissatisfaction with the alternative dominant approach, the psychodynamic model. Dobson and Block (1988) noted that early writings in the area of cognitive-behavioural therapies rejected the psychoanalytic emphases on unconscious processes, the importance of historical events and the need to do long-term therapy that relied heavily on the development of insight. Moreover, increasing attention was being placed on the lack of the empirical evidence supporting the efficacy of long-term psychodynamic therapy. At the same time, research studies, although not without criticisms of the methodology, were demonstrating that cognitive–behavioural treatments were as effective or more effective than strict behavioural approaches or pharmacotherapy.

Developments within cognitive psychology also contributed to the shift towards cognitive-behavioural treatments. Mediational models, particularly cognitive information processing, were being developed, researched and empirically supported in the laboratory. Clinicians were also investigating the role of cognitive processes in clinical constructs such as anxiety and depression. The systematic clinical observations and experimental testing of mediational cognitive processes conducted by Beck and colleagues were particularly influential in increasing awareness of the cognitive-behavioural framework for depression (Beck 1963). Since these initial developments, various treatment approaches have been developed and fall within the broad framework of CBT. Although they have their points of difference, they all share the fundamental premise that cognitions mediate behaviour and, therefore, emotional and behavioural change can be achieved by monitoring and altering cognitions.

RESEARCH CONSIDERATIONS

Psychodynamic psychotherapy

Although the efficacy of long-term psychodynamic therapy has not been examined, several short-term psychodynamic psychotherapies (STPPs) based on psychoanalytic theory have been developed and trialled over the past 35 years. Luborsky et al. (1999) reviewed three meta-analyses focusing on comparing STPPs with other short-term psychotherapies, and concluded that psychodynamic psychotherapy does no better or worse than other psychotherapies.

Barkham et al. (1996) reported on the second Sheffield Psychotherapy Project, which compared psychodynamic interpersonal psychotherapy with CBT and found broadly similar outcomes in patients with depression. Studies examining the efficacy of STPPs compared with CBT in the treatment of depression were reviewed by Leichsenring (2001). The six studies selected for review had used treatment manuals and structured monitoring procedures. These included five different short-term psychodynamic therapies (as developed by Horowitz and Kaltreider, Mann, Rose and Del Maestro, Shapiro and Firth, and IPT by Klerman and Weissman). Although these short-term psychodynamic therapies did have some technical and conceptual differences, they were all based on the general principles of psychodynamic theory. All had features in common, particularly a focus on interpersonal conflicts relevant to the depression and the patients' here-and-now experience. As some researchers would argue against interpersonal therapy being included as a psychodynamic therapy, the results were also assessed excluding IPT. The remaining STPPs were found to be as effective as CBT in the treatment of depression. However, it was emphasised that more research is needed to develop a good evidence base for STPPs in the management of depression.

Interpersonal psychotherapy

IPT has been tested in clinical trials for depression and subsequently modified for the longer-term treatment of depression, for different age groups, and for other psychiatric disorders, including bulimia nervosa, drug dependence, dysthymia, and marital problems (Klerman and Weissman 1993).

The first major, large-scale comparative trial of IPT in the treatment of acute depression was the New Haven–Boston Collaborative study (Weissman et al. 1979). This group found IPT was superior to non-scheduled treatment and equivalent to amitriptyline in the short-term treatment of depression. The combination of IPT with amitriptyline was better than either alone, although this was a non-significant trend. Combination treatment was also more acceptable and better tolerated by patients. In the NIMH Treatment of Depression Study conducted by Elkin and others, acutely depressed patients were randomly assigned to IPT, CBT, or imipramine and clinical management (Elkin et al. 1989). IPT was found to be superior to clinical management and equal to imipramine for mild to moderate depression. IPT was slightly more effective than CBT for severe depression (defined as a Hamilton score >20). The group found no long-term preventive effects for IPT, CBT or imipramine at 6, 12, or 18 months. In the early 1980s, Frank and Kupfer's group in Pittsburgh studied the efficacy of IPT as a maintenance treatment for depression (Frank et al. 1990). After an initial period of treatment with high-dose imipramine and sixteen 1-hour sessions of IPT, remitted patients were randomised to several treatment conditions, one of which included maintenance IPT (IPT-M). IPT-M was less effective than imipramine in reducing relapse rates. The combination of IPT-M and imipramine did not further reduce relapse, but IPT-M alone was superior to placebo treatment in delaying relapse.

Cognitive behaviour therapy

A substantial amount of research has been directed toward investigating cognitive-behavioural approaches to depression, with Beck's cognitive therapy (CT) (Beck et al. 1979) the modality most often studied. In general, CBT is as least as effective as medication in the treatment of unipolar depression (Rush et al. 1977; Hollon et al. 1992). Early studies reported that, compared with medication, CBT may have longer-lasting effects and decreased relapse rates; however, few of these studies were placebo-controlled trials and the adequacy of the medication treatment provided has been criticised (Hollon 1998). There is more recent evidence that CT may reduce relapse. At 12-month follow-up in the NIMH study, the relapse rates were 9 per cent for patients who received CT and 28 per cent for those who received antidepressants plus clinical management (Shea et al. 1992). Hollon and colleagues (1993) found that the relapse rates in the patients receiving CT were not significantly different from those in the continuation antidepressant treatment group. However, CT relapse rates were significantly less compared with those patients whose antidepressant medication was withdrawn at the time their depression remitted. Thus, CBT may have effects beyond the end of a course of treatment.

More recently, there has been considerable debate about the comparative efficacy of CBT and medication for severe depression. The recent large Treatment for Depression Collaborative Research Program found evidence that CBT was less effective than drugs for more severely depressed outpatients, and that overall CBT faired less well than interpersonal psychotherapy (Elkin et al. 1989). There has been considerable debate about the robustness of these findings, which are inconsistent with previous research (Elkin et al. 1996; Jacobson and Hollon 1996). Without replication, definitive conclusions cannot yet be made.

Overall, while a solid evidence base has still to be developed for short-term psychodynamic psychotherapy, there is now substantial evidence supporting the efficacy of both CBT and IPT in the treatment of depression.

PRACTICAL TREATMENT STRATEGIES

Psychodynamic psychotherapy

If psychodynamic therapy is being considered in the treatment of depression, then the more recently developed short-term psychodynamic therapies would appear to be most appropriate (that is, five to forty sessions).

Although there are various models for psychodynamic psychotherapy, common elements are identifiable across therapies. In the assessment phase, the therapist listens carefully and empathetically to the patient's story, building a working alliance with the patient and developing a picture of the interpersonal or developmental context within which the depression began. A key strategy is to help the patient gain insight into these issues to make changes. The therapist is active and uses techniques such as clarification, confrontation and interpretation.

Crucial to the psychodynamic approach is the use of the transferential relationship developed between the therapist and the patient. Within this current relationship, significant issues from the patient's past key relationships are recreated. The patient begins to understand the present with reference to past experiences and relationships.

The therapist attends to any unrealistic responses by the patient that may reflect, for example, previous losses, abandonment, or strivings for nurturance and praise. Through interpretation, the patient gains insight into current maladaptive thoughts and behaviours.

The therapist is also aware of his or her own feelings provoked by the patient, such as helplessness, hopelessness, anger and despair, and is able to process this countertransference as a reflection of what the patient is experiencing. Often this also helps the therapist understand what the patient's loved ones or carers are experiencing (Gabbard 1994). Overall, the patient is helped to understand his or her vulnerability to depression and loss of self-esteem and any maladaptive ways of gaining nurturance or praise, and to learn more positive ways of maintaining a good sense of self.

Interpersonal psychotherapy

IPT is a brief, time-limited psychotherapy developed and defined by Klerman and collaborators (1984). It makes no assumption about the origin of depressive symptoms, but uses the connection between the onset of symptoms and current interpersonal problems as a treatment focus. For depression, the framework of IPT is based on three phases. During the first phase, a detailed history of the depression, current social functioning and interpersonal relationships is obtained. This provides a formulation for the development of the depressive symptoms in an interpersonal context. In other words, the therapist is curious about how the individual relates to others, and psychopathology is defined as what is troubling about the person's relationship with others. The depressive syndrome is then linked to one or more of four interpersonal problem areas: grief, interpersonal role disputes, role transitions, and interpersonal deficits.

In the middle phase of IPT, the therapist addresses here-and-now issues within the chosen problem area. The explicit goal is to improve interpersonal functioning and, by linking this to mood, counter depressive symptoms. The therapist uses a wide variety of nonspecific techniques, including clarification, rephrasing, role play, communication analysis, and decision analysis. Patients tend to be seen for 50-minute sessions, weekly for 12–16 weeks of treatment, and monthly in maintenance IPT.

For *grief*, which is defined as loss through death, sessions focus on the loss and issues in the bereavement period, looking at both the symptoms and history of the environment where the death or loss was experienced. For *interpersonal role disputes*, when the patient and at least one other person have non-reciprocal expectations, the goals of IPT are to identify the dispute and help establish a plan of action by addressing the communication problems. *Role transitions* occur during life changes, for example, the change from full-time work to being unemployed or the change in role from being single to being married. Patients who present with problems in these areas are encouraged to give up the old role by evaluating it, encouraging affective expression and making the transition. Finally, *interpersonal deficits* is an area more difficult to target from an IPT perspective. An individual with deficits may well have a personality disorder, be a poor historian, and have few relationships and limited goals. In terms of treatment, the approach is less clearly defined, but basic techniques such as role play can be useful.

The third and final phase of IPT focuses on relapse prevention, and directly addresses termination, hence constructing the end of therapy as a useful positive model that can be generalised to other relationships. In summary, IPT helps patients to change rather than live with symptoms, and it works on here and now. Providing patients with the sick role clinically validates the depressive symptoms.

Cognitive behaviour therapy

Cognitive behaviour therapy for depression is a brief, present-oriented treatment in which the principle focus is solving current problems and modifying dysfunctional thinking. In CBT, the therapist helps the depressed person learn to identify, evaluate and modify unrealistic thinking and to make behavioural change through the use of both cognitive and behavioural techniques. Cognitive behaviour therapy requires a sound therapeutic alliance. The patient is encouraged to view therapy as an endeavour in which the therapist and patient are working together to overcome the depression. As Beck's cognitive therapy (CT) has received the most attention from researchers interested in CBT for depression, the format and general course of this therapy is described here.

CT begins with an assessment and cognitive case conceptualisation. This conceptualisation provides the framework for the therapist's understanding of the patient, guides therapy and continues to be refined as therapy progresses. The initial focus of therapy is to introduce the patient to the CT model and to establish rapport. The person's expectations and goals are discussed and some education is provided about depression, the cognitive model and the process of therapy. In early CT sessions, the therapist often uses behavioural change strategies to assist the individual to become more active. The therapist's goals during the early sessions are to help the patient select a problem or goal to focus on, to start solving problems and to begin to monitor automatic thoughts. Homework assignments specifically tailored to the patient are a central part of CT for depression. The goal of homework is to extend the opportunities for cognitive and behavioural change throughout the patient's week.

The format of later sessions is similar to earlier treatment. All sessions consist of a brief update and check on mood. An agenda is set for the current session, homework reviewed, discussion of agenda issues conducted and feedback elicited from the patient about the session. The content of the sessions varies according to the patient's problems and goals, and the therapist's goals. Although the therapist initially takes the lead in suggesting agenda items, assisting the patient to identify and monitor automatic thoughts and to develop homework assignments, there is a gradual shift in responsibility from the therapist to the patient for these tasks. As the sessions progress, there is a gradual increase in emphasis to automatic thoughts and underlying beliefs. Behaviour change techniques are used to assist the patient to test certain thoughts and practise new skills. A variety of cognitive and behavioural techniques, including imagery techniques, can be used during CT. The choice of technique depends on factors such as the stage of therapy and the content and goal of a specific session. In the final phases of therapy, there is another shift towards preparing for termination and relapse prevention. It is at this stage that the therapist and patient should discuss the possibility of maintenance sessions.

TREATMENT CONSIDERATIONS

Assessment

A thorough assessment of the patient with depression is not only vital, but often in itself is a reassurance to the patient. It is important to elicit depressive symptoms, any comorbid symptoms, the history of the illness and treatments received, the family history and the effect of the illness on the patient's life and relationships (see also Chapter 14). Alongside understanding the patient's personal and social background and personality style, the therapist needs to explore any issues that may have helped trigger this episode of depression or be contributing to the maintenance of depression.

The therapist is thus developing a picture of the severity and chronicity of the depression, any suicidal thinking, and factors contributing to why this patient might be presenting with a depressive illness at this time. Important also, but too often neglected, is the assessment of the personal strengths of the patient – for example, the positive role of work or relationships in the patient's life. Therapy then may work to build on the patient's pre-existing strengths, rather than concentrating on areas of weakness. Finally, a working case formulation relevant to the chosen psychotherapy needs to be developed, and this will act as a guide and focus for therapy.

Therapeutic alliance

The therapeutic relationship is considered an important ingredient of any psychotherapy. Indeed there is a mounting consensus that a good therapeutic alliance is related to a good outcome for the patient. At least four dimensions are interwoven in the complexity of the therapeutic relationship (Gaston 1990):

- the patient's bond to the therapist and commitment to therapy
- the patient's capacity to work purposefully in therapy
- the therapist's empathic understanding and involvement

- the agreement of the patient and therapist on the tasks and goals of therapy.

If a good therapeutic alliance can be developed early, this bodes for a good outcome. Therefore, it is vital that the therapist investigate and appropriately address a poor alliance or a rupture in the alliance during the progress of therapy.

Choosing a psychotherapy

As yet, there is no definitive evidence as to who does better with which therapy. Patients who appear motivated to change, have good ego strength and have the capacity to relate are likely to do better in any of the time-limited therapies, while those most severely disturbed are not likely to do well. Therefore, many patients may respond to any of the therapies described in this chapter. This may well be because of important common factors across all psychotherapies. These include the importance of the patient–therapist relationship, the expression of feelings and thoughts, self-examination and self-understanding, providing a rationale for the person's problems, strengthening the patient's hope and expectations of change, and encouraging mastery efforts.

Although therapy is effective, it must be remembered that it can also be harmful. The clinician needs to monitor the patient's progress and symptoms of depression and re-evaluate treatment if the patient's mood is deteriorating. For example, more intensive psychotherapy may be detrimental if the patient is severely depressed and engaging in excessive rumination or self-reflection.

Psychotherapy alone or with medication

Whether integrating psychotherapy with medication affords a greater advantage to patients than either alone is an emerging issue in the wake of the efficacy studies. The rationale for combining therapy and medication was that if both were effective then, as they use different techniques and target different mechanisms for change, perhaps both together may be additive. Historically, there has been some controversy over the simultaneous use of antidepressants and psychotherapy. This, in part, has been related to proposed interactions between medications and psychotherapy, and largely promoted by psychoanalysts. The contention was that the presence of medication leads to a state in which individuals are unable to access their deeper emotions and issues. This argument was used to support the avoidance of medication when conducting psychotherapy, but is in fact unfounded.

The practical question asked by clinicians is 'Will a combination of therapy give my patients a better outcome?'. There have now been at least four reviews of the combined approach, which cover thirteen separate articles. These reviews indicate that combined therapy is as effective as medication or psychotherapy alone, but may be superior to psychotherapy alone only in more severe recurrent depression (Thase 1997). So the costs of this approach cannot be routinely justified from the outset of treatment for most patients.

Recent studies suggest that it may be appropriate to have a sequential approach and integrate treatment for patients who fail to respond, partially respond, or have residual symptoms after treatment with either medication or psychotherapy alone. The rationale for integrating medication with psychotherapy after no or partial response to either alone has the following foundations. First, choosing only non- or partial responders will allow for better selection of patients who will benefit from the combined approach. Second, a sequential approach targets residual symptoms that contribute towards an increased risk of recurrence, rapid relapse and poor outcome (Judd et al. 1998). Finally, this approach avoids exposing patients to the potential side effects and extra cost of medication without extra benefit. Several groups have sequentially added cognitive therapy to medication after a partial response. This has led to a decrease in residual symptoms, higher rates of remission, lower rates of relapse and a specific improvement of social and psychological functioning in the group receiving sequential therapy (Paykel et al. 1999). Early results of sequentially adding medication to IPT have also shown higher remission rates in the sequentially treated group (Frank et al. 2000). It is still not clear which sequential approach is superior (that is, medication or psychotherapy first), and whether this is superior to augmenting or switching medication.

Maintenance

The recognition that depression is a chronic or relapsing disorder has led to the study of longer-term use of medication, now a recognised clinical approach. Investigation of longer-term use of psychotherapy, known as continuation or maintenance therapy, has lagged behind. The terms *continuation* and *maintenance* reflect an arbitrary cut-off point in time, usually 6 months of being symptom-free. Thus, acutely depressed patients who recover and remain in therapy are in continuation, and those who are still well after 6 months are considered to be in maintenance therapy.

There is mounting evidence that continuation CBT following acute treatment with the same therapy can reduce relapse rates and recurrences of depression (Jarrett et al. 2001), as can maintenance therapy following recovery with pharmacotherapy (Fava et al. 1998). The addition of CBT to antidepressant medication in patients who have made a partial response (that is, still have residual symptoms) has also been found to significantly reduce rates of relapse (Paykel et al. 1999; Scott et al. 2000). Likewise, continuation treatment with IPT, following acute treatment with medication and IPT, has been shown to decrease relapse and recurrence, or increase time to recurrence (Klerman et al. 1974), as has maintenance treatment (Frank et al. 1990).

The optimal length of continuation or maintenance treatments has not been clearly established; however, most researchers estimate that continuation therapy should carry on until 4–6 months after obtaining remission of the depressive symptoms (Thase 1990). As Fava and Junko (1994) have noted, there is much less agreement on the optimal duration of maintenance therapy, with some authors suggesting maintenance therapies from 1 year to indefinitely. In general, the more adverse the prognosis, the longer the maintenance therapy may need to be.

REFERENCES

Arieti S (1977) Psychotherapy of severe depression. *American Journal of Psychiatry* 134:864-8.

Barkham M, Rees A, Stiles WB, Shapiro DA, Agnew RM, Halstead J, et al. (1996) Outcomes of time-limited psychotherapy in applied settings: Replicating the Second Sheffield Psychotherapy Project. *Journal of Consulting and Clinical Psychology* 64:1079-85.

Beck AT (1963) Thinking and depression I. Idiosyncratic content and cognitive distortions. *Archives of General Psychiatry* 9:324-33.

Beck AT, Rush AJ, Shaw BF, Emery G (1979) *Cognitive Therapy of Depression.* New York: Guilford Press.

Bibring E (1953) The mechanism of depression. In Greenacre P (ed), *Affective Disorders.* New York: International Universities Press.

Dobson KS, Block L (1988) Historical and philosophical bases of the cognitive-behavioral therapies. In Dobson KS (ed), *Handbook of Cognitive-Behavioral Therapies.* New York: Guildford Press, pp. 3-38.

Elkin I, Gibbons RD, Shea MT, Shaw BF (1996) Science is not a trial (but it can sometimes be a tribulation). *Journal of Consulting and Clinical Psychology* 64:92-103.

Elkin I, Shea MT, Watkins JT, Imber SD, Sotsky SM, Collins JF, et al. (1989) National Institute of Mental Health Treatment of Depression Collaborative Research Program. General effectiveness of treatments. *Archives of General Psychiatry* 46:971-82.

Fava GA, Rafanelli C, Grandi S, Conti S, Belluardo P (1998) Prevention of recurrent depression with cognitive behavioral therapy: Preliminary findings. *Archives of General Psychiatry* 55:816-20.

Fava M, Junko K (1994) Continuation and maintenance treatment of major depressive disorder. *Psychiatric Annals* 24:281-90.

Frank E, Grochocinski VJ, Spanier CA, Buysse DJ, Cherry CR, Houck PR, et al. (2000) Interpersonal psychotherapy and antidepressant medication: Evaluation of a sequential treatment strategy in women with recurrent major depression. *Journal of Clinical Psychiatry* 61:51-7.

Frank E, Kupfer DJ, Perel JM, Cornes C, Jarrett DB, Mallinger AG, et al. (1990) Three-year outcomes for maintenance therapies in recurrent depression. *Archives of General Psychiatry* 47:1093-9.

Freud S (1917) Mourning and melancholia. In Strachey J (ed), *The Standard Edition of the Complete Psychological Works of Sigmund Freud*, Vol. 14. London: Hogarth Press, pp. 237-60.

Gabbard GO (1994) Affective disorders. In Gabbard GO (ed), *Psychodynamic Psychiatry in Clinical Practice*, The DSMIV Edition. Washington, DC: American Psychiatric Press Inc, pp. 219-49.

Gaston L (1990) The concept of the alliance and its role in psychotherapy: Theoretical and empirical considerations. *Psychotherapy: Theory, Research, Practice, Training* 27:143-53.

Hirschfeld RM, Keller MB, Panico S, Arons BS, Barlow D, Davidoff F, et al. (1997) The National Depressive and Manic–Depressive Association consensus statement on the undertreatment of depression. *JAMA* 277:333-40.

Hollon SD (1998) What is cognitive behavioural therapy and does it work? *Current Opinion in Neurobiology* 8:289-92.

Hollon SD, Shelton RC, Davis DD (1993) Cognitive therapy for depression: Conceptual issues and clinical efficacy. *Journal of Consulting and Clinical Psychology* 61:270-5.

Hollon SD, DeRubeis RJ, Evans MD, Wiemer MJ, Garvey MJ, Grove WM, et al. (1992) Cognitive therapy and pharmacotherapy for depression: Singly and in combination. *Archives of General Psychiatry* 49:774-81.

Jacobson E (1971) *Depression.* New York: International Universities Press.

Jacobson NS, Hollon SD (1996) Cognitive-behavior therapy versus pharmacotherapy:

Now that the jury's returned its verdict, it's time to present the rest of the evidence. *Journal of Consulting and Clinical Psychology* 64:74-80.

Jarrett RB, Kraft D, Doyle J, Foster BM, Eaves GG, Silver PC (2001) Preventing recurrent depression using cognitive therapy with and without a continuation phase: A randomized clinical trial. *Archives of General Psychiatry* 58:381-8.

Judd LL, Akiskal HS, Maser JD, Zeller PJ, Endicott J, Coryell W, et al. (1998) Major depressive disorder: A prospective study of residual subthreshold depressive symptoms as predictor of rapid relapse. *Journal of Affective Disorders* 50:97-108.

Karasu TB (1990a) Toward a clinical model of psychotherapy for depression, I: Systematic comparison of three psychotherapies. *American Journal of Psychiatry* 147:133-47.

—— (1990b) Toward a clinical model of psychotherapy for depression, II: An integrative and selective treatment approach. *American Journal of Psychiatry* 147:269-78.

Klein M (1934) A contribution to the psychogenesis of manic–depressive states. In *Contributions to Psycho-Analysis*. London: Hogarth Press and Institute of Psycho-Analysis, pp. 1921-45.

Klerman GL, Weissman MM (1993) *New Applications of Interpersonal Psychotherapy*. Washington: American Psychiatric Press.

Klerman GL, Weissman MM, Rounsaville BJ, Chevron ES (1984) *Interpersonal Psychotherapy for Depression*. New York: Basic Books.

Klerman GL, DiMascio A, Weissman MM, Prusoff B, Paykel ES (1974) Treatment of depression by drugs and psychotherapy. *American Journal of Psychiatry* 131:186-91.

Leichsenring F (2001) Comparative effects of short-term psychodynamic psychotherapy and cognitive–behavioral therapy in depression: A meta-analytic approach. *Clinical Psychology Review* 21:401-19.

Luborsky L, Diguer L, Luborsky E, Schmidt K (1999) The efficacy of dynamic versus other psychotherapies. In Janowsky DS (ed), *Psychotherapy. Indications and outcomes*. Washington, DC: American Psychiatric Press, pp. 3-23.

Paykel ES, Scott J, Teasdale JD, Johnson AL, Garland A, Moore R, et al. (1999) Prevention of relapse in residual depression by cognitive therapy: A controlled trial. *Archives of General Psychiatry* 56:829-35.

Rush AJ, Beck AT, Kovacs M, Hollon SD (1977) Comparative efficacy of cognitive therapy and pharmacotherapy in the treatment of depressed outpatients. *Cognitive Therapy and Research* 1:17-37.

Scott J, Teasdale JD, Paykel ES, Johnson AL, Abbott R, Hayhurst H, et al. (2000) Effects of cognitive therapy on psychological symptoms and social functioning in residual depression. *British Journal of Psychiatry* 177:440-6.

Shea MT, Elkin I, Imber SD, Sotsky SM, Watkins JT, Collins JF, et al. (1992) Course of depressive symptoms over follow-up. Findings from the National Institute of Mental Health Treatment of Depression Collaborative Research Program. *Archives of General Psychiatry* 49:782-7.

Thase ME (1990) Relapse and recurrence in unipolar major depression: Short-term and long-term approaches. *Journal of Clinical Psychiatry* 51 Suppl:51-7.

—— (1997) Integrating psychotherapy and pharmacotherapy for treatment of major depressive disorder. Current status and future considerations. *Journal of Psychotherapy Practice and Research* 6:300-6.

Weissman MM, Prusoff BA, DiMascio A (1979) The efficacy of drugs and psychotherapy in the treatment of acute depressive episodes. *American Journal of Psychiatry* 136:555-8.

CHAPTER 21

PSYCHOLOGICAL THERAPIES FOR BIPOLAR DISORDER

Suzanne E Luty
and Janet D Carter

Accumulating evidence has confirmed that psychosocial factors, such as stressful life events, the quality of the family relationship and social supports, all affect the course of bipolar disorder. Moreover, for a large proportion of people, bipolar disorder is associated with significant psychosocial impairment, even when asymptomatic. This has led therapists to explore the role of psychotherapy in the treatment of this illness. The focus on psychotherapy represents a shift from the traditional view that treatment should be biological, as bipolar disorder is strongly biologically determined. Several studies also suggest that chronobiological factors play an important role in relapse. Many of these factors, such as disruption in sleep–wake cycles and stabilising social cues (activity), can be focused on in psychosocial interventions.

When used in combination with medication, psychotherapy for bipolar disorder can address many issues. These include being able to come to terms with the knowledge that the disorder is chronic with a high risk of relapse, understanding the factors that precipitate relapse in order to learn how to modify these, dealing with real and perceived stigmatisation, and accepting a long-term treatment plan that may involve the unpleasant side effects of and compliance with medication. Episodes of depression or mania can also have a strong effect on interpersonal functioning, such as difficulties with social networks, relationship complications, and problems with career pathway or job, which again can be a target in psychotherapy.

GENERAL PSYCHOTHERAPY CONSIDERATIONS

There is a range of general issues with regard to conducting psychotherapy with a patient with bipolar disorder. Many of these centre on the importance of developing a good therapeutic alliance. Owing to the nature of the presenting symptoms of bipolar disorder, it is often more difficult to work with the patient because of mood instability or lack of insight. The therapist can experience a sense of fragility in the working relationship, and undergo strong countertransference reactions against the patient, such as feeling frustrated or overly concerned. Thus, the therapist must learn to control his or her responses (for example, judgmental or paternalistic responses). In addition, non-attendance is common and must be addressed.

Another difficulty therapists face when treating patients with bipolar disorder is how to take into account the stage of the illness when considering the beginning of therapy. In general, patients can present in a variety of different mood states, ranging from euthymia to being acutely unwell with mania or depression, and most often between episodes with residual symptoms. Before beginning psychotherapy, it is important to be clear about the stage of the illness that the patient is experiencing, as the approach may differ for different mood states.

The maintenance phase of psychotherapy of bipolar disorder, defined as the addition of a discrete course of psychotherapy to an already established mood stabilisation regimen such as lithium or sodium valproate, is the most common stage for psychotherapeutic interventions (Perry et al. 1999; Frank et al. 2000).

Psychotherapy is generally not recommended when a patient is acutely manic. At this stage, the therapist's stance is to help the patent maintain a focus and to be crisis-oriented (for example, resolving ambivalence about taking medication). For acute bipolar depression, a focused psychotherapy instead of additional antidepressant pharmacotherapy allows the therapist to avoid medication side effects and minimise the risk of antidepressant-induced mania or rapid cycling.

Patients with bipolar disorder often suffer from additional comorbid disorders, including most common anxiety disorders, substance use disorders and personality disorders (Akiskal et al. 1983; Regier et al. 1990). Each of these comorbid disorders has particular consequences for the patient and increases the overall psychosocial vulnerability of the patient with bipolar disorder. The therapist working with a patient with bipolar disorder should be able to address issues of comorbidity.

DESCRIPTION OF PSYCHOTHERAPY

Psychoeducation

Psychoeducation is a therapy model that uses a practical approach towards understanding the consequences of bipolar disorder. The various psychoeducation packages that have been developed contain common elements. Therapists teach the patient about the disorder by sharing and discussing information in an open, non-judgmental forum. The session focus is on the illness itself, medication and its side effects, course of illness, and obstacles to recovery. Worries about the future are addressed, and written material can be incorporated. Sessions also include in-depth education about the risk factors of bipolar disorder, and how to manage them, including the recognition of early symptoms and the prevention of relapses. The patient is thus regarded as an active collaborator in the therapy, and learns to manage his or her illness. The content of sessions can vary depending on the symptoms present, and issues are discussed with the patient as and when it seems fit. Session length and frequency vary according to the stage of the illness and patient needs.

Interpersonal social rhythm therapy

This therapy is a promising new therapy that has only recently emerged as potentially helpful for patients with bipolar disorder. Ellen Frank and colleagues developed interpersonal social rhythm therapy (IPSRT) from interpersonal psychotherapy (IPT) for depression. This modified form of IPT was strongly influenced by the instability model of bipolar disorder proposed by Goodwin and Jamison (Ehlers et al. 1988). Briefly, this model suggests that psychosocial factors such as stressful life events or interpersonal problems interact with an underlying defect in the circadian pacemaker, which in turn leads to the recurrence of symptoms. The use of a self-monitoring program helps patients initiate and maintain a lifestyle characterised by more regular sleep–wake cycles, meal times, and other *social zeitgebers*. The ultimate goal is to help patients regulate circadian disturbances that may provoke or exaggerate episodes of mood disorder. The therapy also makes links between the active symptoms of bipolar disorder and interpersonal functioning. IPSRT therefore aims to regulate the patient's social rhythms and sleep–wake cycles and to work on interpersonal issues.

There are three stages to IPSRT. In the first stage, much like IPT for depression, the patient is educated about the disorder, and a history of the illness is obtained, as well as a detailed history of the important people in the individual's life – the *interpersonal inventory*. An additional strategy in IPSRT, which is not used in IPT, is the initiation of the social rhythm matrix, where the patient provides a daily written record of his/her social rhythms, including sleep and wake times, meal times, contact with others, and activity levels. The patient and therapist identify imbalances in routines that may be contributing to changes in mood states. Once identified, these are targeted to achieve optimal balance. During the middle phase of therapy, the therapist and patient work together on an identified interpersonal problem area much the same as with IPT for depression. One of four problem areas is chosen from interpersonal disputes, interpersonal role transitions, grief and interpersonal deficits. Unlike the problem area *grief* in IPT for depression, which solely addresses loss by death, the grief of the *lost healthy self* in bipolar disorder is considered an additional issue in IPSRT, as many patients experience a sense of loss of life direction and goals. The social rhythm matrix is reviewed regularly to identify ongoing areas of rhythm disruption, and attempts are made to regulate and balance these by linking them to mood changes.

In the final phase of therapy, the therapist and patient work together to anticipate termination and identify any future stressors, while still actively working on the interpersonal problem area and social rhythm matrix. In contrast to IPT for unipolar depression, the course of IPSRT is over a long period. Sessions tend to be weekly at first then stretch to monthly, with follow-up over at least a whole year (Frank et al. 2000).

Cognitive behaviour therapy

A variety of cognitive-behavioural therapies have been developed for bipolar disorder. Their common goals are to:

- improve the quality of life
- decrease the number and severity of episode
- increase adherence to pharmacological treatment
- enhance psychosocial functioning.

The specific targets of therapy include psychoeducation, medication compliance, teaching cognitive and behavioural skills to cope with prodromes, establishing routines with diet and sleep, and dealing with long-term vulnerabilities. The most effective length and course of therapy has yet to be investigated; current studies typically deliver treatment weekly for about 20 weeks, followed by monthly sessions for at least 6 months. Various texts provide comprehensive guides to the concepts, methods and practice of cognitive behaviour therapy (CBT) in bipolar disorder (Basco and Rush 1996; Lam et al. 1999; Newman et al. 2000).

In the Lam et al. approach, therapy consists of twenty sessions, typically twice weekly and becoming fortnightly as therapy progresses. As in CBT with unipolar depression, a collaborative relationship is an essential element of CBT with bipolar disorder, particularly the importance of a shared responsibility for the therapy focus. There are three phases to cognitive behaviour therapy developed by Lam et al. (1999).

In phase one (sessions 1–5) the focus is on education about mania, depression, the role of CBT, and medication. During the initial phase, a detailed assessment of symptoms and the life history is conducted. The rationale for CBT with bipolar disorder is discussed and the diathesis–stress model is described, in which manic depression is viewed as the result of a combination of genetic predisposition and environmental effects. In addition, the contribution of thoughts and behaviour to functioning is discussed. As a detailed history of symptoms is obtained, the therapist and patient develop a comprehensive list of early warning signs. Patients are asked to monitor activities, mood and thoughts, as well as medication compliance. Homework between sessions is used to assist with optimising treatment outcome. During the initial sessions, the focus is on eliciting the patient's own goals. These goals are returned to and expanded on during phase one and inform the course of therapy. The focus of CBT is on achieving important goals in spite of particular symptoms, rather than always having a strategy of withdrawal or avoidance.

Phase two is the active phase of treatment (session 5–16). The aim of sessions during the second phase is to assist patients to have an understanding of their own specific warning signs for early onset of depression and mania or hypomania. In addition, the patient is assisted to develop strategies to use in response to the warning signs, with the aim of reducing relapse. There is more focus on specific cognitive and behavioural techniques during phase two. These include activity schedules, thought monitoring, thought challenging, behavioural experiments, and addressing underlying dysfunctional assumptions. Information gathered about early warning signs from the symptom history and over the course of treatment is used to create an early warning sign profile, with specific treatment strategies developed that are most likely to alleviate symptoms. Medication compliance continues to be a focus of treatment in most sessions. The patient's experience and feelings about taking medication are elicited, and verbal and written information is provided about medication, including side effects. The costs and benefits of compliance and noncompliance are discussed.

In phase three (sessions 16–20), the focus is on continuing to practise previously learnt techniques. Potential and actual problems are identified. The focus is on reviewing the patient's use of cognitive-behavioural strategies learned earlier in treatment. The importance of routine, diet and sleep is emphasised and the risk of excessive stimulation, substance use or abuse discussed. The consequences of bipolar disorder in the patient's life and the associated issues such as stigma, guilt and grief are also focused on during the third phase.

Family therapies

Family therapy is based on the premise that marital and interpersonal relationships are problematic for bipolar patients, and that the stresses in these relationships can lead to relapse. High expressed emotion characterised by criticism, hostility, rejection, or emotional over-involvement is recognised as playing a particularly important role in relapse. Therapy with families trains the family unit to improve communication skills and re-establish functional relationships. One specific therapy, family-focused therapy, has three defined stages (Miklowitz and Goldstein 1997). In stage one, the initial assessment consists of a structured family interview for expressed emotion, and seven sessions of psychoeducation. In the second stage, which lasts at least seven sessions, the focus is on training in communication enhancement. The final stage concentrates on teaching problem-solving skills to help the family plan ahead for how to deal with issues in the future. Another family intervention model, inpatient family intervention, focuses on coping with hospitalisation, improving functioning, learning to modify unhelpful coping patterns, and identifying stressors within and outside the family (Glick et al. 1985). All types of family therapy acknowledge that the family unit structure and roles are different for a young patient still living at home with the family of origin, compared with an older patient with a spouse and children. Clearly, this approach to the treatment of bipolar disorder relies on the presence and willingness of other family members to participate, so is not suitable in many instances.

RESEARCH CONSIDERATIONS

Overall, the research in this area has been neglected. Of the different psychotherapies for bipolar disorder that have been studied, the commonest include psychoeducation, interpersonal social rhythms therapy, CBT, and family therapy.

The limited research available until recently has had methodological limitations, the most common problems being the small size of the samples studied, and difficulty in defining outcome variables. In general, there is an urgent need for randomised controlled trials.

Psychoeducation

Psychoeducation has been used successfully in other chronic medical illnesses, for example diabetes, to help decrease the impact of the illness. A similar educative approach has been used to help patients develop an understanding of bipolar disorder. Several small studies have examined the effect of psychoeducation on the course of bipolar disorder, although there has been very little long-term follow-up. When compared with standard care, specific psychoeducation has been shown to improve medication compliance in most studies. Psychoeducation also reduces the risk of manic relapse, improves social and vocational functioning, decreases the number of manic episodes and depressive episodes, and decreases hospitalisation (Perry et al. 1999). Similarly, a family-based psychoeducation has been shown to improve outcomes for female (but not male) patients, enhance treatment adherence, and improve global functioning (Haas et al. 1988). The length and type of psychoeducation packages vary for all studies, so it is hard to make definitive comparisons.

Family therapy

Several family therapy interventions have been developed and researched for use with bipolar disorder, and all studies suggest that this approach is efficacious. Family-focused treatment was developed for patients who have recently had an episode of mania or depression (Miklowitz et al. 2000). This therapy uses the combination of communication skills training and problem-solving skills training in addition to psychoeducation, and has shown a substantial decrease in depressive relapse rates when compared with a treatment-as-usual control condition. Other studies of family therapy, such as inpatient family intervention, have shown similar outcomes, with improved overall functioning and better medication adherence at outcome. Most studies of family therapy have included a control group, which has strengthened the results obtained.

Cognitive behaviour therapy

Despite clinical interest, researchers have only recently begun to investigate the utility of CBT in bipolar disorder. To date, most studies have been clinical descriptions or small open pilot studies. In all cases, CBT is seen as an adjunct to mood stabilisers. These preliminary studies suggest that adding a CBT approach to standard medication treatment may help increase medication compliance, reduce hospitalisations, improve psychosocial functioning, and reduce depressive symptoms (Cochran 1984; Palmer et al. 1995; Zaretsky et al. 1999; Patelis-Siotis et al. 2001; Scott et al. 2001). There is also evidence that CBT may promote better coping strategies for bipolar prodromes (Lam et al. 2000) and improve longer-term outcome (Scott et al. 2001).

Lam et al. (2003) have conducted the first randomised controlled trial of CBT in a group of 103 patients with bipolar I who were experiencing frequent relapses. These researchers compared modified cognitive therapy (CT), specifically designed to prevent relapses and promote social functioning, plus mood stabilisers, to mood stabilisers alone. All patients received regular psychiatric follow-up. CT consisted of twelve to eighteen sessions within the first 6 months, followed by two booster sessions within the following 6 months. During the 12-month treatment period, the CT group had significantly fewer and reduced length of bipolar episodes and number of admissions compared with the control group. The CT group also had higher functioning and better ability to cope with the manic prodromes by the end of treatment than the control group.

Overall, although further randomised controlled trials need to be conducted, studies to date support clinical observations that CBT approaches provide a useful tool in conjunction with mood stabilisers for the management of bipolar disorder.

Interpersonal and social rhythms therapy

Researchers have only recently begun to examine the effectiveness of IPSRT for bipolar disorder. IPSRT is clearly effective in stabilising routines, with significant increases in targeted lifestyle regularities. In addition, it has been shown to lead to a reduction of both depressive symptoms and manic or hypomanic symptoms when compared with a clinical management plus pharmacotherapy control group. Preliminary results from ongoing follow-up over 2 years of maintenance IPSRT have shown patients have significantly more days of euthymia during IPSRT when compared with treatment as usual (Frank et al. 2000). Interestingly, a significant increase in relapse rates was evident after withdrawal of IPSRT once patients had been initially stabilised with IPSRT, suggesting the stability of therapy delivery is as important to patients (Frank et al. 1999).

CONCLUSION

Researchers and clinicians have become increasingly aware of the non-biological factors that play a role in the relapse and maintenance of mood episodes in bipolar disorder, and in poor psychosocial functioning even when well. The advent of psychotherapy for bipolar disorder has provided a range of new directions for therapists and patients in being able to collaboratively understand and manage this disabling illness. The research is promising and, although in its early stages, the current indications are that psychotherapy represents a valuable adjunctive treatment for managing the symptoms of bipolar disorder and can contribute towards improving functional outcome.

REFERENCES

Akiskal HS, Hirschfeld RMA, Yerevanian BI (1983) The relationship of personality to affective disorders: A critical review. *Archives of General Psychiatry* 40:801-10.

Basco M, Rush A (1996) *Cognitive-Behaviour Therapy for Bipolar Disorder*. New York: Guilford Press.

Cochran SD (1984) Preventing medical noncompliance in the outpatient treatment of bipolar affective disorders. *Journal of Consulting and Clinical Psychology* 52:873-8.

Ehlers CL, Frank E, Kupfer DJ (1988) Social zeitgebers and biological rhythms. A unified approach to understanding the etiology of depression. *Archives of General Psychiatry*. 45:948-52.

Frank E, Swartz HA, Kupfer DJ (2000) Interpersonal and social rhythm therapy: Managing the chaos of bipolar disorder. *Biological Psychiatry* 48:593-604.

Frank E, Swartz HA, Mallinger AG, Thase ME, Weaver EV, Kupfer DJ (1999) Adjunctive psychotherapy for bipolar disorder: Effects of changing treatment modality. *Journal of Abnormal Psychology* 108:579-87.

Glick ID, Clarkin JF, Spencer JH, Jr, Haas GL, Lewis AB, Peyser J, et al. (1985) A controlled evaluation of inpatient family intervention. I. Preliminary results of the six-month follow-up. *Archives of General Psychiatry* 42:882-6.

Haas GL, Glick ID, Clarkin JF, Spencer JH, Lewis AB, Peyser J, et al. (1988) Inpatient family intervention: A randomized clinical trial. II. Results at hospital discharge. *Archives of General Psychiatry* 45:217-24.

Lam D, Jones S, Hayward P, Bright J (1999) *Cognitive Therapy for Bipolar Disorder: A therapist's guide to concepts, methods and practice*. Chichester: John Wiley & Sons.

Lam DH, Bright J, Jones S, Hayward P, Schuck N, Chisholm D, et al. (2000) Cognitive therapy for bipolar illness – a pilot study of relapse prevention. *Cognitive Therapy and Research* 24:503-20.

Lam DH, Watkins ER, Hayward P, Bright J, Wright K, Kerr N, et al. (2003) A randomized controlled study of cognitive therapy for relapse prevention for bipolar affective disorder: Outcome of the first year. *Archives of General Psychiatry* 60:145-52.

Miklowitz DJ, Goldstein MJ (1997) *Bipolar Disorder: A family-focused treatment approach*. New York: Guilford Press.

Miklowitz DJ, Simoneau TL, George EL, Richards JA, Kalbag A, Sachs-Ericsson N, et al. (2000) Family-focused treatment of bipolar disorder: 1-year effects of a psychoeducational program in conjunction with pharmacotherapy. *Biological Psychiatry* 48:582-92.

Newman C, Leahy R, Beck A, Reilly-Harrington NA (2000) *Bipolar Disorder: A cognitive approach*. Washington: American Psychological Association.

Palmer A, Williams H, Gorsefield D, Adams M (1995) CBT in a group format for bipolar affective disorder. *Behavioural and Cognitive Psychotherapy* 23:153-68.

Patelis-Siotis I, Young LT, Robb JC, Marriott M, Bieling PJ, Cox LC, et al. (2001) Group cognitive behavioral therapy for bipolar disorder: A feasibility and effectiveness study. *Journal of Affective Disorders* 65:145-53.

Perry A, Tarrier N, Morriss R, McCarthy E, Limb K (1999) Randomised controlled trial of efficacy of teaching patients with bipolar disorder to identify early symptoms of relapse and obtain treatment. *BMJ* 318:149-53.

Regier DA, Farmer ME, Rae DS, Locke BZ, Keith SJ, Judd LL, et al. (1990) Comorbidity of mental disorders with alcohol and other drug abuse. Results from the Epidemiologic Catchment Area (ECA) Study. *JAMA* 264:2511-18.

Scott J, Garland A, Moorhead SRJ (2001) A pilot study of cognitive therapy in bipolar disorders. *Psychological Medicine* 31:459-67.

Zaretsky AE, Segal ZV, Gemar M (1999) Cognitive therapy for bipolar depression: A pilot study. *Canadian Journal of Psychiatry* 44:491-4.

CHAPTER 22

MENTAL HEALTH NURSING CARE FOR INDIVIDUALS EXPERIENCING MOOD DISORDERS

Marie T Crowe
and Jane E O'Malley

Mental health nursing practice is concerned with establishing psychotherapeutic relationships and providing facilitative support for people experiencing mood disturbances to manage their day-to-day experiences. Such care requires an understanding of the meaning that the individuals attribute to these experiences and interventions that assist the people to manage their lives in the context of their mood disturbances. The nursing approach emphasises the experience of the individual and the meanings informing that experience. These meanings and how they are signified become available through interpersonal and discursive contexts heavily influenced by culture and history. What is regarded as a mood disorder has a history and context that might be obscured by a psychiatric diagnosis that focuses on current symptomatology. The individual's experiences and his/her narratives of those experiences are important for the mental health nurse to explore in order to help the person understand what is going on.

An understanding of mental distress as situated and developed within a particular cultural context provides a frame of reference for understanding and responding to such people's distress. It provides an opportunity for considering the meaning of the distress within the psychotherapeutic relationship. Parker (1999) proposed that an effective psychotherapeutic relationship involves respect for the meaning the individual attaches to his or her experiences and attention to the contradictions within this. He suggests that, as people come to terms with their distress, there is often tension between different meanings at the same time. Kaye (1999) proposed that a psychotherapeutic role involves reconceptualising the individual's experience to facilitate the development of new meanings and possibilities. For mental health nurses, this involves responses that:

- enable the person to manage his or her life in the context of his or her mood disorder
- bring the person's attention to his or her beliefs and values about his or her self and subjectivity
- encourage the person to explore his or her view of the world from an alternative perspective
- prompt the emergence of new ways of construing experience and changed interpersonal attributes
- promote a questioning of the restraints imposed by cultural beliefs that have been taken for granted as facts or truth
- facilitate the development of self-narratives that acknowledge multiplicity and difference.

The following discussion of mood disorders focuses on the person's experience of the disorder and the nursing interventions that may assist the person at this time.

EXPERIENCES OF MOOD DISORDER

Mental health nursing care needs to focus on consumers' experiences and assisting them to manage these. The following extracts are from the authors' PhD research (Crowe 1998; O'Malley 2002) and reveal some aspects of consumers' experiences. The discussion that follows suggests possible nursing responses.

Making meaning

> My parents would say 'oh she's just depressed' and 'why don't you snap out of it'. I thought they were against me ... that they didn't understand or care about me. I thought that when they said things like that that they didn't really want to help me.

The language and terminology of mood disorders have permeated all aspects of contemporary life in Western cultures. As a consequence, people from all walks of life assume some knowledge. In particular, the term *depression* has pervaded ordinary everyday parlance. Although the language has crossed over to the wider community, there is still only a limited understanding of what constitutes mental disorder, and it is often assumed to be a failure of personal character. This view is derived from earlier historical understandings of mental disorder. The assumption of a character defect leads to the assumption that the person requires only strength of will to overcome what could be regarded as bad behaviour. This has the effect of a double burden for people experiencing a mood disorder – they have to manage not only the disorder itself but also the stigma associated with it. Mental health nurses need to ensure that they do not reinforce this discrimination.

NURSING APPROACH

- Explore the person's experiences of the mood disorder and the meaning that she or he has attached to these experiences.
- Explore the psychosocial precipitants or interpersonal difficulties that have contributed to the current episode.
- Reassure the person that what she or he is experiencing is consistent with other experiences of mood disorders, while acknowledging the uniqueness of this person's particular experiences of the disorder.
- Attempt to understand the experience and how it affects the patient's life.
- Discuss with the person and significant others how the mood disorder interferes with usual functioning and interpersonal relations.
- Provide education about the symptoms of the mood disorder, explain the biochemical and psychosocial causes of mood disorders, emphasise the need for pharmacological and psychosocial interventions, help the person identify psychosocial stressors that may precipitate a future episode and encourage him or her to monitor mood and identify potential signs of relapse.

Withdrawing

> I used to stay in bed all day. I never wanted to do anything. I'd take the children to school, get them their breakfast, get them out of the house, drop them to school and straight back home. I'd jump into bed and lay in bed all day long. I just used to think I wish I could get out of here.

Many people who experience depression in a unipolar or bipolar context describe the difficulties they have in maintaining their daily lifestyle. They often have very low energy and motivation and find that the smallest tasks can be very tiring. The desire to remain in bed could reflect a desire for refuge, confinement, protection and escape. This response could be seen as a loss of interest or motivation, but may also be understood as a retreat within boundaries that are considered safe. Although some people feel a desire to remain in bed, they also describe not being able to sleep. The person may describe this as a semi-wakeful experience where they lose all sense of time.

NURSING APPROACH

- Explore the person's need to withdraw and what this distance provides for the person (for example, a sense of safety, security, and certainty).
- Encourage the person to maintain minimal daily routines. Although these tasks may appear particularly onerous or pointless at first, it is useful to push the patient to engage in usual activities of daily living. When a person is depressed, everyday tasks seem insurmountable, and the nurse should assist the person to complete these (for example, hygiene) until they become more taken for granted. Depressed people may be able to complete only small tasks at a time, but nurses need to actively encourage these tasks despite the resistance they may encounter in the process. Patients are not able to make all decisions for themselves

because of the effects of their depressive symptoms, and need someone to act in their interests. The establishment of even small routines encourages participation in their social world and will eventually require less conscious energy to perform.

- Ensure that the person has adequate nutritional and fluid intake. This may require gentle but firm encouragement the person may be experiencing a lack of appetite and may even find food distasteful. Small amounts of easily digestible food at intervals throughout the day should be encouraged.
- Provide opportunities for the person to opt out of normal social expectations for periods throughout the day.

Feeling overwhelmed

> When I'm down like that I just can't do anything. I can't think straight. Everything seems to pile up around me and I just want to withdraw to my room. It's just horrible everyone else seems to know what they're doing. They know what to do but I can't seem to get myself organised.

A lack of motivation and a lack of energy can impede the patient's ability to do even the simplest of activities. Consequently, the patient may feel overwhelmed by what he or she has to do, and often the inability to act compounds existing problems.

Nursing approach

- Suggest that the person makes lists of things he or she thinks need to be done but is finding it difficult to attend to (for example, making bill payments, addressing work issues, attending to accommodation issues, child care arrangements, financial issues).
- Assist the person to identify the most pressing concern or thing that needs attention and write it down as a goal (for example, 'I need more money to pay bills' rather than 'I never have enough money').
- Help the person clarify the problem.
- Help the person write all the possible solutions he or she can think of. Do not dismiss anything as impractical or unobtainable at this stage. The person might want to talk to family and friends to help come up with suggestions.
- Help the person identify advantages and disadvantages to each possible solution.
- Help the person identify his or her own strengths and weaknesses.
- Assist the person to identify the solution that best fits his or her current situation.
- Encourage the person to identify the steps that need to be undertaken to reach this solution. Include things that need to be done, support needed from others, resources required, potential obstacles and a time frame for achieving the solution.

- Provide the opportunity for the person to rehearse any of the steps (for example, meeting with bank manager to discuss increasing the mortgage).
- Support the person to put the plan into action.
- Review the effectiveness of the solution and encourage the same process for addressing other concerns or problems.

Anxiety

> Sometimes I just can't sit still but I don't know what to do with myself. It's an awful feeling. I feel scared but I don't know what I'm scared about. I worry about things – about my husband, about my family. I can't get the thoughts out of my head. People tell me I don't need to worry but I can't stop myself. I don't want to do anything. I just wander around aimlessly. I can't sit still. I'm in and out.

Many people experience generalised anxiety during a depressive episode. Anxiety is an energy that often overwhelms the person and may not have a specific focus. It is an energy that can be conveyed interpersonally – the nurse may become aware of an anxious energy during interactions with the person even when the person is not discussing what she or he is worried about. The experience of anxiety can precipitate a hyper-alertness and tension that the person is unable to dissipate. It feels to the person as though she or he is under threat, but she or he may not know what the nature of the threat is or its source. The person's perceptual field is often restricted during these periods and she or he may have difficulty paying attention or taking in information. As well as experiencing emotional distress, the person may also experience physiological distress: palpitations, tachycardia, shortness of breath, difficulty swallowing, twitching, fidgeting, tremors, nausea, diarrhoea, and sweating. Nursing approaches need to focus on helping the person dissipate the energy and manage her or his sense of impending threat.

NURSING APPROACH

- Assist the person to either dissipate or focus the anxious energy through exercise or relaxation techniques.
- Assist the person to attain a sense of control over her or his self and environment. This may involve activities that promote a sense of safety.
- Assist the person to identify situations or times when she or he is likely to experience anxiety.
- Encourage diversional activities to help distract the person from her or his worries.
- Assist the person to identify the early signs of anxiety and help the person promote a relaxation response through controlled breathing exercises and progressive muscular relaxation.

Sleep disturbance

> I just feel really tired all the time. I've got no energy. I feel like I'm dragging myself around. But then at night I can't sleep.

Sleep disturbance is often a key feature of a mood disorder. The person may experience difficulty getting to sleep, he or she may wake throughout the night, or may experience early morning wakening. Managing daily activities becomes even more difficult when the person becomes sleep-deprived. This often becomes a vicious cycle, with the person's tiredness and lack of energy contributing to the depression and the depression affecting the sleep pattern. It is important to help the person establish a regular sleep pattern to help him or her manage the other symptoms. The person may need medication to assist with re-establishing a regular sleep pattern, but there are other strategies that he or she could use.

NURSING APPROACH

- Assist the person to establish a regular routine before going to bed (for example, a shower, listening to music) and encourage the person to go to bed at the same time every night.
- Encourage the person to get up at the same time each day. Although he or she may have had little sleep or disturbed sleep, sleeping in may disrupt the sleep pattern further and make it difficult to get to sleep at night.
- Suggest that the person avoid alcohol, cigarettes and stimulants such as tea, coffee and caffeine-based drinks during the evening.
- Suggest a hot milk drink and a shower or bath before bed. Both these can be relaxing and the cooling down process following a bath or shower can aid sleep.
- Encourage the person to have an exercise routine, but, because exercising raises the metabolic rate, it is best avoided in the evening.
- Encourage the person to write down his or her concerns to avoid ruminating about them as he or she goes to sleep.
- Help the person create a comfortable, quiet and undisturbed sleeping environment.
- Suggest that if the person is unable to sleep after 30 minutes he or she should get up and do something relaxing, such as listening to music, until he or she feels sleepy.
- Encourage the person to use his or her bed only for sleeping.

Suicidality

> In hospital they watch you all the time and keep asking you if you are feeling safe. What's that supposed to mean? No one really cares how you are feeling. Then all of a sudden they say you can go on leave ... How come they suddenly decided I was safe? Why did they think I was OK then? When they did that I felt really scared ... really frightened of myself. First they were saying that I couldn't be trusted, that I was a danger to myself, and then it was like everything changed. I could go. They didn't care. It was too much. I ended up taking an overdose in my car in the carpark and I was thinking I'm not any better, nothing's changed, everything's just the same.

The *Diagnostic and Statistical Manual of Mental Disorders*, fourth edition, text revision, notes that completed suicide occurs in 10–15 per cent of individuals with bipolar I disorder. It is important to remember that during a period of acute depression the person's judgment and problem-solving skills will be impaired, and patients may act in ways that they would not normally. As a consequence, they may be overwhelmed by feelings of hopelessness and helplessness. They may not be able to see any future in which they can participate. They may perceive continuing to live as pointless and meaningless.

Talseth et al. (1999) found that, following an attempted suicide, people seek confirming behaviour from nurses, which includes attending to their basic needs, having time for the person, being with the person, listening to the person without prejudice, being open to the person, accepting the person's feelings and communicating hope. The instillation of hope and an orientation to the future requires skills that are subtle, unobtrusive and situated within a therapeutic relationship that acknowledges the person's despair (Cutcliffe and Herth 2002). Surviving a suicide attempt can elicit feelings of blame, anger, guilt, shame and stigma (Barlow and Morrison 2002) that need to be recognised and validated before moving towards more hope-instilling strategies.

NURSING APPROACH The first step in caring for someone who is suicidal is to assess her or his risk. This assessment should include:

- What is the current crisis? What precipitated it? How did the person come to the mental health services' attention? What stresses are present in the person's life?
- Has the person been involved in mental health services before? Has she or he had previous suicide attempts?
- If there was a suicide attempt, was there a note? What did the person understand would happen? What method did the person use and how lethal was it? How specific is the person's suicide plan?
- What plans does the person have for suicide? The potential and deterrents for this to occur? What level of impulsivity does the person have and has this been affected by intoxication, delirium, drug withdrawal, or brain damage?
- How has the person been functioning – mood, sleep, appetite, energy, motivation, concentration, memory, irritability, ability to enjoy her- or himself?
- What is the person's current mental status – appearance, rapport, behaviour, affect, thought form and content, perception, cognition and insight?
- Does the person have other psychiatric symptoms – anxiety, panic, obsessions, hallucinations, delusions?
- Does the person have significant physical impairment? Is she or he taking medication?
- Does the person misuse alcohol and drugs – frequency, amount, types and duration? Was she or he intoxicated at the time of the attempt?

- Is there past psychiatric history in the family?
- What is the person's usual temperament and personality? Has she or he experienced traumatic events in the past?
- What is the person's current social situation – living situation, employment, financial status, social supports, involvement with social agencies?

The initial assessment of the extent of suicidality needs to be repeated regularly because the person's thoughts about suicide may fluctuate.

All interventions need to focus on safety, an effective therapeutic relationship and treatment of mental distress.

Those caring for the suicidal person need to be given all the information about the suicide attempt, the person's current mental status, medication and how to ensure the person is not easily able to access a potential overdose. The environment into which the person is going needs to limit the person's access to hazardous or lethal situations.

If the person is to be cared for at home or with family or friends, the carers need to be comfortable in setting boundaries for the suicidal person, able to provide the necessary level of supervision and know what to do if changes in the person's mental state occur. The carers need to know how to access professional help on a 24-hour basis and when they can expect further contact from mental health services. If an inpatient admission is necessary, the nurse needs to instigate safety checks of the person and her or his environment in conjunction with regular assessment of mental state and level of suicidality. Treatment of mental distress should be the primary focus of an inpatient admission.

Most people who have made suicide attempts will be put on an observation level – on a continuum from within reach, same room and in sight, through to frequent observation (5 minutes to 30 minutes) (New Zealand Ministry of Health 1993). Such observations need to be carried out with respect to the person's rights and need to be in the context of a therapeutic relationship (Horsfall and Cleary 2000).

Regular assessment and review of the treatment plan is important. The nurse needs to be aware of signs that the person's level of suicidality has increased or is fluctuating. Signs to be aware of include increased agitation or distress, marked behavioural change (becoming calm suddenly), expression of intent, becoming increasingly withdrawn, an increased sense of hopelessness and the occurrence of further stressors. This assessment of safety and mental status needs to be carried out in the context of a therapeutic relationship. It is less likely that the nurse will be able to make such an assessment without the establishment of a therapeutic relationship. This is not an easy task, however, as while the nurse may be trying to maintain the person's safety, the person may feel driven to continue attempting suicide. While nurses usually plan care in partnership with people for whom they are caring, the patient's safety has to take priority and it may not be possible to negotiate a course of action. The nurses may need to assume control of the situation but also have to keep the person informed of the reasons for decisions and explain that the nurses need to take control until the person is better able to make her or his own decisions.

The nurse should explore with the person what activities the person can tolerate and what might help soothe or distract her or him from the distress. It may be useful to help the person identify usual strengths and skills and explore ways of using these. The person's social supports should also be involved, and it is useful for the nurse to identify who the person usually feels comfortable with or supported by and encourage the person to make contact with those people. The person will probably be experiencing shame and guilt and may have difficulty initiating such contact, so it may be useful for the nurse to make the initial contact and explain what has happened.

It is also important for nurses to reflect on their own attitudes to suicide and dying. This means being aware of how their own feelings and experiences may affect the care they are able to provide.

Contracting

> They asked me to sign a contract saying I would not kill myself. But that was all I wanted to do and it was all I could think about. It didn't seem very real because they were asking me to do something that if I could do I wouldn't be in hospital.

Some nurses use contracting as an intervention in managing the risk associated with the self-harming behaviour. These contracts identify what the person will do when he or she is distressed and what help he or she can expect. Krawitz and Watson (1999) have identified that some of the advantages of contracting are that it involves nurses and patients in a collaborative process, which may assist with patients feeling more empowered and more in control; it outlines expectations and responsibilities for both parties; and it provides structure, predictability and a reality base from which patients can manage their distress. Miller (1990) has identified potential disadvantages with contracting, which include that it may be an unduly restrictive process that inhibits emotional growth; the nurse may assume an overly parental role; and it may lead to a relaxation of nursing vigilance. It may be difficult for people who have been self-harming to demonstrate the necessary self-control to fulfil a contract when it is their lack of self-control that has brought them into mental health services.

NURSING APPROACH

- If a contract is to be used, the nurse needs to assess the person's ability and motivation to enter into the safety agreement.
- Any contract needs to be collaborative, and the nurse needs to resist compelling the person to enter into any agreement that he or she may be unable to keep.
- The contract needs to outline what the nurse expects the person to do when he or she is experiencing suicidal thoughts and what the person could expect from the nurse when this happens. The nurse needs to be careful about committing other nursing staff to actions which they may not agree with or have the resources to undertake.
- The contract needs to provide options for the person to use, rather than a single course of action.

- The contract needs to balance the person's ability to take responsibility (for example, informing others of his or her distress, taking him- or herself to a safe place) with options that promote empowerment while acknowledging the person's distress (for example, the person may use distraction techniques, self-soothing techniques or relaxation techniques). If these strategies do not alleviate distress, the nurse can be expected to assist the person by helping him or her with other options, including psychopharmacological ones.
- The contract and the person's ability to enter into such an agreement needs to be reviewed regularly.

Elevating

> I had a situation where I knew the nurse and I'd been bought in by the Police so I was obviously fairly elevated ... (at the hospital) they could see that I was in a fairly elevated state. Instead of locking me up straight away they let me have a bath and sort of calm down and they talked to me, you know sort of settled me down, the nurse brought me down to my room and he, sort of, sat and talked to me and said 'what have you been doing and what's been going on' and he spent I suppose about 20 minutes with me then it was time for a jab in the backside and lock the door and I didn't mind at all.

When people experience a manic or hypomanic episode, they are experiencing intense psychological and physiological activation. They usually experience an elevated or irritable mood accompanied by hyperactivity, flight of ideas, distractibility, pressured speech, inflated sense of abilities, and hypersexuality. They often become involved in senseless and risky activities.

The energy and sense of wellbeing experienced during periods of elevation may be highly enjoyable and can be a welcome respite if following a period of depression. The expression of hypomania is not severe enough to cause marked impairment in social and occupational functioning or to necessitate hospitalisation, and there are no psychotic features. During the hypomanic stage, the person may be reluctant to accept a change in environmental, emotional or occupational pace. The mood is cheerful and expansive, but may have an underlying irritability when the inevitable plans and ideas accompanying such an experience are thwarted. Although ideas may be free flowing and patients may perceive themselves as highly capable, their ability to be goal-directed may be compromised by a tendency to be easily distractible and over-stimulated. Because of their increased energy, people may become socially extroverted or hypersexual, leaving themselves vulnerable to behaviour that is out of character.

Mania may show as an intensification of the features experienced during hypomania or it may manifest spontaneously. Euphoria and marked elation coupled with volatility evident as irritability, anger and sadness are all features of the experience of mania. The person experiences a gradual loss of control as ideas, perception, communication and behaviour become fragmented and disorganised. This can be very distressing for the person and those who care about her or him. When people experience mania, their feelings of omnipotence, charm and general ability to act are often irritating or, worse still, threatening to significant others. Relationships may become strained as boundaries of reasonable behaviour are stretched. Past experiences serve to modulate the level of interpersonal difficulty and worry experienced by significant others in the events. In a ward environment, all patients need to feel safe. The nurses' role in mitigating the effect for patients experiencing mania and in managing the environment is important, and patients value nurses who manage disturbance.

Nursing people who experience episodes of mania entails a different focus in the acute phase from when people are relatively symptom-free. In the acute phase, the aim is to minimise the potentially damaging effects of mania: protect the person from harm to self and others; conserve energy; preserve interpersonal relationships and restore balance. During periods of stability, the therapeutic aim is to help the person develop self-awareness and a repertoire of strategies to manage mood shifts and contextual contributors. The strength of goodwill in the nurse–patient relationship will ensure its survival during challenging periods as the person, with support, tries out different strategies in the quest for self-determination.

Self-soothing

> They ran me a bath and gave me a candle in the bath and that was wonderfully therapeutic, a little bit of new age therapy. Some friends gave me some lavender oil and that was really nice, just something like that just purely for your physical senses.

With skill, the nurse can use soothing strategies to assist the person regain a measure of calmness and feel cared for.

NURSING APPROACH

- During periods of heightened elevation, provide a calm, low-stimulus environment to facilitate the person to rest. Assign a single room with simple decor, keep lighting and noise levels low and observe at least every 15 minutes.
- Assist the person to feel calm by modelling calm, consistent behaviour and clear communication.
- Ensure adequate nutritional and fluid intake. This may require direction and supervision if the person is unable to sit still long enough to complete the tasks of eating and drinking or if the person overindulges in fluids.
- Encourage the person to limit caffeine and nicotine intake near bedtime to prepare for sleep.
- Maintain a daily routine: establish a regular time for rising, bathing, eating, activity, rest, and retiring.
- Ensure that people are safe from exploitation and social embarrassment because of their behaviour. If people are unable to manage self-regulation of behaviour, protect them from others and others from them by offering a safe, quiet, alternative space.

- Provide clear, simple feedback and outline expectations. Assist the person to understand the effect on others of his/her behaviour that might be interpreted as intrusive, aggressive, exploitative, sexually inappropriate or frightening.
- Provide people with regular opportunities for appropriate levels of personal contact and physical activity, even during the acute phase when they may be elevated and aroused:neglect of the universal requirement for human contact and an outlet for unspent energy may increase the drive for stimulus that will defeat any structured low stimulus.
- As the person is able to cope with increasing levels of stimuli without becoming overly elevated, provide supervised periods of social, physical and intellectual activity.

Maintaining stability

When I get high I'm full of all this energy and all these ideas. I find lots of things funny and I laugh a lot but no one else seems to understand. I enjoy it for a while but it also scares me.

NURSING APPROACH

- Assist the person to recognise and identify the precursors to the development of mania: identify the environmental and interpersonal triggers and the patterns of change in social and biological rhythms that may herald the onset of mood elevation.
- Have the person identify factors that might exacerbate symptoms of elevation: use of alcohol, caffeine and nicotine; late nights; irregular food or fluid intake; everyday activities such as work, recreation, exercise or shopping that have in the past become excessive as activation increases.
- Acknowledge the heightened experience of energy and wellbeing during the hypomanic phase, while helping the person link the pleasures of hypomanic phase with the understandable temptation to delay early intervention or abandon carefully constructed advanced intervention plans.
- Have the person outline the risks associated with delaying intervention based on past experiences by helping link past acute episodes with consequences for mental health, interpersonal relationships and general functioning.
- Have the person identify effective past strategies and treatments: more careful attendance to circadian rhythms; sleep and other hygiene strategies; balanced and personally manageable patterns of exercise, diet and fluids; management of medications.
- Encourage the construction of an advanced directive (available from the New Zealand Health and Disability Commissioner: <http://www.hdc.org.nz>) to be used during periods of limited competence.
- Have the person identify a trusted family member, partner or close friend who can act as a gauge when early warning signs appear and who will act as an advocate during an acute episode.

CONCLUSION

Mental health nurses can assist individuals experiencing mood disorders in establishing new significance and meaning in their lives by developing their skills in:

- helping people maintain stable social rhythms in an attempt to promote mood stability
- helping people recognise their interpersonal styles that contribute to mood instability
- assisting individuals to recognise the symbolic meaning embedded in their language and behaviour and the role that language plays in constructing these experiences
- developing a discursive approach to mental health nursing practice, which involves an exploration of the sociocultural discourses that underpin the meanings that individuals attribute to their experiences
- accepting difference and promoting multiplicity in individuals' responses to their social world
- promoting social responsibility and connectedness with others as a form of resistance to cultural expectations that promote mental distress.

If mental health nurses recognise the multifaceted experience of mood disorders and the meanings each individual attributes to these experiences, they may be able to provide more client-centred nursing care.

REFERENCES

Barlow CA, Morrison H (2002) Survivors of suicide. Emerging counseling strategies. *Journal of Psychosocial and Mental Health Services* 40:28-39.

Crowe MT (1998) *Doing What No Normal Woman Would Do*. Brisbane: Griffith University.

Cutcliffe J, Herth K (2002) The concept of hope in nursing 2: Hope and mental health nursing. *British Journal of Nursing* 11:885-9.

Horsfall J, Cleary M (2000) Discourse analysis of an 'observation levels' nursing policy. *Journal of Advanced Nursing* 32:1291-7.

Kaye J (1999) Toward a non-regulative practice. In Parker I (ed), *Deconstructing Psychotherapy*. London: Sage.

Krawitz R, Watson C (1999) *Borderline Personality Disorder: Pathways to effective service delivery and clinical treatment options*. Wellington, NZ: Mental Health Commission.

Miller LJ (1990) The formal treatment contract in the inpatient management of borderline personality disorder. *Hospital and Community Psychiatry* 41:985-7.

New Zealand Ministry of Health (1993) *Guidelines on Management of Suicidal Patients*. Wellington, NZ: Ministry of Health.

O'Malley JE (2002) *Critical Social Analysis of Acute Institutionally Based Mental Health Nursing following an Action Research Project, Nursing and Midwifery*. Wellington, NZ: Victoria University.

Parker I (1999) Deconstruction and psychotherapy. In Parker I (ed), *Deconstructing Psychotherapy*. London: Sage.

Talseth A, Lindseth A, Jacobsson L, Norberg A (1999) The meaning of suicidal psychiatric in-patients' experiences of being cared for by mental health nurses. *Journal of Advanced Nursing* 29:1034-41.

SECTION

V

Comorbidity

CHAPTER 23

DEPRESSION AND PERSONALITY DISORDER

Roger T Mulder

Historically, many attempts at classifying depression have included personality variables. These have alluded to the possibility that personality pathology might predispose an individual to develop depression, might denote what form the depression may take, or might predict prognosis and treatment response. The best-known ancient system of psychiatric classification centred on temperament, and considered depressive symptoms largely as an epiphenomenon. Melancholic temperament was associated with individuals who were moody, pessimistic and vulnerable to episodes of depression, and believed to have an excess of black bile. Treatment attempted to restore the balance of black bile by techniques aimed at reducing the humour, including bleeding, vomiting and purging.

The idea that personality is intimately tied up with psychopathology is persistent. Kraepelin, Bleuler, Kretschmer and others tended to regard behavioural abnormalities as variations, or *formes früstes*, of the major psychiatric illnesses. For example, Kraepelin traced two premorbid personalities, claiming that a cyclothymic disposition inclined to manic–depressive insanity and an autistic temperament predisposed to dementia preacox. Kretschmer considered cycloids and cyclothymics as less severely affected variants of manic–depressive psychosis. Most psychoanalysts regarded personality abnormality as an inevitable part of the psychopathology associated with depression. Patients with depression were seen to have undue interpersonal dependency, obsessionality, poor frustration tolerance, and labile self-esteem (Hirschfeld et al. 1983).

In the 1950s and 1960s, the relationship between personality pathology and depression continued to play a major part in attempts to classify depression. A discussion point was differentiating between psychotic and neurotic depressions, or between endogenous and reactive depressions. Psychotic and endogenous depressions consisted of severe unremitting depression, usually with a clear onset and accompanied by retardation, guilt, diurnal variation of mood, severe insomnia, and weight loss. The neurotic or reactive depressions, in contrast, were considered a milder illness, often accompanied by anxiety, prone to fluctuate, and reactive to pleasurable stimuli. Endogenous depression was seen more as a disease process, whereas reactive depression was said to arise out of personality vulnerability, particularly when an individual was stressed.

Various authors attempted to use personality variables to help classify depression. Underlying these efforts was the hope that specific treatments could be found for different depression subtypes. Eysenck claimed that psychotic and neurotic depressions were directly related to his psychoticism and neuroticism dimensions (Eysenck 1970). Overall and his colleagues (1966) proposed three distinct profiles of depression, which they called *anxious depression*, *hostile depression* and *retarded depression*. Paykel and colleagues produced a typology with four categories, called *anxious depressives*, *hostile depressives*, *young depressives with personality disorder*, and a *psychotic cluster*, which corresponded to the traditional psychotic or endogenous subtypes. Paykel claimed some validation for these subtypes by showing a differential response to amitriptyline (Paykel 1972).

American authors also included personality measures as part of the classification of depression. Winokur and colleagues introduced the concept of *depressive spectrum disease*, which they based on the use of familial patterns of mood disorders to define subtypes of depressive disorders (Winokur 1985). Depressive spectrum disease is defined by the presence of alcoholism or antisocial personality disorder in first-degree relatives. In contrast, pure depressive disease is defined by the absence of these disorders. The hypothesis is that the presence and vulnerability to antisocial behaviour or alcoholism is a different type of depression from that suffered by individuals without this predisposition. These differences are claimed to influence treatment response in laboratory findings.

Akiskal identified a character spectrum disorder based on a patient's personality features and lack of depressive biological features, such as rapid eye movement (REM latency) and abnormal dexamethasone suppression test. Another subgroup, subaffective dysthymic disorders, was conceptualised as having secondary personality dysfunction. Akiskal considered that the primary problem is the underlying, largely genetically transmitted, mood disorder, and that personality disorders are the consequence of the mood disorder (Akiskal et al. 1983).

The third edition of the *Diagnostic and Statistical Manual of Mental Disorders* (DSM-III) separated depression and personality pathology into separate axes. DSM-III takes the view that depressive syndromes differ only in severity, rather than there being qualitatively different types. Although it acknowledges that major depression can develop in individuals with personality disorders, it suggests in these cases that two diagnoses should be made on two different axes: major depression on axis I and the appropriate personality disorder on axis II. Its view appears to be that there is no evidence of any particular association of personality and depression and simply describing each diagnosis is the best conceptualisation. This has led to most research being based on the assumption that the separation of axis I and axis II is valid. Although this has been convenient and stimulated research on the relationship between depression and personality disorder, it has largely ended classification systems incorporating personality into subtyping depression.

This chapter will review recent studies on the relationship between depression and personality. Such research is compromised by methodological factors that markedly affect results. The next section will, therefore, examine the ongoing conceptual and theoretical difficulties in studying the relationship between depression and personality. The second section will consider research within the different conceptual frameworks. The third section will summarise and relate the findings to clinical practice.

CONCEPTUAL ISSUES

The relationship between personality pathology and depression may be conceptualised in several ways. Three or four main ones have been proposed by a variety of researchers:

- The *vulnerability*, or *predisposition*, model. This model refers to the tendency for maladaptive personality traits, such as neuroticism or excessive interpersonal sensitivity, to predispose an individual to develop depression. Such an approach is popular in theory and research because it provides an aetiological explanation for depression.
- The *complication*, or *scar*, model. This model describes the development of, or exaggeration in, personality traits as a consequence of depression. This influence is believed to be important if the depression is chronic or of early onset.
- The *spectrum*, or *coaggregation*, model. This model implies that personality disorders and depression overlap phenomenologically and may reflect related vulnerabilities that are simultaneously expressed in the same person. Certain personality disorders may be viewed as *formes früstes* of depression and may result from a common aetiology.
- The *pathoplasty* model. This model emphasises the role of personality disorders in influencing the clinical presentation of depression, its course and, most commonly, its response to treatment. Much recent research has focused on this relationship because of its possible clinical utility.

These models are not mutually exclusive and there has been limited support for each of them at one time or another.

DEFINITION AND MEASUREMENT

There are at least four problems that need to be considered when reviewing studies on depression and personality disorders. First, there are differences in what is meant by personality disorder. This may be a high score on a personality questionnaire, for example, neuroticism or harm avoidance or, more commonly, a personality disorder in a specified category in a diagnostic system such as the *International Classification of Diseases*, tenth edition (ICD-10), or DSM-IV. Most recent studies have used DSM personality disorder categories, and increasingly this is assumed to be the most appropriate measure. Even within the DSM categories there are at least three different standardised interviews, as well as a variety of self-reports to measure them. This seems to matter: how personality disorders are measured significantly affects the rate and type of personality disorder (Zimmerman 1994). For example, Hunt and Andrews (1992) reported that outpatients have nine times the chance of having a personality disorder when diagnosed with the Personality Disorder Questionnaire than with the Personality Disorder Examination Interview.

Second, the validity of DSM personality disorder diagnoses themselves remains open to question. It is not convincingly demonstrated that the operational criteria are robust and valid. The current categories are based on committee consensus, historical precedent, and political argument and opinion. There is a high rate of overlap between personality disorders, and the distribution of symptoms appears to be dimensional and continuous rather than reflecting the ten categories proposed in DSM-IV.

Third, there is an effect of mood on personality disorder measurement. There is reasonable evidence that depressed patients' description of their habitual patterns and tendencies are biased by a negative cognitive set. Depressed people are more likely to endorse unflattering characteristics about themselves than is someone who is not depressed. Structured interviews allow an attempt to disentangle state and trait characteristics. Although some studies report little effect from mood state on results, most do not (Zimmerman 1994).

Fourth, the separation of personality disorders from other psychiatric disorders has enhanced their study. However, this separation is not based on solid evidence. The division appears artificial – the assumption that personality variables are stable and enduring while depressive symptoms are fluctuating and transient has been increasingly challenged.

PREVALENCE OF PERSONALITY DISORDERS IN PATIENTS WITH DEPRESSION

Descriptive studies have reported rates of personality disorder in patients in depression ranging from 9 to 88 per cent. Table 23.1 shows the rates of comorbid personality disorders reported in studies over the past 2 years. The rates vary between 43 and 64 per cent. These rates are similar to those in older studies that used structured interviews (Mulder 2002). It seems reasonable to state that comorbid personality pathology, however defined, is common in depressed patients and is, therefore, potentially important. The most common personality disorders appear to be avoidant, borderline and more variably paranoid and obsessive–compulsive personality disorders. The other personality disorders are generally reported as less common.

Table 23.1
Prevalence of personality disorders in patients with depression

Study	Patients	Instrument*	N	Prevalence
O'Leary and Costello (2001)	Depressed inpatients	Structured assessment of personality	100	43%
Fava et al. (2002)	Depressed outpatients	SCID-II	384	64%
Melartin et al. (2002)	Depressed outpatients and inpatients	SCID-II	269	44%
Brieger et al. (2003)	Depressed inpatients and outpatients	SCID-II	117	51%
Kool et al. (2003)	Depressed outpatients	Questionnaire on personality traits (self-report)	72	58%
Russell et al. (2003)	Depressed outpatients	SCID-II	635	46%
Mulder et al. (2003)	Depressed outpatients	SCID-II	183	45%

*Interview unless noted.

THE VULNERABILITY AND COMPLICATION MODELS

Understanding whether personality pathology may cause depression or be the result of it is difficult for various reasons. First, there is overlap between symptoms of depression and those associated with personality pathology, such as neuroticism, harm avoidance, and avoidant and dependent personality disorder traits. Secondly, the onset of depression is often early, so that in older samples personality pathology may be a mix of risk factors and scar effects from previous depression. Thirdly, most of the data are cross-sectional, reporting an association but with little evidence of causality either from personality to depression or vice-versa.

Assessment of personality before the first depressive episode would obviously be ideal, but requires a very large pool of subjects. One strategy to reduce the need for large numbers is to use high-risk subjects, such as relatives of sufferers. The National Institute of Mental Health psychobiology of depression study looked at 438 relatives of patients with depression who, themselves, had never suffered from a mental disorder. During the next 6 years, twenty-nine suffered their first episode of major depression. When these were compared with the 370 who remained symptom-free, some differences emerged. Those who developed depression were classified as being more neurotic, less emotionally stable and less resilient. However, this effect was confined to older adults, and the differences between subjects who had recovered from major depression and the symptom-free subjects were much smaller. The authors suggested this was due to a scarring effect of repeated major depression episodes and implied that the scar effect might be more significant than any aetiological predisposition (Hirschfeld et al. 1983).

Kendler et al. (1993) used a genetic epidemiological approach to look at the relationship between neuroticism and depression. They reported a strong association between neuroticism and depression, but their model suggested that this was largely mediated through genetic factors common to both traits, rather than a causal pathway. The causal pathway was in the opposite direction:

neuroticism was elevated in depressed subjects because of the effects of depression (via both scar and state). In a recent study, using the same twin registry, Kendler et al. (2002) attempted to construct a comprehensive model of depression. Neuroticism remained an important risk factor and was associated with high genetic risk for depression, as well as with low self-esteem and early onset anxiety disorders. After stressful life events, neuroticism was the strongest predictor of the risk of onset of depression.

One method to study a complication or scar model is by linking age of onset of depression with personality disturbance. Underlying this is the hypothesis that people with earlier onset will have more severe personality pathology, partially, at least, a scar or complication effect of their depressive symptomatology. Rothschild and Zimmerman (2002) recently addressed this and found that depressive episodes of longer duration were associated with an increase in personality disorder diagnoses. The DSM-IV chronic specifier for depression resulted in nearly a two-fold difference in the frequency of any personality disorder (48.6 compared with 28.7 per cent). Russell et al. (2003) also reported that, in chronically depressed patients, early age of onset (before 21 years) was associated with a significantly higher rate of axis II comorbidity, but only for cluster C personality disorders (47.1 compared with 31.9 per cent). Mulder et al. (2003) reported an increased rate of chronic depression in individuals with comorbid personality disorders.

In summary, there is clear evidence of a link between depression and personality pathology. At present, it appears that at least some of this association is explained by a complication or scar effect. Chronic and recurrent depression is associated with higher neuroticism scores and increased rates of personality disorders. Whether personality pathology is a risk factor for depression is less clear. High neuroticism scores appear to predate the onset of depression, although this may reflect common genetic factors rather than a causal pathway. Whether personality pathology conceptualised as personality disorders causes depression is to some degree unresolvable as, by the time a diagnosis of personality disorder can be assigned (at age 18 years), at least 25 per cent of individuals will already have suffered their first depressive episode (Sorenson et al. 1991).

THE SPECTRUM MODEL

The delineation of the phenomenological relationship between depression and personality disorder remains confounded by issues of symptom overlap, mood effects on measurement, and definitional issues. Despite this, recent studies continue to contribute to growing literature with some increasing consistency in findings.

One issue that is becoming clearer is that the assumption that personality dysfunction is pervasive and enduring whereas mood disorders are episodic disturbances is too simplistic. Considerable evidence now exists that many patients with chronic depression have reasonably stable symptoms, while so-called personality symptoms may change over quite short periods. This appears particularly relevant in patients undergoing treatment for depression. Fava et al. (2002) observed a significant reduction in the proportion of patients meeting criteria for avoidant, dependent, passive–aggressive, paranoid and narcissistic personality disorders, and also borderline, obsessive–compulsive and schizotypal traits, over an 8-week trial of fluoxetine. Griens et al. (2002) reported that measures of neuroticism, extraversion and interpersonal sensitivity significantly reduced over 12 weeks of treatment. Du et al. (2002) similarly noted a reversal of high neuroticism scores and low extraversion scores in patients who responded to fluoxetine. These results are consistent with earlier studies.

There are several plausible explanations for these findings. First, personality symptoms may be inherently unstable, and repeating measures will usually result in significant fluctuations. There is evidence to support this view. Seivewright et al. (2002) reported that the measure of agreement between baseline and 12-year personality disorder clusters was slight (κ = 0.14). However, Farabaugh et al. (2002), extending the Fava et al. (2002) study, reported that after the depression had been successfully treated, personality disorder diagnoses remained stable during continuation treatment. They suggested that a personality disorder diagnosis is apt to be unstable when made during a depression episode, but that stability returns once the depression is in remission.

The second explanation is that many so-called personality disorder symptoms are actually features of depression. These would particularly include some avoidant, borderline and dependent traits, as well as neuroticism scores. Treating the depression also causes the personality pathology to reduce. This is related to the third explanation, that such findings are simply an artefact created by depressed individuals over-endorsing negative personality features – which they stop doing when their mood improves. It is difficult to disentangle these reasons. There is consistent evidence that when depressed subjects are no longer depressed, their rates of personality disorder are lower, as are their neuroticism scores (Zimmerman 1994; Mulder 2002).

The fourth possible reason is that treatments for depression are effective in treating personality pathology. The reduction in personality pathology is not due to their overlap with depression symptoms but because there is a direct treatment effect. This is partially supported by the Fava et al. (2002) study, which showed no significant relationship between reduction in personality disorders and the degree of improvement in depression symptoms, leading them to suggest that antidepressant treatment may be accompanied by significant changes in behaviour and attitudes that are part of some personality disorders.

Whatever the explanation, and all may be partially true, it is becoming clear that depression and personality disorder are not simply comorbid independent disorders that happen to be commonly found together.

Another potentially useful way to disentangle depression and personality disorder is via biological measures: the hypothesis being that individuals with depression, personality disorder or both may be different from one another biologically. Abnormal sleep electroencephalogram (EEG) profiles are one of the most consistent abnormalities found in patients with depression. Egyptian workers compared EEG sleep profiles in twenty depressed subjects, twenty borderline subjects (with no comorbid depression) and twenty matched controls (Asaad et al. 2002). They reported highly similar sleep profiles in both patient groups compared with controls, and concluded that their findings suggested a common biological origin for depression and borderline personality disorder. Mulder and Joyce (2002) failed to find any differences in central nervous system serotonin measures in depressed patients with or without comorbid borderline or antisocial personality disorder, or in a variety of other behavioural measures. Biological measures, while limited to small samples and compromised measures, so far show little evidence that depression and personality disorder are separate disorders.

DEPRESSIVE PERSONALITY DISORDER

Mention should also be made about the ongoing debate over the place of depressive personality disorder. DSM-IV includes a provisional set of criteria placed in Appendix B. Depressive personality disorder reinforces the problems alluded to throughout this review, in that the argument revolves around the proper conceptualisation of chronic low to moderate grade depression. Should this be considered an axis I syndrome, an axis II personality disorder, or both? Ryder and Bagby (1999) led a special feature in the *Journal of Personality Disorders* and concluded the depressive personality disorder was not yet sufficiently validated for inclusion in the DSM. They have updated their work in an enlarged review, but with the same conclusion (Ryder et al. 2002). In doing this, they noted that their concerns could be applied to many axis II disorders, particularly as they relate to axis I conditions. This led them to suggest a dimensional reconceptualisation of axis II, placing depressive personality traits dimensionally, rather than as a discrete diagnostic entity. Not surprisingly, they consider that the traits associated with depressive personality disorder are high neuroticism and low extraversion, the same traits that are associated with depression.

THE PATHOPLASTY MODEL

There has been a regular flow of treatment trials in patients with depression which study predictors of outcome. It has been generally believed that patients with comorbid personality pathology have a worse outcome than patients without such difficulties. A recent review has challenged this, pointing out, yet again, that methodological issues may have led to bias (Mulder 2002). The best-designed trials, using structured interviews and randomising patients to treatment, report the least effect of personality disorders on depression treatment outcome. This suggests that comorbid personality pathology should not be seen as an impediment to good treatment response.

Recent studies have partially supported this view. Fava et al. (2002) reported that 64 per cent of 384 outpatients had at least one comorbid personality disorder, but there was no significant relationship between treatment outcome and meeting criteria for any personality disorder at baseline. Similarly, Mulder et al. (2003) reported that in 183 outpatients there was no overall effect on outcome from having a comorbid personality disorder.

Approaching the issue differently, Peterson et al. (2002) studied rigorously defined patients with treatment-resistant depression versus non-treatment-resistant depression, hypothesising that a greater prevalence of axis II conditions would be found in the treatment-resistant patients. They reported no difference in the prevalence of axis II disorders in the two groups. Russell et al. (2003) re-examined the clinical and psychosocial correlates of axis II diagnoses in the largest study yet published: 635 patients diagnosed with chronic major depression or double depression were randomised to 12 weeks of sertraline or imipramine. They reported the presence of axis II personality disorder comorbidity had minimal to no effect on the ability to achieve either an antidepressant response or remission, and had inconsistent effects on the time to response. Interestingly, the presence of axis II personality disorder comorbidity did not appear to reduce functional and quality-of-life improvements among patients responding to acute treatment with sertraline or imipramine.

In contrast, Viinämaki et al. (2002) reported that cluster C personality disorders impaired alleviation of symptoms in major depression, and Meyers et al. (2002) noted that in less depressed subjects, those who met criteria for personality dysfunction had a decreased likelihood of early recovery. O'Leary and Costello (2001) also reported the presence of personality disorder predicted longer times to remission onset, although this was found mainly in a small subgroup with two or more comorbid personality disorders.

Methodological issues again appear to be important. Studies that reported that comorbid personality disorders had no influence on outcome were largely randomised trials. Studies that reported a significant effect were naturalistic studies. Naturalistic studies are likely to introduce bias, as there is strong evidence that not controlling for treatment results in depressed patients with comorbid personality disorders receiving different and possibly less effective treatment. For example, Charney et al. (1981) reported that depressed people with a personality disorder were less likely to receive medication or electroconvulsive therapy, and Black et al. (1988) noted that only 29 per cent of depressed patients with a comorbid personality disorder received an adequate course of drug therapy, compared with 49 per cent of patients without a personality disorder. This potential methodological weakness in uncontrolled studies limits the value of their results. The conclusion that the best-designed studies continue to show the least effect of personality pathology on outcome appears to remain true.

The possibility that there are differential effects with antidepressants is also emerging. As Fava et al. (2002) pointed out, most of the early studies linking personality disorders to poorer outcome use tricyclic antidepressants (TCAs), while more recent studies have tended to use selective serotonin reuptake inhibitors (SSRIs). In their study, all patients were treated with fluoxetine, and although Russell et al. (2003) used sertraline and imipramine, most patients were treated with sertraline. An earlier study reported that the presence of cluster B personality disorder predicted a better response to fluoxetine in depressed outpatients (Fava et al. 1994). This is consistent with several small open studies that reported that borderline personality disorder symptoms respond poorly to TCAs but reasonably well to SSRIs (Mulder and Joyce 2002).

Mulder et al. (2003) looked at differential response. They reported that there was no overall effect of comorbid personality disorder on outcome, but that patients with a comorbid personality disorder did better with an SSRI than with a TCA. This difference was largely explained by the significantly better outcome for patients with a comorbid cluster B personality disorder if they received fluoxetine rather than nortriptyline.

In summary, it appears that well-designed studies using structured interviews and controlling for treatment report little evidence that personality disorders affect outcome for depressed patients. Uncontrolled studies tend to produce the opposite results. It should be noted that this lack of effect on outcome of personality disorders is confined to short-term studies. There may be more significant effects on longer-term outcome. In addition, it appears that drug class may matter: SSRIs may be superior to TCAs, especially in patients with comorbid cluster B personality disorders.

CONCLUSION

Issues around measurement dominate any discussion on the relationship between personality disorder and depression. No matter how it is measured, however, personality pathology is common among patients with depression and is, therefore, potentially important. Recent research has extended some ideas on this relationship.

What appears increasingly likely is that chronic or recurrent depression, particularly if it has an early age of onset, leads to increases in attitudes and behaviours that may be conceptualised as personality pathology. Whether these are measured via neuroticism scores or personality disorder symptoms, there are consistent associations suggesting some type of scar effect from the effects of chronic low mood. Whether personality pathology predisposes individuals to later depression is less clear. High neuroticism is strongly associated with depression and may be a risk factor, although evidence leans toward this being due to common antecedents, notably genes. In addition, neuroticism scores have particular problems in patients with depression. There is a high degree of symptom overlap, particularly if the Hamilton Depression Scores are used to measure depression severity, and neuroticism scores are mood-dependent. Neuroticism is also a broad construct that appears to convey vulnerability in a nonspecific way for a range of distress disorders, and it is not specifically related to depression.

The overlap between personality pathology symptoms and depressed symptoms remains a central concern. Personality disorders respond to treatments for depression even, in some cases, when the depression itself has not been alleviated. Some people with personality disorders improve more than others, suggesting that there may be variable relationships between depression and types of personality pathology. The cold fact is that there are no consistent criteria for deciding what is a symptom of depression and what is a personality trait. Traditional definitions around the stability of personality disorder symptoms and instability of mood symptoms are challenged by recent evidence, making it somewhat arbitrary as to whether disorders are classified on the basis of symptoms or personality traits. The continuing debate around the status of depressive personality disorder illustrates this problem.

The influence of personality pathology on outcome has received ongoing attention. As is often seen in psychiatry, the best-designed studies seem the least likely to report a significant effect. Recent, comparatively large, controlled treatment studies continue to show no overall effect of comorbid personality disorders on treatment outcome for depression, while smaller uncontrolled studies reported a modest negative effect. Overall, comorbid personality disorder, measured using DSM structured interviews, appears to have little effect on short-term outcome if patients are randomised to treatment. In contrast, there may be treatment-specific effects. Patients with comorbid personality disorders, particularly cluster B, appear to respond less well to TCAs. This possibility might have influenced the longstanding belief that comorbid personality pathology predicted poorer outcome, as most of the early studies used TCAs.

The ongoing debate about the effect of mood on assessment of personality disorder has led some authors to encourage clinicians to wait until the depression remits before making a diagnosis of personality disorder (Farabaugh et al. 2002). However, a clinician is interested in making predictions and plans, which usually means studying patients during an acute illness. If measures of personality consistently predict something about outcome or choice of treatment then they are useful. Whether they are actually measuring personality, chronic depression symptoms or current mood is of interest to a researcher rather than a clinician.

In summary, the evidence continues to reinforce the view that the distinction between personality and psychopathology represents a false dichotomy. There is clearly a significant interrelation between personality and depression. The vulnerability model, the complication and scar model and the pathoplasty model all have some empirical support. Perhaps the most compelling model at present is the spectrum model. Many personality traits and disorders may be considered part of the psychopathology of depression, rather than independent factors that contribute to its development, modify its outcome or are caused by it. Much of what is called personality pathology may share a common origin, with a genetic and perhaps environmental aetiology, with what we call depression. The dominance of the current DSM diagnostic system has discouraged exploration of these conceptual issues. A more open-minded approach to the relationship between personality pathology and depression in the future may lead to more useful and clinically relevant studies.

ACKNOWLEDGMENTS

Parts of this chapter are from the article by Mulder RT (2004) Depression and personality disorder. *Current Psychiatry Reports* 6:51-7.

REFERENCES

Akiskal HS, Hirschfeld RMA, Yerevanian BI (1983) The relationship of personality to affective disorders: A critical review. *Archives of General Psychiatry* 40:801-10.

Asaad T, Okasha T, Okasha A (2002) Sleep EEG findings in ICD-10 borderline personality disorder in Egypt. *Journal of Affective Disorders* 71:11-18.
Black DW, Bell S, Hulbert J, Nasrallah A (1988) The importance of axis II in patients with major depression. A controlled study. *Journal of Affective Disorders* 14:115-22.
Brieger P, Ehrt U, Marneros A (2003) Frequency of comorbid personality disorders in bipolar and unipolar affective disorders. *Comprehensive Psychiatry* 44:28-34.
Charney DS, Nelson JC, Quinlan DM (1981) Personality traits and disorder in depression. *American Journal of Psychiatry* 138:1601-4.
Du L, Bakish D, Ravindran AV, Hrdina PD (2002) Does fluoxetine influence major depression by modifying five-factor personality traits? *Journal of Affective Disorders* 71:235-41.
Eysenck HJ (1970) The classification of depressive illnesses. *British Journal of Psychiatry* 117:241-50.
Farabaugh A, Mischoulon D, Yeung A, Alpert J, Matthews J, Pava J, et al. (2002) Predictors of stable personality disorder diagnoses in outpatients with remitted depression. *Journal of Nervous and Mental Disease* 190:248-56.
Fava M, Bouffides E, Pava JA, McCarthy MK, Steingard RJ, Rosenbaum JF (1994) Personality disorder comorbidity with major depression and response to fluoxetine treatment. *Psychotherapy and Psychosomatics* 62:160-7.
Fava M, Farabaugh AH, Sickinger AH, Wright E, Alpert JE, Sonawalla S, et al. (2002) Personality disorders and depression. *Psychological Medicine* 32:1049-57.
Griens AMGF, Jonker K, Spinhoven P, Blom MBJ (2002) The influence of depressive state features on trait measurement. *Journal of Affective Disorders* 70:95-9.
Hirschfeld RM, Klerman GL, Clayton PJ, Keller MB (1983) Personality and depression: Empirical findings. *Archives of General Psychiatry* 40:993-8.
Hunt C, Andrews G (1992) Measuring personality disorder: The use of self-report questionnaires. *Journal of Personality Disorders* 6:125-33.
Kendler KS, Gardner CO, Prescott CA (2002) Toward a comprehensive developmental model for major depression in women. *American Journal of Psychiatry* 159:1133-45.
Kendler KS, Neale MC, Kessler RC, Heath AC, Eaves LJ (1993) A longitudinal twin study of personality and major depression in women. *Archives of General Psychiatry* 50:853-62.
Kool S, Dekker J, Duijsens IJ, de Jonghe F, Puite B (2003) Changes in personality pathology after pharmacotherapy and combined therapy for depressed patients. *Journal of Personality Disorders* 17:60-72.
Melartin TK, Rytsala HJ, Leskela US, Lestela-Mielonen PS, Sokero TP, Isometsa ET (2002) Current comorbidity of psychiatric disorders among DSM-IV major depressive disorder patients in psychiatric care in the Vantaa Depression Study. *Journal of Clinical Psychiatry* 63:126-34.
Meyers BS, Sirey JA, Bruce M, Hamilton M, Raue P, Friedman SJ, et al. (2002) Predictors of early recovery from major depression among persons admitted to community-based clinics: An observational study. *Archives of General Psychiatry* 59:729-35.
Mulder RT (2002) Personality pathology and treatment outcome in major depression: A review. *American Journal of Psychiatry* 159:359-71.
Mulder RT, Joyce PR (2002) Relationship of temperament and behaviour measures to the prolactin response to fenfluramine in depressed men. *Psychiatry Research* 109:221-8.
Mulder RT, Joyce PR, Luty SE (2003) The relationship of personality disorders to treatment outcome in depressed outpatients. *Journal of Clinical Psychiatry* 64:259-76.
O'Leary D, Costello F (2001) Personality and outcome in depression: An 18-month prospective follow-up study. *Journal of Affective Disorders* 63:67-78.
Overall JE, Hollister LE, Johnson M, Pennington V (1966) Nosology of depression and differential response to drugs. *JAMA* 195:946-50.
Paykel ES (1972) Depressive typologies and response to amitriptyline. *British Journal of Psychiatry* 120:147-56.

Peterson T, Hughes M, Papakostas GI, Kant A, Fava M, Rosenbaum JF, et al. (2002) Treatment resistant depression and axis II comorbidity. *Psychotherapy and Psychosomatics* 71:269-74.
Rothschild L, Zimmerman M (2002) Personality disorders and the duration of depressive episode: A retrospective study. *Journal of Personality Disorders* 16:293-303.
Russell JM, Kornstein SG, Shea MT, McCullough JP, Harrison WM, Hirschfeld RMA, et al. (2003) Chronic depression and comorbid personality disorders: Response to sertraline versus imipramine. *Journal of Clinical Psychiatry* 64:554-61.
Ryder AG, Bagby RM (1999) Diagnostic viability of depressive personality disorder: Theoretical and conceptual issues. *Journal of Personality Disorders* 13:99-117.
Ryder AG, Bagby RM, Schuller DR (2002) The overlap of depressive personality disorder and dysthymia: A categorical problem with a dimensional solution. *Harvard Review of Psychiatry* 10:337-52.
Seivewright H, Tyrer P, Johnson T (2002) Change in personality status in neurotic disorders. *Lancet* 359:2253-4.
Sorenson SB, Rutter CM, Aneshensel CS (1991) Depression in the community: An investigation into age of onset. *Journal of Consulting and Clinical Psychology* 59:541-6.
Viinämaki H, Hintikka J, Honkalampi K, Koivumaa-Honkanen H, Kuisma S, Antikainen R, et al. (2002) Cluster C personality disorder impedes alleviation of symptoms in major depression. *Journal of Affective Disorders* 71:35-41.
Winokur G (1985) The validity of neurotic-reactive depression, new data and reappraisal. *Archives of General Psychiatry* 42:1116-22.
Zimmerman M (1994) Diagnosing personality disorders. A review of issues and research methods. *Archives of General Psychiatry* 51:225-45.

CHAPTER 24

ALCOHOL AND DRUG MISUSE AND MOOD DISORDERS

Fraser C Todd and
J Douglas Sellman

Alcohol and drug misuse and mood disorders commonly occur together, both in the general population and in clinical practice. When they do so, they can interact in ways that complicate diagnosis, treatment response and outcome. The aim of this chapter is to provide some up-to-date information to help clinicians deal more effectively with these situations.

The current legal status of nicotine and alcohol in most Western countries and their active promotion through legal commercial activity within these societies makes these two drugs the predominant drugs used. However, with growth in the use of other drugs, especially cannabis, these other drugs are becoming increasingly important for the clinician to be aware of.

Mental health clinicians are often not specifically focused on the assessment of their patients' alcohol and drug problems, or formulation of the nature of psychiatric symptomatology in relation to their patients' alcohol and drug misuse. Alcohol and drug misuse is often swept aside diagnostically as an 'alcohol and drug problem' without further diagnostic elaboration. This is in contrast to patients' 'mood problems', which are almost invariably more precisely formulated and for which appropriate diagnoses are reached. Further, in the case of patients who are also misusing alcohol and other drugs, consideration of the mood difficulties often takes inappropriate precedence over the alcohol and drug component.

DIAGNOSTIC CONSIDERATIONS

The *Diagnostic and Statistical Manual of Mental Disorders*, fourth edition (DSM-IV), divides the substance-related disorders into two sections, both of which are relevant here: the substance, use disorders, and the substance-induced disorders. This structure is the main innovation of DSM-IV over DSM-III-R in terms of the alcohol and drug area.

The substance-use disorders include substance dependence and substance abuse, the latter being excluded by the presence of dependence. Diagnostic strategy should therefore be focused on excluding dependence in the first instance in all patients who appear to be misusing alcohol or other drugs.

The definition of substance dependence is similar to DSM-III-R and the *International Classification of Diseases*, tenth edition (ICD-10), definitions, although somewhat of a departure from that in DSM-III. The current definitions are based on a description of the alcohol dependence syndrome provided by Edwards and Gross in the mid-1970s. DSM-IV specifies that there be a maladaptive pattern of use resulting in clinically significant impairment or distress involving at least three of the seven criteria abbreviated below, occurring at any time in the same 12-month period:

- use is often more than intended (quantity or time)
- unsuccessful attempts to cut down or stop use
- much time is spent in substance use activity
- increased priority given to substance use
- substance use despite knowledge of significant medical or psychological problems
- acquired tolerance
- withdrawal.

Substance abuse refers to a maladaptive pattern of alcohol use, when dependence has been excluded, manifested by at least one of the following features:

- failure to fulfil major role obligations
- recurrent hazardous use
- recurrent substance-related legal problems
- continued use despite having social or interpersonal problems caused or exacerbated by the substance.

For both dependence and abuse, the diagnosis should be made for the specific class of drugs in question: that is, alcohol dependence, cannabis abuse, and so on.

DSM-IV also identifies a diagnosis of substance-induced mood disorder, but includes this as a mood disorder rather than a substance-related disorder. Before DSM-IV, this diagnosis was somewhat submerged in the organic mood disorder category. The diagnosis of substance-induced mood disorder incorporates conditions that appear to develop secondary to the substance use.

Substance-induced mood disorder is defined as a prominent and persistent disturbance in mood that predominates in the clinical picture, results in clinically significant impairment and is characterised by either or both of:

- depressed mood or markedly diminished interest and pleasure in almost all activities
- elevated, expansive or irritable mood.

To make this diagnosis, symptoms need to develop within a month of substance intoxication or withdrawal, need to be in excess of those usually associated with the specific intoxication or withdrawal syndrome for that drug, and should not occur exclusively during the course of a delirium. The symptoms should also not be better accounted for by a mood disorder that is not substance-induced.

Clinicians have tended to use the diagnosis of substance-induced mood disorder in their alcohol and drug patients to refer to mood problems thought to be caused by the substance use, and consider this as being quite different in aetiology and course from primary depression. Studies have clearly shown that, in hospitalised alcoholics, a high proportion will show major depressive symptoms at presentation (up to 70–80 per cent), but that, in most patients, these symptoms dissipate with abstinence over a few weeks without antidepressant medication. Important to note is that, at presentation, these depressive symptoms mimic major depressive disorder in up to a third of patients, carrying a similar risk of suicide.

It is important to be aware that levels of substance use below that commonly associated with a diagnosis of substance abuse or dependence may still affect the course of a mood disorder. Whether this strictly meets the criterion of continued use despite social or interpersonal problems exacerbated by the substance is controversial. The prudent approach in this case is to make a diagnosis of substance abuse on the grounds that the substance is likely to exacerbate likely interpersonal problems associated with the mood disorder.

EPIDEMIOLOGY

The lifetime frequency of alcohol abuse is about 15–20 per cent, other drug abuse around 3–4 per cent, alcohol dependence in the region of 10 per cent, and other drug dependence 2 per cent. These disorders are therefore among the most common of all mental disorders. More than half the people with substance-use problems may have a lifetime history of a co-occurring axis I mental health disorder, the most common being anxiety disorders and mood disorders, which may be found in about 25 per cent of people with substance-use problems.

When we consider people with mood disorders, 25–40 per cent are likely to have a history of a substance-use disorder, and bipolar disorder has frequently been found to be the axis I disorder most strongly associated with a history of substance abuse or dependence. The particular substances that are most-commonly associated with mood disorders are those most widely used in the community: nicotine, alcohol and cannabis.

MOOD DISORDER AND SUBSTANCE-USE DISORDER INTERACTIONS

There are various possible interactions between mood disorders and substance-use disorders:

- Mood symptoms may be part of substance intoxication and withdrawal.
- Mood disorders may arise secondary to drug use (substance-induced disorders).
- Coexisting disorders may interact and influence the course of each other.

Alcohol and other drug misuse might result directly from affective symptoms. There is some evidence that some people with bipolar disorder initiate substance-use disorders because of the dyscontrol of mania rather than any dyscontrol of the particular substance, not infrequently alcohol. However, the existence of this kind of interaction remains controversial and will not be discussed further.

The following section considers interactions between mood disorders and substance-use disorders for five major groups of psychoactive substances: cannabis, alcohol and other depressants, stimulants, opioids, and nicotine.

Cannabis

Cannabis intoxication includes a range of emotional changes characterised by a feeling of euphoria associated with a sense of meaningfulness, wellbeing, relaxation, heightened sexual arousal and a sense of grandiosity. When used in a social setting, the euphoria is often accompanied by infectious laughter, talkativeness and increased sociability. Adverse emotional reactions can occur with acute intoxication. They are most often reported in naïve users who are unfamiliar with the use of cannabis and by some patients given cannabis for therapeutic purposes. One of the most common adverse reactions is anxiety and panic symptoms. Intoxication may also be associated with mild levels of suspiciousness and paranoid ideation.

Cannabis use and depression co-occur frequently. Depressive symptoms attributed to cannabis use are usually mild and transient. Following the euphoria experienced with cannabis intoxication, there may be a period of anxiety or lowered mood, which is usually brief and self-limiting. The relationship between cannabis use and affective disorders is controversial. Several recent large epidemiological studies suggest that cannabis may cause later major depressive disorders, although it may well be that this association is explained by the presence of common vulnerability factors such as adverse early life experiences and disorders such as conduct disorder. On the other hand, clinical anecdote widely reports that cannabis use can relieve symptoms of depression. It is quite possible that the effect of cannabis on depression varies between individuals. There are case series reporting that cannabis can worsen mania, and this would support the experience of many clinicians, but good research evidence supporting this is lacking.

Most people accept the existence of a brief cannabis-induced psychosis, namely a state of delirium secondary to (usually very heavy) cannabis use.

These are most often described as mania with paranoid features or symptoms of a schizophreniform psychosis, and settle within a week or so following cessation of cannabis use, often with minimal pharmacological intervention. There is also some limited evidence that cannabis can precipitate or intensify psychotic symptoms, especially paranoia, in people with psychotic disorders, including depression and bipolar disorder.

Alcohol and other depressants

The three most important groups of drugs in this class are alcohol, benzodiazepines and barbiturates, although alcohols and benzodiazepines are by far the most commonly used. Benzodiazepine misuse occurs in a variety of quite different populations, from adolescents through to the elderly. The most problematic use is found in younger people, in the context of multiple substance use, when it may be very difficult to assess the contribution being made by benzodiazepines to the overall picture. It is important to distinguish this group of benzodiazepine users from those who are dependent on a relatively stable therapeutic dose of benzodiazepines and who do not misuse alcohol or other drugs.

The effects of depressants on mood are quite variable. As for all drug use, many factors are involved, including the expectations of the user, the underlying emotional state, the setting in which the drug is used, and pharmacological factors such as dose, rate of absorption and blood levels achieved. Previous drug experience and conditioning may also be important in determining the final response experienced by the user.

In general, acute administration of depressants is accompanied by signs of central nervous system arousal and a disinhibition euphoria. A second phase is associated with central nervous system depression and accompanying dysphoria and psychomotor retardation. Depressants may also increase tension and, through disinhibition, facilitate the expression of aggressive behaviour. Chronic administration of depressants is typically accompanied by increased depression, anxiety, irritability and social withdrawal, although additional acute doses may temporarily ameliorate these symptoms.

Patients withdrawing from depressant drugs may experience a range of emotional changes such as depression, anxiety and irritability, as well as the other well-recognised symptoms of withdrawal. Anxiety tends to be more a feature of acute withdrawal, although dysphoria and low-level depression are more characteristic of a post-withdrawal syndrome. The post-withdrawal syndrome may last for many months, particularly in patients on long half-life benzodiazepines. Patients who are withdrawing or are on a stable dose of benzodiazepines and exhibit symptoms of depression may pose a difficult diagnostic dilemma as to whether the major depressive syndrome is secondary to the drug use or withdrawal, or whether the patient has a concurrent major depressive disorder.

Heavy alcohol use may be associated with a depressive syndrome indistinguishable from major depression in its presentation. In most cases, these depressive symptoms ameliorate within a few weeks of abstinence from alcohol and are considered secondary to the alcohol use. In a significant minority of cases, however, the depression persists as a primary disorder, requiring specific treatment. There is a suggestion that alcohol may worsen treatment response and increase the speed of cycling of bipolar disorder, and that elevated mood makes relapse to drinking more likely.

Alcohol use has also been associated with a significant increase in the risk of hallucinations and delusions in people with psychotic disorders, and it is reasonable to expect that this will apply to psychotic mood disorders.

Stimulants

The main stimulant drugs of importance here are cocaine, dexamphetamine, methamphetamine and methylphenidate.

Low-dose use of these stimulants results in a magnification of the pleasure experienced from most activities. The user experiences a sense of euphoria, wellbeing and alertness; anxiety levels are reduced; energy, sexuality and self-esteem all increase; and the individual feels more sociable, enthusiastic and productive. There are generally few problems associated with such use, and psychiatric complications are rare. The user often feels encouraged to repeat this pleasant and rewarding experience. Higher doses of the drug enhance the feeling of euphoria and, as the user becomes increasingly preoccupied with this, withdrawal from other social activities may occur. With increased use of high-dose stimulants, the user experiences symptoms that may mimic hypomania and even mania. The symptoms include euphoria, increased energy levels, disinhibition, grandiosity, impulsiveness, decreased need for sleep, increased feelings of sexuality, decreased appetite, impaired judgment, hypervigilance, compulsively repeated actions, and marked psychomotor agitation. With chronic use of high doses, the euphoria is replaced by dysphoric reactions, including agitation, anxiety, irritability, hyperactivity and paranoia. Some people will become psychotic.

An abstinence syndrome on cessation from heavy regular use of stimulants involves three phases: crash, withdrawal and extinction. Depressive symptoms may be a significant feature of each of these states. The crash can last up to 14 days, during which the individual experiences intense feelings of depression, anxiety and agitation, decreased appetite and an intense craving for more stimulants. The craving is then replaced by a desire for sleep, and the individual experiences fatigue and finally exhaustion. An intermediate withdrawal phase then follows over the next few weeks; its severity is dependent on the extent of preceding stimulant use. The mood begins to normalise, as does sleep, and drug cravings are minimal. This state is soon replaced with feelings of fatigue, anxiety and anhedonia, which may induce a renewed craving for the drug. A prolonged period of abstinence for up to 18 weeks generally allows the anhedonia and fatigue to abate. Finally, even after withdrawal symptoms have disappeared, intense drug craving can be precipitated by the same cues or stimuli previously associated with the use of the stimulant drug. Extinction occurs when the conditioned cues lose their effect and the individual no longer uses drugs in response to cravings.

In general, therefore, stimulants appear to elevate mood and induce or precipitate psychosis. Patients with a pre-existing mood disorder may experience a marked improvement in mood, especially early in the course of stimulant use, with a concomitant worsening associated with withdrawal. Similarly, patients with bipolar disorder may experience an exacerbation or even an induction of elevated mood with stimulant use. Both depressed and bipolar patients may be more vulnerable to psychotic symptoms with stimulant use.

Opioids

Although the euphoric effects of these central nervous system depressant drugs are well publicised, the overall picture of opioid intoxication is quite different from that seen with stimulants, which, as described above, may mimic hypomania. Opioid intoxication is typically associated with a very pleasant floating, intoxicated feeling accompanied by euphoria. The usual opioid withdrawal syndrome of a street user is a relatively benign mixture of emotional, behavioural and physical symptoms. A subsequent post-withdrawal syndrome can last up to 6 months and longer. Symptoms include low-level lethargy, irritability and depression, leaving the ex-user vulnerable to relapse.

It is unclear whether opioid use can exacerbate or alleviate the course of mood disorders, although the nature and power of opioid intoxication would suggest that it should make unpleasant experiences more tolerable. There are, however, very high rates of major depression in people in treatment for opioid dependence. It is likely that developmental and social factors that lead to the development of opiate dependence also increase the risk of a person developing depression, and the psychosocial circumstances associated with opioid dependence may also be a significant precipitant of psychiatric disorder in some individuals. However, many people who use opioids do not develop psychiatric illness. Rather, it seems that, for those who do use opioids, the presence of a psychiatric disorder can be a factor in their seeking help.

Other drugs

The psychological effects of nicotine may be less dramatic than with many other drugs, but they remain significant. Nicotine use may alleviate depressive symptoms and anxiety symptoms and enhance memory and other cognitive functions. This is most noticeable during nicotine withdrawal, which can be associated with depressive symptoms and an exacerbation of pre-existing major depressive disorder.

Acute intoxication with LSD (lysergic acid diethylamide-25) – and the group of related hallucinogenic drugs – typically includes alterations in mood and changes in perception. The mood changes may be euphoric, but can also involve feelings of dysphoria, anxiety and panic.

MDMA (3,4-methylene dioxymethamphetamine), or ecstasy, produces a mixture of central nervous stimulant and psychedelic effects; its psychoactive properties are described as being distinct from both stimulants and hallucinogens. Acute effects include euphoria, feelings of wellbeing and increased self-esteem, inner contentment, increased physical and emotional energy, enhanced mental and emotional clarity and insight, heightened sensual awareness, feelings of enhanced communication and emotional intimacy between partners.

Adverse affective symptoms associated with MDMA use can include anxiety, insomnia and panic attacks within 24 hours of drug ingestion, and drowsiness, depressed mood, anxiety and irritability for up to a month following ingestion. Individuals who use high doses of MDMA or have predisposing psychiatric factors are probably more vulnerable to these effects.

Solvent use alone is generally found in early adolescence, before users progress to other drugs. The most consistent finding in relation to solvent use and psychopathology has been the link with antisocial behaviour.

AETIOLOGICAL CONSIDERATIONS

Substance-related disorders and mood disorders are aetiologically complex conditions seldom adequately explained by one or two simple factors. It is therefore highly unlikely that the co-occurrence of these disorders could be explained by one or two causal factors.

The self-medication hypothesis

It has been commonly thought that people who are depressed or elevated in mood self-medicate themselves with psychoactive substances as a way of relieving their low mood. This belief has been important in leading clinicians to downplay the substance use of their depressed patients and to amplify the importance of the depression in their alcoholic patients. However, the evidence does not support this common belief. Patients with depression tend to drink less alcohol than they do when euthymic. Further, whereas many alcoholics get depressed, most people with depression do not develop problematic substance use. In bipolar disorder, increased drinking is associated with the manic phase, probably as part of exuberant disinhibition.

Although it is simplistic and inaccurate to explain problematic substance use in people with mood disorders as being entirely caused by an attempt to self-medicate the depressive symptoms, it must be acknowledged that for many people substance use may improve their mood symptoms. Alcohol may regulate the anxiety and agitation of abnormal mood, cannabis may relieve depressive symptoms in some people, and opioids certainly improve both mood and agitation. As such, the effect of substances on mood symptoms may be an important reason why, once established, substance use is maintained. However, it is unlikely to be main reason for the initiation of substance-use problems.

Genetic linkages between alcoholism and mood disorder

An idea that has had some support for several decades at least has been that of *depression spectrum disease*. This proposes that alcoholism is the male equivalent of depression (predominantly a female problem). However, family and adoption studies have led to the general conclusion that although depression and alcoholism are both significantly influenced by genetics, they are generally not alternative expressions of the same genotype or linked genetically in some other way. Similarly, for most other combinations of substance use and mood disorders, the vulnerability to each disorder seems to be separately inherited. The exception to this may be nicotine dependence and mild depression, where there is some evidence of a common genotype. There is also conflicting evidence regarding the separate heritability of bipolar disorder and moderate-to-severe alcohol dependence.

Depression and alcoholism are commonly seen together in clinical samples. Given the high lifetime prevalence of alcoholism and major depression (both being in the region of 10 per cent), it is likely that significant proportions of people presenting in clinical settings will have both disorders. However, this frequency is probably augmented because a person with two disorders is more likely to present for help than a person with one disorder alone (Berkson's bias). In random community samples, the relative risk of major depression among alcoholics (compared with people with no history of alcoholism) is in the region of 1.8. This contrasts with the considerably higher associations found in clinical samples, indicating that alcoholics with depression are more likely to present for help than are those without depression. Clinicians and researchers studying clinical samples are therefore likely to assume a high association between the two disorders, when in reality the association may be small.

Assortative mating

There is the possibility that assortative mating makes a significant contribution to the observed linkage between alcoholism and depression in clinical samples. It may be that depressed women are more likely than chance alone to bear children of alcoholic men, producing pedigrees in which both disorders are present at higher frequencies than would be predicted by random mating.

Sex differences

The rate of alcohol dependence is about five times greater in men than in women, and for drug dependence the rate is about two to three times greater. Depression as about twice as common in women as in men. The undoubted genetic influence that exists in both sets of disorders appears to be similar for both men and women. No sex-linked genetics have been identified for either of these disorders. Environmental influences are therefore crucial in explaining the observed difference in lifetime prevalence rates by sex.

The higher rate of depression in women compared with men is also found in alcoholic women compared with alcoholic men. The literature further suggests that, although depression is not a risk factor for alcoholic relapse among alcoholic men, it appears to be a significant risk factor for relapse in women.

Neurobiological models

There is growing knowledge of the neurobiology of both mood disorders and alcohol and drug disorders. Of particular interest here are the neurochemical changes induced by drug use, which may mimic those of major depressive disorder, particularly in the brain regions and functional pathways that both depression and addiction share.

All drugs of abuse enhance dopaminergic transmission in the mesolimbic and mesocortical neuronal systems. These pathways are also implicated in the symptoms of depression that appear to be modulated by dopaminergic mechanisms, including anhedonia and amotivation. Furthermore, these pathways are modulated by other neurotransmitters, particularly γ-aminobutyric acid (GABA), serotonin and opioids. It is likely that interactions underpin much of the association between mood disorders and substance use, especially for drugs such as cocaine, amphetamines, alcohol and cannabis. However, most of these drugs also affect other neurotransmitters, such as GABA and serotonin.

Psychosocial variables

Psychosocial factors are important in the aetiology of both substance use and mood disorders, and many of these factors are common to both. Childhood factors such as sexual abuse, physical abuse, childhood hyperactivity and a disadvantaged family background clearly predate the onset of substance use and are found at increased rates in people with mood disorders. Furthermore, peer affiliations play a significant role in the initiation of substance use and subsequent problematic use, and the presence of a mood disorder may be an important factor in the choice of peers more likely to misuse substances, especially in early adolescence.

Comprehensive models

Each of the models mentioned above is likely to play some role in the co-occurrence of substance use and mood disorders, or in the maintenance of these problems once they have become established. However, they all fall short as a complete explanation. Substance use and mood disorders are increasingly seen as arising through a complex interaction of factors acting across all levels of brain–mind organisation, including genes, neurochemicals, temperament and character, psychological, social, cultural and spiritual factors. In any one individual, various aetiological factors interact to lend vulnerability to, precipitate and maintain co-occurring substance use and mood disorders.

TREATMENT

In general, treatment involves the identification and appropriate management of substance-induced mood disorders, followed by the combining of standard treatments for persisting mood disorders and substance-use disorders. As with other combinations of substance use and mental health disorders, a range of systems issues and judgmental attitudes can undermine the delivery of optimal care. It is important therefore that treatment be organised into a coherent package that overcomes the traditional separations between alcohol and drug, mental health and the other systems that a patient may be engaged with. To this end, general principles of organising treatment for coexisting substance use and mental health disorders in a New Zealand context have been identified.

Five key treatment principles

SAFETY Ensuring the safety of the patients and others who may be at risk takes precedence over all other decisions. This involves the assessment of risk of harm to self and to others, reviewing the patients' physical health and dealing with any urgent medical problems, and assessing patients' ability to care for themselves safely.

STABILISATION Once safety is ensured, any acute issues that interfere with further treatment need to be stabilised. Such issues include acute intoxication and withdrawal, psychotic symptoms, psychosocial crises, severe anxiety or depressive symptoms or a combination of these. Stabilisation therefore usually involves detoxification and acute treatments for any persisting severe mental health symptoms.

COMPREHENSIVE ASSESSMENT AND MANAGEMENT PLANNING It is reasonable to expect that all patients presenting with significant alcohol and drug problems be adequately screened for the presence of key mental disorders such as depression, bipolar disorder, antisocial personality disorder, social phobia and anxiety disorders. Similarly, any patient s presenting with a mental health problem should be asked about their alcohol and drug use and screened for abuse and dependence as part of their routine assessment. In any comprehensive assessment of alcohol and drug problems, corroborative history needs to be obtained from a significant other before it can be considered complete.

CLINICAL CASE MANAGEMENT Once the patient is stable and a comprehensive assessment has given rise to a comprehensive treatment plan, clinical case management becomes the focus for ongoing treatment. Essential features include:

- continuity over time
- integration of the case manager within a multidisciplinary team
- skills in a range of interventions such as motivational interviewing, relapse prevention, monitoring of psychiatric symptoms and education of the patient and family
- assertive follow-up and actively enhancing compliance with appointments and medication
- mobile community-based services.

The case manager should be responsible for monitoring the patient's mental state, fostering the therapeutic alliance, liaising with all clinicians involved, coordinating the management of crises, and carrying out as much of the treatment as they are skilled to do.

TREATMENT INTEGRATION Treatment integration aims to integrate the conceptual models and the different systems in which a patient receives care into a coherent package that is easy for the patient to access and understand. Strategies to assist treatment integration include:

- providing a single coordinating point within mental health and alcohol and drug services that delivers 24-hour care
- considering all persisting alcohol and drug and mental health disorders

as primary disorders of multiple aetiology that may follow a chronic, relapsing course.

- using compatible models and conceptual frameworks. Some models used in alcohol and drug treatment are compatible with those used in mental health, while others are not. For example, a strong abstinence-based approach to alcohol and drug problems does not always work well alongside a treatment approach focusing on the need for compliance with psychiatric medications
- harm minimisation. This approach encompasses abstinence of alcohol and drug use and psychiatric symptoms as the ultimate goal of treatment, but accepts degrees of improvement as valid goals in their own right
- the engagement–persuasion model, in which treatment is divided into four stages:

  1. Engagement: to engage the patient in treatment and develop the therapeutic relationship
  2. Persuasion: to help develop motivation to comply with treatment and to change behaviours such as substance use that have negative impact on treatment
  3. Active treatment: to treat both the substance use problems and the mental health symptoms. Medication and cognitive behavioural strategies are the most common approaches, allowing effective integration of treatment
  4. Relapse prevention: to prevent relapse, be it in the substance-use or the mental health disorder. Cognitive behavioural relapse prevention strategies are particularly useful in this context.

Practical issues

SCREENING AND ASSESSMENT It is important that assessments be effective at identifying the presence of mood and substance difficulties when they exist. Screening instruments such as the Alcohol Use Disorders Identification Test may be helpful in picking up alcohol misuse in general settings, in the same way that the Beck Depression Inventory will help identify patients with significant depression in alcohol and drug settings.

IS THE DEPRESSION SUBSTANCE-INDUCED? When it is established that a patient has co-occurring mood and alcohol and drug problems, the critical issue is working out whether the current mood disorder is substance-induced. The odds are that the depression is substance-induced. Three things that point to its not being substance-induced are:

- During significant periods of abstinence (that is, at least 2–3 months), major depression persisted.
- The initial onset of depression was clearly before the onset of regular drug use.
- There is a strong family history of mood disorder in the absence of any family history of alcohol and drug disorder.

However, there are many times when, even taking into account these three aspects of history, the clinician is still unsure about the status of major depressive symptoms. In these cases, a trial of 3–4 weeks' abstinence, while ensuring safety from suicidality and monitoring depressive symptomatology, is an appropriate diagnostic and treatment strategy.

Drug treatment of a substance-induced mood disorder

In patients who are withdrawing from drugs other than alcohol (especially drugs with reasonably long half-lives such as cannabis, long-acting benzodiazepines and methadone), there may be a persistence of major depressive symptoms as part of a post-withdrawal syndrome for several months and longer. Pragmatically, antidepressants can be very useful to ameliorate symptoms and potentially prevent relapse. The purpose of treatment is to relieve suffering. Active intervention with antidepressant medication needs serious consideration if there are no signs of depressive symptoms waning after 3–4 weeks of abstinence. The difficult cases are those in which depressive symptoms and degree of dysfunction are not severe.

Drug treatment of mood disorders in patients with drug dependence

Once a mood disorder has been diagnosed, standard treatment and management should be initiated. It is imperative, however, that the alcohol and drug disorder be kept in mind.

Pharmacological treatment of a mood disorder in patients with alcohol and drug dependence is essentially the same as for those without alcohol and drug complications, with three minor provisos.

First, some of the standard medications used in the treatment of mood disorders may be better than others in substance users. Selective serotonin reuptake inhibitors (SSRIs) are useful in the treatment of depression in people with alcohol dependence, and can not only improve depressive symptoms but may also reduce cannabis use in people with a combination of cannabis use and depression. There is limited evidence that valproate may be more effective than lithium in people with bipolar disorder and substance-use problems, possibly because of the association of substance use with rapid cycling. Evidence is stronger to support the effectiveness of bupropion and nortriptyline in both reducing the symptoms of mood disorder and assisting nicotine cessation, while SSRIs appear to have little effect on nicotine use, although they are undoubtedly effective for depression in smokers.

Second, the use of potentially dependence-producing medications such as benzodiazepines as adjunct treatment for mood disorders is relatively contraindicated.

Third, patients with both an alcohol and drug disorder and a mood disorder may be attending self-help groups, where they may encounter views that could undermine compliance with medication. It is important in such cases to develop a close therapeutic relationship where these difficulties can be openly discussed.

CONCLUSION

Five main points made in this chapter are:

- Mood disorders are commonly associated with alcohol and drug misuse, especially in clinical samples.
- Mood symptoms are frequently associated with intoxication and withdrawal of drug and alcohol use, and can persist as part of post-withdrawal syndromes. These symptoms can mimic those of affective disorders.
- Greater diagnostic clarity in this area has been facilitated by the DSM-IV *substance-induced mood disorder*.
- Depressive symptoms in people with significant drug and alcohol problems usually represent a substance-induced mood disorder, and often completely remit with abstinence.
- Major depressive symptoms which persist for 3–4 weeks despite abstinence should be given serious consideration for treatment with antidepressant medication even if part of a post-withdrawal syndrome.

CHAPTER 25

MOOD DISORDERS AND ANXIETY DISORDERS

Caroline J Bell
and Sean Hood

For a long time, anxiety disorders were considered mild mental illnesses, or even simple personality variants, as opposed to the serious mental illnesses represented by the psychoses and endogenous depression. Even today, treatment for anxiety is difficult to obtain in our communities with shrinking health budgets and where the misnomer *serious mental illness* is often used to exclude patients with anxiety disorders from services, regardless of degree of impairment.

The current nomenclature of anxiety includes panic disorder, social anxiety disorder (SAD), obsessive–compulsive disorder (OCD), post-traumatic stress disorder (PTSD) and generalised anxiety disorder (GAD) – although these diagnostic boundaries are rather recent and in the process of validation.

This chapter reviews the overlap between mood and anxiety disorders and symptoms with respect to diagnostic considerations, epidemiology of the problem, clinical features, aetiological factors and treatment issues.

NOSOLOGY

Valid assessment of comorbidity in anxiety and mood disorders is fraught with difficulties. The reasons for this are multiple and include the following.

First, the term *comorbidity* in psychiatry is used in various contexts, at times leading to a lack of precision and clarity. It is important to distinguish between lifetime co-occurrence and simultaneous (coincident) occurrence, as well as between comorbid disorders and comorbid symptoms.

Second, the relationship between depression and anxiety has a rich history that is still undergoing revision (Himmelhoch et al. 2001; Levine et al. 2001). Its roots lie in the term *melancholia*, which initially was an inclusive concept containing qualities of depression, anxious agitation and epilepsy. Westphal and Freud were among the first to address anxiety specifically. Freud described *anxiety hysteria*; and in later works emphasised the difference between realistic anxiety (*Furcht* or fear) that occurs in the face of actual danger and neurotic anxiety (*Angst*) that occurs when there is no objective danger present. Kraepelin eventually retreated from a rigid categorical position in which he attempted to separate types of affective illnesses (though not individual anxiety disorders) after clinical follow-up showed poor long-term category specificity. Aubrey Lewis proposed a continuum between anxiety and depression and believed that they could not be usefully distinguished. The evolution of the *Diagnostic and Statistical Manual of Mental Disorders* (DSM) similarly reveals difficulties with the concepts of depression and anxiety. Both DSM-I and DSM-II failed to clearly distinguish between anxiety and depression, organising psychiatric problems by severity (neuroses versus psychoses) and precipitants (endogenous versus reactive). DSM-III was a symptom-oriented, atheoretical classification using thresholds and multiple axes; however, anxiety disorders were not codable in the presence of major depression. DSM-III-R and DSM-IV have largely removed this hierarchy, although it still remains for generalised anxiety disorder and is a topical issue (Zimmerman and Chelminski 2003). The changes in DSM's approach to anxiety mean that data obtained before 1980 are difficult to reconcile with current anxiety concepts.

Third, although the categorical classifications such as DSM may reliably aid the diagnosis of depressive and anxiety disorders, this does not confer validity. Many patients are unable to discern whether anxiety or sadness is the core feature of their experience, raising questions about the validity of the distinction. The number and intensity of supra-threshold symptoms, rather than the degree of functional impairment, is used in DSM-IV as a measure of the illness severity, although disturbance of function is of primary concern to many patients. Subsyndromal anxiety and depressive states, partially recognised in the current nomenclature as *mixed anxiety–depression*, are nevertheless attended by significant levels of functional impairment and high use of non-psychiatric medical care, and are a risk factor for more severe psychiatric disorders.

Fourth, there is substantial overlap between rating scales (such as HAM-A and HAM-D), compromising divergent validity. The rating scales themselves have other limitations. For instance, the commonly used HAM-D was intended to measure the severity of depression in previously diagnosed psychiatric inpatients, and may have limited use in other settings. More than eleven different versions are in common use, with the version used frequently miscited in research papers (Williams 2001)! The HAM-D includes three sleep-related items and one relating to weight loss, so it has an inherent bias in favour of tricyclic antidepressants (TCAs) to the disadvantage of selective serotonin reuptake inhibitors (SSRIs).

Finally, the entry criteria used in antidepressant efficacy trials routinely exclude subjects with comorbid anxiety, usually without reporting on the characteristics of those screened but excluded. Analysis of studies that have reported excluded individuals reveals that only about 15 per cent of depressed patients from a routine outpatient practice would be eligible to participate in these trials (Posternak et al. 2002). This substantially limits generalisability of these data to routine practice. Additionally, to our knowledge there have been no randomised controlled trials specifically designed to assess the efficacy of antidepressant medications in patients with a comorbid anxiety disorder; all of our data to date are post hoc.

There have been several theories about the relationship between depression and anxiety. The *separatist* view, supported initially by differential responses of anxiety and depression to benzodiazepines and antidepressants, respectively, considered that co-occurrence was by chance. The *cognitive specificity hypothesis* also distinguished between these conditions by proposing that the cognitions associated with depressive states are absolutist (themes of loss, deprivation and inadequacy) in contrast to the probabilistic (weighing the chances of future harm) patterns seen in anxious states.

The clinical finding of high co-occurrence of depressive and anxiety states and some shared biological abnormalities has prompted revision of these theories. Tyrer's (2001) concept of *cothymia* essentially classifies the comorbid syndromal anxiety and depression group as a new category. However, comorbid models such as this have difficulty accounting for other observations, including the finding that relatives of patients with pure depression are at higher risk of developing anxiety disorders.

Another approach is to consider that depression and anxiety are in fact a *single disease, with variable phenotypes*. The *unitary affect theory* proposes that the high comorbidity, symptomatic overlap, and nonspecific drug response in depressive and anxiety states supports a common general distress factor. This factor, also known as negative affect, is seen as a core feature of a single illness, with other symptoms considered epiphenomena. High correlation in self-report scales of depression and anxiety scores in patient and non-patient populations support this theory. Nevertheless, there is increasing evidence that patients remain within specific anxiety or depression diagnostic classifications over time (Brown et al. 2001), which would not be expected if this were a single disease.

The *tripartite model* attempts to integrate the unitary affect theory with the cognitive specificity theory by proposing three groups of depression and anxiety symptoms: a nonspecific shared group, physiological arousal (unique to anxiety), and anhedonia (unique to depression). Recent evaluation of this model has only partially validated it. In fact, the nonspecific depression and nonspecific anxiety factors seem to be the most valid and specific indicators of depression and anxiety, respectively.

A relatively recent development is the *subsyndromal* view. This recognises that patients with a depression or anxiety diagnosis may also have symptoms of anxiety or depression (respectively) below the threshold level required by DSM or the *International Classification of Diseases* (ICD) for a separate diagnosis to be made. Comorbid symptoms that do not meet formal diagnostic criteria but still cause significant distress are well known to general practitioners, and are now partly accounted for in the ICD-10 and DSM-IV category of *mixed anxiety–depression.*

EPIDEMIOLOGY

The adult component of the 1997 Australian National Survey of Mental Health and Wellbeing reported a 12-month prevalence of 9.7 per cent for an anxiety disorder and 5.8 per cent for a depressive disorder. A comorbid depressive disorder was seen in 22 per cent of women and 8.4 per cent of men having an anxiety disorder in this period. The child and adolescent component of this survey identified 3.5 per cent of all children as anxious or depressed, with no distinction made between these syndromes.

Estimates from other epidemiological studies (Levine et al. 2001) of lifetime major depression comorbidity with anxiety disorders are about 65 per cent for panic disorder; about 65 per cent for generalised anxiety disorder; about 45 per cent for post-traumatic stress disorder; and about 20 per cent for social anxiety disorder. In general, therefore, about half of the individuals with major depression report a lifetime history of an anxiety disorder. Higher rates are generally reported in clinical cohorts. Anxiety disorders and depression are frequently comorbid in children and adolescents, with a quarter to a half of depressed youth having comorbid anxiety disorders and about 15 per cent of anxious youth having major depression. Comorbidity between anxiety disorders themselves occurs in about a third of patients, but further discussion of this is beyond the scope of this chapter.

Analysis of psychiatric outpatient populations shows a high degree of depression and anxiety comorbidity. In a study of psychiatric outpatients with major depressive disorder, a structured clinical interview revealed that 57.4 per cent concurrently met criteria for a specific anxiety disorder and 74 per cent had a lifetime history of an anxiety disorder (Zimmerman et al. 2000). The most frequent current anxiety disorder was social phobia, diagnosed in a third of the patients.

Early reports suggested that comorbid anxiety and depression was less common in the elderly than in younger populations. Healthy survivor effects and age-related catecholamine decline have been used to explain this observation. This view has been challenged more recently, with the finding in one survey that 47.5 per cent of a community sample of elderly people with major depressive disorder had a comorbid anxiety disorder, and 26.1 per cent of those with anxiety disorders had comorbid major depressive disorder (Beekman et al. 2000). It seems that these conditions are more prevalent when geriatric-specific measures are used, although the true prevalence remains unclear.

Comorbidity data for bipolar disorders are rarely reported. Judd et al. (2003) quantified the lifetime anxiety comorbidity in a large sample of bipolar I and II patients. Bipolar II patients had significantly higher lifetime comorbidity of any anxiety disorder (38 compared with 23.7 per cent), OCD

(8.4 compared with 2.2 per cent), SAD (4.2 compared with 0.0 per cent) than the bipolar I cohort, with similar rates of GAD (21.1 compared with 11.8 per cent) and panic disorder (7.0 compared with 5.9 per cent).

CLINICAL FEATURES AND COURSE

The clinical features of the individual anxiety disorders will be familiar to most readers, and will thus be only briefly described here.

The core feature of panic disorder is spontaneous panic attacks, which are sudden episodes of intense fear or discomfort accompanied by physical and cognitive symptoms. Panic disorder was initially differentiated from other disorders on the basis of tricyclic and monoamine oxidase inhibitor responsivity, and more recently on the basis of sensitivity to various pharmacological challenges. Panic disorder is over represented in patient populations with chest pain and normal coronary arteries, irritable bowel syndrome, and unexplained dizziness and vertigo. Patients with asthma and other respiratory illnesses have a four-fold relative risk of developing panic disorder. Agoraphobic avoidance related to panic disorder can sometimes be difficult to discern from the restriction in social repertoire seen in depressive conditions.

Post-traumatic stress disorder is unique in the DSM classification system in that it requires exposure to a stressful event. The stressor must have been extreme, not just severe, and caused powerful subjective responses such as intense fear, helplessness, or horror. The persisting features of PTSD include re-experiencing the traumatic event in some way, avoidance of activities, places, feelings, thoughts or conversations related to the trauma, increased arousal and some degree of emotional numbing. PTSD is a frequently misunderstood condition – the extreme stressor does not have to be 'outside the range of usual human experience' as first conceptualised, only a minority of people exposed go on to develop PTSD, and there is a higher incidence in groups such as women exposed to violent or sexual assault than in combat veterans. Comorbidity with depression is common in patients with PTSD, although it should be appreciated that major depressive disorder itself is a frequent independent sequela of exposure to trauma. For many patients, initial PTSD symptomatology appears to secondarily evolve into a secondary depressive disorder.

Social anxiety disorder (social phobia) is characterised by fear and avoidance of situations in which scrutiny by others is potentially embarrassing and anxiogenic. The person is afraid that he or she may act in an embarrassing and humiliating way; common situations include speaking, eating, drinking or writing in front of others, or meeting people in authority. The sufferer tries to avoid being involved in these situations, and if unable to do so, endures them with great distress. Up to half of patients with social phobia have a lifetime history of major depression. More controversial, however, is the association noted by Akiskal's group between social anxiety disorder and bipolar II disorder (Judd et al. 2003). They suggest that, in most cases, SAD chronologically precedes hypomanic episodes and disappears when the latter episodes supervene – in contrast to OCD and panic disorder, which more often persist during the hypomanic episodes. Severity of social anxiety symptoms, depressive comorbidity, alcohol abuse, and good response to monoamine oxidase inhibitors (MAOIs) have been associated with this bipolar–social anxiety disorder phenotype. Additional validation of this association appears warranted.

The essential features of OCD are *obsessions* (recurrent thoughts, ideas, urges, or images that intrude upon the sufferer's mind and cause anxiety) and *compulsions* (repetitive behaviours or mental acts, which aim at reducing anxiety and distress) that are severe enough to be time consuming, ego dystonic, and impair functioning. It has been long debated whether OCD is primarily a disorder of the intellect (thought) similar to psychosis, a disorder of volition, or one of emotion (anxiety). The emotive view won the argument, and subsequently OCD sits uneasily in classification systems with the other anxiety disorders. OCD *spectrum conditions* include disorders of impulse control (for example, pathological gambling and sexual addiction), neurological disorders with repetitive behaviours (such as Tourette's syndrome and autism), syndromes characterised by exaggerated bodily concerns (for example, body dysmorphic disorder and bulimia), and dissociative disorders. OCD typically also presents before affective illness, but may in time resolve into chronic major depressive illness, bipolar II disorder, or even an organic mood disorder.

An inheritor of the concept of *free floating anxiety*, generalised anxiety disorder emerged in DSM-III as a sort of residual diagnostic category. Despite initial misgivings, GAD is a disorder that has been increasingly validated and is worthy of attention. The central feature of GAD is persistent worry, especially about relatively minor matters and life circumstances such as health, finance, family and work. Sleep disturbance and somatic symptoms such as muscle tension are also common. A study that contrasted cognitions in patients with pure GAD, pure major depression, and comorbid illness showed that an *aimless future* domain was uniquely associated with depressive symptoms, with the comorbid group having a mixed cognitive profile. This is somewhat congruent with the cognitive specificity hypothesis mentioned above. An 8-year follow-up of patients presenting with GAD showed that only 25 per cent never experienced an overlapping episode of major depression (Bruce et al. 2001). Most patients with GAD (58 per cent) had an episode of major depression during follow-up.

Anxiety disorders often precede the onset of major depression. A recent 5-year prospective longitudinal community study of adolescents and young adults with DSM-IV anxiety and depressive disorders confirmed this (Wittchen et al. 2000). At the end of the study, only a minority of patients with anxiety still had pure anxiety; most had developed depression. The risk for onset of secondary depression in the course of the study was increased two- to four-fold above the risk expected in subjects with no previous history of anxiety disorders. A large prospective study found that the presence of SAD in adolescence or early adulthood was a strong risk factor for the subsequent occurrence of depressive illness, and that the combination of depression and SAD in adolescence markedly augments the risk for subsequent depressive disorder, beyond the risk conferred by either disorder alone (Stein et al. 2001).

Anxiety and depression in children are considered *internalising* disorders, or disorders of emotion, in contrast to the *externalising* disorders, or disorders of behaviour. Symptom overlap is so frequent in this area that some authors propose that anxiety/depression is a single construct in children (that is, a single disease, but variable phenotype). Although there is insufficient evidence to confirm this, it does seem that as depressive and anxiety symptoms exceed diagnostic thresholds, separation in cognitive and symptoms sets becomes clearer. The phenomenology of depressive and anxiety symptoms in children differs from adult groups in that children have fewer melancholic symptoms, more somatic complaints, and irritability can be a predominant mood.

Elderly patients with comorbid depression and anxiety have been reported as having more severe somatic symptoms than depressed elderly people without anxiety and poorer social function.

EFFECT OF COMORBIDITY

Comorbidity is seen as a poor prognostic indicator in most psychiatric areas. Conditions that cross existing categorical diagnostic boundaries are likely to have a limited specific evidence base informing treatment, deficits in multiple domains that may act as a marker of severity, and decreased access to local professional resources in an era where limited funding promotes restrictive intake boundaries.

Therefore, it is not surprising that patients with comorbid anxiety and depresssion have a higher rate of mental health service needs (51 per cent) than either patients with pure anxiety disorder (14 per cent) or depression (35 per cent) (Wittchen and Essau 1993). This applies to subsyndromal symptoms as well as anxiety and depressive disorders. Comorbidity is also associated with earlier onset of illness, more severe clinical presentation of both disorders, heavier burden of disability, and increased rates of suicide attempts (see Dunner 2001 for a review). Comorbid anxiety was associated with a lower probability of recovering from dysthymic disorder in a 5-year prospective study.

This generally poor view of comorbidity has begun to be refined recently. For example, although women with PTSD related to violence from an intimate partner were significantly more disabled than women without PTSD, comorbidity with major depression did not increase disability (Stein et al. 2001). A ceiling effect is another explanation for this finding.

There is a strong temporal link between paediatric anxiety disorders and the subsequent development of depression. This link may not be specific to anxiety, however, as other comorbid childhood psychiatric conditions (especially attention deficit hyperactivity disorder) may also precede depression (Axelson and Birmaher 2001).

Anxiety disorders have been poorly studied in the depressed elderly, with little evidence currently available to inform us about the effect of comorbidity in this population. Most authors, however, emphasise that anxious elderly depressed people are more likely to be prescribed benzodiazepines, which carry a potential risk of dependence, falls and impaired cognition.

AETIOLOGICAL FACTORS

A range of different approaches has been used to examine the possible aetiological factors associated with depression and anxiety disorders. As discussed above, clinical observations have reported that anxiety disorders often precede the onset of major depression, suggesting overlap in factors in the aetiological process.

Family studies have also identified this overlap, reporting both that relatives of patients with pure depression are at higher risk of developing anxiety disorders and that relatives of patients with anxiety disorders have an increased risk of depression. A classic genetic study of female twins suggested that there may be a particular association between depression and GAD, with a genetic liability to both being influenced by the same genetic factors. This determines the patient's vulnerability to the conditions, but whether she goes on to develop major depression or GAD is a result of environmental experiences (Kendler et al. 1992).

Positron emission tomography (PET) and other neuroimaging studies have allowed examination of brain function in vivo, and have given us considerable insight into the abnormalities associated with different disorders and areas of overlap. Although the functional neuroanatomy of major depression has not been clearly established, studies have tended to report diminished brain activity in the dorsolateral prefrontal cortex and basal ganglia and elevated activity in the ventrolateral prefrontal cortex. Similar studies in patients with OCD have reported different findings, with elevated activity in the orbitofrontal cortex, anterior cingulate gyrus, caudate nuclei and thalamus. Subcortical areas may be of particular importance to SAD patients, with a PET study finding a relative increase in blood flow to subcortical areas during a public speaking task and other reports of reduced D_2 receptor binding and reduced striatal dopamine reuptake site density. Several studies have now reported MRI evidence of reduced hippocampal volume in PTSD subjects. Regional differences in brain activity have also been noted in patients with GAD. Several studies support the hypothesis that patients with panic disorder are characterised by right frontal hyperactivation, with a [^{11}C]flumazenil PET study by our group showing a global reduction in benzodiazepine site binding (especially right orbitofrontal cortex and right insula) in drug-naïve patients with panic disorder (Malizia et al. 1998).

TREATMENT

The presence of an anxiety disorder (or anxiety symptoms) with depression will affect case formulation and treatment planning. The essence of treatment is that both disorders and symptoms need to be effectively managed. As with depression occurring alone, the choice of treatment options includes both psychological and pharmacological approaches. Tailoring the treatment to the individual patient includes consideration of a variety of factors, including the severity and nature of each of the disorders, patient preference, and the availability of cognitive behaviour therapy (CBT).

Despite the high levels of comorbidity between depression and anxiety, there is only a very limited literature examining the treatment response in these patients. This is because the entry criteria used in antidepressant efficacy trials routinely exclude subjects with comorbid anxiety. Most clinical practice is based on the premise that an appropriate choice of treatment is one that has efficacy in both disorders.

As discussed in Chapter 16, there is a wide range of antidepressants available for the treatment of depression, and a similar range of options for the treatment of anxiety disorders. There is not, however, complete reciprocity of therapeutic profile between the treatment of depression and anxiety disorders with some drugs e.g. benzodiazepines and buspirone being principally used as anxiolytics and having only limited benefit in depression.

Psychological interventions are also effective in the treatment of both depression and anxiety disorders. The techniques use cognitive-behavioural interventions, but emphasise different approaches for the different disorders; the cognitive specificity hypothesis described above exemplifies this. In the treatment of depression, there tends to be an emphasis on cognitive restructuring. In the treatment of the anxiety disorders, in addition to cognitive approaches, there is emphasis on behavioural approaches, such as exposure to treat the phobic avoidance that is often a feature of the condition.

Treatment approaches to depression comorbid with the different anxiety disorders will be discussed in the next section. As there have been very few trials addressing this important issue, our recommendations tend to extrapolate from data examining treatment of both the disorders in isolation.

Depression and OCD

There is considerable evidence that serotonergic reuptake inhibitors (such as clomipramine) and the SSRIs are the most effective medications for treating OCD. These agents have consistently been shown to be more effective than noradrenergic agents. Both serotonergic and noradrenergic agents are effective in treating depression. Although only one study has addressed the question of efficacy in OCD with comorbid depression, this reported a similar pattern of response to that seen in OCD alone, with sertraline being significantly more effective than desipramine (Hoehn-Saric et al. 2000). Studies in OCD patients also report the requirement for higher doses (for example, 60 mg/day paroxetine) and a delay in response (of up to 12 weeks) compared with treatment of depression. One study of depressed patients with comorbid OCD reported a poorer response to fluoxetine than in depressed patients without OCD. This may be explained by the use of a low dose of fluoxetine (20 mg/day) (Sonawalla et al. 2002), perhaps suggesting that where both conditions occur, doses need to be in the higher range used in the treatment of OCD alone.

The psychological treatment of OCD uses a behavioural approach with gradual exposure to the feared situation combined with response prevention (EX/RP). The treatment of obsessional thoughts can be particularly difficult, and can include interventions aimed at thought stopping and other cognitive techniques. Care should be taken not to substitute OCD rituals with cognitive ones, so therapy by an experienced practitioner is highly advised. Although there is little literature directly addressing this issue, these techniques can successfully be used in the treatment of OCD where there is comorbidity with depression.

PET studies in non-depressed patients with OCD have shown that effective treatment with SSRIs decreases the elevated functional activity in orbitofrontal–basal ganglia–thalamocortical circuits. Interestingly, similar responses have been reported in patients with OCD treated with CBT (Baxter et al. 1992). These results add to the evidence that OCD symptoms are mediated by functional activity of these circuits. PET studies of the treatment of depression have reported that treatment response is related to decreasing ventrolateral prefrontal cortex activity. PET studies of patients with concurrent OCD and major depression have reported that treatment of both conditions resulted in decreases in ventrolateral prefrontal cortex but not changes in activity in the orbitofrontal cortex, basal ganglia, or thalamus (seen in patients with OCD alone). This suggests that although both disorders respond to SSRIs, the two syndromes have different neurobiological substrates for response.

In view of this evidence, current recommendations for the treatment of comorbid depression and OCD are to use serotonergic antidepressants at high dosage for at least a year. These should be combined with the cognitive-behavioural techniques outlined above.

Depression and panic disorder

As with OCD, there is evidence (although not quite as strong) that serotonergic agents are more effective than noradrenergic agents in the treatment of panic disorder, with MAOIs also demonstrating efficacy. High, potency benzodiazepines have also been shown to be effective, but are associated with dependence and withdrawal rebound. The studies also report the requirement for moderately high doses (for example, 40 mg/day paroxetine) and a delay in response, with effects often not being seen for about 8 weeks. Exacerbation of panic symptoms and jitteriness on commencement of an antidepressant has been reported. This can be managed by an explanation of the possibility at the start of treatment, using low doses initially (for example, 10 mg/day paroxetine) and covering with a benzodiazepine (such as clonazepam) as needed for a few weeks.

Psychological treatments use a combination of cognitive and behavioural techniques and are effective for treating both depression and panic disorder. Where the two conditions are comorbid, treatment needs to incorporate the treatment of both conditions.

Current recommendations for the treatment of comorbid depression and panic disorder are to use serotonergic antidepressants and to titrate up gradually according to response, with benzodiazepine cover for a few weeks if required to treat any exacerbation in anxiety at the start of treatment. These can be combined with CBT.

Depression and SAD

Pharmacological treatment studies of social anxiety disorder report efficacy for MAOIs (and the reversible MAOI, moclobemide) and several SSRIs, but poor effect of TCAs. The doses used are again typically higher than those used for treating depression, but not as high as those required in OCD (for example, 40 mg/day paroxetine). Similarly, the delay in response is typically between that seen in the treatment of depression and OCD (around 8–10 weeks).

Psychological treatments are also effective. These use a combination of cognitive and behavioural techniques that are delivered in both individual and group settings. The group setting is often a sensitive environment for SAD patients, with the most severely affected patients unable to cope with this format, at least initially.

Current recommendations for the treatment of comorbid depression and social anxiety disorder are to use an SSRI in the first instance (although patients with a treatment-resistant disorder may require an MAOI) and to titrate up according to response. There is some evidence that combining drugs with CBT may have some additional benefits in both the short and long term.

Depression and GAD

Benzodiazepines, buspirone and antidepressants (TCAs, SSRIs and venlafaxine) have all demonstrated efficacy in the treatment of GAD in the absence of depressive symptoms, although, as noted previously, there is frequently overlap between the conditions.

Psychological treatments using CBT approaches have also demonstrated efficacy in GAD and depression.

Current recommendations for the treatment of comorbid depression and GAD disorder are to use an SSRI or venlafaxine and to titrate up according to response. Psychological approaches should incorporate interventions aimed at treating the features of both depression and GAD.

Depression and PTSD

Drug studies of the treatment of PTSD have provided some evidence for benefit of TCAs, MAOIs and SSRIs, although some symptoms (such as nightmares, flashbacks and sleep disturbance) may require other interventions (for example, cyproheptadine and trazodone).

Psychological approaches use CBT, which includes a combination of exposure procedures (both real and in imagination with patient recall and taping a narrative of the trauma), cognitive restructuring and anxiety management techniques.

Current recommendations for the treatment of comorbid depression and PTSD are to use an SSRI and to titrate up according to response. This can be combined with CBT.

PROGNOSIS

Early studies from the literature suggested that depressed patients with a comorbid anxiety disorder had a poorer outcome from treatment that those with depression alone (for example, Lydiard and Brawman-Mintzer 1998).

Two studies investigating the response in depression with comorbid GAD (Silverstone and Salinas 2001) and other anxiety disorders (Sonawalla et al. 2002) reported that the presence of anxiety disorders (apart from OCD) had no effect on the outcome of treatment). Similarly, a study by our group in Christchurch of patients with depression treated with fluoxetine or nortriptyline found that the concurrent diagnosis of panic disorder did not adversely affect outcome. Studies that have examined the treatment response in anxious depression (that is, patients who scored high on anxiety symptoms) reported that antidepressants relieved symptoms of both depression and anxiety (Fava et al. 2000). With regard to anxiety disorder, the results are similarly mixed. The short-term studies tend to report that patients with panic disorder and comorbid depression have similar response rates to those with panic disorder alone, whereas some of the longer-term studies report that comorbid depression predicts a poorer treatment response.

CONCLUSION

It is clear that anxiety disorders have an intimate relationship with mood disorders, especially depressive states. Discerning the boundaries of this relationship has proven historically difficult and is the subject of ongoing review. We do know that these conditions are the most prevalent psychiatric disorders in our communities and are attended by significant morbidity in all age groups. The presence of both disorders is in general a marker of severity, chronicity, or poor prognosis – but nevertheless comorbidity is a common circumstance. Treatments such as SSRIs and CBT are usually effective in these conditions, and although efficacy data from randomised controlled trials specifically relating to comorbid illness are scarce, the clinical reality is that these therapies usually produce substantial benefits in our patients. We look forward to an improved understanding of anxiety and mood disorders in the future.

REFERENCES

Axelson DA, Birmaher B (2001) Relation between anxiety and depressive disorders in childhood and adolescence. *Depression and Anxiety* 14:67-78.

Baxter LR, Jr., Schwartz JM, Bergman KS, Szuba MP, Guze BH, Mazziotta JC, et al. (1992) Caudate glucose metabolic rate changes with both drug and behavior therapy for obsessive-compulsive disorder. *Archives of General Psychiatry* 49:681-9.

Beekman AT, de Beurs E, van Balkom AJ, Deeg DJ, van Dyck R, van Tilburg W (2000) Anxiety and depression in later life: Co-occurrence and communality of risk factors. *American Journal of Psychiatry* 157:89-95.

Brown TA, Di Nardo PA, Lehman CL, Campbell LA (2001) Reliability of DSM-IV anxiety and mood disorders: Implications for the classification of emotional disorders. *Journal of Abnormal Psychology* 110:49-58.

Bruce SE, Machan JT, Dyck I, Keller MB (2001) Infrequency of 'pure' GAD: Impact of psychiatric comorbidity on clinical course. *Depression and Anxiety* 14:219-25.

Dunner DL (2001) Management of anxiety disorders: The added challenge of comorbidity. *Depression and Anxiety* 13:57-71.

Fava M, Rankin MA, Wright EC, Alpert JE, Nierenberg AA, Pava J, et al. (2000) Anxiety disorders in major depression. *Comprehensive Psychiatry* 41:97-102.

Himmelhoch J, Levine J, Gershon S (2001) Historical overview of the relationship between anxiety disorders and affective disorders. *Depression and Anxiety* 14:53-66.

Hoehn-Saric R, Ninan P, Black DW, Stahl S, Griest JH, Lydiard RB, et al. (2000) Multicenter double-blind comparison of sertraline and desipramine for concurrent obsessive-compulsive and major depressive disorders. *Archives of General Psychiatry* 57:76-82.

Judd LL, Akiskal HS, Schettler PJ, Coryell W, Maser JD, Rice JA, et al. (2003) The comparative clinical phenotype and long term longitudinal episode course of bipolar I and II: A clinical spectrum or distinct disorders? *Journal of Affective Disorders* 73:19-32.

Kendler KS, Neale MC, Kessler RC, Heath AC, Eaves LJ (1992) Major depression and generalized anxiety disorder. Same genes, (partly) different environments? *Archives of General Psychiatry* 49:716-22.

Levine J, Cole DP, Chengappa KN, Gershon S (2001) Anxiety disorders and major depression, together or apart. *Depression and Anxiety* 14:94-104.

Lydiard RB, Brawman-Mintzer O (1998) Anxious depression. *Journal of Clinical Psychiatry* 59 Suppl 18:10-17.

Malizia AL, Cunningham VJ, Bell CJ, Liddle PF, Jones T, Nutt DJ (1998) Decreased brain $GABA_A$-benzodiazepine receptor binding in panic disorder: Preliminary results from a quantitative PET study. *Archives of General Psychiatry* 55:715-20.

Posternak MA, Zimmerman M, Keitner GI, Miller IW (2002) A reevaluation of the exclusion criteria used in antidepressant efficacy trials. *American Journal of Psychiatry* 159:191-200.

Silverstone PH, Salinas E (2001) Efficacy of venlafaxine extended release in patients with major depressive disorder and comorbid generalized anxiety disorder. *Journal of Clinical Psychiatry* 62:523-9.

Sonawalla SB, Farabaugh A, Johnson MW, Morray M, Delgado ML, Pingol MG, et al. (2002) Fluoxetine treatment of depressed patients with comorbid anxiety disorders. *Journal of Psychopharmacology* 16:215-19.

Stein MB, Fuetsch M, Müller N, Höfler M, Lieb R, Wittchen HU (2001) Social anxiety disorder and the risk of depression: A prospective community study of adolescents and young adults. *Archives of General Psychiatry* 58:251-6.

Tyrer P (2001) The case for cothymia: Mixed anxiety and depression as a single diagnosis. *British Journal of Psychiatry* 179:191-3.

Williams JB (2001) Standardizing the Hamilton Depression Rating Scale: Past, present, and future. *European Archives of Psychiatry and Clinical Neuroscience* 251 Suppl 2:6-12.

Wittchen HU, Essau CA (1993) Comorbidity and mixed anxiety–depressive disorders: Is there epidemiologic evidence? *Journal of Clinical Psychiatry* 54 Suppl:9-15.

Wittchen HU, Kessler RC, Pfister H, Lieb M (2000) Why do people with anxiety disorders become depressed? A prospective-longitudinal community study. *Acta Psychiatrica Scandinavica. Supplementum* 14-23.

Zimmerman M, Chelminski I (2003) Generalized anxiety disorder in patients with major depresssion: Is DSM-IV's hierarchy correct? *American Journal of Psychiatry* 160:504-12.

Zimmerman M, McDermut W, Mattia JI (2000) Frequency of anxiety disorders in psychiatric outpatients with major depressive disorder. *American Journal of Psychiatry* 157:1337-40.

CHAPTER 26

DEPRESSION IN THE MEDICALLY ILL

Pete M Ellis and
Tracey V Barnfield

A substantial proportion of people who are physically ill also experience psychiatric disorder. About a quarter to a third of medical inpatients and outpatients have some symptoms of depression and nearly 30 per cent of patients in primary care present with some form of psychiatric and physical comorbidity. Some of the variability in these figures reflects the problems of defining depression in the medically ill. Scores on most standard depression rating scales are greatly influenced by somatic symptoms that are common in the medically ill, such as pain, fatigue, anorexia and sleep disturbance. In general, depressive symptomatology in medical populations is milder than among people attending community mental health services, but more prevalent than in community populations.

The prevalence of severe depression in the medically ill is variously reported to be between 4 and 18 per cent, somewhat higher than found in most community studies. Depression is more common in people who are more severely ill, who are bedridden, who have longer hospital stays, who are in pain, and who have been more recently diagnosed. In one study, depression preceded the medical illness in a quarter of subjects and followed it in three-quarters.

Depression is more commonly associated with some disorders than others. Although there is sometimes a tentative causal relationship between the physical disorder and the depressive syndrome, in many cases the evidence for this is conflicting or inadequate. For example, depression may follow infection with a number of viral conditions (for example, glandular fever, herpes simplex, inclusion body encephalitis and influenza) and other infections (for example, brucellosis, toxoplasmosis, typhoid and leptospirosis). However, these conditions are characteristically followed by a period of lassitude and poor concentration that may be mistaken for a depressive syndrome. This exacerbates the difficulty in elucidating the link between infection and affective symptoms. The aetiology of the chronic fatigue syndrome remains unclear, but it may also be viral in some cases.

The association between some neurological disorders and mood disorders is clearer. People with cerebral tumours, particularly involving the frontal lobe, may present with depression. Up to 45 per cent of patients will suffer from depression after experiencing a stroke. This does not appear to be due to physical impairment alone. Depression is more common when the infarcts are more frontal, and perhaps when they affect the dominant hemisphere, although this finding has been controversial. Interestingly, in people with partial complex seizures, depression is found most commonly when their seizures affect the dominant hemisphere.

Subcortical pathways may also be involved in the control of mood. The dopaminergic and serotonergic pathways in the basal ganglia are interrelated. Depression is common in people suffering diseases of the basal ganglia, such as Parkinson's disease (among whom 50 per cent may experience depression) and Huntington's disease, in which depression is sometimes seen as a harbinger of the overt illness. Bilateral damage to the corticobulbar tract caused by stroke or multiple sclerosis may produce emotional incontinence, where the patient experiences incongruous outbursts of distressed behaviour, usually of short duration. This affects at least a fifth of people in the year after a stroke. These observations would suggest that subcortical, as well as cortical, mechanisms may be involved in the expression, and perhaps aetiology, of depressive illnesses.

Endocrine diseases are also associated with depression. Hypo- and hyperthyroidism are the most familiar, and the syndrome of apathetic thyrotoxicosis in the elderly is of particular note. Mood disorders are well described in Cushing's disease, although disturbances of mood in response to steroids are more frequently due to exogenous treatment. Hyper- and hypocalcaemia are of particular interest, as there appears to be a correlation between the degree of metabolic and psychological disturbance. Depression is not infrequent among people suffering from diabetes, although there does not appear to be a direct neuroendocrine mechanism for this.

Depression is common among people with cancer, for psychological reasons and through organic mechanisms. Cancers such as oat cell carcinomas may cause hormonal disturbances, and an otherwise silent cerebral metastasis may contribute to affective symptoms. Pancreatic cancer is reputed to present following some depressive illnesses, although it is not clear if this is a true association or reflects presentation of occult malignancy with symptoms suggestive of depression, such as malaise, weight loss and anorexia.

Depression appears to be more common with connective tissue disorders such as rheumatoid arthritis and systemic lupus erythematosus than with other non-immune-based rheumatic disorders. Cerebral involvement in systemic lupus erythematosus has been demonstrated through striking changes in cerebral blood flow at the time of neuropsychiatric abnormalities.

High rates of major depression (18 per cent of patients) have been reported 8–10 days after myocardial infarction, and 44 per cent of those were still depressed at 3 months. Major depression is an independent risk factor for mortality in the first 6 months after heart attacks, at least equivalent to that of left ventricular dysfunction and a history of previous myocardial infarction (Barefoot and Schroll 1996). The mechanism of this association is unclear (Carney et al. 2002). It may reflect poor compliance, or some instability of the sympathetic nervous system leading to ventricular fibrillation. The latter is suggested by the finding of some increased beat-to-beat variability in otherwise healthy depressed patients. Effective treatment appears to reduce this increased risk, perhaps by reducing the risk of ventricular fibrillation. It has been shown that inadequately treated depressed patients have a higher mortality than adequately treated patients.

Depression has also been reported to be associated with increased mortality in haemodialysis patients, although the mechanisms involved are obscure.

AETIOLOGY

Despite these descriptions, the aetiology of depression in the medically ill is no more clearly understood than when it occurs in other settings. There appears to be a complex interaction between personality characteristics, social conditions, and factors related to the illness and its treatment.

Lipowski emphasised the personal symbolic significance of illness to the sufferer. If the illness is seen as a threat, loss or punishment, it tends to be more disruptive. This may account for the increased incidence of depression in association with AIDS and cancer. The untimely nature of accidents and unexpected trauma appears to contribute to the long-term problems arising from these events. Relatives and friends may also profoundly affect the outcome of an illness, both positively and negatively. For example, overprotection by a concerned and anxious spouse may reinforce dependency in the patient, and the absence of the breadwinner may create lasting changes in the dominance hierarchy of the family. In contrast, the more usual reaction of consistent support, encouragement, and an opportunity to ventilate emotions and fears are valuable and important protective factors.

There are few illnesses, with the possible exception of Parkinson's disease, in which a common pathological mechanism may underlie both the illness and the depression.

The treatment setting may also contribute to distress. The intensive care unit may be perceived as a very frightening environment and the constant observation, activity and noise may contribute to protracted sleeplessness and a degree of sensory deprivation. Good communication, reassurance and psychological support for patients in such settings can ameliorate these factors.

Medication and other treatment for the primary medical condition may directly contribute to depression through side effects. This is a particular problem with steroids, with 18.4 per cent of people without previous psychiatric illness experiencing affective symptoms at doses of prednisone over 80 mg/day (Brown and Suppes 1998). Other drugs causing depression include ß-blockers, antiparkinsonian agents, analgesics and cytotoxic agents. Radiotherapy, particularly to the brain, can also cause depression.

Depression occurring in the course of a medical illness is not fundamentally different from other depressive illnesses. However, in contrast to depression in general, depression in the medically ill is equally distributed across sex, race, and socioeconomic groups, and sufferers are less likely to have a personal or family history of depression.

Most people with a medical illness are able to come to terms with it without professional help. Although they may experience minor affective symptoms, these are not persistent and do not interfere with their daily functioning. They are able to use effective coping strategies and make adjustments in their lives. In these milder reactions to adversity, the patient feels bad about *the situation* (such as being ill, being diagnosed as having cancer, etc), in contrast to the significant loss of self-esteem in more severe depression, when the patient feels bad about *him- or herself*.

DIAGNOSIS

Recognising depression in the medically ill is more difficult because one cannot rely on the biological symptoms of depression. Half to three-quarters of the medically ill report work inhibition, fatigue, anorexia, weight loss, insomnia and somatic preoccupation. Greater reliance has to be placed on the affective and cognitive symptoms of depression: the sense of failure, the loss of social interest, a sense of punishment, suicidal ideation, severe dissatisfaction, severe indecisiveness, frequent crying and anhedonia. These patients are less likely to report anxiety, a distinct quality of depressed mood, hopelessness, helplessness, self-pity, agitation or psychomotor retardation.

In general, the severity of somatic complaints, but not their number, increases with increasing severity of depression. Failure to make the progress expected in rehabilitation despite an improvement in the patient's medical condition may also indicate a significant depressive illness.

DIFFERENTIAL DIAGNOSIS

A variety of organic causes of mood disorder should be considered in the depressed medically ill patient, including infectious diseases, neurological disease, endocrine disease, malignancies and connective tissue diseases. These should be particularly suspected when the depression is of late onset, there is a stable premorbid personality, and there is no family history of mood disorder or apparent psychosocial precipitant.

Assessment of depression in the demented or severely brain-damaged patient is particularly challenging. Although patients may be too demented to give a clear account of their mood state and its development, their affect may still convey this. Feelings of low self-esteem and hopelessness may be evident in statements that family, friends and medical staff 'don't care about me any more'. Feelings of worthlessness may be inferred from statements such as 'don't bother with me, I'm not worth it', and suicidal ideation from protestations that 'I'd be better off dead'. The patients may eat poorly even when a favourite food is provided. The patients' level of agitation is generally constant in depression, in contrast to that in dementia, where it is more clearly related to alterations in what is going on around them or their worsening medical condition.

In the medically ill, symptoms usually considered characteristic of depression may actually indicate other conditions. For example, agitation may reflect delirium, or the effects of cerebral anoxia, or the side effects of drugs such as dopamine or steroids. Retardation may reflect Parkinson's disease or system failure. In such complex situations, it is important to re-evaluate mood over several interviews and to combine this with full discussion with the nursing staff caring for the patient and close cooperation with the appropriate physicians and surgeons.

Pseudodementia has attracted considerable mention in the literature. However, a careful history, corroborated by relatives or others who have known the patient over a long period (such as the general practitioner), will generally distinguish dementia from depression. The diagnosis of depression in the presence of dementia is more difficult.

It is important to also consider other constructs for understanding reactions to acute or chronic stresses. These include burnout, demoralisation and abnormal illness behaviour. It is important that the use of such terms does not preclude an appropriate diagnosis of depression, but they can add significantly to the understanding of a person's presentation and be valuable in considering appropriate management. For example, abnormal illness behaviour is especially common after traumatic injuries sustained in accidents, particularly if the accident has been unpredictable and when culpability, by the patient or others, is a crucial factor. The patient may complain of various somatic symptoms usually linked to the original illness, and fails to return to work or to resume leisure activities as soon as expected. Associated symptoms include depression, anxiety, irritability and poor concentration, and it is unusual for complaints to be entirely somatic. The patient becomes progressively incapacitated without an adequate organic cause for this. Involvement of the family in the overall management of these problems is vital.

Another condition that may coexist with depression is chronic fatigue syndrome (Koschera et al. 1999).

ASSESSMENT

As with any psychiatric disorder, it is essential to assess the severity of the condition and the potential risk for the patient (and others) arising from this. Although it is not clear from the literature whether the rate of suicide among people terminally ill with cancer is elevated, this has been a particular issue for people with HIV/AIDS. Whatever the medical condition, suicide is always a risk for people suffering from depression.

A satisfactory formulation of the predisposing, precipitating and perpetuating factors related to the depression is another essential prerequisite to developing a satisfactory management plan.

MANAGEMENT: GENERAL ISSUES

There is an erroneous belief that organic mood syndromes are relatively unresponsive to treatment. This is not true, and it is important to offer effective treatment as part of an overall treatment plan, including treatment of the physical illness. The Cochrane Collaboration has found antidepressants to be effective in patients with a wide range of physical diseases, with an overall number needed to treat of 4.2 (Gill and Hatcher 2000), and different forms of cognitive therapy have been shown to be effective in treating depression in a range of physical conditions such as multiple sclerosis and HIV/AIDS (Blanch et al. 2002).

The management of depression in the medically ill is broadly the same as that of any other form of depression, although additional factors related to the physical illness and its treatment need to be considered. Information about the illness and empathic discussion of its effect on patients and their families is important. The implications of the prognosis, in terms of alterations in occupational, social and family functioning, will need to be explored. A review of how the patient has previously coped with stressful situations and losses, including previous personal or family illnesses, may reveal strategies for dealing with the present situation. The psychiatrist or physician can then identify the problems which the patient wishes to work on further, with a focus on the 'here and now'. Patients should be supported as they express painful emotions and come to terms with the loss of health, function and roles. Patients may need help to find practical solutions to their difficulties. The family should not be excluded from this process, as they will share many of the same fears and anxieties, and may even fear developing a similar disease themselves.

In addition to these issues, there are often other important factors in the depressed person's life and social network to be considered, as with depressive illnesses arising in other settings.

MANAGEMENT: BIOLOGICAL TREATMENTS

The antidepressant agents currently available differ more in their side-effect profiles than in their efficacy. Most tricyclic antidepressants (TCAs) are potent anticholinergic agents, sedating, and have some degree of noradrenergic and antihistaminic action. Among the monoamine oxidase inhibitors (MAOIs), tranylcypromine is often mildly activating. In contrast, the newer agents are generally less anticholinergic, less sedating and have less antihistaminic action. This is particularly true of the selective serotonin reuptake inhibitors (SSRIs) and the reversible MAOIs.

Despite the extensive literature on the clinical effects of these agents in otherwise healthy depressed subjects, there is a paucity of hard data on their safety in medical disorders. The few trials in the literature often study heterogeneous and poorly described populations of patients. In particular, there are few trials of treatment in the elderly physically ill. This is a particularly important group of patients, and will become more so over the next 30 years. Already 12 per cent of the population of the United States is over 65 years old, and they account for 20–40 per cent of the caseload in primary medical care. Treatment of depression in this group speeds recovery from physical illness and reduces mortality. Treatment needs to be continued for longer than in younger patients before a clinical response emerges, often for 4–6 weeks. The main problem with antidepressants in the elderly physically ill is less their toxicity than that they are underused or not used at all.

Like the elderly, AIDS patients face multiple illnesses. Severe illness itself has significant pharmacokinetic effects, and drug interactions are more likely with the multiple drugs that are often necessary. In one study, only 5 per cent of asymptomatic HIV-positive people suffered severe side effects, as against 25 per cent of those with AIDS.

Clearly, different medical conditions require that particular consideration be given to avoiding certain side effects of antidepressants.

Sedation

Unfortunately, nocturnal sedation with antidepressants is often associated with daytime drowsiness. This is a concern for many, including those with limited functional reserves such as the elderly. The older TCAs are generally sedative while newer agents, such as the SSRIs, serotonin noradrenaline reuptake inhibitors and moclobemide, have fewer effects on psychomotor performance. It is interesting that changes in sleep architecture characteristic of antidepressants have been demonstrated after treatment with the SSRIs. This suggests that the beneficial effects of antidepressants on sleep should not necessarily be associated with sedation.

Cardiovascular system

Orthostatic hypotension is a significant side effect of the TCAs that can lead to falls and fractures, especially in the elderly (Pollock 1999). One large study in the United States found that elderly patients treated with TCAs were at a three-fold increased risk of suffering a fractured hip compared with their age-matched peers. This risk was further increased if they suffered from heart failure, or were being treated with vasodilators, diuretics or benzodiazepines. The postural drop is greater with imipramine than with nortriptyline. In one study of people with left ventricular failure, 50 per cent of those on imipramine, but only 5 per cent on nortriptyline, developed orthostatic hypotension. Unselective MAOIs cause more falls, which is scarcely surprising considering their original use as antihypertensive medication.

Tricyclic antidepressants should never be the initial treatment in depressed patients with cardiac disease, especially ischaemic disease, because of their activity as class 1A antiarrhythmics and thus their potential to induce arrhythmias. The growing data on SSRIs in cardiac disease suggest they are safer alternatives, but there is very limited evidence on their use in the period immediately after myocardial infarction. SSRIs do not block the fast sodium channel and do not prolong either the PR interval or QRS interval, as class 1A antiarrhythmics or TCAs do. Although amoxapine and bupropion do not appear to cause electrocardiographic changes or arrhythmias, maprotiline causes a prolonged QRS interval, which can lead to supraventricular tachycardia, ventricular tachycardia and cardiac arrest, especially in overdose. Trazodone can induce ventricular arrhythmias, but this appears rare. The combination of an MAOI and tyramine can cause a marked pressor response that can lead to arrhythmias and an ectopic ventricular rhythm (Hale 1993; Glassman et al. 1998; Roose 2000, 2001).

The presence of overt or latent damage to the His-Purkinje system or excessive TCA levels can lead to second- or third-degree atrioventricular block, causing asystole and sudden death, bizarre bundle branch blocks, or a re-entry arrhythmia such as Torsade de pointes (a form of ventricular flutter which may progress to fibrillation). It has been recommended that people with left or right bundle branch block or an intraventricular conduction defect with widening of the QRS interval >0.11 should not be prescribed TCAs. Lithium is contraindicated in patients with sick sinus node syndrome.

Cardiac failure presents particular challenges. Although TCAs generally do not have a negative inotropic action, idiosyncratic responses can occur. Lithium is contraindicated in patients with unstable congestive heart failure.

The use of TCAs with thiazide and loop diuretics and angiotensin-converting enzyme inhibitors appears safe. The co-administration of lithium and thiazide diuretics is contraindicated.

The paucity of trials of antidepressants in cardiac patients, particularly elderly cardiac patients, means caution is essential when prescribing for patients with serious cardiac disease and consultation with a cardiologist advisable. Plasma monitoring of antidepressants may be helpful in limiting the risk of toxicity by allowing excessive doses to be avoided.

Dementia

Two double-blind trials indicated a clear antidepressant response to imipramine in depressed patients with Alzheimer's disease. Similar response rates have been reported with other drugs. Interestingly, moclobemide has been reported to improve cognitive functioning in elderly demented patients, but it is difficult to determine whether this reflected genuine memory enhancement or merely nonspecific activation. The anticholinergic effects of the TCAs are best avoided in cognitively impaired elderly people.

Epilepsy

Between 19 and 31 per cent of people who have epilepsy will present for treatment of depression. Evidence-based prescribing is difficult because there is little difference between the low rate of spontaneous first seizures in the community (about 0.08 per cent each year) and the lower end of estimates of antidepressant-related seizures (about 0.1 per cent each year). To have any real power, comparison studies must be much larger than those commonly reported. Such large studies would have to control for predisposing risk factors such as previous epilepsy, a family history of epilepsy, an abnormal electroencephalogram (EEG), brain damage, or concurrent use of other drugs. All these lower seizure threshold, often considerably. For example, seizures occurred in 21 per cent of a group of brain-injured patients treated with antidepressants in one study. This makes the selection of a particular antidepressant for a person with epilepsy difficult. In high-risk groups there may be a place for therapeutic drug level monitoring to avoid excessive blood levels. However, there is no consensus over whether there is a relationship between EEG parameters or TCA blood levels and the likelihood of seizures. In general, antidepressant-related seizures are more likely to occur in the first week of starting treatment or increasing the dose.

The older TCAs rarely cause seizures at therapeutic blood levels. However, the annual cumulative risk of seizures for clomipramine and bupropion is about 1.4 per cent. Maprotiline is also associated with significantly higher risks of seizures, with 42 per cent of these occurring after 6 weeks, suggesting the accumulation of a proconvulsant metabolite. Both maprotiline and amoxapine are associated with a high incidence of seizures after overdose. It is therefore recommended that doses of 225 mg/day for maprotiline, 450 mg/day for bupropion and 250 mg/day for clomipramine not be exceeded. The incidence of seizures with SSRIs appears to be broadly in line with, or less than, that reported for TCAs. The older MAOIs do not appear to have a proconvulsive action, provided tyramine is avoided. Toxic levels of lithium above 3 mEq/L carry a greater risk of seizures, but it is controversial whether lithium is pro- or anticonvulsant at lower doses (Rosenstein et al. 1993).

Antipsychotics, commonly used in treating psychotic depression, also lower seizure threshold. Chlorpromazine appears to be particularly problematic, causing fits in 1 per cent of patients with epilepsy. Haloperidol is probably the drug of choice among the older antipsychotics, but thioridazine, pimozide and fluphenazine could also be considered.

Obviously, overdoses per se are associated with a greater risk of seizures, particularly in the first 6 hours. One substantial review of 2500 patients following overdoses of TCAs found that the incidence of seizures was 8.4 per cent.

When prescribing for patients with an identifiable predisposition to epilepsy or past seizures, it is particularly important to prescribe the minimum effective dose and to avoid sudden large changes of dose.

Eye

Tricyclic antidepressants are contraindicated in narrow-angle glaucoma, and agents without significant anticholinergic action, such as the SSRIs, should be used instead (Lieberman and Stoudemire 1987).

Gastrointestinal system

The more anticholinergic TCAs should be avoided in patients with impaired bowel motility.

Iatrogenic nausea is clearly more common with the SSRIs, although it can occur with other antidepressants too. Taking the antidepressant with food can reduce this. There is generally rapid tolerance to this effect.

Consideration of the use of antidepressants in patients with cirrhosis is important because alcoholism and depression often coexist. The alleged lack of interaction between alcohol and both the SSRIs and moclobemide, and the possible anti-craving effects of the SSRIs, may mean that these drugs are used preferentially in these patients.

Patients with cirrhosis, especially those with subcortical encephalopathy, have an increased susceptibility to the sedative action of psychotropic medication. Single-and multiple-dose studies in patients with cirrhosis indicate that most antidepressants have a longer half-life and decreased plasma clearance. In general, doses should be reduced by 50 per cent in patients with cirrhosis, but the possibility of idiosyncratically higher plasma levels in some individuals with cirrhosis should be borne in mind. In one-single dose study of moclobemide in patients with cirrhosis, three of thirteen patients had particularly high plasma levels. Older MAOIs are contraindicated in liver disease.

Metabolic disorders

Cholinergic agonists, sometimes used to counteract the anticholinergic action of TCAs, are contraindicated in hyperthyroidism.

Fluoxetine appeared well tolerated in non-depressed people with non-insulin-dependent diabetes who were taking this drug for weight control purposes.

Parkinson's disease

Depression is often concomitant with Parkinson's disease. There is sometimes a misguided reluctance to treat it because of a perception that it is organic in origin, with the implication that it is less responsive to treatment. However, nortriptyline has been shown to be effective in a double-blind trial in depressed patients suffering from Parkinson's disease, as has fluvoxamine. The latter exacerbated parkinsonian symptoms in four of twenty patients, which probably reflects the intimate association between the serotonergic and dopaminergic systems. It has also been reported that electroconvulsive therapy appears to help the movement disturbance as well as mood. Amoxapine should be avoided in this condition because of its dopaminergic action (Bhatia et al. 2001).

Respiratory disorders

The anticholinergic action of TCAs can exacerbate respiratory disease by increasing the stickiness of respiratory secretions. Monoamine oxidase inhibitors may interact with sympathomimetic bronchodilators, although other anti-asthma medications appear safe.

Urinary system

From a pharmacokinetic point of view, renal impairment presents fewer challenges than some other disorders. In general, it is only when more than 10 per cent of a drug is excreted renally that problems arise with accumulation. In general, antidepressants are extensively metabolised in the liver and only some 1–5 per cent of the parent drug is excreted unchanged by the kidneys. Several studies have confirmed that the pharmacokinetics of a range of antidepressant drugs are unchanged in renal failure, but it would be prudent to initiate treatment with two-thirds of standard doses and to consider the use of plasma level monitoring.

The anticholinergic side effects of the TCAs make them unsuitable for the treatment of patients with prostatic hypertrophy.

Pregnancy and breastfeeding

These topics are addressed in Chapter 32.

Drug interactions

Many drugs, such as alcohol, barbiturates, cigarette smoking, oral contraceptives, carbamazepine and phenytoin, increase the rate of oxidation of TCAs in the liver and *reduce* TCA levels. Other drugs, such as cimetidine, propranolol, isoniazid, disulfiram, antipsychotics, other tricyclic antidepressants, methylphenidate, and fluoxetine, decrease the rate of oxidation in the liver and *increase* TCA levels. Tricyclic antidepressants may increase phenytoin levels and warfarin levels.

Psychotropic agents, like many other drugs, are metabolised by the cytochrome P450 system. Although the common interactions between psychotropic agents, such as between SSRIs and both TCAs and most antipsychotic agents, may be well known, interactions with other medications may be less familiar. Information on how drugs are metabolised by, and affect, these enzymes is available from various sources, some of which provide full references (such as <http://medicine.iupui.edu/flockhart/>). This allows prediction of likely interactions. It is important to remember that drugs are often metabolised by multiple pathways. Although the therapeutic index for some drugs, such as the SSRIs, is relatively high so that an unexpectedly increased plasma level may put the person taking it at little hazard, this is not so for other antidepressants.

In the elderly, the key pharmacokinetic issue is that the water compartment shrinks and fat compartment expands with age. This means that water-soluble drugs such as lithium and alcohol become more potent in the elderly, and fat-soluble drugs, which include most psychotropic drugs, have a longer half-life. Half of all drugs taken by elderly people are purchased over the counter. This resulting polypharmacy for a variety of different conditions increases the risk of significant drug interactions and adverse events. The risk of an adverse reaction with five drugs is said to be 50 per cent; with eight, 100 per cent. The mean number of drugs taken by the elderly is five.

Drug substitution is now common in both New Zealand and Australia. The bioequivalence requirements of the US Food and Drug Administration are that a generic compound should deliver between 80 and 120 per cent of the dose available from the reference compound. If a patient changes from one form of a drug to another, the dose available to the patient may change quite substantially. Therefore, with drugs with a low or relatively low therapeutic index, it is important that patients not change from one preparation to another of the same drug without the possible implications of this being considered, including implications of interactions with other drugs being taken simultaneously.

MANAGEMENT: PSYCHOLOGICAL TREATMENTS

Treatment of depression in the medically ill with medication is clearly complex, at least at times. This means that alternative evidence-based approaches should also be considered, including structured psychotherapies such as cognitive behaviour therapy (CBT) and interpersonal psychotherapy. At times, clinical experience will support the use of other forms of psychotherapy, even though clear evidence of efficacy in the medically ill is not yet available. Because of limitations of space, only CBT is discussed here.

Cognitive behaviour therapy

Cognitive behaviour therapy is a short-term structured psychotherapy that has demonstrated efficacy in treating depression in a wide range of populations. There is mounting evidence that CBT decreases the emotional distress of illness and increases quality of life, independent of the severity of medical symptoms. CBT complements medical treatment by improving compliance with medication, assists in the associated lifestyle adjustments that are often necessary, and may be an effective treatment for depression in the medically ill. CBT-based groups facilitate adjustment to chronic or life-threatening illness (Sensky and Wright 1993).

Individual responses to illness, such as the development of depression, may be more related to cognitive factors than the particular symptoms or severity of a medical illness. Cognitions are proposed to be a central part of the biopsychosocial response to being diagnosed with an illness, and to mediate the emotional response to this. Depression can be a response to an event that is perceived to be aversive and uncontrollable. CBT helps individuals recognise that how they think about a situation, symptom or event can affect how they feel and behave. CBT for depression aims to identify patterns of unhelpful cognitions and behaviours that maintain depressed mood, and helps individuals learn skills to make changes to these areas of functioning. CBT for depression in medical patients also aims to increase quality of life, reduce risk factors for ill-health by changing behaviours such as diet, exercise and alcohol use, improve coping skills and compliance with medical interventions, and reduce the emotional toll of medical problems. CBT has been demonstrated to reduce dysfunctional ways of responding to illness and to help develop realistic appraisals of ill-health and disability, reduce depression and increase healthy behaviour (Newton and Doron 2000).

CBT interventions have been evaluated in a range of medical illnesses with encouraging results, including cancer, HIV, heart disease, diabetes, multiple sclerosis, and chronic pain. Most research has focused on cancer and chronic pain, which are commonly associated with depression. CBT was found to be effective in reducing the physical and psychosocial disability associated with chronic pain through changing pain-related beliefs and developing appropriate coping strategies (Turner et al. 2001). Individuals with comorbid diagnoses of cancer and depression responded to CBT-based treatments, and CBT groups improved adjustment to their potentially life-threatening diagnoses and developed improved fighting spirit, less hopelessness, reduced anxiety and self-defined life problems compared with control subjects (Moorey et al. 1998). Others found CBT reduced depression and improved self-esteem in patients with metastatic breast cancer, at least in the short term (Edelman et al. 1999).

CBT was effective in treating depressive symptoms and improving blood sugar control (as measured by reduced HbA_{1c}) in people with diabetes (85 per cent of the group achieved remission compared with 27 per cent of controls, with 70 per cent of the treated group free of depression at 6 months) (Culpepper 2000). In contrast, others have identified medical complications and lower compliance with blood glucose monitoring as factors predictive of a poor response to CBT in people with type 2 diabetes (Lustman et al. 1998).

There have been few specific studies into the effectiveness of CBT for depression concurrent with cardiac disease, although effective treatment of such depression lowers mortality rates.

In primary care, CBT is effective in treating physically ill people with depression, with benefits maintained over 1 year. Participants with minor depression and either hypertension, heart disease, diabetes mellitus or osteoarthritis were randomly assigned to an 8-week CBT intervention, or no intervention or information-only control conditions. Those in the CBT group reported fewer somatic symptoms and missed fewer medical appointments than control groups, as well as reporting reduced symptoms of depression (Miranda and Munoz 1994).

CBT is effective not only in treating core symptoms of depression, such as reduced energy, memory problems, reduced self-efficacy, and changes in interpersonal reactions, but also in reducing physical symptoms exacerbated by depression, such as pain and fatigue, and the social and vocational disability associated with the combination of ill-health and depression. It also promotes adherence to medical treatments and self-care (Burg and Abrams 2001).

These studies support the efficacy of referring individuals with concurrent diagnoses of depression and a medical illness for treatment with CBT. Although the evidence base for such treatment is still limited, it is consistent with the substantial evidence for the efficacy of CBT in depression in other settings. It also has the advantage of not introducing further drug interactions into an already pharmacologically complex situation.

The duration of treatment of a depressive illness is currently under review. Although there are increasing data to indicate the need for prolonged prophylactic treatment of recurrent depression in the physically well, the situation in the depressed medically ill with a first episode of depression is less clear. When a mood disturbance responds rapidly to some change in medical management (such as eventual control of disabling pain or resolution of protracted surgical complications), the diagnosis should be reviewed, as should the appropriateness of the treatment for depression.

Appropriate treatment of depression in the medically ill can make a major contribution to a more rapid recovery and, in some circumstances, decreased mortality. Diagnosis, formulation and management are potentially complex and may need to draw on a greater range of disciplines than in some other areas of psychiatry. However, the ability of psychiatrists to draw on an understanding of complex systems and to work effectively in multidisciplinary teams enhances the contribution that can be made to quality patient care in the general hospital.

REFERENCES

Barefoot JC, Schroll M (1996) Symptoms of depression, acute myocardial infarction, and total mortality in a community sample. *Circulation* 93:1976-80.

Bhatia K, Brooks DJ, Burn DJ, Clarke CE, Grosset DG, MacMahon DG, et al. (2001) Updated guidelines for the management of Parkinson's disease. *Hospital Medicine (London)* 62:456-70.

Blanch J, Rousaud A, Hautzinger M, Martinez E, Peri JM, Andres S, et al. (2002) Assessment of the efficacy of a cognitive-behavioural group psychotherapy programme for HIV-infected patients referred to a consultation-liaison psychiatry department. *Psychotherapy and Psychosomatics* 71:77-84.

Brown ES, Suppes T (1998) Mood symptoms during corticosteroid therapy: A review. *Harvard Review of Psychiatry* 5:239-46.

Burg MM, Abrams D (2001) Depression in chronic medical illness: The case of coronary heart disease. *Journal of Clinical Psychology* 57:1323-37.

Carney RM, Freedland KE, Miller GE, Jaffe AS (2002) Depression as a risk factor for cardiac mortality and morbidity: A review of potential mechanisms. *Journal of Psychosomatic Research* 53:897-902.

Culpepper L (2000) Depression and chronic mental illness: Diabetes as a model. *Psychiatric Annals* 32:528-34.

Edelman S, Bell DR, Kidman AD (1999) A group cognitive behaviour therapy programme with metastatic breast cancer patients. *Psycho-Oncology* 8:295-305.

Gill D, Hatcher S (2000) Antidepressants for depression in medical illness. [Update of Cochrane Database Syst. Rev. 2000; (2): CD001312.] *Cochrane Database of Systematic Reviews* (4):CD001312.

Glassman AH, Rodriguez AI, Shapiro PA (1998) The use of antidepressant drugs in patients with heart disease. *Journal of Clinical Psychiatry* 59 Suppl 10:16-21.

Hale AS (1993) New antidepressants: Use in high-risk patients. *Journal of Clinical Psychiatry* 54 Suppl:61-70.

Koschera A, Hickie I, Hadzi-Pavlovic D, Wilson A, Lloyd A (1999) Prolonged fatigue, anxiety and depression: Exploring relationships in a primary care sample. *Australian and New Zealand Journal of Psychiatry* 33:545-52.

Lieberman E, Stoudemire A (1987) Use of tricyclic antidepressants in patients with glaucoma. Assessment and appropriate precautions. *Psychosomatics* 28:145-8.

Lustman PJ, Freedland KE, Griffith LS, Clouse RE (1998) Predicting response to cognitive behavior therapy of depression in type 2 diabetes. *General Hospital Psychiatry* 20:302-6.

Miranda J, Munoz R (1994) Intervention for minor depression in primary care patients. *Psychosomatic Medicine* 56:136-41.

Moorey S, Greer S, Bliss J, Law M (1998) A comparison of adjuvant psychological therapy and supportive counselling in patients with cancer. *Psycho-Oncology* 7:218-28.

Newton TL, Doron SE (2000) Cognitive-behavioral processes in managing the stress and anxiety of medical illness. In Mostofsky DI, Barlow DH (eds), *The Management of Stress and Anxiety in Medical Disorders*. Boston: Allyn & Bacon, pp. 84-99.

Pollock BG (1999) Adverse reactions of antidepressants in elderly patients. *Journal of Clinical Psychiatry* 60 Suppl 20:4-8.

Roose SP (2000) Considerations for the use of antidepressants in patients with cardiovascular disease. *American Heart Journal* 140 (4 Suppl):84-8.

—— (2001) Depression, anxiety, and the cardiovascular system: The psychiatrist's perspective. *Journal of Clinical Psychiatry* 62 Suppl 8:19-22.

Rosenstein DL, Nelson JC, Jacobs SC (1993) Seizures associated with antidepressants: A review. *Journal of Clinical Psychiatry* 54:289-99.

Sensky T, Wright JH (1993) Cognitive therapy with medical patients. In Wright JH, Thase ME, Ludgate JW, Beck AT (eds), *Cognitive Therapy with Inpatients: Developing a cognitive milieu*, pp. 219-46.

Turner JA, Dworkin SF, Mancl L, Huggins KH, Truelove EL (2001) The roles of beliefs, catastrophizing, and coping in the functioning of patients with temporomandibular disorders. *Pain* 92:41-51.

CHAPTER 27

EATING DISORDERS AND DEPRESSION

Janice M McKenzie,
Jennifer Jordan and
Virginia V W McIntosh

Since the earliest reports describing eating disorders, it has been noted that they are frequently associated with depressive illness. Despite clinicians finding that patients with both disorders are often more difficult to treat, there is little guidance as to how best to help these patients.

This chapter reviews theories of the comorbidity of depressive and eating disorders, reports the prevalence of comorbid mood and eating disorders, and considers the clinical significance of the comorbidity. Some practical guidelines are suggested for the assessment and treatment of individuals with combined eating disorders and mood disorders.

RELATIONSHIP BETWEEN EATING DISORDERS AND DEPRESSION

The frequent co-occurrence of depressive and eating disorders has led to various theories about how these two groups of disorders relate. One theory holds that eating disorders are an atypical presentation of an underlying depressive disorder, and that the two disorders share all aetiological features. Other views propose that these disorders are separate, but that one is the primary disturbance, and the other secondary. Another hypothesis is that both share the same aetiological factors, and are merely different manifestations of the same disorder. A further theory views the two disorders as unique, with some shared, and some independent aetiological factors.

Findings from clinical and family studies, and from epidemiological and genetic research, are able to contribute to a discussion about the relationship between eating and depressive disorders. Many depressive symptoms are common in eating disorders. Individuals with eating disorders are more likely to be depressed than those without an eating disorder, and mood disorders are common in the families of individuals with eating disorders. Antidepressants can be effective in the treatment of bulimia nervosa, and may have an effect in helping to maintain treatment gains in individuals with anorexia nervosa. Clinical studies have revealed that both temporal sequences of the development of the disorders occur: depression can predate the eating disorder, and vice versa. Although eating disorders and depression have some shared biological features, many neuroendocrine differences exist. Twin studies suggest that unique gene sets contribute independently to eating disorders and to depression, but also that some shared gene sets may contribute to both disorders.

Based on the current state of knowledge about these two disorder groups, the most likely model of their relationship is that eating disorders and depression result from the reciprocal interplay of different forces at the biological, psychological, familial and sociocultural levels. The two disorder groups appear to be unique, with some shared aetiological factors (Bulik 2002).

RATES OF CO-OCCURRENCE

The association between depression and eating disorders has been investigated from the perspective of each disorder. Although higher rates of eating disorders and symptoms have been reported in samples of individuals with depression than in non-depressed samples (Zaider et al. 2000), more is known about the occurrence of depression in eating disorder samples. This chapter focuses on the presence of comorbid depression among people with eating disorders.

Depression is the most common comorbid condition found in all eating disorders. Prevalences are higher in clinical samples because of referral and other biases such as Berkson's bias (people with more than one disorder are more likely to present for treatment), but even people with eating disorders identified in epidemiological surveys have elevated rates of mood disorder compared with those without eating disorder diagnoses. The prevalence rates reported are variable because of a range of methodological issues. Rates for current comorbid depression in large eating disorder samples have been reported to be around 50 per cent (see O'Brien and Vincent 2003 for a review). About two-thirds of individuals with anorexia nervosa have been found to have a lifetime history of major depressive disorder, with major depression found in up to 50 per cent of individuals with the restricting subtype of anorexia nervosa and up to 90 per cent of individuals with the binge eating/purging subtype. Up to two-thirds of those with bulimia nervosa have been reported to have lifetime major depression. Those with bulimia nervosa and a past history of anorexia nervosa have higher rates of lifetime major depression than those with bulimia nervosa without an anorexia nervosa history. For binge eating disorder, rates of around 50 per cent have been reported for lifetime major depression (for example, Bulik 2002). People with subthreshold eating disorders (eating disorder not otherwise specified) appear to have similar patterns of depression comorbidity to those who meet full diagnostic criteria for one of the specific eating disorders.

THE CLINICAL SIGNIFICANCE OF COMORBIDITY

Although comorbid mood disorders are very common in eating disorders, the effect of this is unclear (Pike 1998). While some studies have reported that comorbid depression at initial presentation does not predict outcome (for example, Steiner et al. 1990; Joyce et al. In press), others have suggested that comorbid depression at intake is associated with a more chronic course and worse prognosis than those with no mood comorbidity at baseline (for example, Agras et al. 2000). However, there is little dispute that the presence of depression at follow-up of patients with an eating disorder is associated with more psychopathology and poorer psychosocial functioning (Schork et al. 1994; Herpertz-Dahlmann et al. 1995).

Mortality in anorexia is high and suicide risk is elevated for people with an eating disorder diagnosis. A large meta-analysis of outcome studies estimated that up to half of the 5.6 per cent mortality per decade of follow-up in anorexia nervosa was due to suicide (Sullivan 1995).

ASSESSMENT CONSIDERATIONS

There are unique problems in the assessment of a patient with an eating disorder and coexisting mood disorder symptoms.

Mood commonly drops in the context of food restriction, irrespective of whether the individual has a history of mood disorder. There is evidence from starvation studies that food restriction in itself can lead to dysphoria, irritability, poor sleep and other mood symptoms (Keys et al. 1950; Vitousek and Manke 1994). Even individuals with bulimia nervosa who are at a normal weight can be restricting severely and suffering from symptoms secondary to malnourishment. Owing to symptom overlap, the use of typical depression measures (clinician-rated or self-report) can be problematic.

Another issue specific to anorexia nervosa is the possibility of denial or distortion in self-reported symptoms during the acute phase of anorexia nervosa. It has been observed that, for some individuals with anorexia nervosa, recovery may lead to greater endorsement of eating disorder symptoms and distress. It may be that once these individuals are healthier they become more aware of their distress, and are less able to ignore or deny eating disorder symptoms. The reality of the need for weight gain may also lead to more distress (Vitousek and Manke 1994).

Binge eating, carbohydrate craving and objective overeating may occur in atypical depression and may be a contributing factor in the onset or exacerbation of bulimia nervosa or binge eating disorder. As the duration and severity of bulimic symptoms increase, the person may feel out of control and demoralisation may set in, adding to depressive symptoms. Increasing severity of bulimic symptoms can then contribute to depressive symptoms and vice versa.

Occasionally individuals with major depression may have such severe weight loss that they are mistakenly diagnosed as having anorexia nervosa despite not having the important associated psychological features of anorexia nervosa – such as disturbed body image and fear of weight gain. Rarely, weight loss secondary to major depression has been reported by patients to apparently trigger the full syndrome of anorexia nervosa.

With the above confounding issues in mind, a full assessment of the eating and mood symptoms, including the appropriate physical investigations, is vital in developing a good formulation and management plan and in beginning to form a therapeutic relationship with the patient. Clarifying the presence of a comorbid mood disorder is important, and can be aided by the following:

- A careful history of the relative onset of the mood and eating disorder symptoms and the presence of a family history of psychiatric disorder may offer important guidance as to whether a major depressive disorder coexists with an eating disorder.
- The presence and severity of current mood symptoms needs to be established. As the somatic symptoms of eating disorders and depression can overlap, careful attention to the cognitive features of depression (such as helplessness, hopelessness, suicidal ideation or suicidal plans) helps further establish the diagnosis of a depressive disorder.
- Assessment of other comorbidity, particularly anxiety and substance-use disorders, and axis II personality disorders, is also important, while bearing in mind the difficulties of diagnosing personality disorders in acute eating disorder and depressive states.

TREATMENT CONSIDERATIONS

A thorough overall assessment, sound formulation, and good clinical judgment is essential in deciding which signs and symptoms are important in prioritising treatment. Important decisions include whether treatment for the comorbid eating and mood problems should be concurrent or sequential.

It is also important to consider the possible influence on treatment of other comorbid disorders such as anxiety, substance use and personality disorders, and to incorporate this into the formulation and treatment planning.

The task of establishing and maintaining a good therapeutic alliance cannot be underestimated in patients with eating disorders. Indeed, the therapeutic relationship is a cornerstone of treatment (Bruch 1986; Pike et al. 1996).

The following section highlights issues important in the treatment of patients with eating disorder and a coexisting mood disorder. It is not intended as a detailed overview of treatments for individuals with eating disorders. A number of excellent reviews and guidelines for treatment of eating disorders are recommended (Wilson and Fairburn 1998; Yager et al. 2000; Beumont et al. In press). Given the absence of evidence-based guidelines for treating comorbid depression and eating disorders, the clinician should expect that the course of treatment may be a series of trials followed by thorough review and reconsideration of the next phase of treatment.

NUTRITIONAL TREATMENT AND STABILISATION

Nutritional treatments for eating disorders emphasise the importance of correcting nutritional status, and providing education and counselling to normalise eating behaviour, allay patients' fears about food, and provide accurate nutritional information (American Dietetic Association 2001). In addition, nutritional treatments aim to help patients develop appropriate responses to hunger and satiety cues (Craighead and Allen 1995).

Anorexia nervosa

Once the clinician is satisfied that the patient has anorexia nervosa together with major depression, the following guidelines for treatment may be considered.

It is important to first tackle the symptoms of starvation in anorexia nervosa, unless they are mild. Clinicians have noted that when patients are in a starved state with a low body mass index (BMI), there may be a poor response to both psychotherapy and psychopharmacology. Hence, refeeding is important to help improve the nutrition, increase the individual's weight, and stabilise physiological, psychological and cognitive changes secondary to starvation.

If the patient's mood is not improving despite improvement in weight (a suggested BMI around 13–15 kg/m^2) and alleviation of the symptoms of starvation, now is the time to consider whether the patient will respond to a psychological therapy, or whether a pharmacological intervention may be indicated.

Bulimia nervosa

As patients with bulimia nervosa may have symptoms of starvation and significant metabolic problems secondary to binge eating and purging, any metabolic abnormalities must be stabilised before proceeding with psychological or pharmacological therapy for depression.

PSYCHOLOGICAL THERAPIES

Anorexia nervosa

Although there is widespread support that weight stabilisation is important in the treatment of anorexia nervosa, good evidence for the use of specific psychotherapies is lacking. In adolescents, family therapy has been shown to be important (Eisler et al. 2000). Cognitive behaviour therapy may well benefit patients with anorexia nervosa (Pike et al. In press), and, given its proven benefits in the treatment of depression, this could be considered the psychotherapeutic treatment of choice when the patient has associated major depression. In a recent Christchurch study (McIntosh et al. In press), supportive psychotherapy with clinical management (nutritional advice and psychoeducation) was effective in treating individuals with spectrum anorexia nervosa (anorexia nervosa diagnosed using a broadened weight criterion).

Bulimia nervosa

Psychotherapy has been found to be helpful in both bulimia nervosa and major depression. Many excellent controlled treatment trials have shown that manual-based cognitive behaviour therapy is currently the first-line treatment for bulimia nervosa. Other psychotherapies also shown to be effective with bulimia nervosa are interpersonal psychotherapy (IPT) and some modified forms of cognitive behaviour therapy (CBT), such as guided self-help. Both CBT and IPT are effective in the treatment of major depression (Elkin et al. 1989). When psychotherapy for concurrent bulimia nervosa and depression is considered, CBT or IPT could be considered the treatment of choice. As patients often prefer psychotherapy to taking medication, it may be advisable to explore this treatment option first.

Binge eating disorder

Many of the treatment strategies found helpful for bulimia nervosa have also, with some modifications, been found useful in binge eating disorder (Wilfley et al. 2002). Both CBT (guided CBT-based self-help) and IPT can be helpful in binge eating disorder along with weight management strategies such as increased exercise and better eating habits.

PSYCHOPHARMACOLOGY

Anorexia nervosa

Modern pharmacotherapy has not been promising as a primary treatment for anorexia nervosa (see Jimerson et al. 1996). Antidepressants, both tricyclic antidepressants and selective serotonin reuptake inhibitors (SSRIs), have been trialled. There is some evidence that fluoxetine may assist with weight maintenance in anorexic women (Kaye et al. 1991). Some antipsychotics have also been studied, with little evidence of success. There is some early evidence that olanzapine may have benefit in assisting with primary weight gain in patients with anorexia nervosa (Powers et al. 2002).

With this in mind, the SSRIs may be considered the initial pharmacological treatment of choice in tackling the symptoms of major depression. The SSRIs are often more acceptable to patients than tricyclic antidepressants because they have fewer side effects – in particular, they do not cause weight gain. SSRIs are also more effective in the younger age group and tend to be safer medically.

Bulimia nervosa

Several different groups of antidepressant medications result in the short-term reduction of bingeing and purging even in the absence of a mood disorder, although the longer-term outcome of these treatments is not established. As low mood can perpetuate ongoing binge eating and purging behaviours, if the patient is not improving with psychotherapy or the symptoms of major depression are significant then antidepressant medication should be considered. There is some evidence that a higher dose of fluoxetine (at least 60 mg/day) is needed for an anti-binge effect. SSRIs are probably the first pharmacological option and, if given at a higher dose, will have an anti-binge effect as well as treat the depression.

Binge eating disorder

Antidepressants (SSRIs at high doses) are also effective in reducing binge frequency in binge eating disorder. However, as with bulimia nervosa, the long-term outcome of treatment has not been established.

CONCLUSION

A high prevalence of depressive comorbidity occurs with eating disorders. Depression can occur before, coincident with, and subsequent to the eating disorder. Various theories have been proposed in attempting to account for the comorbid relationship. Based on evidence to date, it seems most likely that eating and mood disorders are separate entities that have some shared and some independent aetiological factors. Although there have been mixed findings, it seems that the presence of mood disorders may have significant clinical implications over the course of the disorder, with possible increased morbidity and mortality due to suicide risk. While much is still unknown about the most effective treatment of people with depressive and eating comorbidity, some practical guidelines on assessment and treatment have been suggested. Further research is needed in this important but neglected area.

REFERENCES

Agras WS, Crow SJ, Halmi KA, Mitchell JE, Wilson GT, Kraemer HC (2000) Outcome predictors for the cognitive behavior treatment of bulimia nervosa: Data from a multisite study. *American Journal of Psychiatry* 157:1302-8.

American Dietetic Association (2001) Position of the American Dietetic Association: Nutrition intervention in the treatment of anorexia nervosa, bulimia nervosa, and eating disorders not otherwise specified (EDNOS). *Journal of the American Dietetic Association* 101:810-19.

Beumont PJV, Hay P, Beumont RO (In press) Australian and New Zealand Clinical Practice Guideline for the Treatment of Anorexia Nervosa. *Australasian Psychiatry*.

Bruch H (1986) Anorexia nervosa: The therapeutic task. In Brownell KD, Foreyt JP (eds), *Handbook of Eating Disorders: Psychology and treatment of obesity, anorexia and bulimia*. New York: Basic Books, pp. 328-32.

Bulik CM (2002) Anxiety, depression, and eating disorders. In Fairburn CG, Brownell KD (eds), *Eating Disorders and Obesity. A comprehensive handbook*. New York: Guilford Press, pp. 193-8.

Craighead LW, Allen HN (1995) Appetite awareness training: A cognitive behavioral intervention for binge eating. *Cognitive and Behavioral Practice* 2:249-70.

Eisler I, Dare C, Hodes M, Russell G, Dodge E, le Grange D (2000) Family therapy for adolescent anorexia nervosa: The results of a controlled comparison of two family interventions. *Journal of Child Psychology and Psychiatry and Allied Disciplines* 41:727-36.

Elkin I, Shea MT, Watkins JT, Imber SD, Sotsky SM, Collins JF, et al. (1989) National Institute of Mental Health Treatment of Depression Collaborative Research Program. General effectiveness of treatments. *Archives of General Psychiatry* 46:971-82.

Herpertz-Dahlmann BM, Wewetzer C, Remschmidt H (1995) The predictive value of depression in anorexia nervosa: Results of a seven-year follow-up study. *Acta Psychiatrica Scandinavica* 91:114-19.

Jimerson DC, Wolfe BE, Brotman AW, Metzger ED (1996) Medications in the treatment of eating disorders. *Psychiatric Clinics of North America* 10:739-54.

Joyce PR, Luty SE, McKenzie JM, Mulder RT, McIntosh VV, Carter FA, et al. (In press) Bipolar II disorder: Personality and outcome in two clinical samples. *Australian and New Zealand Journal of Psychiatry*.

Kaye WH, Weltzin TE, Hsu LK, Bulik CM (1991) An open trial of fluoxetine in patients with anorexia nervosa. *Journal of Clinical Psychiatry* 52:464-71.

Keys A, Brozek J, Honschel A, Mickelson O, Taylor HL (1950) *The Biology of Human Starvation*. Minneapolis: University of Minnesota Press.

McIntosh VV, Jordan J, Carter FA, McKenzie JM, Luty SE, Bulik CM, et al. (In press) Strict versus lenient weight criterion in anorexia nervosa. *European Eating Disorders Review*.

O'Brien KM, Vincent NK (2003) Psychiatric comorbidity in anorexia and bulimia nervosa: Nature, prevalence, and causal relationships. *Clinical Psychology Review* 23:57-74.

Pike KM (1998) Long-term course of anorexia nervosa: Response, relapse, remission. *Clinical Psychology Review* 18:447-75.

Pike KM, Loeb K, Vitousek KM (1996) Cognitive-behavioral therapy for anorexia nervosa and bulimia nervosa. In Thompson JK (ed), *Eating Disorders, Obesity and Body Image: A practical guide to assessment and treatment*. Washington, DC: APA, pp. 253-302.

Pike KM, Walsh BT, Vitousek K, Wilson GT, Bauer J (In press) Cognitive behavioral therapy in the post-hospital treatment of anorexia nervosa. *American Journal of Psychiatry*.

Powers PS, Santana CA, Bannon YS (2002) Olanzapine in the treatment of anorexia nervosa: An open label trial. *International Journal of Eating Disorders* 32:146-54.

Schork EJ, Eckert ED, Halmi KA (1994) The relationship between psychopathology, eating disorder diagnosis, and clinical outcome at 10-year follow-up in anorexia nervosa. *Comprehensive Psychiatry* 35:113-23.

Steiner H, Mazer C, Litt IF (1990) Compliance and outcome in anorexia nervosa. *Western Journal of Medicine* 153:133-9.

Sullivan PF (1995) Mortality in anorexia nervosa. *American Journal of Psychiatry* 152:1073-4.

Vitousek K, Manke F (1994) Personality variables and disorders in anorexia nervosa and bulimia nervosa. *Journal of Abnormal Psychology* 103:137-47.

Wilfley DE, Welch RR, Stein RI, Spurrell EB, Cohen LR, Saelens BE, et al. (2002) A randomized comparison of group cognitive-behavioral therapy and group interpersonal psychotherapy for the treatment of overweight individuals with binge-eating disorder. *Archives of General Psychiatry* 59:713-21.

Wilson GT, Fairburn CG (1998) Treatments for eating disorders. In Nathan PE, Gorman JM (eds), *A Guide to Treatments That Work*. New York: Oxford University Press, pp. 501-30.

Yager J, Andersen AE, Devlin M, Egger H, Herzog D, Mitchell JE, et al. (2000) Practice guidelines for the treatment of patients with eating disorders (Rev. Ed.). American Psychiatric Association Working Group on Eating Disorders. *American Journal of Psychiatry* 157:1-39.

Zaider TI, Johnson JG, Cockell SJ (2000) Psychiatric comorbidity associated with eating disorder symptomatology among adolescents in the community. *International Journal of Eating Disorders* 28:58-67.

SECTION

VI

Mood Disorders and the Life Cycle

CHAPTER 28

CHILDHOOD DEPRESSION

Graham Martin

Both health care professionals and parents find it hard to believe that children up to the age of 12 years or prior to puberty can be depressed. Despite the pioneering work of Rutter, Kashani and Carlson and Cantwell, the fact that the syndrome may not fully resemble the classic description of adult symptomatology leads to confusion, misdiagnosis and missed opportunities. A recent large study of 8–9-year-old children from Scandinavia provides a good example (Puura et al. 1998). The authors reported that, although parents and teachers had noted depressive symptoms, only a few children received psychiatric assessment and care. Parents described depressed mood, lack of popularity, social withdrawal, disobedience, inattentiveness, and stealing. Teachers were aware of restlessness, poor concentration and school performance, somatic complaints, problems with being bullied, and absenteeism. Those most likely to be referred had asthma or soiling, or behavioural problems – that is, the symptoms were more physical, or troublesome to others.

In part, for all of us, there may be some discomfort to think of children becoming depressed. However, in the past even psychoanalytic theory suggested that small children in particular do not have sufficient superego development to become depressed. This view has now been countered by clinical report and research over many years, and child psychiatry professionals now accept that forms of depression do occur in childhood, and are worthy of careful assessment and treatment. In addition, there is increasing acceptance that childhood depressive illness has a continuity with adolescent and adult major depressive disorder.

THE CLINICAL PICTURE

Depression may be a mood, a syndrome discovered as the result of high scores on depression inventories or scales such as the Children's Depression Inventory (Twenge and Nolen Hoeksema 2002), or an illness. Children with depressive illness may appear persistently sad, may no longer enjoy activities they normally enjoy, or they may frequently appear agitated, hyperactive or irritable. They may appear bored or low in energy, and poor attention and concentration can be key issues. A major change in eating or sleeping patterns may be a sign of depression in children and adolescents. Physical problems such as headaches or stomach aches may be the first complaints indicating a depression, and frequent absences from school or deteriorating academic performance in school may be signals that careful assessment is warranted. An acute onset major depressive disorder occurs (Emslie et al. 1997). In addition, dysthymia is described – a low-grade depression lasting for longer than 6 months (Kovacs et al. 1994). Bipolar disorder is rare in its classic form, though it may occur in families with a strong history (Chang et al. 2000). It is rare in childhood even in the rapid-cycling form – that seen more commonly in adolescents – and clinicians even in inpatient settings are unlikely to see many children with clear-cut hypomania. Comorbidity with other disorders is a major feature of childhood depression (Angold and Costello 1993).

Depressive illness is more complex to diagnose in children, and several issues are worth noting. First, children are not simply small adults – they are developing human beings who may vary markedly among themselves in the same chronological age group. In addition, aspects of development (physical, emotional, psychosexual, cognitive, moral, social) may not all be synchronised in phase. That is, in some, physical development may outstrip cognitive and moral development. In others, cognitive development may be in advance of psychosexual maturity. Individual theorists concerned with development have provided frameworks in which to understand the assessment of a current mental state in the child, but these are guides only, and some tolerance of variability is crucial.

Second, in general, the younger the child the less clear the clinical picture may be. Four- or 5-year-olds are less likely than 8–10-year-olds to be aware of their internal state, may be less able to reflect on this – comparing themselves with where they were last week, or with others – and it is less likely they will have words or concepts to describe their inner world. A linked issue is that the literature suggests children, irrespective of age, may in general present a more diffuse picture of depression, in which classic symptoms and signs are not yet clear. This may well cause doubt about making a formal diagnosis prematurely, with its possible implications for relapse or future episodes. Issues of labelling and possible stigma may also be important concerns.

An important issue is that children live within families. This makes them subject to structural or dynamic forces that may lie behind the presented clinical picture. Intrafamilial experiences may act as stressors and lead to features of depression. Equally, children may reflect or incorporate symptoms from another family member. The implications of this are that it is almost impossible to diagnose a child from individual interview. It is crucial as part of the assessment to meet with the family as a whole to get a sense of how well-functioning each member is, to gauge how each individual interacts with the child, and to assess how the system functions as a whole.

Finally, children spend a large part of their lives at school, and increasingly through their development are influenced not only by their educational and sporting attainment but also through peer interaction in one-to-one situations and as members of small and large groups. No mental health assessment of a child is complete without reports from class and other teachers.

EPIDEMIOLOGY

Significant depressive symptoms may exist in up to a quarter of children up to age 12, but current clinical depression is likely to be present in only about 1–2 per cent per year, although about 5 per cent may report an episode in the past. This increases with age so that about 15 per cent may have experienced an episode by adolescence, with up to a third of these having had a recurrence. Earlier onset of the initial episode may increase the severity or the length of subsequent episodes in young people, and young people with an episode of childhood depression are more likely in adolescence to get depression than another disorder (Orvaschel et al. 1995). Similarly, children who report depression at the age of 8 years are more likely to have depression and suicidal thoughts at 16 years (Sourander et al. 2001). In the Dunedin longitudinal study, depression was less prevalent than behaviour disorders in 11-year-old children and there was often a past history of behavioural problems since the age of 5 years. However, the clinical picture at 11 years had continuity with previously diagnosed depression at age 9 years (McGee and Williams 1988).

AETIOLOGY

Family life

There is clear evidence that socioeconomic adversity, poor parent–child attachment, marital disharmony, and adverse life events (including sexual abuse) may be precursors of depression in childhood severe enough to lead to suicidal thoughts or behaviour in adolescence (Fergusson et al. 2000). Recent work has suggested that psychopathology apparently associated with family type is best explained by compromised quality of the parent–child relationship, parental depression and socioeconomic adversity (O'Connor et al. 2001). The number of adverse childhood experiences is important, with multiple experiences increasing the risks for later depression (Felitti et al. 1998).

Various issues warrant discussion. Early parental loss is a factor, as it is in the longer term (Oakley-Browne et al. 1995), although bereaved depressed children may have a different course from those with classic major depressive disorder (Cerel 2001). Such loss has been postulated to link with genetic vulnerability through enduring changes in hypothalamic–pituitary–adrenal axis function.

Similarly, divorce is a major aetiological factor in childhood depression (Pons Salvador and del Barrio 1993), although cognitive style may modify its expression (Mazur et al. 1999). Part of this picture is likely to be the prior marital discord leading up to the divorce. Children who witness marital violence are prone to exhibit both internalising symptoms such as depression and severe sadness, and externalising symptoms such as aggression, hyperactivity and conduct disorder traits (Perks and Jameson 1999; Norwood 2000).

Another form of family conflict may be between parent and child, 'a robust vulnerability factor for internalising problems like depression' (El Sheikh and Flanagan 2001). Akin to this may be the punitive or overly critical parenting style reported by some young adolescents with depression (Heaven and Goldstein 2001).

Intrafamilial emotional, physical and sexual abuse have all been implicated in childhood depression. Sexually abused children and adolescents seem to be at special risk, and demonstrate significantly more total psychopathology than both community and clinical non-sexually abused control groups, including depression as a major feature. A recent meta-analysis confirms this association and the long-term sequelae of child sexual abuse (Paolucci et al. 2001).

Finally, children of depressed mothers are much more likely to be depressed and to have depressive cognitive schemata (Taylor 1996). Such effects are visible from a very young age in terms of insecure attachment (Cicchetti et al. 1998). The interplay of genetic factors with the environmental risk factor of parental depression is the subject of recent discussion (Silberg and Rutter 2002), research and exploration using twin studies (Rice et al. 2002). At present, it appears that the shared environment is more important in children, but that genetic expression becomes more obvious from adolescence.

School

Children who get depressed are more likely to be struggling with multiple domains of competence, including academic, sporting and social (Seroczynski et al. 1997). Learning difficulties have long been known to be associated with depression (Weinberg et al. 1989). Rejection by peers is an important aetiological factor, as are more serious forms such as bullying (Sourander et al. 2000).

Physical illness

In prospective longitudinal studies, physical ill-health in childhood, independent of family dynamics and socioeconomic status, increases the likelihood of later depressive illness. Children with chronic illnesses, like diabetes, may be more likely to become depressed (Bennett 1994). Similarly, traumatic brain injury may increase the risk of depressive symptoms, especially among more socially disadvantaged children (Kirkwood et al. 2000).

However, chronicity of a medical problem seems to have an inconsistent effect, with asthma (Vila et al. 2000), cystic fibrosis (Geiss et al. 1992), sickle cell anaemia (Yang et al. 1994) and craniofacial deformity (Williamson 1997) not increasing the risk of depression in children. It has been suggested that depression is more likely to occur if there are common immune-mediated vulnerabilities to medical illness and depression (Cohen et al. 1998).

The effect of physical illness in causing childhood depression may be direct or may be mediated through depression of the mother (Mulhern et al. 1992), for instance in childhood cancer. It is notable that being a sibling of a child with chronic illness increases the risk of depression, as does being the sibling of a child with intellectual disability (Rossiter and Sharpe 2001).

With myriad aetiological factors, and their complexity across the environments of the child's life, what is needed is some unifying theoretical framework to bring it together in a coherent and understandable form. This is best provided by the stress vulnerability model (Cicchetti and Toth 1992), which suggests that risk factors from the biological to psychological to family environment through to socioeconomic disadvantage are additive and affect the underlying predisposition to depression.

MANAGEMENT

Given the relatively small contribution of genetic and biological factors to depression in childhood, compared with the apparently large contribution from environmental, family and school factors, it appears rather obvious that pharmacological approaches might not be as useful with children, and that therapy should target specific issues for the child, parent–child interaction and family dynamic factors. However, at this stage, considerably more research is necessary to support such conclusions. Most reviews of the treatment and management of childhood depression agree that specific psychosocial interventions can be shown to have reasonable effect sizes, but that pharmacological intervention should be approached with caution. Lewinsohn and Clarke (1999) in the United States summarised key features common to most cognitive behaviour therapy approaches, including specific treatment components, limited duration and contacts, structured and directive treatment sessions, age modifications, and group versus individual treatments. On the basis of a meta-analysis of studies of cognitive behaviour therapy, the authors estimated an overall effect size of 1.27 and reported that 63 per cent of patients showed clinically significant improvement at the end of treatment. This supports similar British work (Harrington et al. 1998a).

A recent review of family-based approaches noted the key importance of parent–child attachment (Sexson et al. 2001), and suggested therapeutic approaches that target dynamic aspects of family life. However, few studies have assessed the efficacy of family approaches to childhood depression, and even some of the most careful research has shown little that is convincing (Harrington et al. 1998b). There is still a relative lack of response to an early review of psychotherapeutic approaches (Holmes and Wagner 1992), which called for more research and better design of studies.

Psychoeducational approaches to improving understanding for the child and family may have both clinical and preventive implications, although much of the work has been completed in adolescent samples (Brent et al. 1993).

Finally, much of the limited research work on use of antidepressants in young people has examined adolescents rather than children (DeVane and Sallee 1996). What is clear is that there is no place for the use of tricyclic antidepressants in children with depression (Hazell et al. 2000). In addition, there are only non-controlled studies of monoamine oxidase inhibitors in children.

Selective serotonin reuptake inhibitors (SSRIs) may prove useful in childhood depression. Fluoxetine was superior to placebo in randomised controlled studies in children and adolescents (Emslie et al. 1997). Similarly, sertraline was effective with adolescents (McConville et al. 1996). Both pharmaceuticals appear to be well tolerated. However, recent press reports regarding side effects from SSRIs (particularly paroxetine) suggest that caution is warranted until sufficient research is completed that a meta-analysis can be accepted.

Overall, it appears reasonable in work with depressed children to target specific known aetiological factors, to work with the family and school to provide an optimum environment for recovery, and to provide clear psychoeducation and guidelines for families. Given that cognitive behavioural approaches have consistent therapeutic effects and little in the way of adverse effects, at this point they are to be preferred over pharmacological treatments.

CONCLUSION

Children up to the age of 12 years do get depression, and the features may be similar to depression in later life. A case can be made for continuity between childhood, adolescent and adult depression. Overall, childhood depression is likely to persist if not diagnosed and treated, or episodes can recur in adolescence and adulthood. Clinical features may not initially be clear, and this should be no surprise. Children are not little adults, and may have difficulty describing their inner experience without some direct questioning or leading. A key feature is that children are highly influenced by the family environment, and no assessment of childhood depression is complete without thorough assessment of family dynamics and their impact on the child.

Clinical features may initially be construed as denoting some other diagnosis, but over time it becomes clear that depression is more likely; it is important to keep an open mind. Similarly, childhood depression is often comorbid with features of anxiety, behaviour disorders such as attention deficit hyperactivity disorder or oppositional defiant disorder. Treatment of childhood depression with medication has not yet been shown to be more effective than placebo, and cognitive behavioural approaches, counselling or therapy to resolve family conflict, and management of educational difficulties and peer-related problems are the keys to change.

REFERENCES

Angold A, Costello EJ (1993) Depressive comorbidity in children and adolescents: Empirical, theoretical, and methodological issues. *American Journal of Psychiatry* 150:1779-91.

Bennett DS (1994) Depression among children with chronic medical problems: A meta-analysis. *Journal of Pediatric Psychology* 19:149-69.

Brent DA, Poling K, McKain B, Baugher M (1993) A psychoeducational program for families of affectively ill children and adolescents. *Journal of the American Academy of Child and Adolescent Psychiatry* 32:770-4.

Cerel JA (2001) The role of family factors in childhood depression. *Dissertation Abstracts International: Section B; The Sciences and Engineering* 62:2050.

Chang KD, Steiner H, Ketter TA (2000) Psychiatric phenomenology of child and adolescent bipolar offspring. *Journal of the American Academy of Child and Adolescent Psychiatry* 39:453-60.

Cicchetti D, Toth SL (eds) (1992) *Developmental Perspectives on Depression.* Rochester, NY: University of Rochester Press.

Cicchetti D, Rogosch FA, Toth SL (1998) Maternal depressive disorder and contextual risk: Contributions to the development of attachment insecurity and behavior problems in toddlerhood. *Developmental Psychopathology* 10:283-300.

Cohen P, Pine DS, Must A, Kasen S, Brook J (1998) Prospective associations between somatic illness and mental illness from childhood to adulthood. *American Journal of Epidemiology* 147:232-9.

DeVane CL, Sallee FR (1996) Serotonin selective reuptake inhibitors in child and adolescent psychopharmacology: A review of published experience. *Journal of Clinical Psychiatry* 57:55-66.

El Sheikh M, Flanagan E (2001) Parental problem drinking and children's adjustment: Family conflict and parental depression as mediators and moderators of risk. *Journal of Abnormal Child Psychology* 29:417-32.

Emslie GJ, Rush AJ, Weinberg WA, Kowatch RA, Hughes CW, Carmody T, et al. (1997) A double-blind, randomized, placebo-controlled trial of fluoxetine in children and adolescents with depression. *Archives of General Psychiatry* 54:1031-7.

Felitti VJ, Anda RF, Nordenberg D, Williamson DF, Spitz AM, Edwards V, et al. (1998) Relationship of childhood abuse and household dysfunction to many of the leading causes of death in adults. The Adverse Childhood Experiences (ACE) Study. *American Journal of Preventive Medicine* 14:245-58.

Fergusson DM, Woodward LJ, Horwood LJ (2000) Risk factors and life processes associated with the onset of suicidal behaviour during adolescence and early adulthood. *Psychological Medicine* 30:23-39.

Geiss SK, Hobbs SA, Hammersley-Maercklein G, Kramer JC, Henley M (1992) Psychosocial factors related to perceived compliance with cystic fibrosis treatment. *Journal of Clinical Psychology* 48:99-103.

Harrington R, Whittaker J, Shoebridge P, Campbell F (1998a) Systematic review of efficacy of cognitive behaviour therapies in childhood and adolescent depressive disorder. *BMJ* 316:1559-63.

Harrington R, Kerfoot M, Dyer E, McNiven F, Gill J, Harrington V, et al. (1998b) Randomized trial of a home-based family intervention for children who have deliberately poisoned themselves. *Journal of the American Academy of Child and Adolescent Psychiatry* 37:512-18.

Hazell P, O'Connell D, Heathcote D, Henry D (2000) Tricyclic drugs for depression in children and adolescents. *Cochrane Database of Systematic Reviews* (3):CD002317.

Heaven PCL, Goldstein M (2001) Parental influences and mental health among some Australian youth: Crosscultural analysis. *Australian Journal of Psychology* 53:170-5.

Holmes WD, Wagner KD (1992) Psychotherapy treatment for depression in children and adolescents. *Journal of Psychotherapy Practice and Research* 1:313-23.

Kirkwood M, Janusz J, Yeates KO, Taylor HG, Wade SL, Stancin T, et al. (2000) Prevalence and correlates of depressive symptoms following traumatic brain injuries in children. *Neuropsychology, Development, and Cognition. Section C, Child Neuropsychology* 6:195-208.

Kovacs M, Akiskal HS, Gatsonis C, Parrone PL (1994) Childhood-onset dysthymic disorder: Clinical features and prospective naturalistic outcome. *Archives of General Psychiatry* 51:365-74.

Lewinsohn PM, Clarke GN (1999) Psychosocial treatments for adolescent depression. *Clinical Psychology Review* 19:329-42.

Mazur E, Wolchik SA, Virdin L, Sandler IN, West SG (1999) Cognitive moderators of children's adjustment to stressful divorce events: The role of negative cognitive errors and positive illusions. *Child Development* 70:231-45.

McConville BJ, Minnery KL, Sorter MT, West SA, Friedman LM, Christian K (1996) An open study of the effects of sertraline on adolescent major depression. *Journal of Child and Adolescent Psychopharmacology* 6:41-51.

McGee R, Williams S (1988) A longitudinal study of depression in 9 year old children. *Journal of the American Academy of Child and Adolescent Psychiatry* 27:342-8.

Mulhern RK, Fairclough DL, Smith B, Douglas SM (1992) Maternal depression, assessment methods, and physical symptoms affect estimates of depressive symptomatology among children with cancer. *Journal of Pediatric Psychology* 17:313-26.

Norwood WDI (2000) Marital violence and children: A meta-analytic review of the empirical literature. *Dissertation Abstracts International: Section B; The Sciences and Engineering* April; 60 (9 B):4967.

Oakley-Browne MA, Joyce PR, Wells JE, Bushnell JA, Hornblow AR (1995) Disruptions in childhood parental care as risk factors for major depression in adult women. *Australian and New Zealand Journal of Psychiatry* 29:437-48.

O'Connor TG, Dunn J, Jenkins JM, Pickering K, Rasbash J (2001) Family settings and children's adjustment: Differential adjustment within and across families. *British Journal of Psychiatry* 179:110-15.

Orvaschel H, Lewinsohn PM, Seeley JR (1995) Continuity of psychopathology in a community sample of adolescents. *Journal of the American Academy of Child and Adolescent Psychiatry* 34:1525-35.

Paolucci E, Genuis ML, Violato C (2001) A meta-analysis of the published research on the effects of child sexual abuse. *Journal of Psychology* 135:17-36.

Perks SM, Jameson M (1999) The effects of witnessing domestic violence on behavioural problems and depressive symptomatology. A community sample of pupils from St Lucia. *West Indian Medical Journal* 48:208-11.

Pons Salvador G, del Barrio V (1993) Depresion infantil y divorcio. / Child depression and divorce. *Avances en Psicologia Clinica Latinoamericana* 11:95-106.

Puura K, Almqvist F, Tamminen T, Piha J, Kumpulainen K, Raesaenen E, et al. (1998) Children with symptoms of depression – what do adults see? *Journal of Child Psychology and Psychiatry and Allied Disciplines* 39:577-85.

Rice F, Harold GT, Thapar A (2002) Assessing the effects of age, sex and shared environment on the genetic aetiology of depression in childhood and adolescence. *Journal of Child Psychology and Psychiatry and Allied Disciplines* 43:1039-51.

Rossiter L, Sharpe D (2001) The siblings of individuals with mental retardation: A quantitative integration of the literature. *Journal of Child and Family Studies* 10:65-84.

Seroczynski AD, Cole AD, Maxwell SE (1997) Cumulative and compensatory effects of competence and incompetence on depressive symptoms in children. *Journal of Abnormal Psychology* 106:586-97.

Sexson SB, Glanville DN, Kaslow NJ (2001) Attachment and depression: Implications for family therapy. *Child and Adolescent Psychiatric Clinics of North America* 10:465-86.

Silberg J, Rutter M (2002) Nature–nurture interplay in the risks associated with parental depression. In Goodman SH, Gotlib II (eds), *Children of Depressed Parents: Mechanisms of risk and implications for treatment.* Washington, DC: American Psychological Association.

Sourander A, Helstela L, Helenius H, Piha J (2000) Persistence of bullying from childhood to adolescence – a longitudinal 8-year follow-up study. *Child Abuse and Neglect* 24:873-81.

Sourander A, Helstela L, Haavisto A, Bergroth L (2001) Suicidal thoughts and attempts among adolescents: A longitudinal 8-year follow-up study. *Journal of Affective Disorders* 63:59-66.

Taylor LA (1996) Depression vulnerability in high-risk children: The role of the self-schema. *Dissertation Abstracts International: Section B; The Sciences and Engineering* May; 56 (11 B):6423.

Twenge JM, Nolen Hoeksema S (2002) Age, gender, race, socioeconomic status, and birth cohort difference on the children's depression intentory: A meta-analysis. *Journal of Abnormal Psychology* 111:578-88.
Vila G, Nollet Clemencon C, de Blic J, Mouren Simeoni MC, Scheinmann P (2000) Prevalence of DSM IV anxiety and affective disorders in a pediatric population of asthmatic children and adolescents. *Journal of Affective Disorders* 58:223-31.
Weinberg WA, McLean A, Snider RL, Nuckols AS, Rintelmann JW, Erwin PR, et al. (1989) Depression, learning disability, and school behavior problems. *Psychological Reports* 64:275-83.
Williamson LMG (1997) Psychosocial adjustment of children with craniofacial anomalies: Effects of facial appearance, speech quality, and hearing level. *Dissertation Abstracts International: Section B; The Sciences and Engineering* Mar; 57 (9 B):5938.
Yang YM, Cepeda M, Price C, Shah A, Mankad V (1994) Depression in children and adolescents with sickle-cell disease. *Archives of Pediatrics and Adolescent Medicine* 148:457-60.

CHAPTER 29

DEPRESSION IN ADOLESCENTS

Philip Hazell

Adolescent depression plays a central role in our understanding of mood disorders across the life cycle. Most people who will ever suffer from major depression will experience their first depressive episode during the teenage years, with a peak age of onset between 15 and 19 years (Kessler et al. 2001). It is during adolescence that depression becomes more common in girls than boys, suggesting the neurobiological changes underpinning sex differentiation during this period may also be linked to the aetiology of depression. Whereas younger children respond differently to pharmacological treatments, older adolescents respond to antidepressant drugs in a manner similar to adults, again suggesting that the neurobiological architecture mediating depression is established during adolescence. The influence of genes on the expression of depression in adolescents is similar to that in adults, but in children environmental factors seem to play a more important role. Owing to compulsory schooling, the early to mid-teenage years provide the last opportunity within the life cycle to deliver universal preventive programs against depression. Finally, there is the hope that if vulnerable individuals can be protected against the onset of depression during adolescence, their risk of future depression may be reduced.

EPIDEMIOLOGY

The prevalence of major depression among Australian teenagers aged 13–17 years was estimated, from a representative nationwide cross-sectional survey, to be 4.8 per cent in boys and 4.9 per cent in girls (Sawyer et al. 2000). Longitudinal data from New Zealand show that the rate of depression increases more rapidly through the adolescent period in girls than it does in boys (Hankin et al. 1998). Depression occurs more frequently in young people living in single-income or blended families and in families with a low income (Sawyer et al. 2000). In rural areas, depression is more common among boys than girls. The prevalence estimate established by Australian and New Zealand studies is similar to that found in other Western countries (Lewinsohn and Essau 2002) and in developing nations (Chen et al. 1995). Clinical impressions suggest rates of depression may be high in indigenous youth, but neither Australian nor New Zealand studies have involved enough indigenous youth to enable reliable prevalence estimates. Data from a Western Australian epidemiological study of the mental health of Aboriginal children and adolescents are eagerly awaited.

CLINICAL PRESENTATION

Only a minority of adolescents suffering depression are referred for clinical treatment. It appears adults recognise the outward manifestations of depression in young people, but fail to draw the association with depressive disorder (Puura et al. 1998). In fairness to parents and teachers, the accurate diagnosis of depression in young people can be a challenge even for experienced clinicians. A dejected, monosyllabic teenager who avoids eye contact and appears psychomotor-retarded may show a miraculous 'recovery' when he learns not only that the session with the psychiatrist has finally ended but also that he has been excused from school for the remainder of the day. On the other hand, gregariousness and apparent reactivity may mask a significant level of depression. There is a tendency for depression in young people to have an insidious rather than abrupt onset, which makes the condition all the more difficult to identify. Depressed adolescents may come to medical attention because they have harmed themselves, or because they have physical symptoms such as fatigue or headache that cannot be explained by other causes. They may come to the attention of school welfare staff because of bad behaviour, school non-attendance, or an unexpected decline in academic performance. Depressed mood as such is rarely the main presenting complaint, and may be detected only through specific enquiry about symptoms. Although longitudinal data suggest that much of the depression occurring in adolescence is new onset disorder, a significant minority of teenagers will already have experienced problems in their prepubertal years. For some this will be depression, but for others it may include anxiety, obsessive–compulsive disorder, attention deficit hyperactivity disorder or conduct problems (Carlson 2000). Given the overlap of these conditions with depression, clinicians who are treating young people for other psychiatric disorders should, over time, be on the lookout for the emergence of depressive disorder.

By convention, the criteria used to diagnose major depression and dysthymia in adults are also used for adolescents. Many people believe irritability is a more common symptom among depressed adolescents, while features of melancholia and psychosis are less common among teenagers than adults.

COURSE OF ILLNESS

As in adults, depression in adolescents follows a relapsing course. An episode of depression will last, on average, about 7–9 months. There is a 40 per cent probability of relapse within 2 years, increasing to 70 per cent after 5 years. The likelihood of further episodes in adulthood is about 60–70 per cent (Birmaher et al. 1996). The rate of switching to hypomania in young people with depression also seems higher than in adults, with some researchers claiming rates of 20–40 per cent. Depression in young people is not a benign self-limiting disorder.

An episode of depression can be quite devastating to a young person's academic and social development, and can have an adverse effect on family relations, especially if the young person's problems are misunderstood. A third of young people who experience a depressive episode will make a suicide attempt at some stage, and 3–4 per cent will die from suicide.

AETIOLOGY

Depression in adolescents usually arises from a combination of genetic vulnerability, suboptimal early developmental experiences, and exposure to stresses. However, depressive syndromes sometimes occur as sequelae to physical illness such as viral infection, and may overlap with fatigue syndromes (Garralda et al. 1999). The heritability of depression may increase with age (Harrington 2000), but findings from genetics studies are somewhat inconsistent. What is clear is that, unlike chronic medical conditions such as diabetes, very early onset depression is not associated with a greater genetic risk than later onset depression (Rice et al. 2002). Recurrent depression seems to have a stronger familial association than single-episode depression. What exactly is being inherited remains uncertain. At the molecular level, one possible candidate is polymorphism of the serotonin transporter gene. Another may be the regulation of hormones such as dihydroepiandrosterone (Goodyer et al. 2000). At the intrapsychic level, depression-prone individuals may inherit a cognitive style characterised by an overly pessimistic outlook on events (Gladstone and Kaslow 1995). At the interpersonal level, depression-prone individuals may fail to inherit the capacity to use relationships as a protective buffer against adversity.

Stressful life events may trigger the first occurrence of depression, but are rarely sufficient on their own to cause depression. Lower levels of stress are needed to provoke subsequent episodes of illness. This observation has led to the notion of *psychological scarring*, which suggests that the experience of a depressive episode reduces the individual's resilience to adversity. Enduring problems in the relationship with the primary caregivers is an important risk factor for depression, but such difficulties also predispose to other psychiatric disorders. Relationship difficulties that occur early in development may be more important to the development of depression in boys, while for girls recent difficulties, especially in the relationship with the mother, may be more pathogenic.

CLINICAL ASSESSMENT

Obstacles to effective clinical assessment include under recognition of the problem by adults, and low levels of help-seeking by young people. Possible reasons for this low level of help-seeking are summarised in Box 29.1. Any request for the assessment of depression in young people should be taken seriously. Some specialist services offer fast-track appointments to facilitate the engagement of the young person. Although the participation of parents is desirable, it is not essential for people aged 16 years and older. In exceptional circumstances, younger teenagers may need to be seen without their parents or guardians.

BOX 29.1

POSSIBLE REASONS FOR LOW LEVELS OF HELP-SEEKING AMONG YOUNG PEOPLE

- Poor understanding of what a mental health service is or what help it may provide
- A reluctance to consult adults
- Concerns about confidentiality
- Cost of treatment, or lack of understanding of how to access free treatment
- Inconvenient clinic times
- Uninviting clinic environment
- Ambivalence to seeking help arising from the mental disorder itself

SOURCE Abstracted from *Clinical Practice Guidelines for Depression in Young People* (National Health and Medical Research Council, 1997).

The key to the assessment of a teenager with physical or mental health problems is successful engagement. The interviewing techniques required to achieve this may take a little practice. Regardless of the setting, and who has attended the appointment, I recommend the clinician first spend some time alone with the adolescent. This may be the only opportunity to establish a successful rapport with the patient, who will otherwise assume that the clinician is aligned with the parents or authorities. An exception to this rule may occur when a male clinician is required to interview a female patient who has suffered recent sexual abuse. The clinician should avoid being overly solicitous (the teenager will find this intrusive) or authoritarian. Discuss confidentiality, but do not labour the point. I usually state that the detail of our discussion will remain confidential, but clearly parents or caregivers will want to know my conclusions from the interview. Concerns about immediate safety cannot be kept a secret. At the conclusion of the interview I summarise my thoughts about the interview with the adolescent, and ask them if there are any particular details they would not wish to have discussed with the parents. Clinicians may have to be more directive than they would be when interviewing an adult. Young people experience lengthy silences as persecutory. If there is no response to a particular question, move on or say something like, 'I can see that question got you thinking'.

The content of the interview should, if possible, cover the topics summarised in Box 29.2. Bear in mind that, regardless of the time frame specified by the interviewer, adolescents are inclined to describe their symptoms as they have experienced them over the previous day or two. This can lead to discrepancy between the history obtained from the adolescent and the history obtained from adult informants.

BOX 29.2

GUIDE TO THE CONTENT OF CLINICAL INTERVIEW WITH ADOLESCENT

Current level of functioning, established by enquiring about school function, leisure activities, peer relations, and role within the family

Recent stressors: 'Are there things happening at the moment that are worrying or upsetting you?'

Protective factors: 'What helps you cope? Who do you turn to if you have problems?'

Full range of current psychiatric and medical symptoms: 'I would like to ask you about your health'

Past problems, including assessment and treatment

Current and past drug use

Family situation, including whether other family members suffer mental health problems

Intimate relationships, including sexual history and pregnancy

Assessment of suicidality and risk of aggression to others

Mental state examination

I usually invite the adolescent to participate in the interview with the parents or caregivers. Some adolescents choose not to participate because they fear another round of criticism or nagging from their parents. Others may correctly anticipate that their parents would like time alone with the doctor. The interview with the parents provides an opportunity to:

- find out their main concerns and expectations of the assessment
- corroborate the history provided by the adolescent
- obtain information that may be unknown to the adolescent, such as developmental history and family psychiatric history
- gauge the parents' wellbeing
- assess the quality of the relationships within the family.

I ensure that the adolescent is involved in any discussion about treatment.

Further information may be obtained from the school counsellor or student welfare teacher. Important information includes any unexpected decline in academic progress, the results of educational or psychometric assessment if this has been conducted, the quality of relationships with peers and staff, record of conduct and attendance record.

A range of questionnaires may be used to augment the history, and to quantify symptom severity. Self-report measures include the Reynolds Adolescent Depression Scale, the Children's Depression Inventory, and the Reynolds Adolescent Suicide Questionnaire. These self-report scales are better thought of as screening tools than as diagnostic instruments. The Children's Depression Rating Scale is completed by the clinician, using information provided by the young person and the parents. It has value as an aid to diagnosis and as a means of measuring response to treatment. Generic measures such as the Strengths and Difficulties Questionnaire, the Health of the Nation Outcome Scale for Children and Adolescents, and the Clinical Global Assessment Scale are mandated for use in public sector services in some states of Australia. These instruments do not assist with diagnosis, but do offer a means to monitor response to treatment.

Physical examination is an important component of the work-up of a young person thought to suffer depression. Some mental health services request the general practitioner to conduct an examination, but I believe it is preferable that a focused examination be conducted by medical staff working in the psychiatric service. The need for laboratory investigations will be dictated by the history and the findings on physical examination.

TREATMENT

Having established a diagnosis of depression, the first important intervention is psychoeducation for the adolescent and family. The nature of the condition needs to be outlined, including the risks of relapse. Practical advice should be given on how to counter common symptoms such as sleep problems. Attention needs to be given to pathogenic factors such as substance abuse, family conflict and disruption. Adolescents and parents may want to know whether the problem will go away without treatment. The answer is 'eventually yes', but the adolescent may by then have experienced secondary complications such as peer problems and academic decline. It is useful to point out that depression is a noxious psychological state from which people of all ages deserve relief.

The type of treatment that is recommended will be determined by the severity of illness, the pattern of comorbid disorders, the level of suicidality or danger to others, and access to treatment facilities. Most depressive illness in adolescents can be treated on an outpatient basis. Reasons for hospitalisation include a high level of suicidality, the need for complex investigation, a lack of response to outpatient treatment, and a need to provide the young person temporary protection from an adverse social environment. The first objective of treatment is remission of symptoms, followed by protection against relapse of the current illness episode, and then protection against the occurrence of further illness episodes.

The evidence base for the treatment of depression in young people is expanding, but many gaps in our knowledge remain. Although the responsiveness of adolescents to treatment is closer to that of adults than that of younger children, it is still unwise to assume that results obtained from studies conducted in adult samples will generalise to young people. To obtain information on current evidence, the reader is directed to the chapter on child and adolescent depression in *Clinical Evidence*, which can be accessed via the Internet (Hazell 2003). Box 29.3 provides a summary statement of the evidence for treatment current at the time of writing. Controlled trials are needed in the following areas:

- comparative trials of cognitive behaviour therapy versus selective serotonin reuptake inhibitors
- trials of combined psychotherapy and pharmacotherapy versus psychotherapy or pharmacotherapy alone
- trials of inpatient versus outpatient treatment
- trials of the effectiveness of any treatment modality on relapse prevention
- trials of augmentation of antidepressant medication with a mood stabiliser or antipsychotic drug versus antidepressant medication alone for treatment-resistant depression.

BOX 29.3

SUMMARY OF EVIDENCE FOR TREATMENTS FOR DEPRESSION IN ADOLESCENTS, AS OF MARCH 2003

BENEFICIAL

Cognitive therapy (in mild to moderate depression)

LIKELY TO BE BENEFICIAL

Interpersonal therapy in (in mild to moderate depression)

TRADE OFF

Selective serotonin reuptake inhibitors

UNKNOWN EFFECTIVENESS

Intravenous clomipramine

Monoamine oxidase inhibitors

Lithium

St John's wort

Venlafaxine

Electroconvulsive therapy

Family therapy

Group treatments other than cognitive behavioural therapy

Long-term effects of psychotherapy

UNLIKELY TO BE BENEFICIAL

Oral tricyclic antidepressants

SOURCE Abstracted from Hazell (2003).

A systematic review has demonstrated the superiority of cognitive behaviour therapy (CBT) over nonspecific supportive therapies for inducing remission in children and adolescents with mild to moderate depression. The educative approach used in CBT is generally well suited to adolescents, although some complain that participating in CBT is too much like doing schoolwork. Some of the higher-order cognitions required to undertake CBT are developing only in mid-adolescence (Harrington et al. 1998). An example would be the capacity to fully differentiate theory from evidence. For this reason, CBT delivered to adolescents needs to be tailored to individual need. A greater emphasis may need to be given to the behavioural components of the intervention. CBT appears to be equally effective whether it is delivered individually or in a group format. The evidence for other forms of psychotherapy is equivocal.

Selective serotonin reuptake inhibitors (SSRIs) are the only class of antidepressant medication for which there is evidence of efficacy in adolescents. The evidence, however, is weaker than that for adults, with only a small number of published trials involving two agents (fluoxetine and paroxetine), a somewhat smaller risk difference (percentage responding to active treatment minus percentage responding to placebo) than in adult studies, and a tendency for positive responses to be detected on clinician ratings of symptoms, but not ratings made by adolescents. Fluoxetine is longer-acting than the other SSRIs. Although this may expose the patient to a greater risk of side effects, an advantage for teenagers is that the occasional missed dose is less likely to disrupt treatment, or to cause *discontinuation syndrome* (flu-like symptoms associated with a reduction in the dose of SSRI, or to cessation of treatment). Although guidelines recommend cautiously introducing fluoxetine in a dose of 5 or 10 mg/day, I have found that most adolescents will tolerate an adult dose of 20 mg. Owing to the higher rate of switching to mania in young people with depression compared with adults, drug-induced mania is an important risk that should be discussed with the patient and family. It is important to persist with treatment for at least 6 weeks before deciding that it has been ineffective. A trap for the inexperienced is to change a patient to another, possibly less effective treatment, before the first-line treatment has taken effect. Treatment should be continued for at least as long as one would for adults (9–12 months).

A systematic review of tricyclic antidepressants (TCAs) for depression in children and adolescents found evidence of no effect. The findings from an analysis of data from trials involving only adolescents were contradictory, with evidence of a small treatment effect on continuous measures of outcome, but no evidence of effect on categorical measures. One interpretation of this apparent contradiction is that adolescents show a trend towards responding to TCAs in a manner similar to adults.

In the event of a lack of response to an adequate trial of CBT and an SSRI, the diagnosis of depression should be reviewed, and further consideration should be given to the presence of perpetuating factors such as intercurrent substance abuse or environmental stress. This may be an appropriate time to consider hospitalisation, or at least to increase the frequency of outpatient visits. If there is no other explanation for the absence of treatment response, then augmentation of the SSRI with a mood stabiliser or an antipsychotic may be considered, although the efficacy of such strategies has not been evaluated in controlled trials in adolescent patients. Electroconvulsive therapy (ECT) should be considered if symptoms are severe and there has been minimal response to other treatments. Evidence of efficacy is available only from case studies, but it is unlikely that it will ever be possible to conduct randomised controlled trials comparing ECT with sham treatment in young people.

PREVENTION

Strategies to prevent the occurrence of depression among adolescents fall into two major categories. The first is concerned with early intervention directed to mother–infant dyads at risk of attachment difficulties because of problems such as maternal mental illness and economic disadvantage. Such intervention is often seen as being primarily directed to prevention of child abuse and neglect or of the emergence of conduct symptoms in the child. However, it is likely that fostering early attachment is also, indirectly, a protective factor against depression. Such preventive activity has often taken the form of home visiting and supportive counselling. There is some evidence that these interventions reduce the incidence of various social and mental health problems, but the direct effect on the occurrence of depression has yet to be evaluated.

The second group of preventive activities centres on universal and indicated interventions directed to school students. The MindMatters program introduced to some Australian schools combines whole-of-school activities, directed to the reduction of problems such as bullying and harassment, with classroom programs that promote emotional resilience. The Resourceful Adolescent Program (RAP) program is another universal curriculum-based program directed to promoting resilience. In contrast, the Adolescents Coping with Emotions is a targeted intervention for high school students who are already experiencing some symptoms of depression but who do not have the full depressive syndrome. A non-randomised controlled study demonstrated that depressive symptoms at 10-month follow-up were lower in students exposed to RAP than in students who were not exposed to the program (Shochet et al. 2001). Mental health promotion and prevention programs have now been mandated by several Australian states. The effect of such programs on the incidence of mental health problems such as depression has yet to be demonstrated.

While not always considered within a prevention framework, a further important strategy against the development of depression in teenagers is the effective treatment of conditions that may precede the onset of depression. Examples include anxiety disorders (including post-traumatic stress disorder), conduct problems, learning difficulties, chronic medical conditions and substance abuse. It has often been thought that substance abuse arises as a complication of depression (the self-medication hypothesis), but longitudinal research has shown that heavy marijuana use, for example, predisposes to the onset of depression (Patton et al. 2002).

REFERENCES

Birmaher B, Ryan ND, Williamson DE, Brent DA, Kaufman J, Dahl RE, et al. (1996) Childhood and adolescent depression: A review of the past 10 years. Part I. *Journal of the American Academy of Child and Adolescent Psychiatry* 35:1427-39.

Carlson GA (2000) The challenge of diagnosing depression in childhood and adolescence. *Journal of Affective Disorders* 61:3-8.

Chen X, Rubin KH, Li BS (1995) Depressed mood in Chinese children: Relations with school performance and family environment. *Journal of Consulting and Clinical Psychology* 63:938-47.

Garralda E, Rangel L, Levin M, Roberts H, Ukoumunne O (1999) Psychiatric adjustment in adolescents with a history of chronic fatigue syndrome. *Journal of the American Academy of Child and Adolescent Psychiatry* 38:1515-21.

Gladstone TR, Kaslow NJ (1995) Depression and attributions in children and adolescents: A meta-analytic review. *Journal of Abnormal Child Psychology* 23:597-606.

Goodyer IM, Herbert J, Tamplin A, Altham PM (2000) First-episode major depression in adolescents. Affective, cognitive and endocrine characteristics of risk status and predictors of onset. *British Journal of Psychiatry* 176:142-9.

Hankin BL, Abramson LY, Moffitt TE, Silva PA, McGee R, Angell KE (1998) Development of depression from preadolescence to young adulthood: Emerging gender differences in a 10-year longitudinal study. *Journal of Abnormal Child Psychology* 107:128-40.

Harrington R (2000) Childhood depression: Is it the same disorder? In Rapoport JL (ed), *Childhood Onset of 'Adult' Psychopathology*. Washington, DC: American Psychiatric Press.

Harrington R, Wood A, Verduyn C (1998) Clinically depressed adolescents. In Graham P (ed), *Cognitive Behaviour Therapy for Children and Families*. Cambridge: Cambridge University Press.

Hazell P (2003) Depression in Children and Adolescents. Clinical evidence. <http://www.clinicalevidence.org> (accessed March 2003).

Kessler RC, Avenevoli S, Merikangas K (2001) Mood disorders in children and adolescents: An epidemiologic perspective. *Biological Psychiatry* 49:1002-14.

Lewinsohn PM, Essau CA (2002) Depression in adolescents. In Gotlib IH, Hammen CL (eds), *Handbook of Depression*. New York: Guilford Press.

Patton GC, Coffey C, Carlin JB, Degenhardt L, Lynskey MT, Hall W (2002) Cannabis use and mental health in young people: Cohort study. *BMJ* 325:1195-8.

Puura K, Almqvist F, Tamminen T, Piha J, Kumpulainen K, Raesaenen E, et al. (1998) Children with symptoms of depression – what do adults see? *Journal of Child Psychology and Psychiatry and Allied Disciplines* 39:577-85.

Rice F, Harold G, Thaper A (2002) The genetic aetiology of childhood depression: A review. *Journal of Child Psychology and Psychiatry and Allied Disciplines* 43.

Sawyer MG, Arney FM, Baghurst PA, Clark JJ, Graetz BW, Kosky RJ, et al. (2000) The Mental Health of Young People in Australia. Canberra: Mental Health and Special Programs Branch, Commonwealth Department of Health and Aged Care.

Shochet IM, Dadds MR, Holland D, Whitefield K, Harnett PH, Osgarby SM (2001) The efficacy of a universal school-based program to prevent adolescent depression. *Journal of Clinical Child Psychology* 30:303-15.

CHAPTER 30

BIPOLAR DISORDER IN CHILDHOOD AND ADOLESCENCE

Stephanie Moor and
William G A Watkins

Bipolar disorder tends to be an enduring condition requiring management throughout life. It is a particular challenge in childhood and adolescence because of the significant effect it can have on developmental goals that need to be negotiated over this period. In addition, the effect on a family of having a young person with bipolar disorder is usually profound. Parents and other siblings may need support as well as psychoeducation during the course of assessment and treatment. Being alert to these family factors, which in themselves may affect the progress of the young persons' illness, is the task of the child and adolescent psychiatry team.

For an adolescent already experiencing significant physiological and psychological change, the symptoms of bipolar disorder become yet another challenge. If children are ill in primary school, they may miss out on significant building blocks of education, which may impair their ability to attain their full potential at school, despite symptom control. Unwell adolescents may be absent for several terms of the academic year and hence miss crucial examination hurdles. There may be subsequent long-term effects on workplace skills and career choices, far outlasting the period of symptomatic illness. In addition, depression and mania during adolescence are likely to have a huge effect on an adolescent's identity and social development. In summary, early onset bipolar disorder may cause developmental delays in several spheres, and a key role of the child and adolescent mental health team is to help minimise these delays.

Making the initial diagnosis of bipolar disorder may take the clinician some weeks of observation of mood, behaviour and energy levels, in close consultation with the young person, the family and teachers. Clearly, a presentation of mania, with or without a past history of depression, clinches the diagnosis, but atypical presentations are the norm. There is evidence suggesting adolescent mania presents with more mixed mood states and psychoses than adult mania, and that prepubertal mania presents even more atypically, with impulse control and behavioural problems intermixed with affective storms (Geller and Luby 1997). When considering a diagnosis of bipolar spectrum disorder, familiarity with the young person and the family is necessary to understand and disentangle mood symptoms suggestive of emotional dysregulation from other presentations of heightened family emotionality.

The following vignettes illustrate the variety of clinical presentations of early onset bipolar disorder. The questions arising from the vignettes illustrate some of the clinical conundrums that currently exist in this area.

VIGNETTE 1: EMILY

Emily, aged 13 years, was admitted in the middle of the night to a child inpatient unit because of her increasingly bizarre behaviour. Her parents had been called into the school 3 days before because teachers had become concerned about her inappropriate and intrusive behaviour with her classmates and confrontational outbursts with teachers. She had spent the next day at home with her mother, who said Emily became increasingly agitated, overtalkative and abusive over the day. For several nights her parents had heard her up late, but were not too concerned as she often had difficulties getting off to sleep. On the morning before admission, she had left the house after breakfast to collect the mail and, to her parents' consternation, did not return. Despite police assistance, she was not seen for the entire day. She was eventually found in a highly agitated and aroused state, shouting incoherently and scantily clad in the centre of the city at midnight.

Emily's mum had been hospitalised at the age of 16 years with a psychotic depression, and had suffered postnatal depression after the birth of Emily and her brother.

This young girl with first-episode mania raises the following clinical questions:

- What is the likely outcome of childhood-onset bipolar disorder and does early onset predict a more severe course?
- How significant is a family history of mood disorder?
- Which treatments should be used and for how long?
- What is the risk–benefit ratio of early aggressive treatment of children with emerging or early onset bipolar disorder?

Likely outcome

Intuitively, it seems likely that an illness in which we believe genetic vulnerability significantly contributes to risk of disorder will follow a more severe or chronic course, if it occurs early in life. Such a simple hypothesis is not easily answered, for the obvious reasons that we have no genetic markers, it is thought there has been insufficient recognition of early onset bipolar disorder and there is considerable dispute over the appropriate diagnostic criteria to be used. Thus, we desperately need good follow-up studies tracking children not only with uncommon but classic, episodic bipolar I disorder with mania, but also with the proposed broader, more common continuous rapid-cycling forms. The situation is compounded by the fact that in adolescence we are uncertain whether we are seeing the evolution of a disorder that expresses itself as a *prodromal phenotype*, or the same disease process as in adult bipolar disorder, where expression of the disorder is influenced by the stage of brain development. It is clear from adult retrospective studies that many sufferers identify onset during their teenage years, with a lag of up to 10 years between episodic mood changes and a bipolar diagnosis being made (Egeland et al. 2000).

So when should follow-up start? Prospective data are unlikely to yield such strong data for mood instability. Indeed, a 2-year follow-up community study of 14–18-year-old high school students found only a low to moderate level of stability in affective temperaments (Placidi et al. 1998). A higher risk cohort to observe over time is children who have already experienced a mood disorder. For example, in a 10-year follow-up of children with prepubertal major depressive disorder, very high rates of conversion to bipolar disorder of between 33 and 48 per cent were reported (Geller et al. 2001). With hindsight it can be said, for a proportion of this sample, that their bipolar disorder began at the average age of 10 years and was progressive. This is in keeping with the prospective follow-up studies of Kovacs (Kovacs and Pollock 1995), which indicate that dysthymia alone predicts greater risk of subsequent bipolar disorder.

What of those already with identified bipolar disorder? In a large community study (Lewinsohn et al. 1995), adolescents with bipolar disorder were seen just over a year later and compared with adolescents with major depressive disorder followed over a similar period. The bipolar subjects had a poorer outcome with longer duration of episodes and a more prolonged course. The researchers were surprised to find significant impairment occurring as often in those with subthreshold bipolar symptoms as in those with symptoms that met full criteria for bipolar disorder. In a 2-year follow-up of children (mean age of 10 years) with mixed continuously cycling bipolar disorder, Geller et al. (2002) also identified a high probability of relapse within 6 months. These and other more naturalistic studies all point to the strong likelihood of ongoing difficulties for children identified as having bipolar disorder. It needs to be borne in mind that at least some of the impairment and chronicity of these difficulties is attributable to the high rate of comorbid disorders.

In summary, the evidence to date supports concerns about the risk of progression, chronicity and significant impairment in early onset bipolar disorder. This is consistent with the view that bipolar disorder interferes with children's normal developmental trajectories, meaning they attain fewer skills to subsequently fall back on, both when unwell and during times of recovery.

Significance of family history

This is an important clinical question because deciding whether the often ambiguous symptoms are part of a bipolar spectrum disorder may be significantly influenced by whether there is a positive family history of mood disorder. There is ample evidence from several studies of the children of parents with bipolar disorder and a few long-term follow-up studies to show a markedly increased risk of any psychiatric disorder in these high-risk offspring. Around half of the offspring develop a psychiatric disorder, most commonly attention deficit hyperactivity disorder (ADHD), major depressive disorder, dysthymia and bipolar disorder (Chang et al. 2000). The magnitude of the risk for mood disorder is around 25 per cent with one affected parent and up to 74 per cent with two affected parents. Exactly how many will develop bipolar disorder is uncertain, but the follow-up of cohorts is under way. It also appears that early onset bipolar disorder in the parent (possibly particularly in the mother's lineage) increases the risk for the even earlier onset bipolar disorder in their child, akin to genetic anticipation.

Thus, the child and adolescent psychiatrist is often dealing with a *bipolar family*, and a not infrequent dilemma is that of other family members realising for the first time that both they and the presenting child have bipolar disorder. For a parent or sibling to face this diagnosis may place an intolerable burden on an already struggling family system. At these times, one may have an important liaison role in referring the proband's family members to other psychiatric services. In addition, once an older sibling develops bipolar disorder, realistic or undue parental concern may focus on the behaviours of younger children in the family. The clinician may be asked to assess younger family members for the presence of bipolar disorder in a situation where disentangling an underlying mood disorder from instability due to family disruption will be very difficult.

Treatment

ASSESSMENT AND MANAGEMENT Assessment and management is best done in consultation with the family, as they are entering a long-term association with mental health services. Thus, education of the family about bipolar disorder and its treatment is an important component of management to ensure informed participation and aid compliance. Consent to treatment often becomes a difficult issue when treating adolescents, especially when the young person's mental state impairs his or her judgment. At these times, parental authority may be sufficient, along with the adolescent's assent to instigate treatment, but at times resort to the mental health legislation may be required.

Treatment is aimed at symptom reduction, relief of distress and prophylaxis for further episodes, which we believe may worsen the brain pathology and worsen prognosis. Treatment includes the use of psychopharmacology, psychotherapy, and education of both the individual and the extended network of family, school and peers. Currently, there is limited evidence to guide pharmacological intervention, and there are no outcome trials of psychoeducation in childhood and adolescence.

MOOD STABILISERS As with many treatments in this age group, the evidence from adult trials has been extrapolated downwards, often with little modification for body size, brain development and pharmacokinetic differences of childhood. The tricyclic antidepressants (TCAs) were used for childhood and adolescent depression until definitive trials showed a lack of efficacy in this age group. The child literature consists of small studies, often with retrospective data and no adequate control group for comparison of outcome. The use of lithium in this age group is still essentially based on the adult studies for treatment of acute mania and prophylaxis for mania and depression. It is supported by open label studies and one double-blind, randomised controlled trial (RCT) of 10 weeks duration (Geller et al. 1998). In twenty-five adolescents with bipolar disorder and substance abuse, lithium was superior to placebo, but nearly half did not respond to lithium. There have been several studies looking at the characteristics of early presentation bipolar illness, and these suggest that, compared with adults, these younger patients have a more prolonged course, are less responsive to lithium treatment and prophylaxis, are more likely to have a mixed and rapid-cycling presentation and have more psychotic phenomena (Findling et al. 2001). Hence, the role of valproate, which for adults has an established role in mixed and rapid-cycling illness, is currently being investigated. To date, there is one open label study of a comparison of lithium, valproate and carbamazepine in the acute management of bipolar I and II disorders in 8–18-year-olds (Kowatch et al. 2000). Based on an intention-to-treat analysis, the effect sizes were 1.63 for valproate, 1.06 for lithium and 1.00 for carbamazepine (as measured by at least 50 per cent improvements on the clinician-rated Young's Mania Rating Scale and the Clinical Global Impression scale). The investigators concluded that there was a large effect size for all three mood stabilisers in adolescents with mixed or manic episodes. In addition, there are some open label studies of both valproate and carbamazepine in this age group. The results of randomised trials with placebo comparison are awaited.

There are several recent open label trials of all of the atypical neuroleptics alone or with mood stabilisers, and these agents appear promising. One RCT of combined quetiapine and valproate therapy versus valproate plus placebo in acute mania in thirty adolescents showed response rates of 87 per cent and 53 per cent, respectively (DelBello et al. 2002). This supports the open label trials showing the efficacy of valproate in acute mania and that combination therapy with atypical neuroleptics, such as quetiapine, is supported in acute mania at least.

The use of clozapine in children and adolescents with treatment-resistant bipolar disorder is supported only by case reports. There are the obvious concerns regarding blood dyscrasias, especially when used in combination with carbamazepine, and the necessity of haematological monitoring deters its use in this age group.

Carbamazepine has been used more in children with proven or suspected neurological compromise and behavioural problems in the conduct disorder spectrum. However, its efficacy in bipolar disorder has recently been supported by the Kowatch study reported above.

In the United States, there is increasing use of lamotrigine, especially for bipolar depression, as well as gabapentin and other new mood stabilisers. Some supporting evidence exists, at least in adults. However, there is a moderate risk with lamotrigine of skin rash, which may rarely progress to Stevens-Johnson syndrome, and a concern with gabapentin of potential behavioural disinhibition in children. Use of these drugs in Australasia, particularly in the younger age groups, is still novel.

NOVEL TREATMENTS There is preliminary evidence in the management of disruptive behavioural disorders of the use of both omega-3 fatty acid supplements and high-dose vitamin and mineral supplements (micronutrients). If such dietary supplementations gain further scientific support, their use would have great appeal to parents and clinicians alike concerned with the exposure of children's developing brains to medication.

PSYCHOTHERAPIES There is little evidence for improved outcome with family and individual psychotherapy, although there are some promising new treatments and developments in outcome measures.

Some studies have shown that family factors such as *expressed emotion* and *affective style* affect outcome, but interventions using family work or therapy remain descriptive.

Recent work in bipolar adults with interpersonal psychotherapy with social rhythms (IPSRT) and cognitive behaviour therapy (CBT) would justify trials in younger populations, but these are awaited.

ELECTROCONVULSIVE THERAPY Electroconvulsive therapy (ECT) is rarely used in child and adolescent psychiatric practice, but has a place in the treatment of severe depressive and manic symptoms. The reported rates of improvement as well as side effects appear to be similar to those in adult patients (Walter et al. 1999).

Risk–benefit ratio of early aggressive treatment

The ***kindling model*** is derived from rodent experiments, in which intermittent subthreshold stimulation in a brain region leads to full-blown seizures, which then begin to occur spontaneously. This model suggests that, by analogy, repeated affective episodes may predispose to further episodes, which may in turn occur spontaneously and without the stressor, such as life events, that may previously have triggered episodes. The animal models suggest early rather than late anticonvulsant treatment leads to more seizure-free periods and less development of treatment resistance. Would early treatment with full doses of the best available mood stabiliser medication have similar effects? It is plausible, despite little evidence, that young peoples' brains may be best protected from the long-term effects of this disorder by aggressive polypharmacy. The flipside is that, without the evidence to support such hypothesised gains, young peoples' developing brains will be exposed to large doses of pharmaceuticals, which they would need to take for long periods. The only available evidence comes from an 18-month prospective, naturalistic follow-up study of thirty-seven adolescents hospitalised with mania: discontinuation of lithium was associated with a nearly three-fold increased relapse rate (Strober et al. 1990). Current practice is to recommend long-term use of mood stabilisers in severe early onset bipolar disorder. However, as with adults, noncompliance or intermittent compliance is the norm. Young people and their families are likely to conduct their own naturalistic experiments, and part of the challenge of working with families with bipolar disorder is maintaining the therapeutic relationship through such vicissitudes.

PHARMACOKINETICS There is no evidence that children and adolescents are more prone to side effects due to their age, but there are pharmacokinetic differences. For example, lithium's half-life in children is shorter than in adults (18 hours versus 21 hours), as they have a 20 per cent greater renal elimination rate. Thus, steady state for lithium is achieved in a week. Parents need to know the signs of toxicity (such as confusion, altered consciousness, slurred speech and muscle twitching), and how dehydration may easily develop in association with the vomiting or diarrhoea of common childhood illnesses. Lithium toxicity can also develop in children even with lithium levels in the normal range. Common side effects of lithium are tremor, weight gain and acne. Adolescents are understandably acutely sensitive to these because of their potential impact on peer socialisation. It is important to provide information about side effects and give advice on diet and exercise. However, the frequent weight gain of many young people on psychopharmacological medication attests to the difficulties in this area.

Valproate is readily absorbed from the gut, highly protein-bound, metabolised in the liver (by cytochrome P450 system) and has a half-life of 8–16 hours in children and adolescents. The main side effects are gastrointestinal, weight gain, hair loss and tremor. A recent report suggesting anovulatory failure in women raises important questions about the effect valproate has on ovarian function during puberty (Morrell et al. 2002). The place of pelvic ultrasound scanning prior to valproate treatment is uncertain.

CHILDREN AND ADOLESCENTS IN DRUG TRIALS A major impediment to research in this area has been the restriction by regulatory agents on the use of pharmacological treatments of children. However, in a move aimed at increasing research on children to inform practice, the US Food and Drug Administration has made regulatory changes requiring age-relevant research to be undertaken. Another impediment to good data accumulation is the difficulties researchers experience keeping adolescents in drug trials. For example, in a recent trial of valproate versus placebo, only three out of forty-five adolescents completed the placebo arm of the study! Subject retention is vital if phenomena such as the apparent increase in bipolar symptoms around the week 3 mark and a delay in active treatment 'kick-in' in adolescents are to be accurately evaluated.

VIGNETTE 2: TOM

Tom, 15 years old, lives with both his parents and a 13-year-old younger sister. He was admitted from an emergency department because of concerns over his suicidal risk when he began acting on threats to hang himself after an assault on his sister. Tension between all family members has been running high.

Despite a birth weight of 2.83 kg, Tom was thought to be 6 weeks premature. Marked tantrums became apparent from the age of 2 years onwards, and led to significant corporal punishment from his father. In addition, throughout his schooling attentional difficulties, disruptiveness and impulsivity have been apparent. His intellectual functioning is within the borderline range and, given the above multiple difficulties, it is not surprising that he has been experiencing attainment problems, strongly dislikes school and is keen to leave.

Socially, Tom has been isolated from his peers and as he became older has been in conflict with them. He lies, tells fanciful stories, steals, is verbally abusive to all and gets into fights with them. These behaviours led to periods of exclusion from school, which is now permanent.

While his marked attentional and impulsive difficulties have been very responsive to methylphenidate, started at the age of 11 years, it was associated with complete growth cessation in a boy already below the third percentile for height and it had to be stopped. Extensive investigations failed to identify any other cause for his delayed growth. Tom has been very sensitive about his short stature and this has contributed to his explosive feisty outbursts.

Over the past 2 years, Tom has experienced variable anxiety symptoms, periods of low mood and withdrawal. Suicidal ideation is associated with the aftermath of episodes of serious conflict. Two weeks before admission, he was prescribed a serotonin reuptake inhibitor for depression. His behaviour had then deteriorated markedly. He was highly irritable and took offence at little provocation, resulting in verbal and physical fights with his sister. His mother was frightened by his outbursts and yet puzzled by his distressed agitation when he said he was frightened and would not leave her side. He would not go to bed at night because he feared intruders in the house and said he had to stay up and watch for them. His parents were exhausted from trying unsuccessfully to reassure and restrain Tom.

Tom's maternal grandmother has been hospitalised with depression and his paternal grandfather and two uncles have experienced serious alcohol problems.

Tom's combination of attentional problems, educational history and mood symptoms raise the following clinical questions:

- What is the relationship between bipolar disorder and ADHD?
- Is there an increased suicide risk in young people with bipolar disorder?
- What are the special educational issues that need to be considered in early onset bipolar disorder?

Bipolar disorder and ADHD

This really is an 'old wine in new bottles' story. The potential overlap between bipolar disorder and ADHD symptoms, such as attentional and distractibility problems and, of course, overactivity itself has long been noted. Indeed, it led to some early trials of lithium as a potential treatment of ADHD, but these were disappointing, certainly in contrast to the results obtained with stimulants. However, over the past decade the questions of whether bipolar disorder was being misdiagnosed as ADHD, whether ADHD was a prodrome of bipolar disorder, or whether ADHD and bipolar disorder could be comorbidly diagnosed have been revisited. Currently, the reverse question is being asked: 'Is ADHD being misdiagnosed as bipolar disorder?'. Although we lack any tests that can definitively disentangle these questions, they do have important clinical implications, such as whether stimulant treatment could precipitate bipolar disorder or worsen bipolar disorder, leading to psychosis for example, and whether children are being denied, through overlooking bipolar disorder as a diagnosis, effective treatment with mood stabilisers? However, making these diagnostic distinctions and thence such management decisions still comes down to clinical judgment.

Partly this debate has arisen because of the interest in the *bipolar spectrum* concept and the evidence suggesting that bipolar II disorder, bipolar disorder not otherwise specified, cyclothymia, hyperthymia and bipolar temperament are much more common difficulties than bipolar I disorder. How best to distinguish these from a presentation of ADHD comorbid with depression or anxiety disorder or conduct disorder is not clear, especially as the latter common childhood difficulties often endure for years. However, those advocating greater recognition of bipolar disorder in children are suggesting that it is bipolar I disorder in particular that is being missed, despite extraordinarily high rates of comorbidity with ADHD (well in excess of 50 per cent). Diagnostic symptom modification to allow for developmental immaturity has been suggested, notably that irritability, affective storms and prolonged temper tantrums suffice instead of euphoric mood. Further, it is claimed that the most childhood onset bipolar I disorder is presenting in a continuous mixed form. In effect, this dispenses with the DSM-IV criterion A, which requires a distinct period of mood disruption, and this contributes to the risk of bipolar I disorder and ADHD diagnostic confusion or overlap (Geller et al. 2002). The validity of making these diagnostic changes is unresolved, partly because other evidence conveys a mixed or inconsistent picture (Hazell et al. 2003).

Retrospective adolescent and adult bipolar disorder histories often indicate antecedent childhood ADHD or disruptive problems, but long-term prospective ADHD follow-up studies suggest the risk of bipolar disorder is not significantly elevated. The Multisite Multimodal Treatment Study of Children with ADHD (Jensen et al. 2001) identified no children as having bipolar disorder, in contrast to Biederman's Boston research group, which indicated more than 23 per cent of ADHD children have or will develop bipolar disorder (Biederman 1998). A recent review (DelBello and Geller 2001), which included seventeen methodologically sound studies of high-risk offspring of bipolar parents, suggested that major depressive disorder, not ADHD, was the most commonly found antecedent disorder. This is consistent with prospective studies indicating that childhood depressive disorders, including dysthymia, carry significant risk of future bipolar disorder. If bipolar disorder is frequently being missed in ADHD children, then the paucity of evidence showing illness progression, as has been found with the dysthymia studies, is puzzling.

What of community studies? An intriguing 14-year follow-up study of a large epidemiological group of Dutch children (Hofstra et al. 2002) found significant childhood attentional problems did not predict any adult disorders, let alone bipolar disorder! In contrast, rule-breaking behaviour did predict mood disorders.

In all these studies, the question of how thoroughly or effectively bipolar disorder was being identified is crucial. Alternatively, it may be that a continuous non-progressive form of bipolar disorder does affect children, but there is insufficient evidence to decide. Lastly, it is reassuring to note that at least one sizeable long-term study found no evidence that methylphenidate treatment precipitated development of bipolar disorder in young adults. One reviewer has suggested that early onset bipolar disorder may even be responsive to stimulants.

Suicide risk

Young people with bipolar disorder are at greatly increased risk of suicide attempts and completed suicide. Suicidal thoughts are common in both children (23 per cent of a child bipolar population) and adolescents with bipolar disorder. In a large community study, which identified eighteen adolescents with bipolar disorder, 44 per cent had attempted suicide in the previous year. Important predictors of increased suicidal risk are past suicide attempts, major depressive disorder, comorbid substance abuse, family history of major depression and treatment with TCAs (James and Javaloyes 2001). Suicidal thoughts and plans should be asked about routinely, and appropriate intervention taken with families and the young people to minimise risk.

Special educational issues

In the classroom, young people with bipolar disorder may have to contend with the challenges of labile mood, possible comorbid attentional difficulties and cognitive impairment due to disease processes and drug side effects (Ronen et al. 2000). In addition, there is evidence for comorbid learning disabilities with early onset bipolar disorder. A key challenge for the family and the clinician, in conjunction with educationalists, is to optimise educational potential and facilitate vocational options. Also, liaison with the young person's school may be an important component of ongoing management (for example, repairing the social damage of an episode of mania at school). Each school and family will have their own preferences, but generally some education of key staff about the disorder and its treatment is helpful for affected young people when they return to school.

How people decide to discuss the illness with their peer group is an individual matter but requires prior discussion, as casual playground questions can become very threatening and intimidating if a strategy has not been worked out in advance. An extended period of illness around the time of diagnosis of bipolar disorder often means that young people leave school earlier than they planned. Thus, it is important to facilitate links with other training organisations as well as with other rehabilitation agencies.

VIGNETTE 3: ANDREW

Andrew is a 15-year-old boy who in the space of 36 hours became extremely agitated, distractible, dysphoric and quite unable to sleep, even for a few minutes. He began constantly moving around and responding fearfully to perceived threats of knives coming out of the floor or attacks being made on him by his younger brother. He spoke in a garbled way, but insistently describing the objects he was seeing and the sounds he was hearing which others could not. Reassurances had only a fleeting effect. Wearing any clothes, even loose fitting pyjamas, was intolerably uncomfortable. Persuading him to drink was difficult and he had no interest in food.

This dramatic presentation followed 3 years of stability on valproate and risperidone, after Andrew had gradually settled during months of inpatient and day hospital treatment for a similar first presentation when he was 11 years old. Andrew had been developmentally compromised by a severe postnatal cerebral bleed, leaving him with mild hemiparesis, learning difficulties and severe intractable seizures until he was 6 years old. His multiple anti-seizure medications had gradually been withdrawn once he became seizure-free. The last one stopped was valproate (6 weeks before his first episode). For many years his parents and teachers had been concerned over his impulsiveness and attentional difficulties. There was no family history of bipolar disorder.

Andrew's acute presentation raises the following clinical questions:

- What is the relationship between brain injury and early onset bipolar disorder?
- Which differential diagnoses need to be considered?

Brain injury and early onset bipolar disorder

The question of whether brain damage increases the risk of bipolar disorder occurring is difficult to answer. It is likely that brain damage acts as an important nonspecific risk factor for all psychiatric disorder occurring in childhood, especially when it occurs in conjunction with learning difficulties and epilepsy, which we already know are additional risk factors for childhood onset disorder. Follow-up of children who experienced brain damage in road traffic accidents indicated they suffer from a wide range of disorders, but significant attentional problems or symptoms suggestive of ADHD are particularly likely. It may be that brain damage accelerates the age of onset of a disorder, including bipolar disorder.

Differential diagnoses

Mania in childhood is a psychiatric emergency and the individuals usually need to be managed in a child and adolescent inpatient unit. Mental health nurses with expertise in this field using modern pharmacological tranquillisation can usually manage the extremes of behaviour displayed by a floridly manic young person. The presentations of mania are varied and will often raise concern about an underlying organic disorder.

Occasionally a space-occupying lesion, central nervous system infection (including HIV), epilepsy (especially temporal lobe epilepsy) or endocrine abnormality (such as pituitary, thyroid and carcinoid endocrinopathies) may present as a manifestation of bipolar disorder. These are rare presentations, but a thorough medical examination with appropriate investigations should identify these conditions.

When considering the differential diagnosis of schizophrenia/schizoaffective disorder, a period of observation of the phenomenology is prudent. Mood incongruent delusions, cognitive impairment and functional decline may all be seen as part of a manic psychosis, and there is a salutary literature on the dangers of rushing towards a diagnosis with such a heterogeneous phenotype (Joyce 1984). Although initial management may be similar, there are important differences in disease conceptualisation, rehabilitation strategies and treatment decisions (such as whether to use mood stabilisers).

VIGNETTE 4: JENNY

Jenny, a 16-year-old, was seen by her school counsellor because of recent teacher concern about her poor attitude to work, decline in performance and confrontational attitude in class. The counsellor referred her because of Jenny's self-reported low moods associated with suicidal thoughts and multiple superficial cuts to both forearms. Jenny says she has had problems coping with her moods and schoolwork for about a year, although she has had changeable moods since she was 13 years old. She has episodes of feeling sad, emotional and oversensitive. She gets grumpy, picks at her food and cannot be bothered doing anything, just wanting to sleep. The episodes last from an afternoon to 3 days, but occasionally up to 10 days at a time. On direct questioning, she admits to short periods when she feels great, has lots of energy and is in a fun party mood. Her friends complain that she talks too fast, but like her being 'over the top'. During one of these times, she and a couple of friends truanted from school and took two bottles of spirits from one of the boy's parents' liquor cabinet. They all got drunk at her house and she thinks she may have blacked out. These episodes usually last several hours, but have lasted up to a couple of days. She has noticed on the longer episodes that she needs less sleep and gets very grumpy with her friends.

She has used alcohol and marijuana at parties since she was 14 years old, but over the past year she has partied heavily.

She lives at home with her parents, who are worried about their daughter's declining academic performance and attitude problems. Her father is an abstinent alcoholic and her mother reports postnatal depression.

Jenny's story raises important questions about case conceptualisation in contemporary psychiatric practice:

- When is being moody, full of energy and taking risks in adolescence just 'being a teenager with youthful exuberance' or symptomatic of a psychiatric disorder?
- What is the relationship between bipolar disorder and substance abuse in this age group?

Just a teenager or having a psychiatric disorder?

The most debated current controversy in child and adolescent psychiatry is about the diagnostic criteria for bipolar disorder spectrum in young people. There are many adolescents who describe clear episodes of depression and several episodes of 2-day hypomanic periods which do not reach the DSM-IV 4-day criterion for hypomania. However, many would consider this to be sufficient to make the diagnosis of bipolar disorder not otherwise specified. More controversial is the diagnosis of bipolar disorder in children based on chronic non-episodic behaviours, which have been labelled *affective storms* and *ultradian rapid cycling*. A research instrument, the childhood version of the Schedule for Affective Disorders and Schizophrenia (K-SADS) has been modified to include items specific to prepubertal mania, rapid cycling and ADHD. This modified tool, the WASH-U-KSADS, charts the onset and offset of symptoms that the researchers propose enable identification of ultradian cycling in very young children. The phenotype of prepubertal or early onset bipolar disorder is thus said to be validated by instrument reliability, 6-month stability of the diagnoses made, and outcomes that show significant impairment at follow-up consistent with the impairment seen in classic bipolar disorder (Geller et al. 2002). In Australasia, a more conservative view is held over this bipolar phenotype, and whether clinicians should elect to watch and wait or commence mood stabiliser treatment is an open question (Hazell et al. 2003). The outcomes of the American cohorts are awaited with much interest.

Sexual experimentation and risk-taking is often seen in adolescents, but the heightened sexual drive, grandiosity, impaired judgment and impulsivity of hypomania and mania bring increased risks to those with bipolar disorder. In addition to the social sequelae with peers, there is the increased risk of pregnancy and sexually transmitted disease. Also, the pleasure-seeking behaviour of internet-savvy children may result in inadvisable contacts and risk from sexual exploitation from peers and predatory adults.

Bipolar disorder and substance abuse

Substance use is high among the general population of adolescents in Australasia. However, there appears to be a special co-segregation of substance abuse with bipolar disorder. Certainly there is an over representation of substance-abuse disorders in adolescents with bipolar disorder, with comorbidity being around 40 per cent (Wilens et al. 1999). In childhood, substance abuse is much lower, with comorbidity below 10 per cent, probably due to less ease of access. Early cannabis use (before the age of 15 years) has been shown to increase the risk of experiencing psychotic symptoms in community populations, but it appears that, for psychologically vulnerable adolescents, cannabis is a potent risk factor for psychosis (Arseneault et al. 2002). The combination of bipolar disorder and substance abuse is also a potent predictor of poor outcome and it behoves practitioners to ascertain their patients' drug use and factor this into management. Unambiguous information about the destabilising effects of psychoactive substances, including alcohol, on mood needs to be imparted. As with many aspects of a chronic illness, patients may need to experience mood destabilisation on several occasions before the links the clinician is making become pertinent to them and they change their behaviour. There is also a complex multidirectional relationship between bipolar disorder, substance-abuse disorder and conduct disorder in childhood and adolescence. The comorbidity of conduct disorder with bipolar disorder is high (up to 69 per cent) (Faraone et al. 1997), often precedes the bipolar disorder, and is associated with a worse clinical outcome. However, treatment of the mood disorder may markedly reduce the behaviours associated with conduct disorder.

CONCLUSION

When considering the diagnosis of bipolar disorder in childhood and adolescence, it is important to keep in mind the presentation variability illustrated by the vignettes. Although there are many similarities to adult forms, there are also significant differences. Many important long-term prospective studies will be coming to fruition over the next decade, and these will help answer some of the key questions. In the meantime, our goal with children and their families continues to be 'using best practice from available evidence'.

REFERENCES

Arseneault L, Cannon M, Poulton R, Murray R, Caspi A, Moffitt TE (2002) Cannabis use in adolescence and risk for adult psychosis: Longitudinal prospective study. *BMJ* 325:1212-13.

Biederman J (1998) Resolved: Mania is mistaken for ADHD in prepubertal children. *Journal of the American Academy of Child and Adolescent Psychiatry* 37:1091-6.

Chang KD, Steiner H, Ketter TA (2000) Psychiatric phenomenology of child and adolescent bipolar offspring. *Journal of the American Academy of Child and Adolescent Psychiatry* 39:453-60.

DelBello MP, Geller B (2001) Review of studies of child and adolescent offspring of bipolar parents. *Bipolar Disorders* 3:325-34.

DelBello MP, Schwiers MS, Rosenberg BS, Strakowski SM (2002) A double-blind, randomized, placebo-controlled study of quetiapine as adjunctive treatment for adolescent mania. *Journal of the American Academy of Child and Adolescent Psychiatry* 41:1216-23.

Egeland JA, Hostetter AM, Pauls DL, Sussex JN (2000) Prodromal symptoms before onset of manic–depressive disorder suggested by first hospital admission histories. *Journal of the American Academy of Child and Adolescent Psychiatry* 39:1245-52.

Faraone SV, Biederman J, Wozniak J, Mundy E, Mennin D, O'Donnell D (1997) Is comorbidity with ADHD a marker for juvenile-onset mania? *Journal of the American Academy of Child and Adolescent Psychiatry* 36:1046-55.

Findling RL, Gracious BL, McNamara NK, Youngstrom EA, Demeter CA, Branicky LA, et al. (2001) Rapid, continuous cycling and psychiatric co-morbidity in pediatric bipolar I disorder. *Bipolar Disorders* 3:202-10.

Geller B, Luby J (1997) Child and adolescent bipolar disorder: A review of the past 10 years. *Journal of the American Academy of Child and Adolescent Psychiatry* 36:1168-76.

Geller B, Zimerman B, Williams M, Bolhofner K, Craney JL (2001) Bipolar disorder at prospective follow-up of adults who had prepubertal major depressive disorder. *American Journal of Psychiatry* 158:125-7.

Geller B, Craney JL, Bolhofner K, Nickelsburg MJ, Williams M, Zimerman B (2002) Two-year prospective follow-up of children with a prepubertal and early adolescent bipolar disorder phenotype. *American Journal of Psychiatry* 159:927-33.

Geller B, Cooper TB, Sun K, Zimerman B, Frazier J, Williams M, et al. (1998) Double-blind and placebo-controlled study of lithium for adolescent bipolar disorders with secondary substance dependency. *Journal of the American Academy of Child and Adolescent Psychiatry* 37:171-8.

Hazell PL,Carr V, Lewin TJ, Sly K (2003) Manic symptoms in young males with ADHD predict functioning but not diagnosis after 6 years. *Journal of the American Academy of Child and adolescent Psychiatry* 42: 552-60.

Hofstra MB, Van der Ende J, Verhulst FC (2002) Child and adolescent problems predict DSM-IV disorders in adulthood: A 14-year follow-up of a Dutch epidemiological sample. *Journal of the American Academy of Child and Adolescent Psychiatry* 41:182-9.

James AC, Javaloyes A (2001) Practitioner Review: The treatment of bipolar disorder in children and adolescents. *Journal of Child Psychology and Psychiatry and Allied Disciplines* 42:439-49.

Jensen PS, Hinshaw SP, Epstein JN, March JS, Angold A, Wells KC, et al. (2001) ADHD comorbidity findings from the MTA study: Comparing comorbid subgroups. *Journal of the American Academy of Child and Adolescent Psychiatry* 40:159-67.

Joyce PR (1984) Age of onset in bipolar affective disorder and misdiagnosis as schizophrenia. *Psychological Medicine* 14:145-9.

Kovacs M, Pollock M (1995) Bipolar disorder and comorbid conduct disorder in childhood and adolescence. *Journal of the American Academy of Child and Adolescent Psychiatry* 34:715-23.

Kowatch RA, Suppes T, Carmody TJ, Bucci JP, Hume JH, Kromelis M, et al. (2000)

Effect size of lithium, divalproex sodium, and carbamazepine in children and adolescents with bipolar disorder. *Journal of the American Academy of Child and Adolescent Psychiatry* 39:713-20.

Lewinsohn PM, Klein DN, Seeley JR (1995) Bipolar disorders in a community sample of older adolescents: Prevalence, phenomenology, comorbidity, and course. *Journal of the American Academy of Child and Adolescent Psychiatry* 34:454-63.

Morrell MJ, Giudice L, Flynn KL (2002) Valproic acid increases risk of ovulatory failure in epileptic women. *Annals of Neurology* 52:704-11.

Placidi GF, Maremmani I, Signoretta S, Liguori A, Akiskal HS (1998) A prospective study of stability and change over 2 years of affective temperaments in 14-18 year old Italian high school students. *Journal of Affective Disorders* 51:199-208.

Ronen GM, Richards JE, Cunningham C, Secord M, Rosenbloom D (2000) Can sodium valproate improve learning in children with epileptiform bursts but without clinical seizures? *Developmental Medicine and Child Neurology* 42:751-5.

Strober M, Morrell W, Lampert C, Burroughs J (1990) Relapse following discontinuation of lithium maintenance therapy in adolescents with bipolar I illness: A naturalistic study. *American Journal of Psychiatry* 147:457-61.

Walter G, Rey JM, Mitchell PB (1999) Practitioner review: Electroconvulsive therapy in adolescents. *Journal of Child Psychology and Psychiatry and Allied Disciplines* 40:325-34.

Wilens TE, Biederman J, Millstein RB, Wozniak J, Hahesy AL, Spencer TJ (1999) Risk for substance use disorders in youths with child and adolescent onset bipolar disorder. *Journal of the American Academy of Child and Adolescent Psychiatry* 38:680-5.

CHAPTER 31

GENDER AND MOOD DISORDERS

Kay Wilhelm

Mood disorders are common in the community, with significant psychosocial impairment. There has been interest in gender differences in rates and expression of depression over the past three decades, which has produced some useful insights into the gender-related risk factors to onset and maintenance of mood disorders. (Sex describes the biological features that distinguish men and women; gender describes the behavioural and social attributes that define identity in relation to sex.)

WHERE ARE THERE SEX DIFFERENCES?

The early psychoanalytic literature saw men and women as very different in their overall psychological make-up. Some (such as Freud) saw women as more susceptible to their emotions and their reproductive physiology and anatomy; others (for example, Jung) concentrated more on the balance of qualities between men and women. There was a growing sense that women were more emotional and more prone to depression and anxiety – the neurotic disorders.

Weissman and Klerman's (1977) comprehensive review of the available English language literature raised the issue that women are consistently reported with prevalence of one and a half to three times the rates of depression in men. The review laid the groundwork for further enquiry by asking whether such differences were due to biological (for example, X-linked genetic transmission and factors related to women's reproductive system) or psychosocial factors (for example, women's decreased access to income and employment), or due to artefactual factors (such as women's greater help-seeking and subsequent overrepresentation in clinical studies). They concluded that there was a mixture of real and artefactual factors. This influential review emphasised the preponderance of depression in women at a time when the third edition of the *Diagnostic and Statistical Manual of Mental Disorders* (DSM-III) was emerging. The focus then was on establishing a reliable diagnostic instrument, and was then echoed by the *International Classification of Diseases* (ICD) system. In this process, the interest was more on rates of depression than actual experiences of both sexes. These events and the issues voiced at the time largely set the scene for the discussion in the psychiatric research literature over the next three decades. Interestingly, two important pieces of research that did look at individuals reinforced these assumptions in their choice of cohorts: the longitudinal study of Harvard graduates investigating factors leading to success in life studied only men, and a study of the social origins of depression in a working-class suburb in the United Kingdom studied only women.

Much early work investigating gender differences in rates (in the 1960s and 1970s) concentrated on college student groups (where women are in the vulnerable age range) with less severe non-melancholic depression, or in clinical populations (where women are likely to be over-represented because of higher rates of help-seeking). Over the next two decades, a series of community-based epidemiological studies, commencing with the Environmental Catchment Area Study in the United States, was undertaken across a range of countries (including England; a further US study, the National Comorbidity Survey; Canada; New Zealand and Australia) (Kessler et al. 1993). These had the advantage of studying the general population rather than clinical groups, but came to similar conclusions: the rates of depression and anxiety in women were about twice the rates in men. Later studies of community-based studies over a wider age range have demonstrated a smaller difference. In the National Comorbidity Survey, women were 1.7 times more likely to report a lifetime history of depression and 1.6 times more likely to report a 1-month prevalence, and in a recent Australian study with similar methodology the 12-month prevalence for major depression was 1.6 times greater in women than in men (Wilhelm et al. 2003).

THE RANGE OF GENDER DIFFERENCES

While the gender differences were taken as a given, closer examination of the data shows the situation is not quite as straightforward. For bipolar disorder the rates are about equal, although women are more likely to have a rapid-cycling course. For melancholic and psychotic subtypes of major depression there are no differences in rates, age of onset or course. The differences are greatest (in the range of twice the prevalence for women) for mild to moderate severity of major depression, minor depression and dysthymia. Differences in rates are greatest around the ages of 18–55 years, the years of potential childbearing for women.

There have also been findings that gender differences may be related to prevalence of anxiety disorders accompanying or preceding depression, rather than to pure depression. These differences in anxiety disorders are prominent in the childrearing years. Others have differentiated *somatic* depression from *pure* depression, where the somatic presentation is characterised by pronounced appetite and sleep disturbance and fatigue, and found that the *anxious somatic depression* type is the one that is more common in women (Breslau et al. 1995).

For primary school age children there are no gender differences, and the increase in rates occurs in the years after puberty. In older people the rates tend to equalise again: men aged 25–45 years and older men (75 years and older) are at the highest risk of suicide in Australian and New Zealand communities. Community studies report that the gender differences in anxiety and depression diminish in older people (along with a mellowing reflected by decreased rates of neuroticism), with a significant increase in depression rates in older men.

To further add to the complexity of what had seemed a simple picture, there has been a general decrease in sex differences noted in age cohorts over time. A recent British community study of depressive disorders in primary care showed near equality between the sexes (male:female ratio of 1:1.3) for 1-month prevalence rates. This raises the possibility that the gender differences in current prevalence rates are not universal, but vary with age, setting and the time under observation. When considering gender differences in the longer-term course of depression, the National Comorbidity Survey data showed no difference in the probability of being chronically depressed or having an acute relapse in the year following an acute episode, but found that women had higher rates of later recurrence.

We can learn by examining the exceptions. In socially homogeneous groups such as British civil servants and Australian teachers, where subjects were of similar age and educational standing, the sex differences in rates were smaller or nonexistent. Similar findings occurred in close-knit social groups such as the Amish community and a Jewish community in London. This suggests that social factors play a significant role in rates of depression. Gender differences are also reduced when a shorter, more immediate observation period is used, as it seems that men are more likely to forget less severe episodes of depression over time.

Most research into sex differences concentrates on women. However, another intriguing finding is that, although sex differences in rates of depression and anxiety favour women, the total rates of all disorders are the same for both sexes. This means that men may truly have lower rates and are protected in some fashion, possibly by drinking alcohol, or the behaviours involved in drinking and other associated risk-taking behaviours are an equivalent of depression, or that men drink rather than talk and admit their problems and thus are being identified using a different paradigm (Brownhill et al. 2002).

Turning from the rates of episodes to the actual experience, women have generally been found to report more symptoms. Data from the National

Comorbidity Survey suggested a greater severity of illness. Women report more appetite increase and weight change (which may reflect serotonergic mechanisms), while men complain of more self-criticism, social withdrawal and somatic symptoms, but these are not generally picked up as *depression* in the generally accepted self-report measures or depression interviews. However, a study of first episodes of depression found no differences in the rate of recovery, rates of prescription of antidepressants or time to recurrence, suggesting that some gender differences may become more apparent in established episodes of depression. There has been a consistent finding that women have a slightly longer duration of established episodes.

RISK FACTORS TO DEPRESSION

It is important to ask whether we are considering vulnerability, onset, maintenance of episodes, relapse or recurrence, as each of these aspects of depression can have different social or biological risk factors (Frank 2000).

Influence of biology

Family studies have led to a discounting of links between depression and X chromosomes. Although women demonstrate an increased vulnerability to depression and onset of bipolar disorder in the post-partum period, there is no definite link to oestrogen. High neuroticism scores are consistently found to be a risk factor to depression. About 50 per cent of the degree of neuroticism as a trait characteristic is genetically determined, and women tend to score more highly, although men with high neuroticism scores are also prone to depression.

One of the more recent areas of interest has been in the role of oxytocin, a hormone that promotes the birth process and lactation, but also affiliative behaviour (peer bonding as well as pair bonding). Although both sexes have an increase in oxytocin at puberty, it has more effect on affiliative behaviour in girls and may interact with social factors to lead to the significant increase in depression that occurs during the teenage years. There is also a role for testosterone in such male behaviour as aggression, assertiveness and impulsivity. Androgens have an effect on prenatal cerebral organisation, leading to a lower threshold to instigate aggressive behaviour and increased gratification from motor pathways. These differences are accentuated after puberty.

There is an increased risk of depression around the time of childbirth. This includes minor mood changes (post-partum blues) and the rarer (but very significant) onset of post-partum psychosis and melancholic depression. Both of these are at least partly related to hormonal fluctuations.

Although women are less likely than men to abuse alcohol, the effects of alcohol abuse are more significant in terms of cerebral insult, which can in turn lead to a later onset of depression. Smoking tobacco also has an association with incidence and prevalence of major depression, and has a more significant effect on women. Smoking cannabis is now relatively widespread in youth of both sexes, and carries an increased risk of anxiety and depression. This again is greater for adolescent girls, where daily cannabis smoking carries a five-fold increase in rates of anxiety and depression.

Influence of social factors

Women are more likely to report emotional, physical and sexual abuse and dysfunctional childhood environments. This seems to be due to a combination of factors: more accurate reporting, greater likelihood of occurrence, and greater effect on the subject of the abuse. The greater recall of less serious episodes of depression is related to women's tendency to prompt recall of former depressive episodes because they are embedded in a social context ('I remember being depressed at the time that my sister was so ill') whereas men are more likely to simply remember the event ('I was depressed').

There are differences in coping styles that affect behaviour. Women tend to use more internalising, emotion-focused coping. As girls, they are discouraged from risk-taking and, at times, from mastery of their environment. Emotion-focused coping can ameliorate depression and anxiety and lead to help-seeking from friends and professionals, but may lead to longer episodes. Men use more externalising, action-focused coping. As boys, they are given more physical stimulation, encouraged to take more risks and be more active both personally and in terms of mastery over their environment, and higher levels of aggressive behaviour are tolerated. It is thought that such externalising behaviour can diffuse some episodes of anxiety and depression more rapidly (Nolen-Hoeksema 1987).

However, in boys and younger men, bad behaviours (such as truanting, aggression, concentration problems) can be overlooked and not seen as an expression of distress or depression. These may be a masculine method of behaving to similar stressors. The expression of anger is important, as this may also decrease depression for the expressor and transfer the emotional load to the other.

There is an important relationship between anger expression and depression for all ages. Clinically depressed people report greater levels of overall anger and greater suppression of anger (*anger-in*), but no differences in levels of anger expression (*anger-out*). The relationship between anger expression and depression is affected by the perception of self-efficacy, duration of anger and coping style used to defuse the anger. Men also have higher rates of *alexithymia*, which has been construed as a repression of emotion, or anger-in, and men who repress anger are thought to be at higher risk of hypertension and cardiac arrhythmias, which can in turn become risk factors for later vascular depressions. They are also more likely to smoke. All of these problems, particularly for the unemployed, add up to a potent mix of risk factors for depression that are of particular relevance to men. These links are indirect, but are clearly important from a public health perspective.

Anger expression is an area where sex role-typed behaviour is very important. Men are more likely to use action-focused coping styles. Where adaptive, these can involve making plans to resolve the problem and the emotional build-up. When used maladaptively, action-focused coping can involve destructive or impulsive acts and deflecting the anger onto others.

As part of this relationship dynamic, it is thought that submissive behaviour in the face of an aggressor is a style of coping that tends to diminish aggressive behaviour but becomes problematic if the behaviour is frequently adopted. Such submissive behaviour can be related to other important social risk factors for depression, including poor self-esteem and feelings of being trapped and powerless, referred to as the *learned helplessness* model. This model was developed following observations of mammals in situations where they were rendered helpless. Such factors are important in both sexes, but are more common in women. They can cause a chronic low-grade depression (dysthymia) or, when further triggers occur, a superadded acute episode).

GENDER, INTIMATE RELATIONSHIPS AND DEPRESSION

Women are more likely than men to report dysfunctional parenting, a family history of psychiatric disturbance and childhood sexual abuse. Women tend to rate their parental relationships more negatively than men do, and are more likely to rate their spouses as less caring and to rate them as a continuing depressogenic stressor. This may reflect women having greater recall of negative events or greater reactivity to such events, or men's greater ability to repress the effects of negative experiences. It is probably a combination of these factors. Although women have consistently higher rates of neuroticism (reflecting emotional reactivity), they tend to have a greater range of positive as well as negative affect.

Men have been reported as having less tolerance of negative affect. This may result in less flexible coping repertoires for dealing with being depressed (such as increased rigidity, more emotional isolation and social withdrawal), which may be premorbid traits but become more pronounced as a consequence of depression. Men may also demonstrate a more rapid increase in negative affect, which when combined with impulsivity can lead to risk-taking and suicidal behaviour.

Social function in the depressed person's family has been shown to be much slower to normalise after symptomatic relief in the depressive episode. Depressed men can have a powerful effect on others in their family, by becoming more rigid in their personality and their restrictive expectations of their wives. When both husband and wife are depressed, they tend to become more rigid in their sex role-stereotyped interpersonal interactions with the other, which tends to be mutually reinforcing (Hafner 1986; Wilhelm 1995).

GENDER AND TREATMENT

Women characteristically present more for assistance across the range of medical and psychological problems, and this is certainly so for mood disorders. This can lead to stereotyping in terms of case definition, identification methods and arrangement of clinical services, which can favour case identification and access to treatment for women and present barriers to men. This issue is now increasingly being recognised, at least in Western countries.

The well-known reluctance of men in regard to help-seeking for any medical or psychological problems is magnified when they are depressed. This is a major public health issue and of particular relevance to younger men, who tend to disregard the possibility of help from their social network as well as from professionals. Some of the identified barriers to men's help-seeking include difficulties with setting aside the time, doctors (particularly men) overlooking men's emotional problems, perceptions that depression does not fit with traditional notions of masculinity, and lack of awareness of what is available (Moller-Leimkuhler 2002).

When men and women who had been treated were examined, there was little difference in the type of symptoms reported. There were no differences in loss of interest, anger towards self or others, irritability, trouble concentrating, suicidal ideation, sleep disturbance, feelings of hopelessness or helplessness. Women tended to report more appetite disturbance and irritability as a symptom, and men reported more externally directed irritable behaviour, social withdrawal and use of substances and alcohol as self-medication. There were no differences in duration of episode, or severity as measured by clinician-rated or self-report measures, but higher comorbid anxiety symptoms were found in women. This suggests that men and women with an established history of depression experience the episode in a very similar fashion, although women experience more symptoms of anxiety and physiological arousal, consistent with the frequently reported higher levels of neuroticism and anxiety disorders in women (Wilhelm et al. 2002).

There are some differences in treatment response. There is said to be a modest difference in response to antidepressants: the selective serotonin reuptake inhibitors are better tolerated and more effective in women, and the tricyclic antidepressants better tolerated and more effective in men, but the findings are modest and not universal. The gender differences are greater for younger men and women, with post-menopausal women behaving (physiologically speaking) more like older men.

Cognitive behaviour therapy has been thought to be more suited to men, who prefer a more structured, problem-based approach, and interpersonal therapy may be more relevant for women's more interpersonal framework, which focuses on social roles. These recommendations sound reasonable, but can work in two ways, acknowledging differences in style but also building to sex role stereotypes. However, the opposite may apply. To continue the sex role-stereotype argument, perhaps men who have few interpersonal skills would do better to learn to understand their emotional expression and relationships, and women who have few problem-solving and assertion skills would do better to develop a thicker skin and learn to use a more structured therapeutic approach.

CONCLUSION

When unpacking the various elements of mood disorders in relation to gender, we find some consistent reports. Rates of melancholic depression and bipolar disorder are similar for both sexes and the experience of these episodes is not significantly gender-related. The higher lifetime rates of depression in women are related partly to the increased levels of neuroticism and anxiety disorders in women in the childbearing years. In general, women do seem to have greater affiliative needs and awareness of social issues in their networks, which renders them more interpersonally aware and leaves them more socially and psychologically vulnerable to depression. Such differences are amplified by the sociocultural context within which they negotiate the years of potential and actual childrearing. Men and women who live in a more egalitarian social environment (and have more equal sex roles) have more equal rates of depression. There has been less emphasis on men's experience of depression, despite higher rates of suicide. It is still unclear about the relationship between men's experience of anger and substance and alcohol abuse and how this relates to mood disorders.

Once men and women have established episodes of depression and have sought treatment, the actual experience of depression is similar. There are a few differences: women are more likely to experience appetite disturbance, put on weight, and demonstrate care-eliciting responses that are more specific to depression (crying, telling their friends and doctor they are depressed), whereas men tend to withdraw, become irritable, and demonstrate distress in manners that are less likely to communicate their depression (taking risks, drinking alcohol). Men can experience a rapid escalation of negative affect, feel they are losing control and become impulsive, and this can lead to suicidal behaviour.

Women's greater experience of depression is related to a higher rate of anxiety disorders during the childrearing years. It has been hypothesised that women's high arousal levels during those years have an adaptive function: women are better at multitasking and need simultaneously to be alert to problems in their offspring. The greater prevalence is related to some increased onset and greater duration of episodes, which is related to women's greater use of emotion-focused coping, which helps in the short term but may not bring closure to the episode. Men's episodes tend to be shorter because of their more action-focused approach, but men also demonstrate greater impulsivity and risk-taking, so that they may have an accident or repress the negative emotions.

As rates of depression in men are thought to be increasing, the importance of looking at how depressed men cope and affect their social network will grow in importance. First, men need to be encouraged to attend for preventive and actual treatment for depression, which implies addressing both the stigma involved and the various barriers to presentation. Men may require assistance in dealing with increasing rigidity of style both in their own personality structure and how they deal with significant others. If this is recognised, there may be preventive strategies, such as placing emphasis on maintenance of activities and social contacts away from the family. As women appear to be more sensitive to the interpersonal effects of people in their social environment, they may require skills aimed at building up interpersonal resilience in the areas of self-esteem and assertion. The findings also draw attention to a need to recognise couples where both are depressed and the effects that the presence of chronic or repeated episodes can have on each other, and by implication on their family.

Implications for men and women

As well as considering depression type, predisposing, precipitating and perpetuating factors, there are benefits in considering how these interact with gender. Although there are more similarities than differences in how men and women experience mood disorders, the differences are illuminating. There are differences in risk factors, help-seeking behaviours, and coping styles of particular relevance to both sexes. It is important that they be recognised to maximise effective identification and management of mood disorders. Although specific factors may be more relevant to one sex, it is likely that they are still relevant to some people of the other sex (unless specifically related to biology unique to one sex).

REFERENCES

Breslau N, Schultz L, Peterson E (1995) Sex differences in depression: A role for preexisting anxiety. *Psychiatry Research* 58:1-12.

Brownhill S, Wilhelm K, Barclay L, Parker G (2002) Detecting depression in men: A matter of guesswork. *International Journal of Men's Health* 1:259-80.

Frank E (2000) *Gender and its Effects on Psychopathology*. Washington, DC: American Psychopathological Association.

Hafner RJ (1986) *Marriage and Mental Illness: A sex roles perspective*. New York: Guilford Press.

Kessler RC, McGonagle KA, Swartz M, Blazer DG, Nelson CB (1993) Sex and depression in the National Comorbidity Survey. I: Lifetime prevalence, chronicity and recurrence. *Journal of Affective Disorders* 29:85-96.

Moller-Leimkuhler AM (2002) Barriers to help-seeking by men: A review of sociocultural and clinical literature with particular reference to depression. *Journal of Affective Disorders* 71:1-9.

Nolen-Hoeksema S (1987) Sex differences in unipolar depression: Evidence and theory. *Psychological Bulletin* 101:259-82.

Weissman MM, Klerman GL (1977) Sex differences and the epidemiology of depression. *Archives of General Psychiatry* 34:98-111.

Wilhelm K (1995) The effects of husbands on the mental health of their wives. In Jorm AF (ed), *Men and Mental Health*. Canberra: Australian Government Publishing Service.

Wilhelm K, Roy K, Mitchell P, Brownhill S, Parker G (2002) Gender differences in depression risk and coping factors in a clinical sample. *Acta Psychiatrica Scandinavica* 106:45-53.

Wilhelm K, Mitchell P, Slade T, Brownhill S, Andrews G (2003) Prevalence and correlates of DSM-IV major depression in an Australian national survey. *Journal of Affective Disorders* 75:155-62.

CHAPTER 32

MOOD DISORDERS IN PREGNANCY AND THE PUERPERIUM

Philip M Boyce
and John T Condon

For most women, the experience of pregnancy, childbirth and looking after their new infant is an enriching and fulfilling experience. However, up to 15 per cent of women experience a mood disorder either during pregnancy or in the first 6 months after giving birth. For many of these women, this is the first experience of a mood disorder; for others, it is a recurrence of a pre-existing disorder. These disorders occur at a time when women are regularly in contact with health professionals and so, in theory, any mood disorders ought to be identified and treated. However, this is not the case, and many women do not have their disorder recognised or treated.

There are essentially three mood disorders that can occur during the puerperium (pregnancy and following childbirth): puerperal psychosis, bipolar disorder (both manic and depressive phases) and major depression (postnatal depression and antenatal depression). *The blues* is often considered a mood disorder; however, given its ubiquity (up to 70 per cent of woman will experience the blues), it is probably best considered a part of normal response to the stress of childbirth. Its symptoms need to be recognised, as it can often herald the emergence of a full mood disorder.

Mood disorders following childbirth are of great public health and clinical importance for the following reasons (Boyce and Stubbs 1994):

- They are common.
- They are predictable (arising within the 6 months following childbirth).

- Pregnancy and the post-partum period are an ideal time for prevention and early intervention.
- These disorders are often not recognised (and hence not treated), despite there being good screening instruments to identify postnatal depression (Buist et al. 2002).
- They are disabling and can contribute to the start of a chronic depression or be the first episode of a lifetime of recurrent depression.
- Postnatal depression can have a negative effect on the quality of the woman's key relationships, especially with her partner and infant, as well as possibly having a detrimental effect on infant development.
- In their severe form, they may jeopardise the safety of the woman or her infant.

Before discussing the clinical characteristics and treatment of the disorders that arise during the puerperium, we will describe a conceptual framework for understanding. First, all of these disorders need to be understood using a broad biopsychosocial approach. There is a strong biological component to some disorders (perhaps linked to the changes in oestrogen and progesterone); for others, the disorder is more determined by social and psychological factors. Notwithstanding this, the clinical management of these disorders needs to take into account biological, psychological and social factors contributing to the woman's illness.

Second, in considering these disorders, one has to always take into account the developing fetus or the infant. The clinical management, especially pharmacological interventions, of these disorders can have an effect on both the fetus and a breastfed infant.

Third, it is important to distinguish disorders arising de novo during the puerperium from disorders that recur or relapse during the puerperium. Similarly, it is important to distinguish between disorders that are uniquely linked to pregnancy and childbirth and those that can relapse or recur with any psychosocial stressor. With disorders that do recur, the emphasis is on prevention.

In this chapter we discuss each of the major mood disorders, examining the background and epidemiological factors, clinical features, possible causal factors, and clinical management of the disorder.

PREGNANCY

In Western society, there is a widespread tendency to idealise both pregnancy and parenthood (Condon et al. 2001). Positive aspects of pregnancy tend to be overestimated, especially by adolescents, while negative aspects are underestimated. The importance of this observation is that, if the reality of pregnancy falls short of idealised expectation, some degree of disillusionment is inevitable. For example, many women expect the second trimester of pregnancy to be a time of enhanced psychological wellbeing; in reality, only 10–15 per cent of Australian women reported increased psychological wellbeing during the second trimester (Condon and Esuvaranathan 1990). Thus, disillusionment can be one factor that contributes to antenatal depression.

In many Western societies, the age of first pregnancy has increased substantially over the past few decades. Rates of voluntary childlessness are also on the increase. In an Australian study, 40 per cent of pregnancies were neither totally planned nor totally unplanned. These observations suggest ambivalence towards childbearing, driven in part by the competing demands placed on women in modern society. Ambivalence may also contribute to dysphoria during pregnancy for some women.

Recent research suggests that the incidence and prevalence of antenatal depression are equivalent to those of the postnatal period (Evans et al. 2001). Depression at any time in a woman's life is, of course, significant. However, there are specific factors that render depression during pregnancy of particular significance and concern. First, pregnancy has been conceptualised as a period of preparation for parenthood. Many authors have described the *psychological tasks* of pregnancy. All of these can be significantly impeded by a depressive episode, especially of substantial duration. An important task during pregnancy is the development of an attachment relationship to the unborn baby (Condon 1993). In normal pregnancy, there is a progressive increase in attachment, especially following the experience of quickening. In the post-quickening period, the fetus is increasingly conceptualised as *child*, and this in turn triggers a variety of protective behaviours, including participation in antenatal care and cessation of behaviours (such as smoking and drinking alcohol) that could potentially damage the fetus. Depression can significantly interfere with the development of antenatal attachment, and depressed women often describe a feeling of detachment from the fetus and even a sense of unreality about its existence. Research has shown that a high degree of antenatal attachment is predictive of a high level of attachment in the early postnatal period (Condon and Dunn 1988).

A second psychological task during first pregnancy is the adjustment of the dyadic couple relationship to accommodate a child (that is, to become a triadic relationship). For many men, their partner's evolving attachment to the unborn baby is their first experience of her becoming emotionally invested outside of the couple relationship. Some men find this threatening. A decrease in sexual intimacy, which is not uncommon during pregnancy, can further exacerbate male insecurities. Recent research has shown that pregnancy is a significantly more stressful time for the male partner than any other time during the entire postnatal year. If the woman is depressed, this can impose very substantial additional strain on the partner relationship, and the adjustments that would normally take part during pregnancy are potentially impeded.

Depression can also interfere with the changes in self-concept that may be important for both members of the couple and begin during pregnancy. Relinquishing the child role and accepting the restrictions and responsibilities that accompany the parent role normally begins during pregnancy. Women who are depressed can often lose perspective on the magnitude of the losses involved and feel threatened or overwhelmed by both the pregnancy state and impending parenthood. This loss of perspective can sometimes cause women to seek termination of pregnancy, a decision that may be greatly regretted once the depression remits. Thus, depression can significantly interfere with the reshaping of the self-concept to accommodate the parenthood role. Parents who have not relinquished the child role are at risk of looking to the baby to gratify their own needs. When the infant fails to do so, anger and resentment often surface, and this is a common dynamic underlying physical infant abuse.

Finally, first pregnancy is a time when both men and women often re-examine and re-evaluate the quality of the parenting they received themselves. This is especially so in the case of the same-sex parent. Thus, pregnant women often become more preoccupied with their own mothers and begin to grapple with the notion of whether they wish to follow in their mother's footsteps in terms of childrearing practices or whether they wish to forge a different pathway. Women (and men) who lack a good role model in their same-sex parent often begin during pregnancy to develop a new model compatible with the kind of parent they wish to be. Depression can interfere with this process and cause women who have not had good parenting from their own mothers to feel overwhelmed by the prospect of motherhood.

In summary, the special significance of depression during pregnancy lies in its potential to disrupt the early psychological adjustments involved in developing a relationship to the unborn baby, adopting a changed style in the couple relationship and the transition in the self-concept to that of *parent*.

Risk factors for depression arising during pregnancy have not, as yet, been clarified, but may not be very different from those for depression at any other time in a woman's life. The one possible exception, although the evidence is equivocal, is that women who have a history of severe premenstrual syndrome may be more prone to depression both during pregnancy and the postnatal period.

It is important to realise that there is often a distinction between an *unplanned* pregnancy and an *unwanted* pregnancy. Unplanned pregnancies often become much wanted. However, unwanted pregnancy, which the woman feels unable to terminate either because of her own views or her family's views, is certainly a risk factor for antenatal depression.

CLINICAL FEATURES AND ASSESSMENT

Antenatal depression has received far less research attention than postnatal depression. In assessing a woman who may be depressed during pregnancy, four areas warrant consideration. The results of this exploration can then guide the clinician towards the most appropriate treatment plan.

First, the danger of self-harm needs to be explored, together with the possibility of harm to the fetus. The latter lies along a spectrum extending from fetal neglect to physical fetal abuse (Condon 1993). If depression is present, safety issues must always be explicitly probed.

Second, the quality of the woman's mood should be explored. In particular, anhedonia, feelings of hopelessness and worthlessness, feelings of guilt (especially ruminating over past events) and a sense of inner numbness all point to severe depression that may require pharmacological treatments.

Third, neurovegetative changes should be explored. Allowance must be made for the potential influence of the physiological state of pregnancy. For example, sleep disturbance is common in late pregnancy because of discomfort or urinary frequency; however, consistent early morning wakening would be of concern. Diurnal mood variation in which the woman describes consistently feeling worse in the morning with improvement over the course of the day is a further pointer towards biological depression. Obviously, appetite, weight change and constipation are less reliable indicators of biological depression in a pregnant woman.

Fourth, the clinician can usefully explore each of the four psychological tasks described in the previous section, and assess the possibility that depression is interfering with these tasks. More specifically, feelings towards the fetus should be explored, relationship issues with the partner can often be usefully discussed, and the woman can be encouraged to talk about her feelings about the forthcoming parenthood role and perhaps the extent to which she can comfortably embrace the role model of parenting provided by her own mother.

Every effort should be made to involve the male partner in both the assessment and treatment of antenatal depression. Men in this situation will often feel perplexed and bewildered by the emotional difficulties that their partners are experiencing. In the absence of explanation and understanding, an initially supportive attitude may give way to a more critical and punitive one, which in turn can both worsen and perpetuate the woman's depression. Men often cling to the explanation that it's 'just hormones' and may withdraw or distance themselves emotionally from their partners. This can further exacerbate the woman's distress and impede recovery.

Assuming that there are reasonable strengths in the couple relationship, the clinician should seriously consider involving the male partner in all aspects of management, provided that this is acceptable to the woman.

MANAGEMENT OF DEPRESSION DURING PREGNANCY

Experienced doctors and mental health professionals often feel unsure of their knowledge and skills to manage a significantly depressed pregnant woman. The origin of this lack of confidence is multifactorial and probably involves uncertainties about the risks of prescribing during pregnancy as well as concern about suicide, with the possibility that two deaths would result. A further source of unease is sometimes the realisation that, regardless of pharmacological intervention, a potentially time-consuming psychosocial intervention is almost always indicated when a crisis occurs at such an important life transition point. These anxieties and lack of confidence can sometimes lead to avoidance and denial of the severity of the woman's depression and thus undertreatment or no meaningful treatment at all. Anxiety can also sometimes lead to unnecessary specialist referral of women whom the practitioner would normally feel completely comfortable to manage if they were not pregnant. Unfortunately, in many modern mental health settings, this kind of referral can lead to unnecessary delay in initiating treatment.

We argue that there are only two acceptable approaches to the management of antenatal depression: either a combination of pharmacological and psychosocial intervention, or psychosocial intervention alone. There is no place in this setting for pharmacological intervention in isolation.

There are two aspects of making the decision whether to use pharmacological interventions in depressed pregnant women.

Assessment of the depression

Use of pharmacological therapies should be seriously considered if there are substantial neurovegetative changes, the quality of mood is characterised by the features described above, and, in particular, if there is any evidence of psychomotor retardation (slowing of motor movements and thinking) or severe agitation.

Risk–benefit analysis of prescribing

The risk–benefit analysis of the consequences of prescribing compared with not prescribing is summarised in Table 32.1.

Table 32.1
Prescribing in pregnancy: risk–benefit analysis

	Fetus	Mother
Risk of prescribing	1 Death 2 Congenital abnormality 3 Growth retardation 4 Neonatal toxicity 5 Long-term neurodevelopmental effects ('behavioural neurotoxicity')	Overdose Adverse effects Possible negative effect on therapeutic alliance
Risk of NOT prescribing	Fetal abuse or neglect Adverse effect of maternal mental state on the fetus	Distress and morbidity Suicide or self-harm Family or relationship deterioration Use of harmful substitutes

The table can provide a framework for the practitioner to address the decision whether or not to prescribe a psychotropic drug during pregnancy. It can also guide discussion with the woman, preferably in conjunction with her partner.

A categorisation of harmful effects to the fetus has been developed using five classes as shown in the table. For the first four classes, evidence (albeit of variable quality) is available for the more commonly used psychotropic medications. Class 5 is largely unexplored, but should not deter prescription where this is otherwise indicated. The relevance of the unknown risk in class 5 is to impress on the practitioner that no psychotropic agent can be considered completely safe in pregnancy, non-pharmacological interventions always warrant consideration, and unnecessarily high dosage and duration of treatment should be avoided. However, in relation to dosage, there are increases in total body water during pregnancy, as well as alterations in protein binding. Some pregnant women may require higher dosages of some medications (such as antidepressants) for an effective response.

Caution is warranted in prescribing only on the basis of preventing a condition (especially unipolar depression) which is not currently present (for example, postnatal depression).

A more detailed description of the use of this table is contained in *Therapeutic Guidelines: Psychotropic*, which also includes a simple protocol for prescribing during pregnancy, as well as a discussion of the use of various specific antidepressants.

source Reproduced with permission from *Therapeutic Guidelines: Psychotropic*, 5th edition, 2003.

As a general rule, if there is a reasonable likelihood of success of a psychological intervention, then this would be the treatment of choice, especially in the first trimester. However, clinicians should be aware that antidepressants can be safely prescribed at all stages of pregnancy, and there is substantial evidence that many classes of antidepressants are not significant human teratogens (Altshuler et al. 1996). In many cases, the risk of not prescribing will outweigh those of the use of effective antidepressant treatment.

Non-pharmacological interventions are similar to those commonly used in non-pregnant depressed patients. These include cognitive behaviour therapy, interpersonal psychotherapy, family or relationship therapy, and analytically oriented psychotherapy. The value of simple supportive psychotherapy (involving empathic listening, education and explanation, problem solving, and similar interventions) should not be underestimated. The four areas outlined above as tasks can help focus supportive therapy upon the areas of greatest relevance to a depressed pregnant woman.

Prevention

If a woman has had a previous episode of depression during pregnancy, she is at increased risk of recurrence on subsequent pregnancies. This is especially so if depressive episodes have occurred only during pregnancy.

However, we would not advocate prophylactic use of antidepressants in this situation. The woman (and her partner) should be advised of the early warning signs of recurrence and advised to seek assessment should these emerge. Treatment should be initiated only after proper assessment (as above) indicates that relapse has occurred.

THE BLUES

The blues is perhaps the best-known mood disturbance following childbirth. The term *blues*, or *baby blues*, is often misused to mean postnatal depression (it is a catchy name), whereas it is in fact describing a common set of symptoms women experience in the third to fifth day following childbirth. Up to 70 per cent of women will experience some transient mood symptoms at this time. Characteristic symptoms include tearfulness, anxiety, irritability, and lability of mood. The ubiquitous nature of these symptoms suggests that this condition represents a normal response following childbirth and should not be classified formally as a mood disorder. The clinical importance of the blues is twofold. First, it is important for clinicians to recognise that this is a common experience for women following childbirth and that for most women these symptoms have no prognostic significance. Women experiencing the blues need to be reassured that the symptoms will settle quickly and that there are no adverse outcomes from it. Second, for some women, the blues may be an indicator that they may go on to develop a subsequent mood disorder in the weeks or months after childbirth. Not all women who experience the blues go on to develop a post-partum mood disorder, but most women who have a post-partum mood disorder will have had the blues.

No definitive mechanism for the blues has yet been identified. Hormonal swings have been one postulated mechanism. However, it is recognised that the blues are more common among women who have high levels of neuroticism, previous history of depression, associated with unplanned pregnancy, a difficult labour and being anxious or depressed during pregnancy (Henshaw 2003). It is noteworthy that these are much the same as the risk factors for developing a depressive disorder following childbirth.

PUERPERAL PSYCHOSIS

An association between childbirth and the onset of a severe psychosis has been recognised throughout history. The link between such illness and the tragic fact that some such women may kill their infant (as a result of their psychosis) has led to special legislation to deal with such acts (infanticide) in some countries (but not the United States) (Oberman 2003).

In a pioneering study examining the relationship between psychiatric disorder and childbirth, Kendell et al. (1987) were able to link together obstetric and psychiatric hospital admission records. They found a close association between childbirth and admissions to a psychiatric hospital, particularly for psychosis, with a twenty-fold increased risk of admission within 30 days of delivery. Puerperal psychosis is a severe psychotic disorder that affects between one and two women per 1000 live deliveries (Brockington 1996). Although there has been considerable debate about the nosological status of this condition, the current consensus is that puerperal psychosis is a variant of bipolar disorder. It has many symptoms in common with bipolar disorder and a similar outcome. Its uniqueness lies in the close association with childbirth.

The causes of puerperal psychosis are not fully known, but there is clearly an underpinning biological (probably genetically determined) process occurring that contributes to the women's psychotic features. There is also the common observation that puerperal psychosis is common among women who have a perfectionist or obsessional personality style.

This underpinning biological basis of the disorders is not clearly understood; however, it is likely that falling levels of oestrogen may trigger off a cascade of events in neurotransmitters that contribute to the disorder's onset (Wieck et al. 1991).

Clinical features and assessment

Puerperal psychosis generally has its onset within the first 3 weeks following childbirth. Patients may present with a wide variety of symptoms with features of mania, major depression, or, as is often the case, a mix of the two. In addition to these symptoms, there will be evidence of a psychosis with hallucinations or delusions. Such hallucinations or delusions are generally mood congruent or, in many instances, delusional ideas about their infant. There are some unique features of puerperal psychosis, and women with this disorder will often present as confused or perplexed. Women with puerperal psychosis often appear indecisive, particularly when it relates to activities related to looking after their infant.

The symptoms of puerperal psychosis wax and wane; women may have periods in which they appear quite well, yet may relapse fairly quickly with a re-emergence of their psychotic symptoms.

If women have delusions, these will often be delusions about their infants. For example, women with a manic presentation may believe that their infant is the saviour of the world, or the devil, or have other grandiose delusions about their infant. Of great concern are women who have paranoid ideas about the infant, believing the infant may be out to cause harm. In such situations there is a high degree of risk, and the women will usually need to be placed in hospital for their own and the infants' protection.

Assessment of women suffering from a puerperal psychosis will involve:

- A comprehensive psychiatric history and mental state examination. In collecting this history, it is important to assess aspects of safety to the woman, to her baby and to others. History and mental state items that should raise concerns about safety are delusions about the baby, particularly if the woman believes the baby has special powers (such as that her baby is the devil or has come to save the world); command hallucinations; and hopelessness.
- An assessment of ability to care for the infant. If a woman is disorganised it will be difficult for her to manage routine activities associated with childcare.
- Medical and obstetric assessment.

Management of acute episodes

The management of puerperal psychosis involves, first, ensuring the safety of the mother and her infant, and second, providing symptomatic control of her symptoms of puerperal psychosis. Women should be admitted to a psychiatric unit if there are concerns about either their safety or their infants' safety.

Ideally, such a unit should specialise in mothers and babies, and there are a few specialised mother and baby units available for such women. This allows the mother to be in hospital with her infant, thus minimising the chances of any disruption of the mother–infant relationship during the mother's illness. There are also safety considerations for the mother, as she may be suicidal and may harm herself under the effect of her psychosis. It is therefore prudent that such women be observed closely.

Treatment issues

Women suffering from a puerperal psychosis need to be treated assertively with the appropriate medication. Psychotic symptoms need to be treated with an appropriate antipsychotic agent. There are no specifically preferred antipsychotic agents; the choice of agent will depend on whether the mother is breastfeeding, responses to previous treatment and patient preference. There is much known about the effects of the conventional antipsychotics on breast milk, and there do not appear to be any contraindications for their use. There is less information about the safety of using the newer antipsychotics for breastfeeding mothers (Austin and Mitchell 1998).

If the woman is depressed, she will need to be treated assertively with antidepressant medication. When women are profoundly depressed, particularly if they have marked psychomotor change, electroconvulsive therapy may be indicated, as it is a safe and effective treatment for puerperal psychosis.

Women will often also need to be treated with a mood stabiliser (lithium, valproate, or carbamazepine). If women are breastfeeding, caution in using mood stabilisers is required. Details about the use of mood stabilisers and breastfeeding can be found in *Therapeutic Guidelines: Psychotropic*. In some circumstances, it might be appropriate to recommend that mothers do not breastfeed if they have a puerperal psychosis, as the demand on them having to breastfeed can be very stressful. It is also much easier for the care of the infant, as the mother may be quite sedated at a time when she needs to feed the infant and there are risks associated with that. However, every effort should be made to support the mother in breastfeeding.

Prevention

There is a high risk of relapse of puerperal psychosis in any subsequent pregnancies. This will need to be explained at an appropriate time, generally when the woman is recovering from the first episode of puerperal psychosis. These discussions will also need to include contraceptive advice, as the risk of relapse is higher the closer together the pregnancies are.

There will then need to be discussion with the woman (and partner if appropriate) about the pros and cons of having further children, with the knowledge that there is a 50 per cent chance of relapse.

If women decide they would like further children, preventive strategies for relapse can be put in place. These could include the following features:

- It is important to ensure that the woman has regular psychiatric contact and support during the course of the pregnancy.
- There should be discussion about using preventive medication to reduce the risk of relapse. There is evidence that mood stabilisers introduced into the later part of the pregnancy, generally during the late second trimester, are effective in preventing relapse. Discussions should involve the pros and cons of taking preventive medication, which include balancing the risks and benefits for the mother taking medication, the developing fetus or the breastfeeding infant..
- An alternative strategy is a *watch, wait and see* strategy. In this approach, the woman will need to be seen regularly during the pregnancy. During this time an inventory needs to be made of the early symptoms she had of her psychosis. If a partner is available, he can perform a useful monitoring role and be an important treatment ally. The woman will then need to be seen very regularly during the first 3 weeks after giving birth, with regular checks to see if she is developing any early symptoms of her puerperal psychosis. Assertive treatment will then need to be implemented immediately any symptoms start to occur. In managing such symptoms, it is necessary that the woman can have 24-hour contact with the treatment team.

Whatever approach is taken, women need to be seen very regularly in the first month after they have had the baby. It is recommended that they have additional support over this period, and it is crucial that they get adequate sleep, as sleep deprivation may be a significant triggering factor for puerperal psychosis.

BIPOLAR DISORDER

Although pregnancy appears to confer some protection against psychosis, bipolar disorder in both the manic and depressive form can recur during pregnancy and, in rare instances, may have its first presentation during pregnancy. When bipolar disorder does occur during pregnancy in either the manic or depressive form, it needs to be treated as at any other time in the life cycle. However, there are some caveats in this, particularly the use of mood-stabilising drugs, which may be teratogenic. It is safer to use antipsychotic or antidepressant medication, as the risk of harm to the fetus is lower. The use of mood-stabilising drugs should be confined to the later stages of pregnancy (Mitchell et al. In press).

As we have noted above, childbirth is a significant life stressor and, in women who have bipolar disorder, can precipitate episodes of mania or depression in the first month after they have had a baby. Thus, it is important to provide counselling to women with bipolar disorder about the risks of having an episode of illness after childbirth.

The key to managing women suffering from bipolar disorder during pregnancy and the post-partum period is ensuring there is a careful management plan in place, and that the issues of safety to the mother, developing fetus and infant are taken into account.

Women who are planning to have children and suffer from bipolar disorder should have a psychiatric assessment before they become pregnant, to ensure that they do not become pregnant while taking a potentially teratogenic mood stabiliser. If the woman decides to have a baby, then she will need to come off her mood stabiliser before conceiving. Withdrawal from the mood stabiliser needs to be under psychiatric care, as there is a high risk of relapse upon cessation of mood stabilisers. It is therefore prudent to ensure that the woman has appropriate support when her mood stabilisers are withdrawn, and that the mood stabiliser is withdrawn at a time of the year when she is under the least stress, and at the time of the year when she is least likely to have a bipolar relapse. Withdrawal, if possible, should be gradual.

In the planning to cease the mood stabiliser, an inventory of the woman's bipolar symptoms should be recorded, so that if she starts to develop emergent symptoms, appropriate treatment can be instituted quickly, generally with an antipsychotic or an antidepressant.

If the woman has been well maintained on a mood stabiliser, the mood stabiliser can be reintroduced late in the second trimester of pregnancy, and continued for the remainder of the pregnancy and post-partum period.

If the woman is being treated with lithium, the dose will need to be reduced in the later part of the pregnancy, generally to about a third of the normal dose (serum levels of around 0.2 mmol/L) to prevent any possible lithium toxicity arising during labour when the woman may become dehydrated, and to avoid any complications for the infant (as lithium passes through the placenta). The full dose of lithium should be reintroduced immediately after the birth.

The risks and benefits of breastfeeding and taking a mood stabiliser will need to be discussed with the woman so she can make an informed decision.

Any episodes of bipolar disorder arising after giving birth will need to be treated in the conventional manner; however, particular care should be taken about safety to the woman and to her infant.

POSTNATAL DEPRESSION

Over the past 30 years, there has been increasing interest in postnatal depression. Postnatal depression is an episode of major depression that arises in the first 6 months following childbirth. It is not a specific type of depression, as had originally been suggested by Pitt (1968), nor does it have unique symptoms. Its importance lies in its proximity to childbirth and its possible effect on the developing infant.

Postnatal depression is common, with there now being a consensus that postnatal depression affects between 10 and 15 per cent of women in the first 6 months following childbirth (O'Hara and Swain 1996). Postnatal depression is no different symptomatically from non-psychotic, non-melancholic major depression arising at any other time in the life cycle, although there may be more anxiety symptoms present. Furthermore, the prevalence of postnatal depression, while recognised as being high, has been shown in various studies to be no higher than depression arising among non-childbearing women (Cox et al. 1993).

Given its association with childbirth, postnatal depression has been considered related to some hormonal change. However, despite considerable research, no clear association has been demonstrated, although for a small group of women there may be a link between oestrogen sensitivity and the onset of depression (Bloch et al. 2000).

The main causes of postnatal depression are psychosocial: that is, the disorder is precipitated by the stress of childbirth among vulnerable women.

A range of vulnerability factors to postnatal depression has been identified; these have been summarised in two meta-analyses (Beck 1996; O'Hara and Swain 1996) and in one comprehensive literature review (Pope et al. 2000).

Vulnerability to postnatal depression lies in several domains. Sociodemographic factors such as socially disadvantaged women, and young (teenage) first-time mothers, have been shown to have increased risk. Adverse early life experiences, particularly child sexual abuse or experiencing poor parenting (characterised by a lack of care), also increase the risk of postnatal depression.

Women who have poor social support networks, particularly emotional support, also have an increased risk of developing postnatal depression. Support from partners is critical at this time, and women in non-supportive relationships are at high risk of developing postnatal depression (Boyce

1994). It should be noted that many women will shift their social network after childbirth so, when they have the new baby, they do not have the same access to their social network as previously. This may increase their vulnerability to postnatal depression.

A woman's personality style has an influence. In particular, women who are anxious worriers, overly sensitive or high on neuroticism have an increased risk of postnatal depression (Boyce 1994).

There is very clear evidence that women with previous psychopathology (anxiety or depression) are at increased risk of developing postnatal depression. Women who are depressed or anxious during pregnancy also have an increased risk. Obstetric variables such as having a traumatic delivery may increase the risk of postnatal depression. When there has been a traumatic delivery (such as a high forceps delivery), post-traumatic stress disorder can arise and may mimic postnatal depression. It is important to recognise post-traumatic disorder and to be aware it can coexist with postnatal depression.

Clinical features

Postnatal depression is, in general, no different from major depression arising at other times in the life cycle. However, many women with postnatal depression also report a variety of anxiety symptoms, most notably irritability. The assessment of postnatal depression has to take into account that many women may experience symptoms that appear to be similar to depression that arise by virtue of looking after a small infant. Such symptoms include weight loss, tiredness, loss of libido and sleep disturbance.

Women often report that symptoms emerge gradually over the first 6 months following childbirth, with most women experiencing the symptoms between 6 weeks and 3 months after giving birth. Common symptoms include loss of self-esteem, particularly with regard to their role in being a mother. Fatigue is a common symptom; although this might be the result of a lack of sleep because of the baby's routine, the fatigue of depression is more than just tiredness. These women often report difficulty in getting to sleep (frequently lying awake worrying about their baby) despite feeling tired. A lack of interest or enjoyment in activities is other common symptom of postnatal depression.

Anxiety symptoms commonly accompany postnatal depression, with the most prominent symptom being irritability. This is a particularly troublesome symptom as women may become irritable with people around them, especially their partners. This can lead to increasing difficulty in the marital relationship, especially if the partner withdraws support because of the irritability. Many women with postnatal depression report anxiety surrounding care of their infant.

Women often mask their symptoms of postnatal depression because they feel shame about not coping at a time when they are supposed to be happy. They will often ensure that they are well groomed, and that the infant is well cared for, despite feeling depressed. They will often talk about themselves as being the only ones who have ever experienced such symptoms, and do not realise that many other women have postnatal depression as well.

Assessment and management

The assessment of women with postnatal depression follows the pattern of conducting a routine psychiatric assessment. There are some special features that need to be conducted in assessing women with postnatal depression. These are outlined below.

In eliciting the normal depression and anxiety symptoms, care must be taken to ensure that the symptoms are due to depression and not arising by virtue of having to care for the infant (symptoms such as weight loss, loss of libido, and fatigue).

In assessing women with postnatal depression, the health professional has to take into account the safety of both the mother and the infant. It was thought that suicide rates were lower among nursing mothers; however, a recent study has shown that suicide is the commonest cause of maternal death (Oates 2003). Suicidal feelings need to be explored very carefully among women with postnatal depression, particularly examining for thoughts such as 'the baby will be better off without me'. Suicide risk is high among women who feel hopeless, who have experienced abuse or neglect themselves, or who have a past history of suicide attempts.

A careful assessment needs to be made about the potential harm to the infant. This may be harm by neglect, in which the woman does not care for the infant or look after it properly because of her depression, or it may be more direct harm to the infant, including physical abuse. This can be associated with irritability, particularly when the woman becomes frustrated with an infant who will not settle. Women who have been abused or are in a relationship characterised by domestic violence are at high risk of abusing their infants. When there is domestic violence, it is important to remember the infant is at risk of abuse from the father. He may take out his frustrations at his partner's depression or her paying more attention to the baby than to him and abuse the infant. Whenever there are concerns about potential abuse for the infant, the appropriate child protection agencies have to be notified.

The quality of the woman's social support network and, in particular, the quality of relationship with her partner has to be examined thoroughly, as this may be a major factor contributing to her depression. Where there are difficulties in the marital relationship, these need to be dealt with. It may take some time to explore thoroughly with the woman the quality of her relationship. It is noteworthy that many women suffering from postnatal depression are still victims of domestic violence in various forms.

There needs to be a careful assessment of the quality of the mother–infant relationship. Women who are depressed may not be able to cue appropriately to their infants, and may not be able to respond appropriately. When this arises, there needs to be further work to assist the mother with her mothercraft skills at both a practical and emotional level.

The assessment should always take into account the woman's obstetric history, her experiences of childbirth and her current contraception.

The assessment should examine the woman's feelings about breastfeeding and whether she is breastfeeding, as this may affect treatment choices.

In many ways, the clinical management of postnatal depression follows the management of depression at other times in the life cycle, and as described earlier for depression arising during pregnancy. The major difference is the consideration of the choice of medication for the breastfeeding mother if medication is required (Table 32.1) (Austin and Mitchell 1998). Treatments always need to include a psychosocial component, which may be supplemented by pharmacotherapy and specific psychological intervention.

The general approach to treatment is first to obtain a comprehensive assessment of the woman, and explain to her about postnatal depression. Many women do not have knowledge about postnatal depression, and they believe the way they are feeling is what is expected of healthy nursing mothers. Women need to be told that they are suffering from a common treatable illness (a figure of one in ten mothers suffering from postnatal depression is a useful thing to explain to them) and that they will get better.

At a basic level, allowing the woman to talk about her experiences, the difficulties she is having with the baby, any disappointments she has about her new role as a mother and taking a supportive psychotherapeutic stance will be helpful for many women, particularly when this is coupled with some psychoeducation about postnatal depression.

The standard treatments that have been used at other times in the life cycle, such as cognitive behaviour therapy, interpersonal therapy and supportive counselling, are all of benefit in postnatal depression. The specific treatment for an individual woman will be determined by the factors that have contributed to her depression, her preferences and the treating doctor's skill. Pharmacotherapy can also be used for postnatal depression, but the risks and benefits need to be discussed carefully with the mother, particularly if she is breastfeeding. The pharmacological approach will be indicated under the following circumstances:

- where the woman is suffering from a biologically determined depression, characterised by neurovegetative symptoms and psychomotor change
- in women suffering from a moderate to severe form of depression
- where there may be overwhelming anxiety and panic attacks associated with the depression that does not respond to non-pharmacological interventions
- where a woman may have had a successful treatment with antidepressant medication previously, and is requesting antidepressant medication again.

Prevention

Postnatal depression is a condition in which preventive strategies would seem appropriate, given the proximity between a specific life event and the onset of depression. Preventive intervention has been offered to women in antenatal clinics, often coupled with antenatal classes. However, these tend to be more universal preventive interventions and have not shown great benefit in reducing the risk of postnatal depression.

A more practical approach to prevention will be to individually target factors that may have contributed to a woman developing postnatal depression in the past, dealing with those risk factors prior to the baby being born, so that the risk of her relapsing is much reduced. Such interventions would include strategies such as stress inoculation, ensuring appropriate supports are available for her after the baby has been born, and dealing with any marital difficulties that may arise before the birth of the baby.

REFERENCES

Altshuler LL, Cohen L, Szuba MP, Burt VK, Gitlin M, Mintz J (1996) Pharmacologic management of psychiatric illness during pregnancy: Dilemmas and guidelines. *American Journal of Psychiatry* 153:592-606.

Austin MP, Mitchell PB (1998) Use of psychotropic medications in breast-feeding women: Acute and prophylactic treatment. *Australian and New Zealand Journal of Psychiatry* 32:778-84.

Beck CT (1996) A meta-analysis of predictors of postpartum depression. *Nursing Research* 45:297-303.

Bloch M, Schmidt PJ, Danaceau M, Murphy J, Nieman L, Rubinow DR (2000) Effects of gonadal steroids in women with a history of postpartum depression. *American Journal of Psychiatry* 157:924-30.

Boyce PM (1994) Personality dysfunction, marital problems and postnatal depression. In Cox J, Holden J (eds), *Perinatal Psychiatry: Use and misuse of the Edinburgh Postnatal Depression Scale*. London: Gaskell, pp. 82-102.

Boyce PM, Stubbs JM (1994) The importance of postnatal depression. *Medical Journal of Australia* 161:471-2.

Brockington I (1996) *Motherhood and Mental Health*. New York: Oxford Medical Publications.

Buist AE, Barnett BE, Milgrom J, Pope S, Condon JT, Ellwood DA, et al. (2002) To screen or not to screen – that is the question in perinatal depression. *Medical Journal of Australia* 177 (7 Suppl):S101-5.

Condon JT (1993) The assessment of antenatal emotional attachment: Development of a questionnaire instrument. *British Journal of Medical Psychology* 66:167-83.

Condon JT, Dunn DJ (1988) Nature and determinants of parent-to-infant attachment in the early postnatal period. *Journal of the American Academy of Child and Adolescent Psychiatry* 27:293-9.

Condon JT, Esuvaranathan V (1990) The influence of parity on the experience of pregnancy: A comparison of first- and second-time expectant couples. *British Journal of Medical Psychology* 63:369-77.

Condon JT, Donovan J, Corkindale CJ (2001) Australian adolescents' attitudes and beliefs concerning pregnancy, childbirth and parenthood: The development, psychometric testing and results of a new scale. *Journal of Adolescence* 24:729-42.

Cox JL, Murray D, Chapman G (1993) A controlled study of the onset, duration and prevalence of postnatal depression. *British Journal of Psychiatry* 163:27-31.

Evans J, Heron J, Francomb H, Oke S, Golding J (2001) Cohort study of depressed mood during pregnancy and after childbirth. *BMJ* 323:257-60.

Henshaw C (2003) Mood disturbance in the early puerperium: A review. *Archives of Women's Mental Health* 6 Suppl 2:s33-42.

Kendell RE, Chalmers JC, Platz C (1987) Epidemiology of puerperal psychoses. *British Journal of Psychiatry* 150:662-73.

Mitchell PB, Malhi GS, Redwood BL, Ball J (In press) Australian and New Zealand Clinical Practice Guideline for the Treatment of Bipolar Disorder. *Australian and New Zealand Journal of Psychiatry*.

Oates M (2003) Suicide: The leading cause of maternal death. *British Journal of Psychiatry* 183:279-81.

Oberman M (2003) A brief history of infanticide and the law. In Spinelli MG (ed), *Infanticide: Psychosocial and legal perspectives on mothers who kill*. Washington, DC: American Psychiatric Publishing.
O'Hara MW, Swain AM (1996) Rates and risk of postpartum depression – a meta-analysis. *International Review of Psychiatry* 8:37-54.
Pitt B (1968) 'Atypical' depression following childbirth. *British Journal of Psychiatry* 114:1325-35.
Pope S, Watts J, Evans S, McDonald S, Henderson S (2000) An Information Paper. Postnatal Depression: A systematic review of published scientific literature to 1999. Canberra: National Health and Medical Research Council.
Wieck A, Kumar R, Hirst AD, Marks MN, Campbell IC, Checkley SA (1991) Increased sensitivity of dopamine receptors and recurrence of affective psychosis after childbirth. *BMJ* 303:613-16.

CHAPTER 33

DEPRESSION IN OLDER PEOPLE

Gerard J A Byrne

In most developed countries, decades of falling mortality rates have led to increased numbers of older people. During 2002, people over the age of 65 years accounted for about 12 per cent of the population in both Australia and New Zealand, and this proportion is projected to rise to more than 25 per cent over the next few decades. Interestingly, the fastest-growing component of the population is people aged 85 years and over. Falling birth rates have meant that the mean age of populations has also increased. As the population ages, gender differentials in mortality mean that older people are increasingly likely to be female. Similar trends are beginning to emerge in developing countries.

Culture and language are important issues in ageing populations. Many Maori and indigenous women have had prejudicial experiences earlier in life that may predispose them to depression. Many immigrant women have not had the opportunity to work outside the home and have not acquired a good grasp of English. Assessment and management of depression in older patients from non-English-speaking backgrounds may be assisted by involving a transcultural mental health worker or experienced translator.

EPIDEMIOLOGY

The epidemiology of depression in older people has been the subject of considerable debate over recent years. Data from community surveys generally indicate that the prevalence of serious depressive illness declines with advancing age. For example, the 1997 Australian National Survey of Mental Health and Wellbeing of Adults found that less than 1 per cent of men and less than 2 per cent of women aged 65 years and older living in the community met diagnostic criteria for a depressive disorder. The New Zealand Mental Health and General Practice Investigation found that the prevalence of depressive disorder in general practice attendees aged 65 years and older was 2.1 per cent for men and 4.8 per cent for women (MaGPIe Research Group 2003).

However, surveys that do not include older people in residential care settings are likely to seriously underestimate the true prevalence of depression in older people. It is now well established that older people living in supported accommodation have a much higher prevalence of depressive illness. Between 6 and 18 per cent of older people living in aged hostels and nursing homes have been found to suffer from depressive disorders. The prevalence of depression in older people receiving domiciliary nursing care and in older hospital inpatients is even higher. The association of depressive disorders with physical illnesses such as stroke, cancer and myocardial infarction, and with spousal bereavement, raises important questions about the low prevalence rates found in community surveys of older people. In the Cache County Study, which surveyed community and institutionalised older people, the point prevalence of major depression was 2.7 per cent in men and 4.4 per cent in women, and the estimated lifetime prevalence of depression was 9.6 per cent in men and 20.4 per cent in women. Regardless of the true prevalence of depressive disorders in older people, it is clear that older women are almost twice as likely as older men to suffer a depressive disorder.

Depressive states that do not meet diagnostic criteria for major depression also occur in older people, although the prevalence of such states is unclear. In the Cache County Study, dysthymia (chronic low-grade depression), uncomplicated bereavement, subsyndromal depression and monosymptomatic depression were each relatively uncommon. However, earlier work using different diagnostic criteria found quite high rates of so-called minor depression in older people (Steffens et al. 2000).

Surveys of depressive symptoms rather than disorders show a similar age-related decline in prevalence, although some of this apparent decline is likely to be due to response bias, with fewer older people responding to surveys based on census tracts or the electoral roll.

CLINICAL FEATURES

There is little firm evidence that the phenomenology of depressive disorder in older people is systematically different to that in younger adults. However, clinical experience suggests that mixed anxiety and depressive states occur commonly in older people. These mixed states are often termed *agitated* depression.

Anhedonia (from the Greek *an*, without, and *hédoné*, pleasure), demoralisation, pessimism, worthlessness, hopelessness and guilt are common symptoms of depression in older people. Sleep and appetite disturbance also occur commonly in depressed older people, but are not particularly discriminating as they also occur in older people who are not depressed. Psychomotor retardation and agitation, including the combination of gross motor retardation and fine motor agitation, frequently accompany depression in older people. Some older people with depression exhibit *Weltschmerz* (from the German *Welt*, world, and *Schmerz*, pain; pronounced vĕlt' shmĕrts), an exaggerated sadness over the real or perceived evils of the world. Although crying is uncommon, depressed older people commonly react with exaggerated distress to the vicissitudes of life, despite having been rather stoical previously. Importuning behaviour may accompany depressive illness, but its presence should not automatically lead to the assumption that the older person suffers from serious character pathology.

Somatic presentations of depression mimicking cardiorespiratory, gastrointestinal and neurological illness may lead to extensive investigation for underlying physical illness. However, the trap for the clinician is that many older people both experience and report a marked amplification of symptoms of actual physical illness when they develop a depressive disorder.

Old age psychiatrists frequently report that many of their older depressed patients smile, albeit rather superficially, at them during assessment interviews. Such displays of socially sanctioned smiling by older people should not be taken as evidence against the diagnosis of a depressive disorder. These presentations have been referred to as *smiling depression*.

DIFFERENTIAL DIAGNOSIS

In older people, the syndrome of depression needs to be distinguished from several other common conditions, including anxiety, delirium, dementia, parkinsonism and excessive sedation due to prescribed medication. Occasionally, serious physical illness such as malignancy or chronic infection may masquerade as depression. Stroke may be associated with emotionalism, including tearfulness that can be confused with depression. However, to complicate matters further, stroke is also commonly associated with depressed mood and depressive disorder. Depression must also be distinguished from grief that occurs following loss and from demoralisation that occurs in a variety of situations, including serious physical illness. The differential diagnosis of depression in older people can be satisfactorily dissected following detailed history-taking, age-specific mental state examination, careful physical examination, and judicious use of laboratory investigations and imaging studies.

Grief versus depression

In older people, it is important to be able to distinguish *grief* from *depression*. Grief is a normal response to loss and, unless prolonged, severe or complicated by psychiatric disorder, should not normally come to psychiatric attention. Gender and culture have major effects on the manifestations of normal grief, and it is important to appreciate culturally sanctioned expressions of grief so as to avoid medicalising a normal phenomenon. Within a particular culture, the nature of grief reactions is a reflection of the nature of the attachment that has been lost and the manner in which the attachment has been lost. Thus, ambivalent attachments and sudden or unexpected losses often presage pathological grief. Pathological grief includes severe and prolonged grief reactions and grief complicated by substance abuse or other psychiatric disorder.

Symptoms of grief are generally experienced in waves – *the pangs of grief* – and tend to diminish gradually over several months without treatment. Common symptoms of grief in Western cultures include crying, insomnia, somatic symptoms, thoughts about the deceased and a sense of presence of the deceased. Hallucinations of the deceased and thoughts of death also occur relatively commonly. When grief is complicated by persistent anhedonia or suicidal thoughts or when severe grief persists for more than a few months, the clinician should consider whether a depressive disorder might have developed (Byrne and Raphael 1994).

COMORBIDITY

The US National Comorbidity Study found high levels of comorbidity among mental disorders in adults, but did not sample older people. However, it is likely that similar levels of comorbidity affect older people with mental disorders. The available evidence certainly indicates that depressive disorders are often accompanied by comorbid anxiety disorders, with the association between the *Diagnostic and Statistical Manual of Mental Disorders*, fourth edition (DSM-IV), major depressive disorder and generalised anxiety disorder being particularly strong. Approximately 35 per cent of older people with major depressive disorder also meet diagnostic criteria for generalised anxiety disorder. This has implications for treatment, as treatment of major depressive disorder without concomitant treatment of generalised anxiety disorder is likely to increase the risk of early relapse or recurrence.

The relationship between depression and dementia is also strong, although the nature of the association is still the subject of debate. Depressive symptoms occur commonly among people with dementia, particularly those with a vascular component to their dementia. For instance, the US Cache County Study found that the prevalence of depressive symptoms in patients with Alzheimer's disease was 20 per cent, whereas the prevalence of depressive symptoms in patients with vascular dementia was 32 per cent (Lyketsos et al. 2000).

Although depressive symptoms are common in mild, moderate and severe dementia, they have a tendency to decline slightly in prevalence with increasing severity of the dementia. Depressive disorders precede dementia more often than expected, raising questions about the relationship between the two disorders. It is possible that neurodegenerative changes in the ageing brain lead first to late onset depression and then to dementia.

Substance-use disorders are uncommon in older people, and when present may indicate the presence of serious psychopathology. It is important to realise that substance abuse is often limited by income in later life. Substance-abuse disorders may complicate mood disorders. In older people, abuse of prescription drugs, mainly benzodiazepines, and abuse of alcohol are the most common forms of substance abuse.

In older people, depression commonly accompanies physical disorders such as stroke, heart attack and cancer. These common serious physical disorders are associated with excess morbidity from depression, and the outcome of these conditions is adversely affected by untreated depression. For myocardial infarction at least, outcome is significantly improved if depression is treated effectively.

DEPRESSION IN CAREGIVERS

Many older people care for a physically or mentally impaired spouse or sibling, and some older people care for an impaired adult child. Although the caregiving role brings with it certain rewards, many older carers experience a great sense of burden. Some older carers develop depressive symptoms and depressive disorders that can at least partially be attributed to their caring role. When assessing an older person for a mental disorder such as depression or dementia it is important to also briefly assess his/her spouse or other carer for the presence of depression.

SUICIDE

There is a strong relationship between depressive disorders and suicide, although not all completed suicide is related to depressive disorder. Over recent decades there has been a slow fall in the overall mortality rate from suicide among older people, although rates among men aged 75 years and older remain high. Older men tend to use hanging, firearms and carbon monoxide poisoning to commit suicide. In contrast, older women tend to use drug overdose, hanging, carbon monoxide poisoning and drowning.

In 1996, the prevalence rate of completed suicide among Australian men aged 65 years and older was 26 per 100 000 per year, whereas the rate among older women was 5 per 100 000 per year, with an overall rate for older people of 14 per 100 000 per year. Very similar prevalence rates have been found in New Zealand.

Isolation, recent losses, physical illness, mood disorders and other psychopathology are the main risk factors for completed suicide in older people. There is some evidence also that a personality style characterised by hopelessness, anhedonia, anger and antisocial traits may predispose to completed suicide (DeLeo et al. 2001).

RISK FACTORS

Risk factors for depression in older people may vary according to whether the patient's first episode of depression occurred early or late in life. There is evidence that personality factors, family history of mood disorder, and self-reported difficulties with maternal relationships are more common in early onset depression. Premorbid personality, particularly neuroticism, is an important risk factor for both depressive and anxiety disorders in older people. Bereavement is associated with an increased risk of depressive disorders.

Stroke and other types of cerebrovascular disease are increasingly recognised as causal factors in late onset depressive disorders. Cerebrovascular disease affecting the dorsolateral prefrontal cortex or subcortical structures seems important in the aetiology of many cases of late onset depression, and makes effective treatment of depression more difficult. There is also an increased risk of depression following acute myocardial infarction, with people who have untreated depression showing a higher subsequent mortality rate from heart disease.

Certain medications used to treat general medical conditions have been associated with the development of depression in vulnerable older people. In particular, corticosteroids, interferon and gonadotrophin-releasing hormone agonists are associated with depression. Reserpine, propranolol and alpha methyldopa, although no longer commonly prescribed, may also cause depression. Drugs used to treat Parkinson's disease, particularly levodopa, may be associated with a variety of adverse neuropsychiatric effects, including depression.

PREVENTION

The evidence base for the prevention of depression in older people is rather poor. However, there are several straightforward preventive interventions that are worthy of consideration. These include the recognition and treatment of pathological grief, the aggressive control of risk factors for cerebrovascular disease and the use of combination pharmacotherapy and psychotherapy to prevent depressive relapses (Byrne 1995).

ASSESSMENT

It is usually appropriate to see depressed older people alone and then with selected family members or other supporters. Sometimes, the older person will ask to be accompanied throughout the assessment by a family member. However, it is important to be able to ask the older person about domestic violence and other forms of elder abuse, and this may be difficult if the entire interview is completed in the presence of another person.

There is often considerable value in interviewing someone other than the older person with depression. Corroborative history may uncover essential information that can be used for both diagnosis and treatment. Sensory impairment (problems with eyesight and hearing) and cognitive impairment (including depressive pseudodementia) may limit the patient's ability to provide a comprehensive history.

When taking the history from an older person who may be depressed, it is important to consider both the developmental and family contexts. From a developmental point of view, it is necessary to place patients within the context of the whole of their life. As this may extend to eight decades or more, sufficient time must be set aside during clinical assessment to obtain this history. Older people have often experienced considerable adversity earlier in life. It is important to inquire about wartime experiences, economic depression and poverty. It is also necessary to consider the various family contexts that might be relevant, including the older persons' family of origin and family of procreation. Their current relationship to siblings and adult children should be assessed. Some older depressed people may even have very elderly parents still alive, some of whom might enjoy better health than the patient. The older patient should be asked about elder abuse, which may involve physical, emotional, sexual or financial abuse. Always consider the possibility of psychotic symptoms and have a high index of suspicion for psychotic symptoms in mute patients and those with bizarre behaviour.

Although clinical assessment necessarily focuses on current deficits, it is important to allow time to assess the older person's strengths. These may include, for example, high premorbid intelligence, good social support, low neuroticism, good general health, financial security and religious beliefs.

It is important to formally assess cognitive performance at some point. It may be necessary to allow additional time for the slow responses sometimes seen in severely depressed older people. If sufficient time is allowed, it should be possible to distinguish between the increased speech latency and indecisiveness often seen in severe depression and the incorrect responses given in dementia. The use of a brief objective scale such as the Mini-Mental State Examination (MMSE) is recommended.

Affect can be deceptive in well-socialised older people. As previously noted, the term *smiling depressive* refers to older people who are still able to maintain a social smile despite the presence of clinically significant depressed mood.

Although rating scales should not generally be used as diagnostic tools, they can be useful adjuncts to clinical assessment. The best self-rating scale for assessing the severity of depression in older people is the Geriatric Depression Scale, which comes in several forms. Its yes/no responses make it particularly suitable for use in very old people. The Cornell Scale for Depression in Dementia is also useful when assessing the extent of any depression complicating dementia.

MANAGEMENT PRINCIPLES

The management of depressive disorders in older people requires time and patience on the part of the clinician. It is essential to allow sufficient time to explain to the patient the nature of the depressive disorder and the rationale behind its treatment. Many older people will be quite fearful of the implications of a psychiatric diagnosis and will feel particularly stigmatised by it. They may fear being consigned to an asylum or being rejected by their family as a result of such a diagnosis. Alternatively, they may welcome the explanation for their symptoms and the provision of effective treatment. Just as the assessment of older depressed people requires adopting developmental and family perspectives, so does treatment planning. Treatment responses in older people often take much longer than in younger people, and the clinician must be prepared to take a multimodal approach and persist with this approach until the symptoms resolve. Therapeutic nihilism must be actively avoided.

BIOLOGICAL TREATMENTS

There are particular pharmacokinetic and pharmacodynamic considerations when prescribing antidepressant medication to older people. The main pharmacokinetic changes in later life include an increased volume of distribution for fat-soluble drugs (all psychotropic medications other than lithium), reduced liver metabolism, and reduced renal excretion. The main pharmacodynamic change is increased susceptibility to central nervous system adverse effects. The practical implication of these changes with age is that older people usually require lower doses of antidepressant medication than middle-aged people and tend to be more susceptible to adverse effects. Thus, the usual advice when prescribing to older people is to start low, go slow, and check frequently for adverse effects. Other considerations when prescribing to older depressed patients include the older person's propensity to constipation and urinary retention, and the serious consequences of falls due to postural hypotension.

The selective serotonin reuptake inhibitor (SSRI) antidepressants are now considered the most appropriate agents for first-line treatment of depressive disorders in older people. SSRIs with shorter half-lives and better adverse effect profiles (for example, sertraline or citalopram) are generally preferred in this situation. However, the more sedating drug, fluvoxamine, may be preferred in agitated patients or in those with marked sleep disturbance. The older tricyclic and tetracyclic antidepressants (for example, nortriptyline and mianserin), and the newer serotonin and noradrenaline reuptake inhibitor (SNRI) medications (for example, venlafaxine) are generally considered second-line agents because of their adverse effect profiles, the need for dose titration and the frequent need for twice-daily dosing.

The usual starting dose of sertraline in older people is 25 mg daily, and the usual final dose is 50–100 mg daily. The usual starting dose for citalopram in older people is 10 mg daily and the usual final dose is 20–40 mg daily. Higher doses are sometimes used. There is a risk of hyponatraemia with all centrally acting drugs, but particularly with the SSRI and SNRI antidepressants. Female gender, cerebrovascular disease and diuretic therapy are additional risk factors for hyponatraemia. Hyponatraemia may present with an apparent worsening of depressive symptoms or with agitation. Prudent prescribers check the serum sodium concentration before and about 1 week after commencing antidepressant medication in older people. However, hyponatraemia may occur unexpectedly later in the course of treatment, so clinicians need to keep a high index of suspicion for this effect.

Mood stabilisers, including lithium, valproate and carbamazepine, are frequently used to good effect in older patients. Mood stabilisers are an essential component of the treatment of depressive episodes in older patients with bipolar disorder and are sometimes used as adjuncts to treatment with antidepressant medication in older patients with treatment-resistant depression. Of the three mood stabilisers in common use, valproate is probably the safest to use in older people, although both lithium and carbamazepine are effective and do have a place. Lithium has a narrow margin of safety in older people, particularly for those living in warmer climates, and carbamazepine has a greater tendency to interact with other drugs.

Very little research has investigated the use of antidepressant medication to treat depression occurring in the context of dementia. However, there is good evidence for the efficacy of antidepressant medications when used to treat depression complicating serious physical disorders such as stroke or cancer. A Cochrane review has found that the number needed to treat is 4.2.

There is evidence for the greater efficacy of antidepressant medication when combined with psychotherapy in middle-aged people and, although similar evidence in older people is lacking, there is no obvious reason why the combination should not be better than either treatment given alone in older people as well. However, there is good evidence in older people for the value of combination treatment with antidepressant medication and psychotherapy for preventing depressive relapses following successful treatment of an index episode of depression. In addition, there is evidence of superior outcome when treatment with antidepressant medication is supported by a care manager who is able to provide education, support and help with problem solving (Gill and Hatcher 2003).

Electroconvulsive therapy (ECT) is a well-established treatment for depression in older adults. In fact, there are certain clinical situations in which ECT is the preferred treatment for older depressed patients. When depression is complicated by psychotic symptoms, marked suicidality or inadequate intake of food or fluid, ECT is often the most appropriate treatment. Older people, particularly those with pre-existing cognitive impairment, are at increased risk of both ECT-related delirium and ECT-related amnesia. When ECT is used in older people, it is generally preferable to apply the electrical stimulus to the non-dominant hemisphere to minimise the cognitive adverse effects of the treatment. Maintenance ECT, where a single treatment is given every few weeks, usually on an outpatient basis, is also useful for older people with severe, recurrent depressive disorders. The main impediment to the use of ECT is the stigma associated with its use. Unfortunately, health workers who are insufficiently informed about the efficacy and safety of this treatment sometimes contribute to maintaining this stigma.

Transcranial magnetic stimulation is currently being used as a research tool, and there are insufficient efficacy data to enable it to be recommended as a treatment for depression in older people.

PSYCHOLOGICAL TREATMENTS

Although formal psychotherapy is not commonly used in the management of depression in older people, this has more to do with the sociology of medicine (and clinical psychology) than with efficacy data. Cognitive behaviour therapy (CBT), suitably modified for older people, has been demonstrated to be more effective than a no-treatment comparison condition for treating mild to moderate depression in older outpatients. Similarly, interpersonal psychotherapy (IPT) has been found to prevent relapse in older people who have recovered from an index episode of depression. In practice, old age psychiatrists generally combine antidepressant medication with aspects of psychotherapy selected from CBT, IPT and psychodynamic psychotherapy traditions.

OTHER TREATMENTS

Several other treatments have been suggested for late life depression. Although thyroid hormone and psychostimulants such as dexamphetamine have been used in treatment-resistant depressed older patients, the evidence base for these interventions is poor. St John's wort (*Hypericum perforatum*) has been found superior to placebo in middle-aged patients with mild to moderate depression, but there is little formal evidence of its efficacy and tolerability in older people. Although treatment with bright light might relieve depression in patients with both seasonal and non-seasonal depressive disorders, the effect seems not to persist very long. More encouragingly, there is now evidence that both aerobic exercise and weight training may be useful treatments for older patients with depression.

ADVOCACY AND OTHER BROADER ROLES

It is appropriate for doctors and other health workers to advocate on behalf of older people with depression and other mental disorders. This advocacy may take various forms, including negotiating with relatives, residential care providers and guardianship boards. It may also involve the provision of education and training for workers providing housing, income support, domiciliary care and other community services to older people. Well-informed health workers should be able to engage in public debate to reduce the stigma often associated with mental disorder in older people.

CONCLUSION

As the population ages, increasing numbers of older people will require treatment for depressive disorders. Good treatments are available and should be used. Clinicians should adopt an optimistic, assertive and persistent approach to the treatment of depression in older people, as delayed treatment responses commonly occur. The most effective approaches to treatment and relapse prevention involve the combination of antidepressant medication with some form of psychological treatment (Unutzer et al. 2002).

REFERENCES

Byrne GJA (1995) Opportunities for preventive intervention for mental disorders in the elderly. In Raphael B, Burrows G (eds), *Handbook of Preventive Psychiatry*. Amsterdam: Elsevier, pp. 185-202.

Byrne GJA, Raphael B (1994) A longitudinal study of bereavement phenomena in elderly men. *Psychological Medicine* 24:411-21.

DeLeo D, Hickey PA, Neulinger K, Cantor CH (2001) Ageing and suicide. Canberra: Commonwealth Department of Health and Aged Care.

Gill D, Hatcher S (2003) Antidepressants for depression in medical illness (Cochrane Review). *The Cochrane Library* Issue 2. Oxford: Update Software.

Lyketsos CG, Steinberg M, Tschanz JT, Norton MC, Steffens DC, Breitner JC (2000) Mental and behavioral disturbances in dementia: Findings from the Cache County Study of Memory in Aging. *American Journal of Psychiatry* 157:708-14.

MaGPIe Research Group (2003) The nature and prevalence of psychological problems in New Zealand primary healthcare: A report on Mental Health and General Practice Investigation (MaGPIe). *New Zealand Medical Journal* 116:U379.

Steffens DC, Skoog I, Norton MC, Hart AD, Tschanz JT, Plassman BL, et al. (2000) Prevalence of depression and its treatment in an elderly population. The Cache County Study. *Archives of General Psychiatry* 57:601-7.

Unutzer J, Katon W, Callahan CM, Williams JW, Hunkeler E, Harpole L, et al. (2002) Collaborative care management of late-life depression in the primary care setting: A randomized controlled trial. *JAMA* 288:2836-45.

SECTION

VII

Impact, Outcome and Burden of Mood Disorders

CHAPTER 34

LONG-TERM OUTCOME OF DEPRESSION

Roger T Mulder

The long-term outcome of depression has been studied in two major ways. The first is by naturalistic studies, in which a cohort of patients is either followed up prospectively or recontacted after some time and the course of illness retrospectively constructed. The second is through treatment studies, in which patients are treated until in remission and then randomised to continuation of treatment or placebo. Sometimes these models are blurred: patients who were given a controlled treatment for a short period are then enrolled in a longer-term naturalistic follow-up. These different study designs and other aspects of methodology (such as the nature of the sample, length of follow-up and definition of outcome) vary considerably, making direct comparison of such studies very difficult.

This chapter reviews studies from 1960 onwards. Modern drugs for depression were introduced in the late 1950s in the form of tricyclic antidepressants (TCAs) and monoamine oxidase inhibitors (MAOIs). Lithium became widely used in the 1960s and selective serotonin reuptake inhibitors (SSRIs) and other novel antidepressants have been developed from the 1970s onwards. Although there is reasonable evidence that such drugs have an immediate and sometimes dramatic effect on the short-term course of depression, their effect on recurrence and the longer-term course of the illness is less clear (Paykel 1994). There are surprisingly few long-term studies in depressed patients. It may be that the apparent initial success of antidepressants and the prevailing air of optimism reduced interest in long-term studies. If patients did not appear to respond to treatment, there was a tendency to label them as having *depressive personality* or *characterological depression*, suggesting that their problems reflected personality rather than illness (Scott 1988).

REVIEW OF STUDIES

The 1960s and 1970s

There were four major long-term treatment outcome studies published during the 1960s and 1970s. The first showed that continuation of imipramine after treatment of depressed patients with electroconvulsive therapy was clearly superior to placebo (Seager and Bird 1962). Similar studies reported that continuing antidepressant treatment after remission resulted in a significantly better outcome (Mindham et al. 1973). Klerman et al. (1974) reported that both drug therapy and psychotherapy reduced the relapse rate compared with placebo. These studies consistently established that many patients who demonstrated a good initial response would relapse if treatment did not continue for at least 6 months.

Two naturalistic follow-up studies were also published in the 1970s. Morrison et al. (1973) noted that 22 per cent of 225 unipolar depression patients from the 'Iowa 500' remained ill or never fully recovered over the average 4-year follow-up. Murphy et al. (1974) followed up thirty-seven patients for a mean of 4 years, and reported that 25 per cent had no recurrence of depression and that 16 per cent remained chronically ill. The remainder had between one and nine depressive episodes.

These studies sporadically looked for factors that might predict long-term prognosis. Mindham et al. (1973) reported that previous episodes and initial severity appeared to have no effect. In the study by Murphy et al. (1974), 22 per cent of subjects had regular psychiatric follow-up, which did not alter outcome.

The 1980s

Studies in the early 1980s continued to demonstrate that ongoing treatment was superior to placebo in preventing relapse in patients who had had an initial response to treatment. Recovered outpatients on placebo had a 69 per cent relapse rate, compared with 28 per cent on amitriptyline over 6 months (Stein et al. 1980). Lithium, but not imipramine, was effective in reducing relapse in patients with major depression over a 12-month period (Kane et al. 1982). Prien et al. (1984) reported equal efficacy between the two drugs, with imipramine more effective if the index episode was severe, and Glen et al. (1984) reported that amitriptyline and lithium were equally effective in preventing relapse. All reported studies showed that an active drug was significantly better at preventing relapse than placebo.

In 1988, two important long-term follow-up studies were published in the same issue of the *British Journal of Psychiatry*. Lee and Murray (1988) reported on the 18-year outcome of eighty-nine consecutive inpatients (the Maudsley sample). Kiloh et al. (1988) reported on 145 inpatients followed up an average of 15 years later (the Sydney sample). Both studies reported similar findings: in essence, that the prognosis for inpatients treated for depression was quite bleak. Only a minority (15 per cent in the Maudsley sample, 39 per cent in the Sydney sample) remained well. The Maudsley sample in particular found that patients often did very badly; 34 per cent had a very poor outcome, including suicide. Based on the Maudsley sample outcome criteria, the Sydney sample did a little better, but still had 11 per cent of patients classified as having a very poor outcome.

The 1980s also saw publication of the first papers from the National Institute of Mental Health (NIMH) long-term outcome study. Keller et al. (1984) reported on the 2-year follow-up of ninety-seven patients with major depression. The major findings were that 21 per cent never recovered and that 64 per cent of patients recovered at 6 months, but from that point recovery rate slowed. Of the patients still depressed at 6 months, only 28 per cent recovered by 1 year. Subsequent recovery over the next two 6-month periods was 15 and 10 per cent.

Some of the studies reported on predictors of relapse but, like earlier studies, produced few consistent predictors. Past history, response to acute treatment and presenting symptoms appeared to have no effect (Stein et al. 1980). The NIMH study reported that long duration of index episode and low family income predicted poorer recovery. However, severity, previous episodes, comorbidity, sociodemographic variables and treatment given did not (Keller et al. 1984). Nor did age, number of episodes or hopelessness (Simons et al. 1986). In the Maudsley study, classification of depression subtype added little to prediction (Duggan et al. 1991). High neuroticism at baseline predicted a poorer outcome, but this was much less important once mood severity was allowed for (Duggan et al. 1990). Andrews et al. (1990) reported that previous illness and personality disorder weakly related to poor outcome.

The 1990s

The 1990s witnessed a significant increase in the number of reports on all aspects of depression, including longer-term follow-up studies. There were several trials sponsored by drug companies, and these appeared to re-establish what researchers had discovered in the 1960s and 1970s. They again reported that, once patients have recovered, continuing their medication for 6 months to a year is superior to switching them to placebo. Doogan and Caillard (1992), for example, reported that patients taking sertraline had less than a one-third chance of relapsing compared with those taking placebo, in a 44-week study. Montgomery et al. (1993) reported that citalopram at doses of 20 mg and 40 mg was superior to placebo over a 6-month follow-up. Anton et al. (1994) showed that nefazodone and imipramine were superior to placebo during a 1-year follow-up. There were virtually identical studies using most of the new antidepressants.

More importantly, further results from the NIMH naturalistic study were reported. The 5-year outcome data were that subjects had only a 22 per cent chance of sustained recovery (Lavori et al. 1994). Most (around two-thirds) recovered but relapsed at least once, and 12 per cent remained chronically depressed throughout the 5 years (Keller et al. 1992). After a 15-year follow-up, a cumulative proportion of 85 per cent of subjects experienced a recurrence of their depression. Even the 105 subjects who remained well for 5 years after recovery had a 58 per cent recurrence rate over the next 10 years (Mueller et al. 1999).

A seminal study treating patients with recurrent depression also appeared. Patients who had at least three previous episodes, including one in the past 30 months, were treated with imipramine and interpersonal psychotherapy (IPT). Those who remitted (that is, were symptom-free for 20 weeks) were randomised to a long-term maintenance treatment for 3 years. The study showed that maintenance with imipramine provided protection to nearly 80 per cent of patients over this period. There was also a significant effect from IPT, but this was weaker than that found with imipramine, and combining IPT and imipramine did not enhance the effect of imipramine alone (Frank et al. 1990). The authors also reported that the effect of imipramine was maintained for at least 5 years (Kupfer et al. 1992) and that continued full dosage was required (Frank et al. 1993).

A British study also followed up a depressed cohort from Cambridge for 1 year and reported that, although 70 per cent were in remission at 6 months, 40 per cent relapsed over the subsequent 15 months (Ramana et al. 1995). They reported that residual symptoms were strong predictors of subsequent early relapse, but that this was not related to length of illness, dysthymia or worse treatment (Paykel et al. 1995). They also noted that psychosocial factors did not predict the subsequent course of depression. Similarly, an Edinburgh cohort of eighty patients followed for 12 years reported a 60 per cent recurrence rate, with around a third experiencing a very poor outcome (Surtees and Barkley 1994).

Twenty-first century

The trend to report on the longer-term outcome of previous cohorts continued. The Cambridge cohort was re-contacted after 8–11 years. Ninety-two per cent had recovered during this time; two-thirds subsequently suffered a recurrence (Kennedy et al. 2003). The Sydney sample was also extended out to 25 years. Brodaty et al. (2001) reported that only 22 per cent of recovered subjects remained continuously well. Slightly more promising was that, in the decade since the 15-year follow-up, 27 per cent improved in clinical outcome (including four out of the five previously chronically depressed subjects), but 55 per cent remained unchanged and 18 per cent worsened. A Japanese sample was followed up for 6 years after recovery from an episode of major depression (Kanai et al. 2003). Their outcomes were better: 35 per cent had no significant depressive symptoms over the next 5 years and 42 per cent relapsed, while the remaining 23 per cent had some subthreshold symptoms.

Community studies

Community surveys have also confirmed the chronic relapsing nature of major depression. In the Australian National Mental Health Survey, people who met the criteria for depression during the previous year dated the onset of the first episode an average of 5.4 years earlier (range 1–54 years). Nearly half (44 per cent) reported a previous episode within 12 months of their latest episode, and 39 per cent had met criteria for a full remission between the two episodes (Andrews et al. 2001). The US National Comorbidity Survey showed that three-quarters of people aged 15–54 years who had ever met criteria for depression had had more than one episode (Kessler et al. 1997).

DISCUSSION

The results from the studies discussed above lead to three important conclusions. The first is that the long-term outcome of depression is not benign. The idea that depression is a psychiatric disorder with discrete episodes of illness (or even a single episode) alternating with recovery to a state of complete wellbeing is not true for most patients. Failure to remit, delayed remission, partial remission with residual symptoms, relapse and recurrence are common outcomes of depressive illness.

The 'end of innocence', as Paykel (1994) has put it, began with the NIMH study in the early 1980s and was effectively reinforced by the Sydney and Maudsley long-term follow-up studies in 1988. Subsequent studies have supported their results as discussed above.

The findings may be summarised as follows:

- Depending on the sample studied, 10–20 per cent of depressed patients appear not to recover at all and have chronic symptoms of fluctuating severity.
- Over 5 years, 80–90 per cent of patients do recover at some point, but, of those, 70–80 per cent subsequently relapse.
- Over 10 years, only 25 per cent of patients have a single episode or, to put it another way, there is only a 20–25 per cent chance of sustained recovery following an episode of major depression.

One note of caution is that these figures are almost exclusively based on inpatient samples, who are presumably more severe, recurrent and have significant comorbidity. It may be that outcomes are better in cohorts of moderate or first-episode patients. The Japanese cohort had a 5-year recurrence rate of 42 per cent in their sample of first-visit patients, of whom two-thirds had only a single episode (Kanai et al. 2003). This rate is 10–20 per cent lower than most other samples. A Canadian cohort that restricted itself to first-episode cases also suggested that 40 per cent experienced only a single episode of depression in the next 12–18 years (Bland and Orn 1982). Similar estimates are reported in primary care and community samples (Van Weel-Baumgarten et al. 2000). These studies generally contain small samples, high attrition rates and shorter follow-ups, so these estimates may be overly optimistic. However, it is possible that as many as 40 per cent of patients presenting as outpatients to psychiatrists may experience only a single episode.

The second conclusion is that discontinuation of antidepressant treatment is associated with a return of depressive symptoms in a large proportion of patients. This is certainly true after a response to treatment of the acute episode. If antidepressants are not continued after the first 6–12 weeks, around 40–60 per cent of patients will relapse over the next 6 months. This is two to three times the rate in patients whose medication is continued over the same period. There are a few studies that suggest a similar effect extends out to 12 months, but beyond this point the data are sparse. The study by Frank et al. (1990) implies this effect continues for 3 or even 5 years in patients with what they call *recurrent depression*, but the numbers are very small. A recent systematic review concluded that continuing treatment with antidepressants reduces the odds of relapse by 70 per cent (95% CI, 62–78 per cent; $P < 0.00001$). It calculated the average rate of relapse on placebo was 41 per cent, compared with 18 per cent on active treatment. The authors noted that most trials were of 6–12 months' duration (Geddes et al. 2003). As epidemiological studies report that at least half of depressed subjects have recurrent depression, long-term treatment might be appropriate for a much larger group of patients than clinical wisdom currently suggests. Possibly the most troubling consideration is that no study, to my knowledge, has reported a time when randomising subjects to placebo does not result in an increased relapse rate.

The third conclusion is that there are very few consistent predictors about which patients have a sustained recovery, who relapses and who remains unwell. No demographic factors appear to predict outcome. Mood severity and chronicity and number of episodes have little if any ability to predict outcome. Even neuroticism has little effect, particularly if mood severity is allowed for. Comorbidity also has little effect. There is some evidence that residual symptoms predict relapse, but this may be related to non-recovery from the initial episode. In the few studies that looked at life events, social support and marital status, these factors also did not predict outcome.

Perhaps of more concern is the lack of evidence that treatment particularly affects long-term outcome in the naturalistic studies. In the study by Murphy et al. (1974), 22 per cent of subjects had regular psychiatric follow-up, but this made no difference to outcome. Stein et al. (1980) reported that response to acute treatment was not related to 6-month outcome, which was also reported at 2 years by Keller et al. (1984). Similarly, Ramana et al. (1995) found outcome unrelated to adequacy of treatment. Only Ceroni et al. (1984) found an association between lack of adequate treatment and worse outcome. This is in contrast to the controlled treatment studies. Here relapse rates on acute treatment over 6–12 months ranged from 8 to 29 per cent. Even at 3 years, nearly 80 per cent of patients remained well if they continued on the active drug (Frank et al. 1990). One reason for the apparent discrepancy may be that the follow-up period (with the exception of the study by Frank et al.) is relatively short. Another may be that only patients who initially respond to treatment are entered into these treatment studies. This means that the 30–40 per cent of patients who typically do not respond are not followed up. These may be the very patients with the worst outcome in the long term.

CLINICAL IMPLICATIONS

Most patients with major depression, followed up for a reasonable period, have a relapsing or chronic illness. There are few useful predictors of long-term outcome in patients with major depression. Efficacious treatments for depression are available and appear to work well in controlled treatment studies for at least 6 months and possibly up to 3 years.

If the long-term outcome is relatively bleak when efficacious treatments are available, then either such treatments are not being used effectively or many depressed people do not seek treatment. There is surprisingly little research into these issues. There is some evidence that, despite successful treatment of an episode, many people do not return to treatment with the onset of new symptoms (Keller et al. 1984). Andrews (2001) has pointed out that our current model of practice, in which depressed patients seek help only when they deem it necessary, is inappropriate for an episodic but lifelong condition that affects hope, volition, reduces compliance and predisposes to suicide. He and others advocate a proactive shared model of treatment using case registers, patient education, clinical practice guidelines for care, and active follow-up, similar to that used in other chronic medical conditions such as asthma and diabetes.

Whether such an approach would be useful for managing depression is uncertain. The evidence, such as it is, suggests our current models of practice are not particularly successful. Advocating a proactive approach generates further research questions. First, should all patients be managed in this way or can we find useful predictors of the 20–25 per cent (and possibly up to 50 per cent in first-episode patients) who will recover and remain well? Second, is it fair to tell a patient recovering from weeks or months of despair, insomnia and anergia that his/her condition is likely to recur? Third, will a proactive disease model serve our patients better than our current practice?

There is very little information to help guide us. Predictors have been haphazardly sought without any consistent useful ones emerging. We seem to be spending much time and energy collecting clinical material that has little effect on what happens to our patients. It is time to look for other measures, including genetic and neuroendocrine ones, that may actually be clinically helpful. Although many clinicians are concerned that telling depressed people their real prognosis may worsen their depression, there is no evidence at present. Research is needed, but surely the most ethical way to proceed is to tell people the truth. Whether proactive treatment works is also not clear. Enhanced treatment produced better outcomes in primary care, but the effects were short-term (Lin et al. 1999). Proactive care for people with subsyndromal depression was not considered cost-effective (Sturm and Wells 1995). Clearly, proactive care will cost more than usual care, but the potential to reduce suffering and disability may outweigh this. In addition, the persistence of chronic conditions produces direct treatment costs as well as overall burden of disease. It is reported that people with depression generate twice the direct healthcare costs of other primary care attenders, even after controlling for the effect of comorbid conditions (Simon et al. 1995). Proactive care may, therefore, be cost-effective even though the direct cost per patient is higher than usual for care.

In summary, it is now well established that, in the long term, depression is usually a chronic relapsing condition which is responsive to treatment in controlled settings. We need to learn the effect of telling our patients this, try to more accurately predict which patients need proactive treatment, and research whether such a treatment works.

REFERENCES

Andrews G (2001) Should depression be managed as a chronic disease? *BMJ* 322:419-21.

Andrews G, Henderson S, Hall W (2001) Prevalence, comorbidity, disability and service utilisation: Overview of the Australian National Mental Health Survey. *British Journal of Psychiatry* 178:145-53.

Andrews G, Neilson M, Hunt C, Stewart G, Kiloh LG (1990) Diagnosis, personality and the long-term outcome of depression. *British Journal of Psychiatry* 157:13-18.

Anton SF, Robinson DS, Roberts DL, Kensler TT, English PA, Archibald DG (1994) Long-term treatment of depression with nefazodone. *Psychopharmacology Bulletin* 30:165-9.

Bland RC, Orn H (1982) Course and outcome in affective disorders. *Canadian Journal of Psychiatry* 27:573-8.

Brodaty H, Luscombe G, Peisah C, Anstey K, Andrews G (2001) A 25-year longitudinal, comparison study of the outcome of depression. *Psychological Medicine* 31:1347-59.

Ceroni GB, Neri C, Pezzoli A (1984) Chronicity in major depression: A naturalistic prospective study. *Journal of Affective Disorders* 7:123-32.

Doogan DP, Caillard V (1992) Sertraline in the prevention of depression. *British Journal of Psychiatry* 160:217-22.

Duggan CF, Lee AS, Murray RM (1990) Does personality predict long-term outcome in depression? *British Journal of Psychiatry* 157:19-24.

—— (1991) Do different subtypes of hospitalized depressives have different long-term outcomes? *Archives of General Psychiatry* 48:308-12.

Frank E, Kupfer DJ, Perel JM, Cornes C, Mallinger AG, Thase ME, et al. (1993) Comparison of full-dose versus half-dose pharmacotherapy in the maintenance treatment of recurrent depression. *Journal of Affective Disorders* 27:139-45.

Frank E, Kupfer DJ, Perel JM, Cornes C, Jarrett DB, Mallinger AG, et al. (1990) Three-year outcomes for maintenance therapies in recurrent depression. *Archives of General Psychiatry* 47:1093-9.

Geddes JR, Carney SM, Davies C, Furukawa TA, Kupfer DJ, Frank E, et al. (2003) Relapse prevention with antidepressant drug treatment in depressive disorders: A systematic review. *Lancet* 361:653-61.

Glen AI, Johnson AL, Shepherd M (1984) Continuation therapy with lithium and amitriptyline in unipolar depressive illness: A randomized, double-blind, controlled trial. *Psychological Medicine* 14:37-50.

Kanai T, Takeuchi H, Furukawa TA, Yoshimura R, Imaizumi T, Kitamura T, et al. (2003) Time to recurrence after recovery from major depressive episodes and its predictors. *Psychological Medicine* 33:839-45.

Kane JM, Quitkin FM, Rifkin A, Ramos-Lorenzi JR, Nayak DD, Howard A (1982) Lithium carbonate and imipramine in the prophylaxis of unipolar and bipolar II illness: A prospective, placebo-controlled comparison. *Archives of General Psychiatry* 39:1065-9.

Keller MB, Klerman GL, Lavori P, Coryell W, Endicott J, Taylor J (1984) Long-term outcome of episodes of major depression. *JAMA* 252:788-92.

Keller MB, Lavori PW, Mueller TI, Endicott J, Coryell W, Hirschfeld RMA, et al. (1992) Time to recovery, chronicity, and levels of psychopathology in major depression: A 5-year prospective follow-up of 431 subjects. *Archives of General Psychiatry* 49:809-16.

Kennedy N, Abbott R, Paykel ES (2003) Remission and recurrence of depression in the maintenance era: Long-term outcome in a Cambridge cohort. *Psychological Medicine* 33:827-38.

Kessler RC, Zhao S, Blazer DG, Swartz M (1997) Prevalence, correlates, and course of minor depression and major depression in the National Comorbidity Survey. *Journal of Affective Disorders* 45:19-30.

Kiloh LG, Andrews G, Neilson M (1988) The long-term outcome of depressive illness. *British Journal of Psychiatry* 153:752-7.

Klerman GL, DiMascio A, Weissman MM, Prusoff B, Paykel ES (1974) Treatment of depression by drugs and psychotherapy. *American Journal of Psychiatry* 131:186-91.

Kupfer DJ, Frank E, Perel JM, Cornes C, Mallinger AG, Thase ME, et al. (1992) Five-year outcome for maintenance therapies in recurrent depression. *Archives of General Psychiatry* 49:769-73.

Lavori P, Keller MB, Mueller TI, Scheftner WA, Fawcett J, Coryell W (1994) Recurrence after recovery in unipolar MDD: An observational follow-up study of clinical predictors and somatic treatment as a mediating factor. *International Journal of Methods in Psychiatric Research* 4:211-99.

Lee AS, Murray RM (1988) The long-term outcome of Maudsley depressives. *British Journal of Psychiatry* 153:741-51.

Lin EH, Simon GE, Katon W, Russo JE, Van Korff M, Bush TM, et al. (1999) Can enhanced acute-phase treatment of depression improve long-term outcomes? A report of randomized trials in primary care. *American Journal of Psychiatry* 156:643-5.

Mindham RH, Howland C, Shepherd M (1973) An evaluation of continuation therapy with tricyclic antidepressants in depressive illness. *Psychological Medicine* 3:5-17.

Montgomery SA, Rasmussen JG, Tanghoj P (1993) A 24-week study of 20 mg citalopram, 40 mg citalopram, and placebo in the prevention of relapse of major depression. *International Clinical Psychopharmacology* 8:181-8.

Morrison J, Winokur G, Crowe R, Clancy J (1973) The Iowa 500. The first follow-up. *Archives of General Psychiatry* 29:678-82.

Mueller TI, Leon AC, Keller MB, Solomon DA, Endicott J, Coryell W, et al. (1999) Recurrence after recovery from major depressive disorder during 15 years of observational follow-up. *American Journal of Psychiatry* 156:1000-6.

Murphy GE, Woodruff RA, Jr, Herjanic M, Super G (1974) Variability of the clinical course of primary affective disorder. *Archives of General Psychiatry* 30:757-61.

Paykel ES (1994) Historical overview of outcome of depression. *British Journal of Psychiatry Supplement* 6-8.

Paykel ES, Ramana R, Cooper Z, Hayhurst H, Kerr J, Barocka A (1995) Residual symptoms after partial remission: An important outcome in depression. *Psychological Medicine* 25:1171-80.

Prien RF, Kupfer DJ, Mansky PA, Small JG, Tuason VB, Voss CB, et al. (1984) Drug therapy in the prevention of recurrences in unipolar and bipolar affective disorders. Report of the NIMH Collaborative Study Group comparing lithium carbonate, imipramine, and a lithium carbonate-imipramine combination. *Archives of General Psychiatry* 41:1096-104.

Ramana R, Paykel ES, Cooper Z, Hayhurst H, Saxty M, Surtees PG (1995) Remission and relapse in major depression: A two-year prospective follow-up study. *Psychological Medicine* 25:1161-70.

Scott J (1988) Chronic depression. *British Journal of Psychiatry* 153:287-97.

Seager CP, Bird RL (1962) Imipramine with electrical treatment in depression – a controlled trial. *Journal of Mental Science* 108:704-7.

Simon GE, Von Korff M, Barlow W (1995) Health care cost of primary care patients with recognized depression. *Archives of General Psychiatry* 52:850-6.

Simons AD, Murphy GE, Levine JL, Wetzel RD (1986) Cognitive therapy and pharmacotherapy for depression. Sustained improvement over one year. *Archives of General Psychiatry* 43:43-8.

Stein MK, Rickels K, Weise CC (1980) Maintenance therapy with amitriptyline: A controlled trial. *American Journal of Psychiatry* 137:370-1.

Sturm R, Wells KB (1995) How can care for depression become more cost effective? *JAMA* 273:51-8.

Surtees P, Barkley C (1994) Future imperfect: The long-term outcome of depression. *British Journal of Psychiatry* 164:327-41.

Van Weel-Baumgarten EM, Schers HJ, Van Den Bosch WJ, Van Den Hoogen HJ, Zitman FG (2000) Long-term follow-up of depression among patients in the community and in family practice settings. *Journal of Family Practice* 49:1113-20.

CHAPTER 35

NATURAL HISTORY AND OUTCOME OF BIPOLAR DISORDER

Philip B Mitchell

Our knowledge of the course of this unpredictable and capricious illness comes from a relatively small number of major longitudinal studies, some of which are referred to in this chapter. The main long-term investigations have been those of the National Institute of Mental Health (NIMH) Collaborative Depression Study, the Zurich study and the Iowa 500 Research Project. Other studies have been carried out in Naples, Cologne, Chicago and at the University of California, Los Angeles (UCLA). Apart from the Iowa study, all have been undertaken since the introduction of modern biological therapies, and are therefore potentially prone to the contaminating effect of such treatments.

The best prospective data on the natural course of bipolar disorder before the introduction of modern therapies were those collected in the Iowa 500 Study, which also examined the course of unipolar depression and schizophrenia. Using files from the Iowa Psychopathic Hospital, Winokur and colleagues obtained clinical details on 100 bipolar disorder patients admitted between 1934 and 1944 (Winokur and Tsuang 1996). As that hospital had routinely collected follow-up information from patients, relatives or clinicians each 6–12 months, it was possible for Winokur's group to determine the progress of this condition in the era prior to the advent of electroconvulsive therapy, lithium, neuroleptics, antidepressants and psychosurgery. Informative data was obtained on eighty-seven bipolar patients, who were followed up for between 6 months and 20 years (an average of 2.2 years). Over that period of time, 54 per cent recovered fully at some stage, while

21 per cent were continuously symptomatic over the follow-up period. This pattern was not distinguishable from unipolar depression, but contrasted markedly with schizophrenia, in which 78 per cent showed continuous illness and a further 13 per cent had deteriorated. Most bipolar patients took 2–3 years to recover from their index episode (of mania or depression); however, for those able to be followed up over 10–20 years, all had fully recovered at some stage. Interestingly, about 5 per cent of those initially diagnosed with depression went on to develop mania over the follow-up period, mostly within 3 years of the index admission.

PRODROMAL SYMPTOMS AND PREMORBID PERSONALITY

Unlike for schizophrenia, there is no universal acceptance that there is a definite prodromal phase for bipolar disorder. There have been some reports suggestive of a prodrome, manifesting in particular with increased rates of mood lability, low energy, worrying, attentional problems, school role impairment, excitability, sensitivity, somatic complaints and stubbornness (Egeland et al. 2003).

Similarly, there have been no consistent findings of distinct premorbid personality traits or disorder in people who develop bipolar disorder, although advocates of the *soft bipolar spectrum* include temperamental characteristics such as hyperthymia and cyclothymia in that concept.

ONSET OF ILLNESS

Age and polarity of onset

Although the onset of bipolar disorder can occur in late childhood or early adolescence, this is uncommon, with most illness presenting for the first time in mid- to late teenage years or 20s. The peak age of onset is in the 20s. Various studies have suggested that a depressive onset is more common than mania, but this has not been consistently demonstrated.

There is currently significant controversy about the presentation of bipolar disorder in childhood and adolescence, with a considerable increase in the diagnosis of childhood and adolescent bipolar disorder being made in contemporary US practice. This issue is addressed further in Chapter 30.

Onset is earlier in people with a family history of bipolar disorder. Refining the age of onset distinction further, Bellivier et al. (2003) have reported three (apparently genetically determined) age of onset subtypes: early (mean 17 years), intermediate (25 years), and late (40 years).

A very early onset, occurring in late childhood or early adolescence, tends to be associated with a more severe illness. Very late onset, in the 60s or later, is less likely to be associated with genetic factors, and is often related to neurological conditions such as cerebrovascular disease or traumatic brain injury. Furthermore, mania initially presenting in that older age group has a high mortality, for example when compared with depression.

Bipolar disorder in women not infrequently presents for the first time in the post-partum period (see Chapter 32). In addition, there have been reports of a more malignant form of illness presenting for the first time in perimenopausal women (Freeman et al. 2002).

First-episode mania

There have been few studies of first-episode mania, although it has been consistently reported from retrospective investigations that the first presentation of later-established bipolar disorder is frequently diagnosed as schizophrenia (Joyce 1984). One of the largest relevant studies of first-onset psychosis is the McLean–Harvard First-Episode Project (Tohen et al. 2000), which found that although 86 per cent of manic episodes had resolved within 6 months, only a third of patients had functionally recovered over that time, suggesting that even first-episode mania is often slow to recover.

COURSE OF BIPOLAR DISORDER

Subtypes and courses

BIPOLAR I AND II Dunner and Fieve (1974) distinguished between bipolar I and II disorder on the basis of the severity of the elevated phase of the condition, defining bipolar I disorder by the occurrence of manic episodes, and bipolar II disorder by the presence of only episodes of hypomania and depression. The clinical distinction between bipolar I and II appears to remain consistent over time (Coryell et al. 1989). However, the clinical and heuristic value of separating these two syndromes has been controversial, with varying opinions over whether they represent a difference in illness severity or rather distinct nosological entities.

RAPID CYCLING Rapid-cycling bipolar disorder is defined by the occurrence of four or more separate episodes of hypomania, mania, depression or mixed episodes over 12 months. It probably represents a transient phase of the condition for most patients, but for some individuals this is the ongoing manifestation of their illness. It is more common in women, who comprise about three-quarters of those with this form of bipolar disorder. It is sometimes caused by antidepressants or hypothyroidism.

NATURE OF CYCLE Many patients have circumscribed cycles in which they move from depression to mania prior to recovery (the *depression–mania–interval*, or DMI, pattern); on the other hand, some cycles move from mania to depression before recovery (the *mania–depression–interval*, or MDI, pattern). The MDI pattern appears to indicate a greater likelihood of response to lithium. Furthermore, MacQueen et al. (2002) reported that patients who become depressed following a period of euthymia are more likely to respond to treatment than those who become depressed following a period of hypomania or mania. Other patients have distinct but separated episodes of mania and depression. About 10 per cent of subjects only have manic episodes, although subtle depressive episodes are frequently apparent on more detailed clinical inquiry.

OTHER PATTERNS Some patients demonstrate a *seasonal* predilection, most commonly evidencing winter depressions and spring or summer manic episodes. For most patients, however, episodes are not seasonally related. Many patients have *psychotic* features during their manic or depressed episodes. This indicates more severe illness, and a lesser likelihood of response to treatments such as lithium.

Proportions of depressive and manic phases

PREDOMINANCE OF DEPRESSION Although the pathologically elevated mood of mania and hypomania is the distinctive hallmark of bipolar disorder, it is becoming increasingly apparent that depression is the predominant affect of this condition. Such recognition has major implications for service delivery, as the major emphasis in management hitherto has focused on acute control of manic episodes – usually in response to the marked disruption resulting from that phase of the illness.

Two recent reports from the NIMH Collaborative Depression Study (Judd et al. 2002; Judd et al. 2003b) have convincingly demonstrated that bipolar disorder patients experience depression much more frequently than hypomania or mania. First, in a study focusing on patients with bipolar I disorder, Judd et al. (2002) reported on a follow-up of 146 patients over an average period of 12.8 years. Assessing weekly symptom status, the authors found that patients experienced depressive symptoms for 32 per cent of weeks over that period. This compared with only 9 per cent of the time accounted for by hypomanic or manic symptoms, and 6 per cent for cycling or mixed presentations. When the depressive symptoms were examined in detail, it was apparent that most of this was not related to major depression, with 14 per cent of weeks being due to minor depression or dysthymia, and 9 per cent to subsyndromal depression. Only 9 per cent of the time was experienced in major depression. It was also apparent that a prolonged depressive or mixed/cycling episode at intake into the study was one of the major indicators of chronicity during follow-up, a finding consistent with an earlier report from this study (Coryell et al. 1998).

In the second paper, Judd et al. (2003b) reported on weekly symptomatic status in bipolar II patients from the same cohort. Eighty-six patients were followed up for a mean of 13.4 years. In this population, depression was even more prevalent than in the bipolar I sample, accounting for 50 per cent of weeks, compared with 1 per cent of weeks in hypomania and 12 per cent cycling or mixed. When the specific form of depression was examined, 24 per cent of weeks were experienced in minor depression or dysthymia, and 14 per cent in subsyndromal depression. Again, major depression was relatively less common, accounting for only 13 per cent of time.

Comparing the bipolar I and II groups, Judd et al. (2003a) reported in a subsequent paper that bipolar II patients were statistically more likely to experience both major and minor depressive episodes. They were also more likely to have both a chronic course and shorter intervals between episodes.

This report of a high prevalence of minor and subsyndromal depressive syndromes in bipolar disorder is consistent with findings from other samples. For example, in two national epidemiological studies (Kessler et al. 1997; Mitchell et al. 2003), dysthymia was found to be commonly comorbid with bipolar disorder. In the 12-month Australian prevalence survey of Mitchell et al. (2004), dysthymia was eight times more common in those with bipolar disorder.

GENDER EFFECTS AND PATTERN STABILITY The Zurich study demonstrated that females experience more depressed episodes and males more cyclic episodes (mania and depression), whereas purely manic and mixed episodes are equally prevalent across genders (Angst and Sellaro 2000). These patterns remain stable over time, indicating no variance with increasing age.

Duration of episodes

In the Zurich longitudinal study, the average episode duration for pure depression, mania or mixed episodes was 3 months, whereas cyclic episodes (mania and depression) lasted almost 50 per cent longer (Angst and Sellaro 2000). The Epidemiological Catchment Area study reported shorter episodes (2–3 months).

Two reports from the NIMH Collaborative Depression Study are relevant to this issue (Keller et al. 1986; Keller 1988). After 8 weeks, only 44 per cent of patients with bipolar depression had recovered, compared with 61 per cent of those with mania and 33 per cent of subjects in a mixed or cycling episode (Keller et al. 1986). After 1 year, 78 per cent had recovered from an initial bipolar depressive episode, compared with 93 per cent of those who were manic and 68 per cent of those in a mixed or cycling presentation (Keller 1988).

There have been contradictory accounts concerning any change in length of episodes with increasing age or episode number. Some studies have reported a greater episode length with time, whereas others have found no change in duration.

Recurrence rates and episode length

Most patients who experience an episode of mania go on to have future episodes of mania or depression, although recurrence rates vary substantially between studies. In a naturalistic study of patients followed after treatment for mania (most subjects had established bipolar disorder), only 28 per cent of patients had not relapsed into at least one episode of depression or mania in the subsequent 4 years (Tohen et al. 1990).

Kraepelin (1921) reported an increasing frequency of episodes with age, that is, a progressive shortening of cycle length. However, controlling for the number of episodes, Angst et al. have found from their large-scale longitudinal studies that although there is an initial shortening of cycle length (in their data over the first three cycles), there is no predictable pattern after that, with a subsequent median cycling of 18 months. Examining the US Collaborative Study of the Psychobiology of Depression cohort, Coryell et al. (1994) reported no shortening of cycle length in a 10-year prospective follow-up.

Effect of comorbidity

Recurrence rates are also greater in people with comorbid anxiety disorders and substance abuse (Suppes et al. 2000), both of which are more common in patients with bipolar disorder (see Chapters 24 and 25). Better outcome of bipolar disorder has also been linked to fewer personality disorder symptoms, particularly cluster A (Bieling et al. 2003).

Switch rates

As recently reviewed by Angst and Sellaro (2000), follow-up studies from both Europe and the United States have reported switch rates from unipolar depression to bipolar disorder of about 1 per cent per year of observation. Akiskal et al. (1995) found that, although people who switched to bipolar I disorder were not clinically distinguishable from depressed patients who remained stable, those who switched to bipolar II disorder had an early age of depression onset, pleomorphic psychopathology, high rates of substance abuse, and disrupted careers and relationships.

Predictors of outcome

There have been few studies of clinical or other predictors of the outcome of bipolar disorder. Several relevant reports have arisen from the NIMH Collaborative Study of Depression. Examining predictors of the 15-year outcome of bipolar I disorder, Coryell et al. (1998) reported that, after logistic regression, the only correlates of poor outcome were poor optimal functioning in the 5 years before baseline assessment and the persistence of depressive symptoms in the subsequent 2 years.

Although there is a well-documented delay in appropriate diagnosis and initiation of treatment, the only report examining the effect of such a delay in treatment initiation has not demonstrated any relationship between this and the outcome of prophylactic treatment (Baethge et al. 2003). This contrasts with the situation in schizophrenia, where there is some indication of poorer outcome when time to treatment onset is prolonged.

Precipitants of episodes

Although many episodes of bipolar disorder occur autonomously (that is, they appear to be independent of any apparent environmental triggers), particularly in people with multiple prior episodes, there are undoubtedly frequently demonstrable precipitants for relapses. It is well established that stressful life events (usually negative but sometimes even positive, for example due to increased but overwhelming responsibilities) are common precipitants for both manic and depressed relapses in bipolar disorder (Ellicott et al. 1990). This is particularly pertinent in the early episodes of the illness, but may be relevant also for later recurrences. Other related environmental triggers are disruptions in social rhythms and sleep–wake cycles, for example due to insufficient sleep, travel across time zones, or jobs involving shift work. Biological precipitants of mania include antidepressants, and illicit substances such as marijuana or stimulants.

There has been a recent emphasis on the early recognition of features of the prodrome to relapse, and the identification of potential causes for these (such as disturbed social rhythms). Prodromal features for mania (such as reduced sleep or increased busyness) are more readily identified by patients than prodromes for bipolar depression.

FUNCTIONAL OUTCOME

Bipolar disorder remains a disabling illness for most sufferers. Keck et al. (1998) investigated the 12-month course of illness of 134 patients following hospitalisation for the treatment of a manic or mixed episode. Outcome was examined in terms of syndromic (resolution of the DSM-III-R syndrome), symptomatic and functional recovery, and was considerably less favourable than is usually appreciated by clinicians. Syndromic recovery occurred in only 48 per cent of subjects but, even more dramatically, full symptom resolution was found in only 26 per cent and functional recovery in 24 per cent over the year.

Similar results have been demonstrated in cross-sectional epidemiological studies. For example, Mitchell et al. (2004) found lower employment rates and higher levels of disrupted relationships in people with bipolar disorder. Disability (defined in terms of days out of role) was greater even than that seen in those with depression. Bipolar disorder subjects identified through a community survey had more frequent difficulties in work-related performance, social and leisure activities, and social and family interactions than the rest of the sample (Calabrese et al. 2003). Women with bipolar disorder reported more disruption in social and family life, whereas men reported higher rates of being gaoled, arrested and being convicted of crimes.

Disability due to bipolar depression

It is becoming increasingly apparent that much of the disability due to bipolar disorder is related to the depressed component of this condition. First, in a US Veterans Affairs sample, Bauer's group reported that the functional outcome of forty-three bipolar disorder outpatients correlated significantly with their depressive but not manic symptoms (Leverich et al. 2001). Second, in a healthcare utilisation study of a large US private insurer, Bryant-Comstock et al. (2002) found that bipolar disorder patients used three to four times the healthcare costs of the average patient in the organisation, with bipolar depression incurring the highest expenditure – higher even than that due to mania or mixed episodes. Furthermore, this disability appears not to be related only to major depression. Altshuler et al. (2002), examining a sample of bipolar I disorder patients with subsyndromal depressive symptoms, recently reported that the functional level of the subjects still correlated inversely with the severity of the depression.

MORTALITY

As highlighted in a recent follow-up of over 30 years, the mortality associated with bipolar disorder is high, 58 per cent above general population rates (Angst et al. 2002). Rates are substantially lower in people receiving treatment, in terms of deaths due to both suicide and natural causes.

Suicide

Lifetime rates of attempted suicide are more common in bipolar disorder than in major depressive disorder (ranges of 26–29 per cent compared with 14–16 per cent) (Chen and Dilsaver 1996; Mitchell et al. 2004), with Kessler et al. (1997) reporting a rate of 48 per cent in a bipolar I population. Rates of completed suicide are also high, varying from 10 to 19 per cent. A meta-analysis of suicide studies in a range of psychiatric conditions reported that the suicide rate for bipolar disorder was fifteen times that of the general population, a rate only less than the twenty-fold increase for major depressive disorder (Harris and Barraclough 1997).

Suicidal ideation is reported by 79 per cent of people with bipolar depression, occurring much more commonly in that phase of the illness than during mania or mixed episodes (Dilsaver et al. 1997). Completed suicide also occurs predominantly during the depressed phase of the illness (79 per cent) (Isometsa et al. 1994), as do suicide attempts (Lopez et al. 2001). Patients with bipolar II disorder are at a higher risk of suicide than those with bipolar I disorder, possibly related to the more frequent periods of depression found in bipolar II disorder.

A recent study reported that serious suicide attempts were most strongly related to a history of sexual abuse, lack of a confidant prior to illness onset, more prior hospitalisations for depression, suicidal thoughts when depressed, and cluster B personality disorder (Leverich et al. 2003).

Consistent with prior reports, a study of suicide attempts and completed suicides of bipolar disorder patients in two large US integrated health plans found that rates were lower among patients taking lithium than those taking divalproex (Goodwin et al. 2003). Although not specifically examined in that study, prior reports had suggested that this apparent anti-suicide effect was independent of lithium's antidepressant activity (Baldessarini et al. 2001).

Death from 'natural causes'

Angst et al. (2002) found death from cardiovascular disease and all vascular disease to be significantly elevated. Rates were significantly higher in people not receiving treatment. Similar results were seen in their unipolar depressed sample. The nature of this relationship between bipolar disorder and a greater mortality due to cardiovascular disease is yet to be understood.

CONCLUSION

Bipolar disorder is a frequently recurrent condition for most sufferers. Its functional impact on employment and relationships is considerable, with marked disability continuing despite resolution of the individual episodes of mania, major depression or mixed episodes. Rates of major and subsyndromal depression are higher than previously considered, and appear to be closely related to the likelihood of disability, as well as to attempted and completed suicide.

REFERENCES

Akiskal HS, Maser JD, Zeller PJ, Endicott J, Coryell W, Keller M, et al. (1995) Switching from 'unipolar' to bipolar II. An 11-year prospective study of clinical and temperamental predictors in 559 patients. *Archives of General Psychiatry* 52:114-23.

Altshuler LL, Gitlin MJ, Mintz J, Leight KL, Frye MA (2002) Subsyndromal depression is associated with functional impairment inpatients with bipolar disorder. *Journal of Clinical Psychiatry* 63:807-11.

Angst F, Stassen HH, Clayton PJ, Angst J (2002) Mortality of patients with mood disorders: Follow-up over 34-38 years. *Journal of Affective Disorders* 68:167-81.

Angst J, Sellaro R (2000) Historical perspectives and natural history of bipolar disorder. *Biological Psychiatry* 48:445-57.

Baethge C, Smolka MN, Gruschka P, Berghofer A, Schlattmann P, Bauer M, et al. (2003) Does prophylaxis-delay in bipolar disorder influence outcome? Results from a long-term study of 147 patients. *Acta Psychiatrica Scandinavica* 107:260-7.

Baldessarini RJ, Tondo L, Hennen J (2001) Treating the suicidal patient with bipolar disorder: Reducing suicide risk with lithium. *Annals of the New York Academy of Sciences* 932:24-38.

Bellivier F, Golmard J-L, Rietschel M, Schulze TG, Malafosse A, Preisig M, et al. (2003) Age of onset in bipolar I affective disorder: Further evidence for three subgroups. *American Journal of Psychiatry* 160:999-1001.

Bieling PJ, MacQueen GM, Marriot MJ, Robb JC, Begin H, Joffe RT, et al. (2003) Longitudinal outcome in patients with bipolar disorder assessed by life-charting is influenced by DSM-IV personality disorder symptoms. *Bipolar Disorders* 5:14-21.

Bryant-Comstock L, Stender M, Devercelli G (2002) Health care utilization and costs among privately insured patients with bipolar I disorder. *Bipolar Disorder* 6:398-405.

Calabrese JR, Hirschfeld RMA, Reed M, Davies MA, Frye MA, Keck PEJ, et al. (2003) Impact of bipolar disorder on a U.S. community sample. *Journal of Clinical Psychiatry* 64:425-32.

Chen Y-W, Dilsaver SC (1996) Lifetime rates of suicide attempts among subjects with bipolar and unipolar disorders relative to subjects with other axis I disorders. *Biological Psychiatry* 39:896-9.

Coryell W, Keller M, Endicott J, Andreasen N, Clayton P, Hirschfeld RMA (1989) Bipolar II illness: Course and outcome over a five year period. *Psychological Medicine* 19:129-41.

Coryell W, Turvey C, Endicott J, Leon AC, Mueller T, Solomon D, et al. (1998) Bipolar I affective disorder: Predictors of outcome after 15 years. *Journal of Affective Disorders* 50:109-16.

Coryell WG, Akistal HS, Endicott J, Keller M, Mueller T (1994) Manic–depressive (bipolar) disorder: The course in light of a prospective ten-year follow up of 131 patients. *Acta Psychiatrica Scandinavica* 89:102-10.

Dilsaver SC, Chen Y-W, Swann AC, Shoaib AM, Tsai-Dilsaver Y, Krajewski KJ (1997) Suicidality, panic disorder and psychosis in bipolar depression, depressive-mania and pure-mania. *Psychiatry Research* 73:47-56.

Dunner DL, Fieve RR (1974) Clinical factors in lithium carbonate prophylaxis failure. *Archives of General Psychiatry* 30:229-33.

Egeland JA, Shaw JA, Endicott J, Pauls DL, Allen CR, Hostetter AM, et al. (2003) Prospective study of prodromal features of bipolarity in well Amish children. *Journal of the American Academy of Child and Adolescent Psychiatry* 42:786-96.

Ellicott A, Hammen C, Gitlin M, Brown G, Jamison K (1990) Life events and the course of bipolar disorder. *American Journal of Psychiatry* 147:1194-8.

Freeman MP, Wisonitzer Smith K, Freeman SA (2002) The impact of reproductive events on the course of bipolar disorder in women. *Journal of Clinical Psychiatry* 63:284-7.

Goodwin FK, Fireman B, Simon GE, Hunkeler EM, Lee J, Revicki D (2003) Suicide risk in bipolar disorder during treatment with lithium and divalproex. *JAMA* 290:1467-73.

Harris EC, Barraclough B (1997) Suicide as an outcome for mental disorders: A meta-analysis. *British Journal of Psychiatry* 170:205-28.

Isometsa ET, Henriksson MM, Aro HM, Lonnqvist JK (1994) Suicide in bipolar disorder in Finland. *American Journal of Psychiatry* 151:1020-4.

Joyce PR (1984) Age of onset in bipolar affective disorder and misdiagnosis as schizophrenia. *Psychological Medicine* 14:145-9.

Judd LL, Akiskal HS, Schettler PJ, Coryell W, Maser JD, Rice JA, et al. (2003a) The comparative clinical phenotype and long term longitudinal episode course of bipolar I and II: A clinical spectrum or distinct disorders? *Journal of Affective Disorders* 73:19-32.

Judd LL, Akiskal HS, Schttler PJ, Endicott J, Maser J, Solomon DA, et al. (2002) The long-term natural history of the weekly symptomatic status of bipolar I disorder. *Archives of General Psychiatry* 59:530-7.

Judd LL, Akiskal HS, Schttler PJ, Coryell W, Endicott J, Maser JD, et al. (2003b) A prospective investigation of the natural history of the long-term weekly symptomatic status of bipolar II disorder. *Archives of General Psychiatry* 60:261-9.

Keck PE, Jr, McElroy SL, Strakowski SM (1998) 12-month outcome of patients with bipolar disorder following hospitalization for a manic or mixed episode. *American Journal of Psychiatry* 155:646-52.

Keller MB (1988) The course of manic–depressive illness. *Journal of Clinical Psychiatry* 49:4-6.

Keller MB, Lavori PW, Coryell W, Andreasen NC, Endicott J, Clayton PJ, et al. (1986) Differential outcome of pure manic, mixed/cycling, and pure depressive episodes in patients with bipolar illness. *JAMA* 255:3138-42.

Kessler RC, Rubinow DR, Holmes C, Abelson JM, Zhao S (1997) The epidemiology of DSM-III-R bipolar I disorder in a general population survey. *Psychological Medicine* 27:1079-89.

Kraepelin E (1921) Translated by R. Mary Barcley. In Robertson GM (ed), *Manic–depressive Insanity and Paranoia*. Edinburgh: E.S. Livingston.

Leverich GS, Altshuler LL, Frye MA, Suppes T, Keck PE, McElroy SL, et al. (2003) Factors associated with suicide attempts in 648 patients with bipolar disorder in the Stanley Foundation Bipolar Network. *Journal of Clinical Psychiatry* 64:506-15.

—— (2001) Determinants of functional outcome and healthcare costs in bipolar disorder: A high-intensity follow-up study. *Journal of Affective Disorders* 65:231-41.

Lopez P, Mosquera F, de Leon J, Gutierrez M, Ezcurra J, Ramirex F, et al. (2001) Suicide attempts in bipolar patients. *Journal of Clinical Psychiatry* 62:963-6.

MacQueen GM, Young LT, Marriot M, Robb J, Begin H, Joffe RT (2002) Previous mood state predicts response and switch rates in patients with bipolar depression. *Acta Psychiatrica Scandinavica* 105:414-18.

Mitchell PB, Slade T, Andrews G (2004) Twelve-month prevalence and disability of DSM-IV bipolar disorder in an Australian general population survey. *Psychological Medicine* (In press).

Suppes T, Dennehy EB, Gibbons EW (2000) The longitudinal course of bipolar disorder. *Journal of Clinical Psychiatry* 61:23-30.

Tohen KN, Waternaux CM, Tsuang MT (1990) Outcome in mania: A 4-year prospective follow-up of 75 patients utilizing survival analysis. *Archives of General Psychiatry* 47:1106-11.

Tohen KN, Strakowski SM, Zarate C, Hennen JJ, Stoll AL, Suppes T, et al. (2000) The McLean-Harvard First-Episode Project: 6 month symptomatic and functional outcome in affective and non-affective psychosis. *Biological Psychiatry* 48:467-76.

Winokur G, Tsuang MT (1996) *The Natural History of Mania, Depression, and Schizophrenia*. Washington, DC: American Psychiatric Press.

CHAPTER 36

DEPRESSIVE DISORDERS IN PRIMARY CARE SETTINGS

Ian B Hickie and
Tracey A Davenport

Although the burden of depression in our communities is substantial (Table 36.1), the potential effect of currently available pharmacological and non-pharmacological treatments on short- and long-term illness course is considerable. However, two major barriers stand in the way of rapid progress in the delivery of effective treatments to those in need. The first is the fact that almost half the people with depressive disorders do not present for any form of medical or psychological care (Andrews et al. 2001). The second is that our primary medical systems are poorly structured, resourced or supported by secondary and other specialist care systems to deliver treatments that work (Hickie et al. 2001b). The result in Australia is that only 15 per cent of people with depression currently receive an evidence-based treatment. Any change will depend on a fundamental recognition that the challenges faced by primary care practitioners are different from those experienced by mental health specialists.

REDUCING BARRIERS TO EFFECTIVE CARE

Primary care health systems have the capacity to dramatically affect these major barriers to reducing the burden of depression in our countries. Most obviously, an improvement in the quantity and quality of effective treatments in primary care settings could be achieved. However, such improvements depend on a wide range of professional, educational and health service

Table 36.1
Prevalence of common psychiatric disorders in the community and primary care

Common psychiatric disorders	International primary care[a] (%)	United States community[b] (%)	Australian community (1997)[c] (%)
Depressive disorders			
Major depression	10.4	2.1	5.1
Dysthymia	10.3	2.5	1.1
Anxiety disorders			
Generalised anxiety disorder	7.9	3.1	3.1
Panic disorder/agoraphobia	2.6	5.1	2.4
Somatic disorders			
Somatisation	2.7	—	—
Neurasthenia	5.4	—	—
Hypochondriasis	0.8	—	—
Alcohol disorders	6.0	9.7	6.5
Any psychological diagnosis	24.0	29.5	17.7
Two or more mental disorders	9.5	14.0	4.8

NOTES [a] ICD-10: Goldberg and Lecrubier (1995). [b] DSM-III-R: Kessler et al. (1994). [c] Andrews et al. (1999). [d] Hickie et al. (2002).

SOURCE Adapted from Hickie et al. (2002b), p. 7.

reforms. Although these may seem overwhelming, we now have good evidence from recent Australian experience that such widespread change is possible (Hickie et al. 2004) and that a decade of prior expansion of treatments has already resulted in a fall in suicide in those people who reach primary care (Hall et al. 2003).

PROMOTING GOOD HEALTH

Additionally, we now recognise that depression leads to death and disability not just through its direct contributions to unemployment, poor performance in education and training, reduced social function and increased accidental injuries, deliberate self-harm and suicide, but also through its contribution to increased other physical health problems. Notably, these include cardiovascular disease and associated other health risk factors such as obesity, tobacco smoking and harmful patterns of cannabis and alcohol use. Better health outcomes for people with depression depend, therefore, not only on earlier provision of evidence-based treatments but also better integration of medical and psychological care (Box 36.1). Primary care-based mental health services offer real opportunities for earlier intervention as well as continuation of effective treatments, implementation of depression relapse prevention strategies and promotion of other health risk factor reduction strategies such as tobacco cessation and reduction of harmful drinking patterns.

BOX 36.1

BRINGING DOWN THE WALL OF DEPRESSION AND ANXIETY: THE PUBLIC HEALTH PERSPECTIVE ON REDUCING THE PREVALENCE OF DEPRESSION AND ANXIETY

Not yet assessed

- Decrease the length of time before treatment.
- Encourage presentation to GPs. Dependent on previous experience; public awareness; language and cultural barriers.

Contact with GP but no diagnosis

- Increase identification rate by the doctor.
- Encourage use of improved self-report instruments and interview style.

Diagnosed but not receiving effective treatment

- Provide effective treatment to decrease recovery time.
- Increase knowledge base of effective treatment options.

Treated but relapsed

- Actively prevent relapse.
- Implement a disease management approach.

SOURCE Hickie et al. (2002b), p. 6. Reproduced with permission from Educational Health Solutions.

REDUCING STIGMA IN PRIMARY CARE

It is often less obvious to many mental health experts that not only will expanded primary care services affect the quantity and quality of services currently provided in our communities but they will also offer one of our most effective methods for promoting the belief that depression is a major health problem deserving treatment. Much of the stigma that surrounds mental illness – often just as profound for people with common disorders such as depression and anxiety as for people with other psychiatric disorders – springs from the belief that it is not a real medical problem, that medical services do not want to treat people with these conditions, that people who receive treatment are at risk from those interventions (Highet et al. 2002), or that they will not respond to available interventions (Jorm et al. 2000). Patients with depression, and their families, have often reported dismissive interactions with their primary care practitioners or a sense that they did not deserve the time and effort involved in providing effective treatments (Highet et al. 2002). If we are able to change our primary care systems to deliver such treatments efficiently then it is highly likely that community attitudes towards treatments, and the providers of those treatments, will also change rapidly. When people believe that a treatment is available, effective and not likely to cause them further harm, they are much more likely to present for care.

INTERNATIONAL EVIDENCE

Throughout the world, most of the management of people with depression and anxiety occurs in primary care settings. The prevalence of depressive disorders in primary care settings varies as a consequence of cultural, patient and local service organisation factors (Table 36.2). What is more relevant is the abundance of psychological disorders in primary care and the general estimates that one-third of people presenting have significant psychological difficulties and about one-fifth have a formal psychiatric diagnosis – typically of depression or anxiety. Further, studies have repeatedly demonstrated that busy medical practitioners probably identify only about half of these patients during their visit to the clinic. While illness-related factors such as severity and duration contribute to recognition rates, it is also clear that a large range of non-illness factors (for example, patients' sociodemographics and education status, doctors' interest and training in mental health, and practice organisation factors such as the amount of time spent with each patient) have big effects.

Table 36.2
Prevalence and physician identification rates of current depression as defined by the ICD-10

	Prevalence (%)	Recognition as a psychological case by treating physician (%)
Santiago	29.5	74.0
Rio de Janeiro	15.8	43.9
Paris	13.7	61.5
Manchester	16.9	69.6
Groningen	15.9	59.6
Mainz	11.2	55.6
Bangalore	9.1	45.7
Athens	6.4	22.2
Berlin	6.1	56.7
Ankara	11.6	28.4
Seattle	6.3	56.7
Verona	4.7	70.0
Ibadan	4.2	39.7
Nagasaki	2.6	19.3
Shanghai	4.0	21.0
TOTAL	10.4	54.2

SOURCE Adapted from Üstün and Sartorius (1995, pp. 326, 354).

Evidence about delivery of treatments internationally may be seen to be headed in two quite divergent directions. One is to study the effects of delivering common treatments through routine general practice methods (Üstün and Sartorius 1995). This appears to result in short-term benefits to the patients but little long-term gain (Goldberg et al. 1998). The other is to construct new healthcare delivery systems or so-called *stepped-care* models (Katon et al. 1999). These seek to bring the right mix of primary and specialist care treatments together at appropriate points in the illness course, as well as focusing on treatment continuing until the person is fully recovered (back at school or work) and then preventing relapse. Although such ideal systems have only really been possible within specific clinical trial settings, they do appear to point the way to delivering effective treatments in the future. If such patterns of service delivery were extended to the Australian healthcare system, we could achieve twice the gains for the same amount of health expenditure (Sanderson et al. 2003).

RECENT AUSTRALIAN AND NEW ZEALAND EVIDENCE

As the Australian and New Zealand health care systems have strong historical links with the British system, both have traditionally involved a highly medicalised form of primary care – namely, general or family practice by specifically credentialled medical practitioners. In recent years, the systems in Australia and New Zealand have become increasingly different, with the Australian system maintaining notions of universal access, coverage and functioning as a primary gatekeeper to other specialist medical systems. Within both countries, such systems have not served our indigenous populations well, leading to new models of primary care for those subpopulations. By comparison with other international primary care systems, less emphasis has also been placed on the doctor working collaboratively as part of a primary care team with nurses and other non-medical health practitioners. Within the Australian system, the traditional fee-for-service model of payment has also meant that doctors who see more patients for shorter periods are also likely to derive the maximum financial benefit.

Systematic data have now been kept within the Australian general practice system for over a decade (Britt and Miller 2000). As a consequence, we know that general practitioners (GPs) are now diagnosing more depression and providing more treatments that they were in the 1990s. Depression is now the fourth most common disorder identified and treated in general practice. Most evidence-based treatments provided by GPs are now the newer antidepressant agents. Importantly, however, GPs recognise as many people again with other common psychological disorders such as anxiety, and are far less likely to provide them with antidepressant medication.

FACTORS AFFECTING QUALITY OF CARE

With regard to the quality of psychological practice in Australian general practice, we now also have access to another large database that examined more than 46 000 individual patient consultations (Hickie et al. 2001a). The key messages were not only that psychological problems were common, but also that there was great variability in the ways in which patients were recognised and managed. This variability is underpinned by a large number of patient, doctor and practice organisation factors (Box 36.2). Currently, it is clear that young educated women who present to their female doctor (who works part-time and has a mental health interest and training), come when they are less ill, and are more likely to receive the forms of psychological and medical care they prefer. By contrast, men, older people, people from non-English-speaking backgrounds and those who present to very busy, fast-turnover medical practices that have little interest in mental health are likely to receive less care, and less quality or choice of care.

BOX 36.2

PATIENT, DOCTOR AND ORGANISATION FACTORS INFLUENCING QUALITY OF PRACTICE IN AUSTRALIA

Patient factors

Young people with mental disorders are particularly poorly served by our current general practice system. By contrast, middle-aged, female, Australian-born, and unemployed patients are more likely to have their needs met, even though they may have less severe disorders.

Doctor factors

Certain characteristics of GPs are associated with provision of mental health services. These include being female, having an interest in mental health and having obtained mental health training.

Organisation factors

Characteristics of practice organisation that predict increased detection and management rates include being in part-time practice, shared practices and location of practices in regional Australia. Higher-quality mental health service is also predicted by practices with fewer patients and those in which GPs see fewer patients per week.

source Hickie et al. (2001a). Reproduced with permission from the *Medical Journal of Australia*.

IMPROVING THE QUANTITY AND QUALITY OF CARE

Mental health training that targets GPs' needs may have a significant effect on the quantity and quality of treatment provided. Such education, however, needs to be backed by real system reform to have any actual effect (Hickie and Groom 2002). Limited educational interventions without system reform have no demonstrable effect on patient outcomes (Thompson et al. 2000).

Introduction of practice-based reforms offer greater potential for lifting the quality and quantity of treatments. One common method proposed has been to introduce screening tools such that all those who come to primary care are asked about their mental health – in much the same way that people are asked about smoking or alcohol use or have their blood pressure regularly checked. Such opportunistic screening would result in detection of more cases but also brings potential hazards. A recent review (Table 36.3, see pp. 452–3) of major reviews indicated that screening is viable only when it is linked other processes that deliver more effective care (Hickie et al. 2002a).

Other components that might result in better care can be summarised as:

- better patient information procedures; for example, access to books, websites (Box 36.3), discussion with other patients, discussion with health practitioners (Box 36.4)
- better clinical assessment by trained professionals
- promotion of a wider range of pharmacological and non-pharmacological strategies
- better working relationships between GPs and other mental health specialists (such as nurses and clinical psychologists)
- better patient-tracking procedures and more assertive follow-up procedures (including patient reminders, telephone contacts and in-person outreach services)
- more active collaboration between services, patients, and their families in joint management strategies (for example, tracking of medication side effects and use of patient-outcome tools such as a worksheet for activity planning and sleep–wake cycle management).

BOX 36.3

GUIDE TO AUSTRALIAN DEPRESSION WEBSITES

RECOMMENDED SITES OVERALL (ALPHABETICAL ORDER)

- beyondblue http://www.beyondblue.org.au
- BluePages http://bluepages.anu.edu.au
- CRUfAD http://www.crufad.unsw.edu.au
- Infrapsych http://www.infrapsych.com.au

RECOMMENDED SUBSECTIONS OR ASPECTS OF SITES (ALPHABETICAL ORDER OF FEATURES)

Accessible and above-average quality

- Dark side of the mood <http://www.abc.net.au/health/depression/default.htm>

Antidepressants

Management of depression

- Infrapsych
- depression doctor.com (http://www.depressiondoctor.com)

Side effects

- myDr <http://www.mydr.com.au>

Ways of coping with side effects

- depression doctor.com

Cognitive behaviour strategies

- beyondblue
- CRUfAD

Evidence-based information about treatments

- BluePages

Focused search of other depression sites

- BluePages

Online consumer support

- DepressioNet <http://www.depressionet.com.au>

Online depression screening

- BluePages
- CRUfAD
- Infrapsych

source Griffiths and Christensen (2002). Reproduced with permission from the *Medical Journal of Australia*.

BOX 36.4

IS IT DEPRESSION?

For more than *two weeks* have you:

1 Felt sad, down or miserable most of the time?

2 Lost interest or pleasure in most of your usual activities?

If you answered 'yes' to either of these questions, complete the symptom checklist below.

Behaviours	**Thoughts**
Stopped going out	'I'm a failure'
Not getting things done at work	'It's all my fault'
Withdrawn from close family and friends	'Nothing good ever happens to me'
Relying on alcohol and sedatives	'I'm worthless'
Stopped doing things you enjoy	'Life is not worth living'
Unable to concentrate	

Feelings		**Physical**
Overwhelmed	Guilty	Tired all the time
Unhappy, depressed	Indecisive	Sick and run down
Irritable	Disappointed	Headaches and muscle pains
Frustrated	Miserable	Churning gut
No confidence	Sad	Can't sleep
Poor appetite/weight loss		

If you answered 'yes' to question 1 and/or 2 and ticked 3 or more of the above symptoms, you probably have a depressive illness.

source Hickie et al. (2001c), p. 1. Reproduced with permission from Educational Health Solutions.

Interestingly, people's willingness to consult their family doctor for a psychological problem is strongly linked to age. Younger people are much more likely to consult family and friends, whereas older people who often see their GP regularly for other medical problems are more likely to consult them for a psychological problem. This is a challenge for primary care in the future, as the greatest need for psychological care is in younger people and the greatest opportunity for early intervention is often in the teenage years.

SOMATIC PRESENTATIONS FOR CARE

One of the most important issues that complicates the identification and management of depression and anxiety in primary care settings is the extent to which patients discuss preferentially their physical rather than psychological symptoms. Doctors often respond to such symptoms by commencing a search for a medical rather than psychological cause. This can lead to unnecessary or prolonged medical consultations and laboratory tests. Many factors contribute to this phenomenon, including:

- the difficulty patients experience discussing any highly stigmatised condition
- the relative lack of knowledge in the community about the physical and psychological symptoms of many mental disorders
- patient reluctance to waste doctors' time with psychological problems
- doctors' reluctance to identify and manage common psychological disorders and the overlap between the nonspecific physical symptoms that accompany depression and anxiety (such as tiredness, headaches, muscle aches and pains, palpitations, gut disturbance)
- other common physical illnesses.

Much effort has been spent in recent years in attempts to improve family doctor interviewing and diagnostic skills so that psychological disorders can be more efficiently managed (Gask and Goldberg 1993). Although improved skills are one key component, other important factors may well include use of appropriate screening tools, provision of more illness-related information, and reorganisation of key practice characteristics to encourage both doctor and patient to spend sufficient time together to both identify and commence management of the relevant psychological problem.

Another important factor is that many of the common psychological disorders seen by family doctors do not fit easily into conventional specialist psychiatry classification systems. Patients are more likely to experience a mix of physical and psychological symptoms that do not easily add up to a simple diagnosis of major depression or panic disorder. A more dimensional view of symptoms is often appropriate. Within this model, a case for treatment is often conceptualised as a person who has sufficient psychological and nonspecific somatic symptoms, is disabled by them, is at risk of harm (through comorbid factors such as alcohol or drug misuse, or risk of self-injury) and is seeking help for these problems. Specific screening instruments have been developed for these conditions, including the Somatic and

Table 36.3
Review of reviews: summary of four key reviews focused on screening for depression in general practice and related medical settings

Mulrow et al. 1995	**Gilbody et al. 2001**
Years covered by studies within the review	
1977–1994	1976–1996
Study factors	
Depression; case-finding instruments.	Screening and outcome questionnaires; depression and anxiety; recognition rates; management; clinical outcome; non-psychiatric settings.
Number and type of studies	
18 prospective studies in primary care.	Nine randomised trials in primary care and general medical settings (screening and feedback to clinician vs screening with no feedback to clinician).
Outcomes/end points	
Characteristics of case-finding questionnaires for depression: length; administration time; sensitivity and specificity for detecting depression.	Rates of detection. Number of patients treated or referred for treatment. Outcome of psychiatric disorders.
Measures of association/statistical results	
Nine case-finding instruments were assessed. No significant differences were found between instruments: overall sensitivity 84%; overall specificity 72%.	Four (of nine) studies were combined in a meta-analysis: suggests routine screening and feedback to clinicians did not increase overall detection rate. Two (of nine) studies showed routine administration and selective feedback for high scores increased recognition rate. This did not lead to increased rate of intervention.
Findings	
Several questionnaires are available with reasonable operating characteristics to assist clinicians with the identification of patients with depression. Screening improve recognition of depression in primary care.	Studies of routine administration of psychiatric measures with feedback to clinicians have no effect on patient outcome and do not influence clinicians' behaviour.

SOURCE Hickie et al. (2002a). Reproduced with permission from the *Medical Journal of Australia*.

Pignone et al. 2002	Williams et al. 2002
1976–2001	1977–1999
Screening; depression; recognition rates; treatment rates; clinical outcomes; primary care.	Case-finding questionnaires for depression; recognition rates; primary care.
14 randomised trials in primary care (routine screening vs usual care).	28 prospective studies in primary care.
Differences in clinicians' rate of detection. Proportion of patients with depression who were treated or referred for treatment. Clinical outcomes of depression.	Characteristics of case-finding questionnaires for depression: administration time; likelihood ratios (positive and negative) for depression.
Seven (of 14) studies were combined in a meta-analysis: suggests screening and feedback provides a 13% reduction in relative risk for depression.	11 case-finding questionnaires were assessed. No significant differences between questionnaires were found.
Screening for depression can improve patient outcome in primary care, particularly when screening is integrated with the aim to improve treatment provision and clinic systems (coordinated and timely follow-up of diagnosis and treatment). Screening with feedback to clinicians generally increases recognition of depression by a factor of two to three.	Several questionnaires with reasonable performance characteristics are available to assist clinicians in identifying and diagnosing patients with depression. may

Psychological HEalth REport (SPHERE) (Hickie et al. 2001b), and are an alternative to traditional brief screening instruments such as the Kessler Psychological Distress Scale (K10) (Kessler et al. 2000) for depressive disorders. Traditional specialist classification systems often refer to these disorders as mixed depression and anxiety, subsyndromal disorders, and somatoform disorders.

Another way of conceptualising this model is revealed by statistical modelling of the common psychological and nonspecific somatic symptoms that are presented in primary care settings. Within this model, seven classes that lie along two dimensions of symptoms (fatigue, and anxiety/depression) are presented. One of these dimensions essentially describes a psychological dimension of sleep disturbance, irritability and later depression and anxiety with somatic symptoms. The other has a more somatic profile, emphasising chronic pain and prolonged fatigue states.

Family practitioners often deal with patients who present primarily with prolonged fatigue or chronic pain. Although these patients often have major depressive or anxiety symptoms, they rarely respond to interventions in the same way as patients with classical mood disorders. Aetiological research suggests that they are genetically different (Hickie et al. 1999b) and treatment research highlights that they do not respond readily to antidepressant therapies (Working Group of the Royal Australasian College of Physicians 2002). Much behavioural work has been done, and it emphasises the need for use of appropriate psychological and behavioural techniques. Modification of the sleep–wake cycle is particularly important (Box 36.5).

BOX 36.5

DEPRESSION AND SLEEP

Depression usually leads to:

- Difficulty getting to sleep
- Poor-quality sleep
- Fewer hours of sleep
- More awakenings during the night
- In severe cases, waking very early in the morning and being unable to get back to sleep
- Daytime tiredness.

Poor quality of deep sleep leads to:

- Daytime fatigue
- Poor concentration
- Irritability
- Musculoskeletal aches and pains
- Reduced immune function
- Prolonged depression.

SOURCE Hickie et al. (2001c, p. 8). Reproduced with permission from Educational Health Solutions.

MEDICAL AND PSYCHOLOGICAL COMORBIDITY

At least half of the depressive disorders that family practitioners encounter will be in the setting of another significant medical illness. Some of those disorders will be the direct cause of the depression (for example, secondary to stroke, cancer, central nervous system infection, hypothyroidism or use of corticosteroid drugs; Box 36.6), while others will fluctuate in association with the course of the medical disorder (for example, in association with multiple sclerosis or other autoimmune disorders). Some medical and psychological problems become entwined over time, such as development of depression in association with chronic pain secondary to musculoskeletal injury or chronic arthritis, or in the context of the personal and social losses that occur secondary to chronic disability.

BOX 36.6

COMMON MEDICAL CAUSES OF DEPRESSION

- Low thyroid function
- Brain injuries and diseases (such as stroke, head injury, epilepsy, Parkinson's disease)
- Some forms of cancer
- Blood vessel disease in the brain due to diabetes or hypertension
- Infectious diseases
- Some steroid and hormonal treatments
- Chronic pain
- Poor physical health due to smoking, obesity, lack of exercise.

SOURCE Hickie et al. (2001c p. 2). Reproduced with permission from Educational Health Solutions.

Many doctors place an overemphasis on the understandability of depressive reactions in patients who have serious medical conditions. This notion that because depression has a medical context it does not need to be treated has an adverse effect on the outcome of both the depression and the related medical disorder. That is, patients with stroke and depression have a worse outcome and remain more disabled than those with stroke alone. Second, the mechanisms by which physical illnesses give rise to depression are more complex than simplistic notions of psychological reactions to adversity. For example, stroke may disrupt critical frontal and temporal lobe circuits regulating mood. Some cancers and infectious diseases are associated with the production of pro-inflammatory cytokines that can induce depression. Chronic pain often disrupts sleep, and this gives rise to later depression. The emphasis in assessment in such situations should be on determining the likely pattern of association and attempting to modify factors that can be adjusted. For example, with chronic arthritis, better nocturnal pain management may lead to better sleep and less depression.

OUTCOMES IN PRIMARY CARE

One of the most important but poorly understood areas of depression research is the long-term outcome of patients who are identified and treated within primary care settings. On one hand, they may be less severely or less chronically ill than patients who reach secondary care services. Consequently, they may require less intensive first-line therapies and greater use of non-pharmacological and informational strategies. On the other hand, depression is often a relapsing or chronic illness with considerable effects on long-term disability, social factors (for example, marital breakdown) and other physical health problems (such as heart disease). Most patients who present to primary care have actually been unwell for some months (Hickie et al. 1999a), although they may present to see the doctor on the pretext of some more immediate crisis (such as sleep disturbance due to job loss) or some other intercurrent medical problem.

Formal longitudinal or treatment studies of depression in primary care are still rare. Much public health commentary and education for GPs still relies on evidence collected in secondary care settings. For more severe depressive disorders (melancholia, psychotic depression, depression in the context of bipolar disorder, depression with severe predisposing or complicating anxiety, depression compounded by alcohol or substance misuse), treatment should be as intensive as in any other setting and a commitment to long-term medical and psychological care should be clear. For less severe or less enduring disorders, a proactive attitude to appropriate psychological and medical treatments is still needed, but there may be less need for continued treatments, particularly continued pharmacological treatments.

CONCLUSION

We know that the general public prefers their family doctor as the first point of contact for assessment of emotional problems (Highet et al. 2002). As depression awareness increases, one would expect increased presentations for care within family practice environments. Although GP identification and active management of depression has increased substantially (Britt and Miller 2000), structural, professional and financial barriers to the further expansion of quality care have been identified. The lack of access to effective non-pharmacological forms of treatment has been emphasised by both consumers and carers (McNair et al. 2002), evidence-based guidelines and professional associations. The need to prioritise integration of medical and psychological care, treatment across a whole episode of illness, continuity of care for recurring and chronic conditions, comorbidity between drug and alcohol misuse and mental disorders, changes in attitudes among people who provide mental health interventions, and provision of appropriate psychoeducational resources have all been highlighted by those whose lives are directly affected by these conditions (McNair et al. 2002).

Primary care services are changing in Australia and New Zealand, with an increasing emphasis on providing more services, better services and continuity of medical and psychological care. Mental health specialists need to be more responsive to these changes and participate more actively in the long-term management of these patients in association with their primary care practitioners.

REFERENCES

Andrews G, Slade T, Peters L (1999) Classification in psychiatry: ICD-10 versus DSM-IV. *British Journal of Psychiatry* 174:3-5.

Andrews G, Henderson S, Hall W (2001) Prevalence, comorbidity, disability and service utilisation: Overview of the Australian National Mental Health Survey. *British Journal of Psychiatry* 178:145-53.

Britt HC, Miller GC (2000) The BEACH study of general practice. *Medical Journal of Australia* 173:63-4.

Gask K, Goldberg D (1993) Impact on patient care, satisfaction and clinical outcome of improving the psychiatric skills of general practitioners. *European Journal of Psychiatry* 7:203-18.

Goldberg D, Lecrubier Y (1995) Forms and frequency of mental disorders across centres. In Üstün TB, Sartorius N (eds), *Mental Illness in General Health Care. An international study*. New York: John Wiley & Sons, pp. 324-34.

Goldberg D, Privett M, Ustun B, Simon G, Linden M (1998) The effects of detection and treatment on the outcome of major depression in primary care: A naturalistic study in 15 cities. *British Journal of General Practice* 48:1840-4.

Griffiths KM, Christensen H (2002) The quality and accessibility of Australian depression sites on the World Wide Web. *Medical Journal of Australia* 176 (10 Suppl):S97-S104.

Hall WD, Mant A, Mitchell PB, Rendle VA, Hickie IB, McManus P (2003) Association between antidepressant prescribing and suicide in Australia, 1991–2000: Trend analysis. *BMJ* 326:1008-11.

Hickie IB, Groom G (2002) Primary care-led mental health service reform: An outline of the Better Outcomes in Mental Health Care initative. *Australasian Psychiatry* 10:376-82.

Hickie IB, Kirk K, Martin N (1999a) Unique genetic and environmental determinants of prolonged fatigue: A twin study. *Psychological Medicine* 29:259-68.

Hickie IB, Davenport TA, Ricci CS (2002a) Screening for depression in general practice and related medical settings. *Medical Journal of Australia* 177 (7 Suppl):S111-16.

Hickie IB, Scott E, Davenport T (2002b) *Treating depression and anxiety: A training manual for general practitioners*. Melbourne: Educational Health Solutions.

Hickie IB, Davenport T, Issakidis C, Andrews G (2002c) Neurasthenia: Prevalence, disability and health care characteristics in the Australian community. *British Journal of Psychiatry* 181:56-61.

Hickie IB, Davenport TA, Naismith SL, Scott EM (2001a) Conclusions about the assessment and management of common mental disorders in Australian general practice. *Medical Journal of Australia* 175 (2 Suppl):s52-5.

Hickie IB, Bennett B, Lloyd A, Heath A, Martin N (1999b) Complex genetic and environmental relationships between psychological distress, fatigue and immune functioning: A twin study. *Psychological Medicine* 29:269-77.

Hickie IB, Pirkis J, Blashki G, Groom G, Davenport TA (2004) 'All hands to the pump!': General practitioners' response to mental health needs in Australia. *Medical Journal of Australia*. In press.

Hickie IB, Davenport TA, Hadzi-Pavlovic D, Koschera A, Naismith SL, Scott EM, et al. (2001b) Development of a simple screening tool for common mental disorders in general practice. *Medical Journal of Australia* 175 (2 Suppl):s10-17.

Hickie IB, Scott E, Morgan H, Sumich H, Naismith S, Davenport T, et al. (2001c) *A Brief Guide to Depression Management, second revision*. Melbourne: Educational Health Solutions.

Highet NJ, Hickie IB, Davenport TA (2002) Monitoring awareness of and attitudes to depression in Australia. *Medical Journal of Australia* 176 (10 Suppl):S63-8.

Jorm AF, Medway J, Christensen H, Korten AE, Jacomb PA, Rodgers B (2000) Public beliefs about the helpfulness of interventions for depression: Effects on actions taken when experiencing anxiety and depression symptoms. *Australian and New Zealand Journal of Psychiatry* 34:619-26.

Katon W, Von Korff M, Lin E, Simon G, Walker E, Unutzer J, et al. (1999) Stepped collaborative care for primary care patients with persistent symptoms of depression: A randomized trial. *Archives of General Psychiatry* 56:1109-15.

Kessler RC, Andrews G, Colpe L (2000) Short screening scales to monitor population prevalences and trends in nonspecific psychological distress. Cambridge, MA: Department of Health Care Policy, Harvard Medical School.

Kessler RC, McGonagle KA, Zhao S, Nelson CB, Hughes M, Eshleman S, et al. (1994) Lifetime and 12-month prevalence of DSM-III-R psychiatric disorders in the United States. *Archives of General Psychiatry* 51:8-19.

McNair BG, Highet NJ, Hickie IB, Davenport TA (2002) Exploring the perspectives of people whose lives have been affected by depression. *Medical Journal of Australia* 176 (10 Suppl):S69-76.

Sanderson K, Andrews G, Corry J, Lapsley H (2003) Reducing the burden of affective disorders: Is evidence-based health care affordable? *Journal of Affective Disorders* 77: 109-25.

Thompson C, Kinmonth AL, Stevens L, Peveler RC, Stevens A, Ostler KJ, et al. (2000) Effects of a clinical-practice guideline and practice-based education on detection and outcome of depression in primary care: Hampshire Depression Project randomised controlled trial. *Lancet* 355:185-91.

Üstün TB, Sartorius N (1995) *Mental Illness in General Health Care: An international study*. Chichester: John Wiley & Sons.

Working Group of the Royal Australasian College of Physicians (2002) Chronic Fatigue Syndrome Clinical Practice Guidelines – 2002. *Medical Journal of Australia* 176 (9 Suppl):S17-55.

CHAPTER 37

SUICIDAL BEHAVIOUR AND MOOD DISORDERS

Robert D Goldney

The acknowledged importance of mood disorders in relation to suicidal behaviour has varied over time. For example, the psychiatric illness model of suicide enjoyed favour in the early and mid-nineteenth century and then more sociological views predominated until well into the twentieth century, with the influence of psychiatric illness, including mood disorders, being minimised. However, in the past three or four decades in particular, the illness model with specific focus on depression has again predominated, although not without its critics.

This chapter provides a brief historical review before referring to suicide in mood disorders and then mood disorders in association with suicide, attempted suicide, and suicidal ideation. The issues of comorbidity, other risk factors, and the potential impact on suicidal behaviours by adequate recognition and treatment of mood disorders are then addressed. Finally, comment on the neurobiology of suicide and future research directions is made.

HISTORICAL REVIEW

The Dutch historian van Hoof (1990) reviewed more than 1000 examples of suicide in ancient texts and considered that two-thirds were related to what he described as *pudor*, *dolor*, or *desperata salus*. These terms are synonymous with shame, grief, and despair, respectively, and give a good indication of the emotions that we would now equate to various forms of mood disorder and recognise as being associated with suicide.

Probably the earliest clear delineation of the emotional state associated with suicide in the English language literature is that provided by Sym in 1637 in his publication 'Life preservative against self-killing' (Goldney and Schioldann 2002). He referred to the 'signs of self-murder' as being 'solitariness ... sudden neglect of necessary duties ... a regardlessness of those persons, and things in the world that he most affected ... change in outward behaviour, with gastly lookes, wilde frights and flaights ... restlesse behaviour'. Such words fit easily with our current description of a person with major depressive disorder with melancholia, and this is an illustration of the early association of such symptoms with suicidal behaviour. It is further of note that Sym went on to state that 'self-murder is prevented, not so much by arguments against the fact; which disswades from the conclusion; as by the discovery and removall of the motives and causes, whereupon they are tempted to do the same; as diseases are cured by removing the causes, rather than of their symptoms'. Sym was surprisingly modern in his description of the prevention of suicide by alleviating antecedent causes, including what we would now refer to as the mood disorders.

In 1828, Burrows in England noted that suicide was 'a feature of melancholia', and he also observed, 'Mania and melancholia are hereditary; but melancholia may beget mania in the next generation, and mania melancholia; but the propensity to suicide will propagate its own type through successive races'. He went on to state that 'the medical treatment of the propensity to suicide, whether prophylactic or therapeutic, differs not from that which is applicable in cases of ordinary insanity' (Goldney and Schioldann 2002). Again, this is a clear description of the need to treat the underlying condition.

There was increasing recognition in the nineteenth-century literature of the importance of the association between mood disorders and suicide. For example, in 1877 in a report from the American New England Psychological Society, Tyler noted of melancholia that there was a 'nearly unanimous feeling that the suicidal impulse is inherent in this form of illness and should be assumed in every case'. Furthermore, in England in 1890, Mercier referred to 'the tendency to suicide which so often accompanies' melancholia, and Savage in 1892 stated that 'all melancholic patients must be considered suicidal till they are fully known' and that even 'simple melancholia of very slight depth is a very common cause of suicide' (Goldney and Schioldann 2002).

In the early twentieth century, there was a more sociological and psychological view of suicide, which tended to minimise the importance of mood disorders, or indeed psychiatric illness in general, in regard to suicidal behaviour. This culminated in Hawton and Catalan (1982) noting in relation to suicide attempters that 'only a minority of patients suffer from formal psychiatric disorders requiring psychiatric treatment'. However, in the last three or four decades of the twentieth century, the close association between mood disorders and suicidal behaviour was increasingly recognised.

SUICIDAL BEHAVIOUR IN MOOD DISORDERS

Early follow-up studies of people with mood disorders led to standard psychiatric texts reporting a 15 per cent lifetime risk of suicide for people with major depressive disorders. However, such a figure was challenged by Blair-West et al. (1997), who demonstrated that there was a 3.5 per cent lifetime risk, with the previous higher figure being due to the bias of early studies involving hospitalised subjects with high suicide risk, rather than patients generally seen in clinical practice. Other researchers have confirmed this revised figure (Lonnqvist 2000), and Boardman and Healy (2001) recently presented data which suggest that, for people with mood disorders without comorbid conditions and who have not had mental health service contact, the lifetime suicide rate may be as low as 1.1 per cent. However, bearing in mind the prevalence of mood disorders in the community, this still represents a major contribution to suicide at the population level.

That there is an elevated risk not only for major depression but also for other mood disorders has been demonstrated by Harris and Barraclough (1997), who used meta-analysis to demonstrate increased standardised mortality ratios for people with different mood disorders. Their results indicated that patients with major depression, bipolar disorders, dysthymia and mood disorders not otherwise specified had twenty, fifteen, twelve and sixteen times the standardised mortality ratio due to suicide of those without mood disorders.

MOOD DISORDERS IN SUICIDE

An alternative way of examining the association between suicidal behaviour and mood disorders is to examine the presence of the disorders in people who engage in such behaviour. The *psychological autopsy* was devised to address this issue in people who had suicided, in a manner analogous to that of the autopsy in general medical practice. At least a dozen studies from no fewer than ten countries have now published their results, and about two-thirds of people who suicided were reported to have had major depressive disorders (Lonnqvist 2000). This has been illustrated well by the Taiwanese study of Cheng (1995), in which a standardised instrument was used to assess depression in three different groups, two of aboriginal Taiwanese people and the third of Han Chinese immigrants from mainland China. In each group, about 80 per cent of those who had suicided could have been diagnosed with a major depressive disorder before their suicide. Indeed, this led Cheng to state, 'These findings strongly indicate that the psychiatric antecedents of suicide are the same in the east and the west. This work reveals a more universal nature of suicide than could previously have been assumed', a reference to the previous belief that mood disorders were not so prominent in Chinese suicide as had been demonstrated in Western studies.

A common theme in these studies is that mood disorders had often not been diagnosed in many of the people who suicided, and that even when they had been, those people had often not received adequate treatment for their depressive conditions (Lonnqvist 2000).

It is sometimes asserted that mood disorders may be of less relevance in suicide in young people. However, Shaffer et al. (1996), in a study of 120 suicides under the age of 20 years in New York, reported that two-thirds had a mood disorder and 50 per cent had had a duration of symptoms for more than 3 years, with less than 5 per cent having symptoms for less than 3 months. This study is particularly important, as it indicates that there is almost invariably a window of opportunity during which the mood disorder could be recognised and treated.

MOOD DISORDERS AND ATTEMPTED SUICIDE

The association of mood disorders with attempted suicide is sometimes considered less clear-cut. This probably arose from early studies, which reported that less than 10 per cent of people who attempted suicide had depressive conditions, although a more comprehensive review concluded that between 35 and 79 per cent of people who attempted suicide had a mood disorder (Weissman 1974). It became apparent that when standardised instruments were used, more depression was delineated than had been the case with clinical reports. For example, in an early international study, Goldney et al. (1981) examined the nature of depression in young women aged between 18 and 30 years who had attempted suicide in Australia, New Zealand and Canada, and found that two-thirds had a mood disorder, and that a half of those had symptoms consistent with endogenous depression, as delineated by a depression questionnaire.

More recently, a New Zealand case control study of 'serious' suicide attempts demonstrated that those with a mood disorder were thirty-three times more likely to have attempted suicide than comparison subjects (Beautrais et al. 1996). This study was also probably the first to use the *population attributable risk* (PAR) to examine the importance of mood disorders in suicidal behaviour.

It is pertinent to digress and describe the PAR, as it is a singularly appropriate statistic for research because it has the potential to place different risk factors in perspective at the population level. The PAR provides a measure of the proportion of a condition that can be associated with exposure to a risk factor, or the proportion of that condition which would be eliminated if the risk factor were not present. This can be illustrated by considering the association between smoking and lung cancer, as it is well recognised that, although there is a causal relationship, not all succumb. The PAR of smoking for lung cancer is about 80 per cent, which means that if all smoking could be eliminated, about 80 per cent of lung cancer would be eliminated.

Beautrais et al. (1996) used the PAR and noted that mood disorders made the greatest contribution to the risk of a suicide attempt. Indeed, they concluded that, 'The population attributable risk estimates suggest that elimination of mood disorders would result in very substantial reductions, up to 80%, in risk of a serious suicide attempt'. They also reported that the PAR showed variations depending on age and gender, and a more recent study of older adults led Beautrais (2002) to conclude that, 'The predominant role of mood disorders was confirmed by population attributable risk (PAR) estimates (73.6%), suggesting that the improved detection, treatment and management of mood disorders should be the primary focus of suicide prevention strategies for older adults'.

MOOD DISORDERS AND SUICIDAL IDEATION

Although it is beyond dispute that mood disorders are associated with suicide and attempted suicide, it is not generally recognised that such an association also holds for suicidal ideation. Indeed, suicidal ideation appears to be minimised and considered normal by many in the community. This is particularly so for the elderly, where expressions of wishing to die may be accepted by family and friends, and even by some clinicians, despite findings such as those of Waern et al. (1999), who conducted a psychological autopsy study on 100 suicides over the age of 65 years, and confirmed earlier reports that feelings of life-weariness and death wishes were strongly related to depression.

Recent community surveys using the PAR statistic have confirmed the importance of mood disorders in suicidal ideation. For example, random and representative community studies using two different methods of delineation of both depression and suicidal ideation have demonstrated PARs of 47 and 57 per cent, respectively (Goldney et al. 2000; Goldney et al. 2003). These findings are consistent with results from the Australian National Survey of Mental Health and Wellbeing, where in an examination of more then 10 000 respondents there was a PAR of 38.8 per cent of mood disorders for suicidal ideation and 39.5 per cent for attempted suicide (Pirkis et al. 2000).

It is acknowledged that not all who are suicidal are necessarily depressed, and that there are other well-recognised psychosocial and traumatic stressors. Their relative importance has been demonstrated in a recent study of factors contributing to suicidal ideation in a community sample (Goldney et al. 2000). In an initial univariate statistical analysis, stressors such as marital breakdown, serious illness, and the death of someone close (for convenience referred to collectively as *psychosocial events*), as well as the more dramatic stressors of sexual molestation, assault and life-threatening accidents (referred to as *traumatic events*), were statistically significant stressors, along with clinical depression as delineated by the short-form health survey (SF-12). However, when allowance was made for the interaction between the various significant factors by using multivariate analysis, none of the individual stressors remained statistically significant, whereas clinical depression did, contributing 46.9 per cent PAR to suicidal ideation. Indeed, although the lifetime summation of traumatic events remained a significant contributor to suicidal ideation, even the effect of the total of all current psychosocial stressors was no longer statistically significant. Such results challenge the commonsense view of focusing on current psychosocial stressors in therapy with people who are suicidal.

It is important to reflect that these results can be considered valid only for the populations studied (that is, in Western countries with well-developed health and social services), and they may not be applicable to, for example, developing countries where there could be alternative public health priorities. However, the PAR statistic could be used to tease out the relative importance of depression in relation to other contributing factors to suicidal behaviour in other populations.

It is evident that there is a consistency of findings in relation to the importance of mood disorders, not only for suicide but also for attempted suicide and suicidal ideation. However, there is also a consistent tendency for the association to be minimised in clinical and community settings, and it has only been by using objective methods of assessment that the strength of the association has been appreciated.

COMORBIDITY

Depression is often associated with other conditions, both emotional and physical, and comorbidity has been well recognised as a factor in suicidal behaviour. Henriksson et al. (1993), in a psychological autopsy study of 229 Finnish suicides, reported that the most prevalent axis I diagnoses were depressive disorders (59 per cent), but 43 per cent also had alcohol dependence or abuse. Furthermore, 31 per cent had an axis II or personality diagnosis, and 46 per cent had at least one axis III (physical illness) diagnosis. Similar findings have been reported for people with suicidal ideation and behaviour, as illustrated by Beautrais et al. (1996), who noted that 56.6 per cent of people who had made serious suicide attempts had had two or more disorders. Furthermore, although the odds ratio for people with a mood disorder to make a serious suicide attempt was 33.4 compared with people with no psychiatric disorder, when subjects had had two or more disorders, the odds of a serious suicide attempt increased to 89.7 times the odds of those with no psychiatric disorder (Beautrais et al. 1996).

Similar findings of comorbidity were found in adolescent suicides by Shaffer et al. (1996), who noted that 'a limited range of diagnoses – most commonly a mood disorder alone or in combination with conduct disorder and/or substance abuse – characterises most suicides among teenagers'.

OTHER RISK FACTORS

Although depressive disorders are undoubtedly important in the evolution of suicidal behaviour, in themselves they lack specificity in regard to the development of such behaviour. This has been illustrated well by longitudinal research. For example, in a New Zealand study, although young people who developed major depression had fifty-four and twelve times the likelihood of suicidal ideation and suicide attempt, respectively, compared with those who were not depressed, most who were depressed did not develop suicidal ideation or attempt suicide (Fergusson et al. 2003). Other factors of importance were a family history of suicide, childhood sexual abuse, neuroticism, novelty seeking, self-esteem, peer affiliations, and school achievement. Fergusson et al. (2003) noted that 'positive configurations of these factors confer increased resiliency, whereas negative configurations increase vulnerability', and the influences operated similarly for those who were depressed and non-depressed.

NEUROBIOLOGY, DEPRESSION AND SUICIDE

In 1976, Asberg et al. in Sweden demonstrated a lowered level of 5-hydroxyindole acetic acid (5-HIAA) in the cerebrospinal fluid (CSF) of suicide attempters who had used violent methods. This was important, as CSF 5-HIAA is a breakdown product of serotonin, one of the neurotransmitters associated with mood disorders. This finding has been replicated in other centres, and it is a predictor (albeit at the research level) of subsequent suicide. Indeed, it remains one of the most robust neurobiological results in psychiatry. It is also of note that binding to serotonin transporter sites in the ventral prefrontal cortex of the brain of completed suicides is reduced compared with binding in people who have died from other causes (Arango et al. 1995).

The activity of another neurotransmitter, dopamine, has also been examined, by measuring the growth hormone response to apomorphine in depressed people, some of whom later suicided. Pitchot et al. (2001) reported a significantly lower response in eight male depressed patients who suicided compared with eighteen depressed patients who had never attempted suicide. This suggests that dopamine may also be involved in the biology of suicide in mood disorders.

EFFECT OF TREATMENT

Although it has been noted correctly that 'no single intervention has been shown in a well-conducted randomised controlled trial to reduce suicide' (Gunnel and Frankel 1994), the challenge to such a conclusive demonstration of a cause and effect relationship is that, although suicidal behaviour is dramatic and sometimes said to be common, the reality is that it has a low base rate. Indeed, because of the numbers required, and the ethical constraints of not treating some suicidal subjects, it is unlikely that conventional trials will ever be able to clinch the association. Therefore, large community analyses will offer the best hope of demonstrating the effectiveness of intervention strategies.

Probably the first such study was on the Swedish island of Gotland, where, following a program to enhance the recognition and treatment of depression by general practitioners, there was a decrease in suicide, as well as a greater use of antidepressants, a decrease in prescribing of neuroleptics and hypnotics, and a decrease in hospitalisation for depression (Rutz et al. 1992). Although there has been debate about the significance of the reduction in suicide, Rihmer et al. (1995) further analysed their data and reported that before the program 43 per cent of suicides had major depression, whereas after the program only 15 per cent of the fewer number were so diagnosed, a statistically significant difference.

These encouraging findings have been supported by national data. In a study of suicide and the prescription of antidepressants in Sweden between 1978 and 1996, Isacsson (2000) concluded that, 'The increased use of antidepressants appears ... to be one of the contributing factors to the decrease in the suicide rate'. In contrast to the relationship with antidepressants, there was no association between suicide rates and alcohol consumption or unemployment. Similar results were found in Denmark, Norway and Finland.

Isacsson acknowledged that 'This naturalistic study is not conclusive', and that the increased use of antidepressants could reflect other aspects of improved diagnosis and management of depression. It is also fair to note that other Swedish work has demonstrated that, although the major reduction in suicide coincided with the introduction of selective serotonin reuptake inhibitor (SSRI) antidepressants, a lesser decline had commenced before their availability (Carlsten et al. 2001).

Notwithstanding these caveats, the association between increased SSRI prescribing and a decline in youth suicide has been commented on by Joyce (2001) in New Zealand, and a recent Australian study has provided results consistent with the original Swedish research (Hall et al. 2003). As Joyce (2001) noted, such results add 'further support to the hypothesis that better recognition and treatment of depression is having a detectable effect on suicide rates, and especially youth suicide rates'.

FUTURE RESEARCH DIRECTIONS

Research into the association between suicidal behaviour and mood disorders is multifaceted. Further elucidation and replication of the psychosocial variables reported by Fergusson et al. (2003) is indicated, and issues such as the mental health literacy of people who may be depressed and suicidal should be clarified. For example, Goldney et al. (2002) found that the knowledge and beliefs about depression and its treatment were similar for people with major depression with and without suicidal ideation, despite the latter groups having had significantly more treatment and professional contact than those who were not depressed, and this suggests that specific educational programs may be needed for those who are depressed and suicidal.

The effect of personality disorders on depression is also a fertile area for enquiry. Thus, Joyce et al. (2003) reported that depressed patients with borderline personality disorders 'did poorly in the short term if treated with nortriptyline rather than fluoxetine', compared with depressed patients with other personality disorders. Indeed, they noted that the response for depressed patients with borderline personality disorder was similar to that for depressed patients with no personality disorder. This is of potential importance because of the increased frequency of suicidal behaviour in borderline personality disorder.

Although such clinical studies are important, the most dramatic advances may well be made in neurobiological research, where compelling findings in regard to the actions of antidepressants and their possible effect on the brain are emerging. Thus, Gurevich et al. (2002) have found altered editing of serotonin 2C receptor pre-mRNA in the prefrontal cortex of depressed suicide victims. Furthermore, they noted that treatment of mice with fluoxetine causes changes in editing that are opposite to those seen in suicide victims, and they concluded that 'one outcome of fluoxetine treatment may be to reverse the abnormalities in 5-HT_{2C} pre-mRNA editing seen in depressed suicide victims'.

Clearly we are still some distance from fully understanding the significance of such findings. Furthermore, no matter what emerges with regard to the neurobiology of mood disorders and suicide, the challenge will remain to incorporate those findings into our broader psychosocial understanding of these conditions.

CONCLUSION

There is a strong association between mood disorders and suicidal behaviour. However, it must not be forgotten that although mood disorders per se may be a necessary precondition for many suicides, they are not a sufficient explanation. Indeed, it is important to avoid having a unidimensional view of suicidal behaviour and mood disorders. Nevertheless, in terms of a clinician's ability to influence the course of people who have mood disorders and who may be suicidal, the imperative remains not only to ensure that mood disorders are recognised but that people afflicted have the best available treatment. In this manner, the clinician can be assured that the most important antecedent of suicidal behaviour has been addressed.

REFERENCES

Arango V, Underwood MD, Mann JJ (1995) Postmortem findings in suicide victims: Implications for in vivo imaging studies. *Annals of the New York Academy of Sciences* 8365:269-87.

Asberg M, Traskman L, Thoren P (1976) 5-HIAA in the cerebrospinal fluid: A biochemical suicide predictor? *Archives of General Psychiatry* 33:1193-7.

Beautrais AL (2002) A case control study of suicide and attempted suicide in older adults. *Suicide and Life-Threatening Behavior* 32:1-9.

Beautrais AL, Joyce PR, Mulder RT, Fergusson DM, Deavoll BJ, Nightingale SK (1996) Prevalence and comorbidity of mental disorders in persons making serious suicide attempts: A case–control study. *American Journal of Psychiatry* 153:1009-14.

Blair-West GW, Mellsop GW, Eyeson-Annan ML (1997) Down-rating lifetime suicide risk in major depression. *Acta Psychiatrica Scandinavica* 95:259-63.

Boardman AP, Healy D (2001) Modelling suicide risk in affective disorders. *European Psychiatry* 16:400-5.

Carlsten A, Waern M, Ekedahl A, Ranstam J (2001) Antidepressant medication and suicide in Sweden. *Pharmacoepidemiology and Drug Safety* 10:525-30.

Cheng AT (1995) Mental illness and suicide. A case–control study in east Taiwan. *Archives of General Psychiatry* 52:594-603.

Fergusson DM, Beautrais AL, Horwood LJ (2003) Vulnerability and resiliency to suicidal behaviours in young people. *Psychological Medicine* 33:61-73.

Goldney RD, Schioldann JA (2002) *Pre-Durkheim Suicidology: The 1892 Reviews of Tuke and Savage*. Burnside: Adelaide Academic Press.

Goldney RD, Adam KS, O'Brien JC, Termansen P (1981) Depression in young women who have attempted suicide. An international replication study. *Journal of Affective Disorders* 3:327-37.

Goldney RD, Fisher LJ, Wilson DH, Cheok F (2002) Mental health literacy of those with major depression and suicidal ideation: An impediment to help seeking. *Suicide and Life-Threatening Behavior* 32:394-403.

Goldney RD, Dal Grande E, Fisher LJ, Wilson D (2003) Population attributable risk of major depression for suicidal ideation in a random and representative community sample. *Journal of Affective Disorders* 74:267-72.

Goldney RD, Wilson D, Dal Grande E, Fisher LJ, McFarlane AC (2000) Suicidal ideation in a random community sample: Attributable risk due to depression and psychosocial and traumatic events. *Australian and New Zealand Journal of Psychiatry* 34:98-106.

Gunnel D, Frankel S (1994) prevention of suicide: Aspirations and evidence. *British Medical Journal* 308:1227-33.
Gurevich I, Tamir H, Arango V, Dwork AJ, Mann JJ, Schmauss C (2002) Altered editing of serotonin 2C receptor pre-mRNA in the prefrontal cortex of depressed suicide victims. *Neuron* 34:349-56.
Hall WD, Mant A, Mitchell PB, Rendle VA, Hickie IB, McManus P (2003) Association between antidepressant prescribing and suicide in Australia, 1991–2000: Trend analysis. *British Medical Journal* 326:1008-11.
Harris EC, Barraclough B (1997) Suicide as an outcome for mental disorders: A meta-analysis. *British Journal of Psychiatry* 170:205-28.
Hawton K, Catalan J (1982) *Attempted Suicide*. Oxford: Oxford University Press.
Henriksson MM, Aro H, Marttunen MJ, Heikkinen ME, Isometsa ET, Kuoppasalmi KI, et al. (1993) Mental disorders and comorbidity in suicide. *American Journal of Psychiatry* 150:935-40.
Isacsson G (2000) Suicide prevention – a medical breakthrough? *Acta Psychiatrica Scandinavica* 102:113-17.
Joyce PR (2001) Improvements in the recognition and treatment of depression and decreasing suicide rates. *New Zealand Medical Journal* 114:535-6.
Joyce PR, Mulder RT, Luty SE, McKenzie JM, Sullivan PF, Cloninger RC (2003) Borderline personality disorder in major depression: Symptomatology, temperament, character, differential drug response and six month outcome. *Comprehensive Psychiatry* 44:35-43.
Lonnqvist JK (2000) Psychiatric aspects of suicidal behaviour: Depression. In Hawton K, van Heeringen K (eds), *The International Handbook of Suicide and Attempted Suicide*. Chichester: John Wiley & Sons, pp. 107-20.
Pirkis J, Burgess P, Dunt D (2000) Suicidal ideation and suicide attempts among Australian adults. *Crisis* 21:16-25.
Pitchot W, Reggers J, Pinto E, Hansenne M, Fuchs S, Pirard S, et al. (2001) Reduced dopaminergic activity in depressed suicides. *Psychoneuroendocrinology* 26:331-5.
Rihmer Z, Rutz W, Pihlgren H (1995) Depression and suicide on Gotland. An intensive study of all suicides before and after a depression-training programme for general practitioners. *Journal of Affective Disorders* 35:147-52.
Rutz W, von Knorring L, Walinder J (1992) Long-term effects of an educational program for general practitioners given by the Swedish Committee for the Prevention and Treatment of Depression. *Acta Psychiatrica Scandinavica* 85:83-8.
Shaffer D, Gould MS, Fisher P, Trautman P, Moreau D, Kleinman M, et al. (1996) Psychiatric diagnosis in child and adolescent suicide. *Archives of General Psychiatry* 53:339-48.
van Hoof AJL (1990) *From Autothanasia to Suicide. Self-killing in classical antiquity*. London: Routledge.
Waern M, Beskow J, Runeson B, Skoog I (1999) Suicidal feelings in the last year of life in elderly people who commit suicide. *Lancet* 354:917-18.
Weissman MM (1974) The epidemiology of suicide attempts, 1960 to 1971. *Archives of General Psychiatry* 30:737-46.

CHAPTER 38

MOOD DISORDERS AND FORENSIC PSYCHIATRY

Philip M J Brinded
and Mark Earthrowl

Forensic psychiatry is that branch of the specialty that deals largely with the assessment and treatment of people who, by virtue of the mental illness, pose a significant danger to others. For many years, leaders in this field held the view that mentally disordered people were no more likely to offend or to be violent than any member of the general population (Monahan 1984). Slowly, this view has been moderated as researchers have more closely studied specific groups of people and specific offences, finding that certain diagnostic groups of mentally disordered people do, in fact, offend more frequently when compared both with other diagnostic groups and with the general population. Evidence now supports the proposition that patients with schizophrenia are generally overrepresented in groups of violent offenders and are more likely to offend in this way than patients with mood disorders. However, what of the association between mood disorders and offending, particularly violent offending? It is certainly clear that, although patients with schizophrenia are the most likely to offend violently, there are numerous occasions in forensic psychiatry in which the existence of a mood disorder is doubtless the precipitating factor in offending. It is vital that undiagnosed mood disorder be considered an important differential diagnosis in the assessment and treatment of offenders, particularly those who have been violent. The scope for therapeutic intervention and, therefore, prevention of future violent incidents is enormous. As Mullen (1988) so cogently said, 'The importance of recognizing the link, rare though it be, between serious violence and mental disorder, is that it offers the chance for effective prevention'.

OFFENDER POPULATIONS

Epidemiological studies into the prevalence rates of mental disorders within prisons worldwide were few and far between before 1980. More recently, greater interest has been shown in the identification of the level of psychiatric disturbance within prisons, results of which have been published from the United States, Canada, Australia, the United Kingdom and other countries in Europe and Australasia. Greater concern has also been expressed over the suicide rate in prisons, which has been reported in many countries throughout the world as exceeding the rate found in the general population. Interestingly, few of these studies discuss diagnosis but tend to focus on other aspects of the inmates' presentation, such as charge, length of sentence, when they arrived at jail, and time of day of attempt. This lack of diagnostic focus is of some concern, and perhaps exemplifies the fact that depressed people in prison are probably less likely to receive adequate treatment than if they are floridly psychotic or behaviourally difficult. The isolative, quiet and undemanding prisoner in the grip of a mood disorder is much less trouble to manage in a penal institute and, therefore, more likely to have treatment needs overlooked.

Many of the recent studies describing prevalence rates of major psychiatric disorder in prisons highlight the high rates of personality disorder, substance abuse or dependence, and schizophrenia. However, those that have relied on the use of semi-structured or structured clinical interviews (as opposed to retrospective analyses of prison medical files, which are subject to diagnostic bias) have demonstrated that rates for mood disorders in prison populations are elevated compared with the general population, thus constituting a significant treatment problem. Retrospective studies have shown a significant reluctance to diagnose mood disorders (particularly unipolar depression) in the prison setting. One such study of 362 inmates in Winchester Prison in the United Kingdom, who were identified over a 4-year period as mentally disordered, diagnosed only eight as suffering for a depression requiring clinical treatment (Faulk 1976). It is now clear from current epidemiological literature that such figures represent significant lack of recognition of depressive symptoms in the prison setting. The level of psychosis (including affective psychosis) in prisons would now appear to be greater than that found in class-matched community populations. In the United States, Teplin (1990) demonstrated point prevalence rates for mania and major depressive illness of 1 and 4 per cent, respectively, and in Canada, Hodgins and Coté (1990) found rates of major depression twice and bipolar disorder four times those in the general population. In the United Kingdom, Gunn and his colleagues (1991) found point prevalence rates of 0.4 per cent for affective psychoses and 6 per cent for major depression, while a study from Melbourne discovered 12 per cent of its cohort suffering from undiagnosed, and therefore untreated, major depressive disorder (Hermann et al. 1991). In a national prison study in New Zealand, Brinded et al. (2001) demonstrated prevalence rates (in the previous month) for incarcerated women, remand and sentenced males of 11, 10.7 and 6 per cent, respectively, for major depression. Self-report showed that only 46 per cent were in receipt of treatment. This finding contrasted with 81 per cent of all prisoners shown to be suffering from bipolar disorder (last month prevalence, 1 per cent of total prison population) who were receiving treatment. Higher rates have been found in remand prisoner populations, as such people are usually intensely involved in the court process and trial proceedings, are experiencing the first shocks of incarceration and separation from normal life, and have often not yet been screened for the possible existence of psychiatric disturbance.

The elderly population in prison also seems to be a distinct group with regard to the prevalence of major psychiatric disorder. Studies have shown mood disorders and, in particular, psychosis to be much more prevalent in male prisoners over 55 years than in younger offender populations.

NEUROBIOLOGY AND THEORIES OF AGGRESSION

In the past decade, researchers have become increasingly interested in the possible neurochemical associations between aggression and depression, suicidal behaviour and violent outbursts. Psychoanalytic theory has long associated the two, conceptualising depression as anger turned against the self, with violent behaviour being the external manifestation aimed towards others. It has been shown that reduced concentrations of 5-hydroxyindole acetic acid (5-HIAA) in the cerebrospinal fluid of psychiatric patients appears to be related to a history of previous suicide attempts. It has also been shown that the behavioural correlates of reduced central serotonin function (through prolactin response to fenfluramine challenge) are different in patients with personality disorders compared with those with major depressive disorder. The important variable appears to be the existence of irritable, impulsive and aggressive behaviour in patients with personality disorder. Self-directed aggression may well be more common in patients with a primary major depressive disorder uncomplicated by coexistent personality disorder, although this picture is somewhat complicated by other research findings that have demonstrated increased hostile aggressive or antisocial behaviour in suicidal depressives with low 5-HIAA levels in cerebrospinal fluid (CSF). It is, however, accepted that both self-directed and externally directed aggression in patients with personality disorder and self-directed aggression in patients with major mood disorder are associated with reduced central serotonin function, as reflected by the prolactin response to fenfluramine challenge. Other studies have highlighted interesting differences between suicidal, violent and non-violent patient groups. Of most interest has been the finding that, in such a study, levels of depression and sadness correlated positively with suicidal behaviour in the non-violent group, but not in the violent group. Suicidal behaviour in this group was positively correlated with anger, lack of impulse control, suspiciousness, rebelliousness and anxiety. Happiness correlated negatively with suicide in the non-violent depressed group, but not in the violent group. One suggested reason for this finding is the apparently low prevalence of mood disorder often found in violent patient groups. This may be due to underdiagnosis of mood disorders, but some authors have postulated different theories. They suggest that violent patients suffer from an ego deficit that inhibits the expression of depressive symptoms. Effectively, they may act out sad feelings through acts of violence, in the form of self-inflicted injury or aggression towards others. This is supported by findings that show significant correlations between anger and suicide risk in violent patients, but not in the non-violent patient group. This suggests that the therapeutic approach to depressed suicidal non-violent patients could be different from that used to manage suicidal violent patients. For suicidal violent patients the treatment focus should be on behavioural intervention and medication to reduce impulsiveness, rather than antidepressant medication and psychotherapy.

Linnoila and his associates found low levels of CSF 5-HIAA in patients who had murdered their sexual partners, compared with patients who had attempted suicide and with normal controls. Such findings have also been linked to increased risk of suicidal behaviour or relapse of depressive symptoms. Animal studies suggest that a propensity for aggression is governed by excitatory and inhibitory centres, including the orbitofrontal cortex, septal area, hippocampus, amygdala, caudate, thalamus, hypothalamus, mid-brain and the cerebellum. Dopamine, γ-aminobutyric acid (GABA) and norepinephrine, in addition to hypothalamic and gonadal hormones, are suggested as mediating aggression. Dopamine is said to have a positive correlation with affective aggression but a negative one with predatory aggression. Acetylcholine has also been implicated in the activation of aggressive behaviour. In general, research in this area also suggests that aggressive behaviour cannot be explained purely by neurobiological factors without considering psychosocial influences.

Fine (2002) described the case reports of treatment-emergent violent behaviour of patients prescribed selective serotonin reuptake inhibitors (SSRIs), particularly fluoxetine, since its introduction in 1987. These behaviours include homicide and suicide. Cases such as this remain extremely rare with no compelling evidence of a substantiated link. A review article by Walsh and Dinan (2001) undertook a literature review of serotonin, SSRIs and aggression. They concluded that no increased susceptibility to aggression or suicidality could be connected with fluoxetine or any other SSRI; in fact, SSRI treatment served to reduce aggression.

MENTAL DISORDER AND VIOLENCE

Until recently, it was generally accepted that mentally ill people did commit violent acts or offend against the law in other ways, but they did so no more frequently than the general population. Recent research now suggests that this is not the case. By focusing on certain groups of mentally ill people and on certain types of crime, it has been shown that certain mentally disordered people are more likely to perpetrate acts of violence than people without mental illness. Patients in the acute phase of a paranoid schizophrenic illness, for example, are greatly overrepresented in populations charged with violent offences. Before discussing in any further detail the association between mood disorders and violence, it is perhaps important to place this issue in some sort of perspective. There are six important points:

- Mental illness appears to be a risk factor for violence in the community. A body of research taken as a whole supports the idea that an association exists between mental illness and violence in the general population.
- The size of the association between mental illness and violence, while statistically significant, does not appear to be very large. Also, the absolute risk for violence posed by mental illness is small.
- The combination of a serious mental illness and a substance abuse disorder significantly increases the risk of involvement in violent acts.
- The association between mental illness and violence is probably significant, even when demographic characteristics are taken into account.
- Active symptoms are probably more important as a risk factor than is simply the presence of an identifiable disorder.
- No clear information about the causal paths that produce the association between mental illness and violence is available.

Although much of the literature in this area deals with schizophrenia and substance abuse, patients presenting with mood disorders are common in forensic psychiatric practice. In bipolar disorder, many studies have shown that there is an increased risk of violence in patients who are manic.

Newman et al. (1996) followed a birth cohort to age 21 years and found that 31.6 per cent of the young adults with mania had a criminal record. Other community follow-up studies have found that people with mood disorders have a higher rate of aggressive behaviour and offending during the follow-up period than do those with schizophrenia (Hodgins and Coté 1990; Monahan et al. 2001). Several factors that have been shown to predict violence in manic patients recently admitted to an inpatient unit have been the degree of psychosis (as measured by the Brief Psychiatric Rating Scale), the severity of the manic state, degree of violence prior to admission, and a history of severe childhood discipline. On occasion, manic patients do perpetrate violent offences, and community surveys have shown bipolar patients to be several times more likely to be violent than the general population. However, Gunn (1991) pointed out that the theme of the rarity of serious harm following a manic episode is consistent throughout the literature, although it can occur. Nevertheless, manic patients often appear to be highly irritable, confrontational and threatening, which in an institutional setting can rapidly develop into a violent confrontation with other patients, prisoners or staff. Feldmann (2001) pointed to the risk of violence being greater in the manic phase, although such violence is random and rarely goal-directed. He emphasised that early diagnosis and pharmacological intervention are the key to preventing violence in manic patients.

Depression is perhaps more often associated with violence and other types of offending than one might imagine from a cursory perusal of the forensic literature. However, there appear to be certain offence types in which depressive illness is central to the offending behaviour, high levels of illness being found, for example, in populations perpetrating murder–suicide (extended suicide), infanticide and filicide. These are discussed later in this chapter. Occasionally, it appears that undiagnosed mood disorder can present to the forensic psychiatrist in the form of a patient charged with a single violent assault. The following case vignettes highlight the presenting features of two such cases.

Mr A was a 22-year-old single man, living at home with his mother and younger brother. Although the elder, he was the less successful of the two siblings, both socially and academically. He had become a target for taunts and ridicule by his brother and his friend and this had resulted in an increasing self-imposed isolation and removal from the day-to-day activities of the family, to the extent that he would spend most of his time in his room, eat all of his meals alone, and avoid his brother as much as possible. Following a derogatory remark from his brother, Mr A brooded as to what to do, before bursting into his brother's bedroom and threatening him with a knife. A fight ensued between the two brothers, during which Mr A remembers punching his brother, but was unaware that he had stabbed him. The wound required minor surgery, but the brother survived. On examination, Mr A presented with clear symptoms of major depressive disorder, probably present for the previous 2 years at least.

Mr B was a 16-year-old adolescent who lived with his parents and elder brother. He enjoyed a happy and supportive family life and had a close relationship with all members of his family. He performed well at school, both academically and in sport, until the age of about 14 years, when a change became apparent. He began to behave antisocially at school and was disciplined for smoking and fighting. He began to truant as well. His demeanour at home became increasingly sullen, he was unresponsive to his parents and brother and rapidly alienated himself from his family and school friends. This continued for 18 months prior to his offence. One night, he sat and watched a particularly violent film and, at its completion, reported feeling that his head was 'full of violent thoughts'. He had not ingested any alcohol or drugs. He went to his room, where he picked up a large screwdriver, sat on his bed and attempted to 'control' his thoughts. He then went through to his brother's bedroom where his brother was sleeping and struck him twice on the head with the screwdriver handle. The brother required several sutures to a large scalp wound. On examination, Mr B had symptoms of major depressive disorder that appeared to have been present for some 18 months. He made an excellent recovery following antidepressant treatment. Neither Mr A nor Mr B had any prior history of depressive illness.

These case vignettes serve to illustrate the importance of considering major depressive disorder in the forensic evaluation of people who have acted violently and of performing careful risk assessment of patients with mood symptoms, because of the distinct possibility of aggressive outbursts as part of the symptom complex.

Just as it has been highlighted that major depressive disorder is often underdiagnosed in the prison population, so it is also the case that major mood disorders can often be overlooked at the time of serious offending and certainly during the trial process. The defence of insanity in New Zealand is the major mechanism in court for establishing lack of criminal responsibility because of mental illness. It is more commonly used in New Zealand than many other countries that also have provision for 'diminished responsibility' in their statutes. Insanity, as defined in Section 23 of the *Crimes Act 1961*, is modelled on the concept of 'McNaughten Rules', whereby the presence of a 'disease of the mind' has first to be established. If this is established to the satisfaction of the court then, for the insanity defence to succeed, the defence must further establish that, by virtue of this 'disease of the mind', the person either 'did not know the nature and quality of their actions' or, if they did, they were 'incapable of knowing that such actions were morally wrong'. There is rarely any difficulty in establishing that major depressive disorder constitutes a 'disease of the mind'. The problem usually arises over the fact that a patient frequently has to be psychotic to satisfy the other limbs of Section 23. Suffering from major depression, no matter its severity, does not usually suffice, and will often result in a conviction. Prior to the *Sentencing Act 2002*, only one sentence was available to the court for a major charge such as murder, the resulting disposition appearing to completely ignore the existence of mental illness and its likely contribution to the offence – a life sentence. This has been mitigated somewhat by the Sentencing Act, which allows the imposition of non-parole periods instead of a single life sentence. The introduction of a defence of diminished responsibility for murder would assist offenders who are suffering from major mood disorders but who do not satisfy criteria for legal insanity.

MOOD IN RISK ASSESSMENT

The assessment of the risks for self-harm or suicide among their patients is an established part of routine clinical practice for mental health professionals. Forensic psychiatric practice in the past few years has led a change away from considering people dangerous to the evaluation of risk and planning risk management strategies. Several factors have driven these developments:

- Dangerousness as a concept suggests a static attribute. The concept of risk, on the other hand, implies more dynamic factors that can be evaluated and managed.

- The power to predict a single event (violence) occurring in the future is limited. Clinicians are much more able to evaluate the risk factors, environmental factors etc. that led to a particular event and then develop a management plan to control these risks to prevent recurrence.

Studies to date have identified that a combination of clinical examination, assisted by use of an actuarial risk assessment tool, is the most accurate and successful approach to risk formulation. There is a more varied attitude and approach to the assessment of the risk of interpersonal violence. What is apparent from the more recent literature in the field is that the pessimistic views of the 1970s and 1980s (Monahan 1984) regarding a clinician's ability to reliably predict future risk of interpersonal violence was misinformed. If certain types of mental disorder or more specific groups of symptoms are targeted and the assessment includes a thorough clinical assessment with the additional use of one of the currently available actuarial tools, these predictions are improved with increased reliability in the short-term expression of risk. A risk assessment is, of course, most valuable if it informs a comprehensive risk management plan. As well as the risk of interpersonal violence, mood may be relevant in the assessment of other risks, including recklessness or omissions within a patient's behaviour. Violence is a complex interaction of social, environmental, characterological and clinical variables coming together within specific contexts. Affect or mood disorder may feature in one or more of these categories. What has emerged from recent inquiries internationally following tragic events perpetrated by people with mental disorder is that mental health professionals are placed under increasing obligation in risk management reduction, and this is a tool of the trade that is viewed as part of routine clinical practice in the same way as the assessment of risk of suicide (Petch and Bradley 1997).

Specific mood disorders are not strongly represented within commonly used actuarial tools, although they are encompassed within broader categories. In the Psychopathy Checklist, Revised Version (Hare 1991), a superficial or shallow affect is referred to being linked with the assessment of a person's empathic style. In the HCR-20 (Webster et al. 1997), mood disorder is subsumed within the categories of historical or current major mental disorder and active symptomatology. In the Violence Risk Appraisal Guide (Harris et al. 1993), there is no specific reference to mood disorder. In the MacArthur Violence Risk Assessment Study, anger and major mental disorder are referred to.

Apart from specific clinical diagnoses and symptoms, affect is inextricably bound up within other domains of risk assessment, including its relationship to impulsivity, the labile affect within personality disorder, and the subjective and objective view of the affective response to symptoms, situations or contexts. This would include symptoms suggestive of physiological arousal, anger, suspiciousness or fear, in addition to depressed or elevated mood. In terms of risk assessment these features may be important negatives to note.

The Epidemiological Catchment Area study provided a survey of more than 10 000 people living in a community in the United States regarding self-reported violence in the previous year (Swanson et al. 1990). By diagnosis, where no diagnosis of mental disorder was made, a baseline rate for the community was 2 per cent. This was increased in diagnosis of major depressive disorder to 12 per cent, and for bipolar disorder or mania, 11 per cent, similar to that for a diagnosis of schizophrenia (13 per cent). One reason that interpersonal violence within mood disorders, particularly depression, may be overlooked is that it is often an omission in the major psychiatric texts discussing violence and associated psychiatric disorders.

DEPRESSION

Depression has suggested links with a range of specific offences, including homicide and suicide, maternal and paternal filicide, and infanticide in postnatal depression or puerperal psychosis. Altruistic violent offending may be associated with nihilistic delusions. Depressive disorder is more likely to result in violence towards previously identified individuals, particularly family members, carers or other intimates. Serious depressive interpersonal violence may be the result of an acute catathymic process and is more often seen in individuals who may not have prominent prior records of violent behaviour. In the catathymic process, as depression intensifies, dormant conflicts regarding competency and self-esteem may be rekindled, and this leads to pronounced feelings of failure and hopelessness. It is in these cases that a patient without apparent motive may resort to extreme violence directed at an intimate. Malphurs et al. (2001) established that depression was a prominent premorbid feature in older men who perpetrated spousal homicide–suicide. Half of these individuals were in caregiving roles, highlighting the raised degree of risk for those who are in close relationships with people who have serious mood disorders. Interesting, none of the perpetrators tested positive for antidepressants at autopsy, highlighting the role of intensive risk management planning. In murder–suicide, premorbid elements of narcissism within the perpetrator's personality are often present. Male perpetrators have a higher than average history of domestic violence in spousal assault or homicide.

A link has been suggested between a history of violent suicide attempts and subsequent serious interpersonal violence or homicidal incidents. Although each individual case must be specifically addressed, as a general rule, risk of interpersonal violence may be increased in depression with marked psychomotor agitation and, as in the assessment of suicide risk, patients with major depressive disorder present more risk of violent behaviour in the early stages of treatment response as motivation and drive returns. As for other syndromes or symptoms, risk factors around mood disorders are cumulative and greatly increased by comorbidity, particularly with alcohol and substance abuse and by environmental and social factors. As in the psychoses, it is active symptoms rather than the mere presence of the illness that are more pertinent to the risk assessment and subsequent management. In the assessment of any constellation of symptoms, it is important to extrapolate from this both the subjective and objective affective or emotional response, followed by consideration of perpetuating or ameliorating factors, any likelihood of recurrence, and the likely effect on degree of self-control or impulsiveness.

Common features noted with hindsight following a depressed individual engaging in homicidal behaviour have been that people close to the individual note a prolonged sense of dejection, worthlessness or irritability, and attempts at reassurance fail. Anger and provocation then allow the externalisation of the self-hatred that immobilises the depressed person. As a result, it is not uncommon for a severely depressed person to engage in behaviour that is provocative (for example, pointing a weapon at the police) as a means of suicide.

MANIA

Patients with mania are more likely to present risks of interpersonal violence across a broader range of behaviours, which includes recklessness as well as direct assault. This is likely to be accompanied by prominent anger and irritability and may often be precipitated or aimed at people who are seen as setting limits or boundaries around these people. Patients with acute mania are more violent than patients with schizophrenia in the first 24 hours of hospital admission. However, this is not sustained after hospital discharge. Violence is more likely to be disorganised, poorly planned and impulsive. Victims are more likely to be people in the immediate environment and, unlike with depression, less likely to be those specifically in a caring role. McNiel and Binder (1989) suggested that manic patients are more likely to have a history of pre-admission violence followed by increased rates of inpatient violence in the first 24 hours of admission. They are also more likely to perpetrate assaults without prior threats. Severe interpersonal violence and mania is more likely to be of a reactive and impulsive type, and is often accompanied by intense sympathetic arousal of the autonomic nervous system. Aggression is often rapidly displaced. Generally, people with mania are far less likely than those with depression to present risks of planned and well-organised violence. Patients with bipolar disorder are more likely to be violent during a manic phase than in their depressed phase.

One other area where affect may be important in risk assessment is that of emotional blunting as a negative feature in schizophrenia, which may result in callous and damaging behaviour. Ordinarily, these are more minor acts of property damage, but on occasion may result in more serious offending. Generally, however, emotional blunting and its accompanying loss of drive or motivation militate against planned or persistent aggression.

HOMICIDE

There do not appear to be increased numbers of people suffering major mood disorders in populations convicted of homicide over and above what would be expected by chance. This is not the case if certain types of homicide are studied.

Infanticide

This legal term refers to the killing of a child in the first 12 months of its life by its biological mother. A successful finding of infanticide following such a killing allows a variety of dispositions from the court and, rather than being imprisoned, the defendant is often placed on a community supervision order. The history of infanticide extends far back into English legal history, to the Act to Prevent the Murthering of Bastard Children of 1624. It provides for the situation in which a killing would in other circumstances be considered murder, but at the time 'the balance of her mind was disturbed by reason of her not having fully recovered from the effect of giving birth to the child or by reason of the effect of lactation consequent upon the birth of the child' (referring to the mother). d'Orbán (1979) has pointed to the fact that social and psychological stresses are often factors, but there is no doubt that the mood changes consequent on childbirth, postnatal depression or puerperal psychosis can and often do appear to be central to the motivation for such killings. However, this is perhaps not true as frequently as medicolegal tradition would have us believe. It is also the case that in neonaticide – a term coined by Resnick to describe the killing of a child in the first 24 hours of life (see d'Orbán 1979) – mothers have been shown rarely to suffer from psychiatric disorder, but more frequently have personality disorders or are suffering intellectual deficits.

Maternal filicide

The killing of a child through an impulsive violent act is probably the most common form of filicide. These mothers have been shown to be overwhelmed by their chaotic social situation and by psychological stress, rather than the killing being directly due to the existence of mental illness. In one such study, this group represented about 40 per cent of cases of maternal filicide (Resnick 1969). The same study, however, identified 27 per cent of the deaths as being perpetrated by mothers suffering from mental illness, most of whom were suffering some form of depressive symptomatology. This group of women frequently contemplated or attempted simultaneous suicide. It was not uncommon for there to be more than one child victim, as the mother endeavoured to kill all her children. Psychosis was diagnosed in 16 per cent of the group, 8 per cent had puerperal psychosis with mixed schizoaffective symptomatology, 10.5 per cent had schizophrenia, 5 per cent had paranoid psychosis, and one individual had psychotic depression.

Paternal filicide

Stanton and Simpson (2002) reviewed the sparse literature in this area. Neonaticides by fathers are extremely rare. Paternal filicide is characterised by a lower rate of major mental illness and a higher rate of accidental killing, often associated with premorbid child abuse. Motives are described as including extended suicide, altruism, hostility and sexual jealousy. In a series of 29 men, none had a diagnosis of major mental disorder; personality disorder and high psychosocial stressors were common. Most children had been previously injured. More than half the men were not the biological fathers. The described interpretation of the child's behaviour is extremely important in the assessment of these cases – the child is often seen as a threat capable of adult thinking and of acting wilfully. Other case series have described high rates of mood disorder; misinterpretation of a child's behaviour is again highlighted as an important motivational factor. In several cases this was delusional.

Murder–suicide

This tragic event, also referred to as *extended suicide*, is characterised by the perpetrator of a murder subsequently killing or attempting to kill themselves. The following case describes a typical example.

> Mr C was 68 when he was charged with the murder of his wife. He said, 'I felt dreadfully depressed that morning. I was washing my hands. She had her back to me and it just happened. I thought I would kill both of us. I didn't commit suicide. I knew it would upset my wife that's why I didn't do it before. Quick as a flash, it came to me – kill myself and take her with me. Her last words to me were "stop trembling". I strangled her so that she didn't feel what I did after'. He cut his wrists and throat and drank chloral. He was found unconscious and revived; she died. His childhood was unremarkable; he had no previous criminal history and had apparently lived the life of a devoted family man and successful skilled worker until retirement. He had had previous psychiatric treatment for depression when aged 50 and again when he was 57 years, with apparently good recovery. About a year previously, he had presented again as depressed and his general practitioner had started to treat him. His wife had previously given a good account of his depression to family and friends, who became informants after her death. He was convicted of manslaughter on the grounds of diminished responsibility and, after several months on remand in prison, went to a local psychiatric hospital under a hospital order.

It is estimated that murder–suicide accounts for about 1500 deaths annually in the United States, and the annual incidence of 0.2–0.3 per 100 000 person-years is relatively constant across industrialised nations. It has also been shown that these are a phenomenologically distinct group when compared with mass murderers (an offender who wilfully injures five or more people, three or more of whom die) and serial murderers (an offender who kills others in three or more separate incidents) regardless of whether there are multiple victims. The principal perpetrators are young men with intense sexual jealousy, depressed mothers, or depressed and despairing elderly people, often with an ailing spouse. Up to 75 per cent of these people suffer from a major mood disorder, with 95 per cent being male. This contrasts strongly with comparable groups of homicide perpetrators, most of whom were not found to be depressed. West (1965) observed that 'the greatest risk of murder suicide would occur in paranoids ... especially those in whom emotional distress takes the depressive form'. When a sufferer is a mother, then it is not uncommon to find her children being victims, killed to protect them from perceived threat that is vested only in the mother's illness.

AMNESIA

The phenomenon of amnesia following homicide and its association with possible depressive illness has been described several times in the forensic psychiatric literature. One study showed that *amnesic* killers had significantly increased scores on the depression scale of the Minnesota Multiphasic Personality Inventory when compared with *confessed* killers (Parwatikar et al. 1985). However, the consistent finding appears to be that, while symptoms may not reach the required level for confirming a clinical diagnosis of major depressive disorder, there is usually evidence that depressed mood has been present for weeks or months prior to the offence in the amnesic group.

THEFT

Of all theft, perhaps shoplifting has maintained the highest profile in medicolegal circles as being the most likely form of theft to be associated with mental illness. It is likely, however, that such a profile is unjustified, given that there are a multitude of reasons for theft and shoplifting and psychiatric illness is an uncommon one. The cases of shoplifting often reported in this context are reasonably affluent people (usually women in middle age) who steal something that they probably do not need and can certainly pay for. The view that this occurs more frequently in women is probably more to do with previous research that has reported on cohorts of women only, rather than fact. Gibbens and his colleagues (1971) found that, of 525 women followed up 10 years after their original offence, 20 per cent re-offended; forty-four had been admitted to psychiatric hospitals. This represents about three times the expected rate, most (twenty-four) being admitted because of high risk of suicide. Another study from Canada compared fifty shoplifters referred to forensic psychiatric services by the courts with fifty other people remanded for pre-trial psychiatric reports (Bradford and Balmaceda 1983). The typical shoplifter profile in this group was a 37-year-old, relatively affluent, professional woman who was suffering psychological stress, anxiety and depression with symptoms of dissociation. The shoplifter group were more like the general psychiatric population than they were like offender populations. Bluglass (1990) in the United Kingdom has also studied the rate of psychiatric disorder in populations of shoplifters referred to psychiatrists by the courts. Over a 10-year period, 675 women were referred, 34 per cent of whom were shoplifters. Of these women, 33 per cent were shown to be depressed, with 30 per cent having personality 'problems'. Only forty male shoplifters were identified, 9 per cent showing depressive symptomatology. The association between the activity of shoplifting (or theft) and the existence of psychiatric disorder, particularly depression, is unclear. It has often been viewed as analogous to parasuicidal behaviour, a cry for help by people under severe psychological stress, perhaps exacerbated by mental illness. It is perhaps interesting that so much emphasis has been placed on shoplifting as the premier medicolegal theft, given that many of the same features can be found in white-collar crime, including fraud. Certainly, there are cases where, like the depressed shoplifter, no attempt at concealment takes place, as if the perpetrator wished to be apprehended. The problem appears to be that while the courts will accept an affluent woman stealing a packet of biscuits in an obvious fashion as evidence of psychological distress or psychiatric disorder and act accordingly, they have more trouble if a person has blatantly defrauded his employer of $50 000, even if his symptomatology is the same as that of the depressed female shoplifter.

MORBID JEALOUSY

There is a close association between mood disorders and morbid jealousy, with depressive disorders being common in this group. It is important to recognise several factors when assessing jealousy. First, jealousy can be a normal emotion and should not be necessarily seen as pathological. The accuracy or otherwise of a person's jealous belief is no guide as to whether the belief is morbid. For example, some delusions of infidelity may indeed have some basis in fact; however, it is the patient's behaviour and thought processes that identify them as morbid or pathological. The accurate and careful assessment of such symptoms can be vital to the safety of the patient and others who are the subject of their jealousy. Morbid jealousy can occur in a wide variety of psychiatric disorders, including organic brain disorders, alcohol and drug abuse, obsessional disorders, personality disorders, schizophrenia and depression. The association with depression is very important, given the frequency with which the two conditions coexist and the therapeutic opportunities to intervene in a potentially very dangerous situation. Mullen has stated that:

> The presence of significant mood disorder in association with the jealousy complex should be treated vigorously in its own right, even if it is considered secondary or reactive. Depression is too dangerous in jealousy to be ignored and its treatment should have priority whatever the theoretical assumptions of the therapist about its origins and relationship to the jealousy.

In one series, 50 per cent of patients with morbid jealousy were found to be suffering from depression. It appears that depression may not be an altogether uncommon event following continuous relationship disharmony and suspicion, and the depressive syndromes also appear to be a frequent breeding ground for morbidly jealous symptoms. Depression should always be considered in the diagnostic assessment of people presenting with morbid jealousy. People whose jealousy may well be within normal bounds may progress from increasing suspicions to florid delusional jealousy following the onset of a major depressive disorder. To be reassured by an apparent explanation for the jealous thoughts in that they are understandable from the patient's perspective is to court disaster if this reassurance leads to therapeutic inertia.

REFERENCES

Bluglass R (1990). In Bluglass R, Bowden P (eds), *Principles and Practice of Forensic Psychiatry*. London: Churchill Livingstone.

Bradford J, Balmaceda R (1983) Shoplifting – Is there a specific psychiatric syndrome? *Canadian Journal of Psychiatry* 28:248-53.

Brinded PM, Simpson AI, Laidlaw TM, Fairley N, Malcolm F (2001) Prevalence of psychiatric disorders in New Zealand prisons: A national study. *Australian and New Zealand Journal of Psychiatry* 35:166-73.

d'Orbán PT (1979) Women who kill their children. *British Journal of Psychiatry* 134:560-71.

Faulk M (1976) A psychiatric survey of men serving a sentence in Winchester Prison. *Medicine, Science and the Law* 16:244-51.

Feldmann TB (2001) Bipolar disorder and violence. *Psychiatry Quarterly* 72:119-29.

Fine EW (2002) Selective serotonin reuptake inhibitors (SSRIs) and cases of alleged related violence. *American Journal of Forensic Psychiatry* 23:5-38.

Gibbens TCN, Palmer C, Prince J (1971) Mental health aspects of shoplifting. *BMJ* iii:612-15.

Gunn J, Maden A, Swinton M (1991) Treatment needs of prisoners with psychiatric disorders. *BMJ* 303:338-41.

Hare R (1991) The Hare Psychopathy Checklist – Revised. Toronto, Ontario, Canada: Multi-Health Systems.

Harris GT, Rice ME, Quinsey VL (1993) Violent recidivism of mentally disordered offenders: The development of a statistical prediction instrument. *Criminal Justice and Behaviour* 20:315-35.

Hermann H, McGorry P, Mills J, Singh B (1991) Hidden severe psychiatric morbidity in sentenced inmates: An Australian study. *American Journal of Psychiatry* 1489:236-9.

Hodgins S, Coté G (1990) Prevalence of mental disorder among penitentiary inmates in Quebec. *Canada's Mental Health* 3:1-4.

Malphurs JE, Eisdorfer C, Cohen D (2001) A comparison of antecedents of homicide-suicide and suicide in older married men. *American Journal of Geriatric Psychiatry* 9:49-57.

McNiel DE, Binder RL (1989) The relationship between preadmission threats and later violent behaviour by acute psychiatric patients. *Hospital and Community Psychiatry* 40:605-8.

Monahan J (1984) The prediction of violent behaviour: Toward a second generation of theory and policy. *American Journal of Psychiatry* 141:10-15.

Monahan J, Steadman HJ, Silver E, Appelbaum PS, Robbins C, Mulvey EP, et al. (eds) (2001) *Rethinking Risk Assessment: The MacArthur study of mental disorder*. Bew Tirj: Oxford University Press.

Mullen P (1988) Violence and mental disorder. *British Journal of Hospital Medicine* 40:460-3.

Newman DL, Moffitt TE, Caspi A, Magdol L, Silva PA, Stanton WR (1996) Psychiatric disorder in a birth cohort of young adults. *Journal of Consulting and Clinical Psychology* 64:552-62.

Parwatikar SD, Holcomb WR, Meninger KA (1985) The detection of malingered amnesia in accused murders. *Bulletin of the American Academy of Psychiatry and the Law* 13:97-103.

Petch E, Bradley C (1997) Learning the lessons from homicide inquiries: Adding insult to injury? *Journal of Forensic Psychiatry* 8:161-84.

Resnick PJ (1969) Child murder by parents: A psychiatric review of filicide. *American Journal of Psychiatry* 126:325-34.

Stanton J, Simpson A (2002) Filicide: A review. *International Journal of Law and Psychiatry* 25:1-14.

Swanson JW, Holtzer CE, Ganju VK, Jonjo RT (1990) Violence and psychiatric disorder in the community: Evidence from the E.C.A. surveys. *Hospital and Community Psychiatry* 41:761-70.

Teplin LA (1990) The prevalence of severe mental disorder amongst male urban jail detainees. Comparison with the Epidemiologic Catchment Area Programme. *American Journal of Public Health* 80:663-8.

Walsh M, Dinan TG (2001) Selective serotonin reuptake inhibitors and violence: A review of the available evidence. *Acta Psychiatrica Scandinavica* 104:84-91.

Webster C, Douglas K, Eaves D, Hart S (1997) HCR-20 Assessing risk for violence – Version 2. Vancouver, Canada: Mental Health, Law and Policy Institute, Simon Fraser Univesity.

West DJ (1965) *Murder Followed by Suicide*. London: Heinmann.

CHAPTER 39

PUBLIC AND PROFESSIONAL UNDERSTANDING OF DEPRESSION

Anthony F Jorm
and Claire M Kelly

People take a major role in managing their own health, and those who have greater understanding of how to prevent, recognise and treat illnesses are likely to have an advantage. In the area of physical health, the public have quite a lot of knowledge. For example, many people know that they can prevent cancers by not smoking and by keeping protected from the sun, they know the advantages of physical activity and eating certain types of food, they may know the early warning signs of cancer and heart disease, and some people have done first aid courses so they can assist in an emergency. While there is considerable public understanding of major physical illnesses, public understanding of mental health (what has been called *mental health literacy*) has lagged. A lack of mental health literacy has some important consequences, as listed below.

The first consequence of a lack of mental health literacy is that some people will not recognise that they have a mental disorder and will not get appropriate professional help. We know that many people who suffer from common mental disorders like depression do not receive any professional help, and that delayed help-seeking is associated with worse outcomes (Parslow and Jorm 2002). It is also known that general practitioners (GPs) often fail to recognise depression in their patients, but they show better recognition when the patient self-labels as depressed and specifically consults for psychological symptoms (Parslow and Jorm 2002).

Poor mental health literacy of the public also places a limit on the implementation of evidence-based medicine. The idea behind evidence-based medicine is that patients will benefit if health care practitioners can be educated to provide care that is supported by scientific evidence as effective. However, this approach will work only if patients are willing to accept evidence-based care. For example, if patients falsely believe that a new psychotropic medication is addictive, then they will be less likely to accept and use this treatment, regardless of the strength of the scientific evidence. For the implementation of evidence-based medicine, the education of health practitioners is necessary but is not sufficient. There needs to be a concordance between the health practitioner and patient in how they think about the patient's illness, and this requires that the public be given evidence-based information as well.

Another consequence of poor mental health literacy is that it limits the family and community support provided to people with mental disorders. The prevalence of mental disorders is so high that everybody in the community will at some time have close contact with a person who suffers from a mental disorder. However, community ignorance and the stigma of mental disorders means that members of the public often do not provide appropriate support, and this can have negative consequences. We know that people suffering from disorders such as depression are more likely to seek professional help if relatives or friends suggest it (Parslow and Jorm 2002). There is also substantial evidence that if family members are supportive and not critical of the sufferer, this can assist recovery and reduce the risk of relapse (Parslow and Jorm 2002). Improving the mental health literacy of the public can help produce a more supportive community.

Mental health has been very much a Cinderella area, with a poor image, a relatively low level of funding for services, greater difficulty in recruiting healthcare professionals and less attention from researchers. If this situation is to improve, it will require the support of the community in general, which will be facilitated by greater mental health literacy. Political leaders and policy makers will be assign a higher priority to an issue that has widespread community interest and support.

PUBLIC UNDERSTANDING

There has been a range of community surveys assessing knowledge and attitudes to depression in Australia, but none so far in New Zealand. These surveys are described below.

National Survey of Mental Health Literacy

This was a household survey of more than 2000 adults carried out in 1995. Half the participants were shown a vignette of a person suffering from depression, and the other half a vignette of schizophrenia. Only the results from the depression vignette are described here. The vignette was:

> John is 30 years old. He has been feeling unusually sad and miserable for the last few weeks. Even though he is tired all the time, he has trouble sleeping nearly every night. John doesn't feel like eating and has lost weight. He can't keep his mind on his work and puts off making decisions. Even day-to-day tasks seem too much for him. This has come to the attention of John's boss, who is concerned about his lowered productivity.

After they had read the vignette, participants were asked what, if anything, they thought was wrong with the person described. There were 39 per cent who mentioned the conventional psychiatric label of depression, 22 per cent mentioned stress, and most of the others mentioned a mental health problem of some kind. Only 11 per cent mentioned a physical disorder. Thus, most people recognised that some sort of mental health problem was present, although only a minority gave the conventional psychiatric label.

Next, participants were given a long list of potential interventions for depression, including seeking help from various professions, a range of medications, psychological treatments and lifestyle changes. They were asked to say whether each of these interventions was likely to be helpful, harmful or neither for the person described in the vignette. The interventions most likely to be rated as helpful were seeing a GP, a counsellor, help from close friends, becoming physically more active, getting out and about more, and attending courses on relaxation, stress management, meditation or yoga. Two standard medical interventions for depression, antidepressants and electroconvulsive therapy, were more often rated as likely to be harmful than helpful. In fact, even vitamins and herbal remedies were rated higher than antidepressants. In general, the public preferred lifestyle and psychological treatments, with medical treatments the least preferred.

Participants were next asked, 'What would be the likely result if John had the sort of professional help you think is most appropriate?' and 'What would be the likely result if John did not have any professional help?'. The public was found to be very optimistic about the outcome following professional help, with most expecting a full recovery. However, most expected the person would get worse without professional help.

The survey also asked participants about what they thought were the likely causes of the condition of the person in the vignette and whether they thought certain groups in the population were at higher or lower risk of developing this problem. Social environmental factors were seen as the most likely causes (for example, some recent traumatic event, or day-to-day stressors at work or in the family). The highest risk-groups were seen to be the unemployed, divorced, the poor and young people. These views accord well with the research evidence showing the importance of the social environment in depression, but the public underrate the importance of genetic vulnerability.

Finally, the survey asked a range of questions to assess stigmatising attitudes. One of these questions asked whether the person in the vignette would be discriminated against by others in the community after he had received treatment. There were 54 per cent who thought there would be discrimination (compared with 75 per cent for schizophrenia).

South Australian Health Omnibus Survey

A mental health literacy survey was subsequently carried out in 1998 as part of the Health Omnibus Survey in South Australia (Goldney et al. 2001). This survey involved about 3000 participants aged over 15 years. The same vignette of a depressed person was used as in the earlier national survey, and many of the survey questions were the same. However, an innovation was that participants were assessed for depression to see if personal experience of depression had an effect on knowledge and beliefs. The results were similar to the earlier national survey. In particular, more people believed that antidepressants would be harmful than believed they would be helpful. Again, vitamins and herbal remedies were more likely than antidepressants to be rated as helpful. Participants who were depressed were more likely to rate antidepressants as potentially helpful. However, this proportion was still only 40 per cent, and an equal proportion of depressed participants rated antidepressants as likely to be harmful. An analysis was also carried out looking at participants who had suicidal ideation, but few differences in mental health literacy were found (Goldney et al. 2002).

beyondblue survey

The most recent Australian survey was carried out in 2001 for *beyondblue: the national depression initiative* (Highet et al. 2002). This survey involved a national sample of 900 adults. The aim was to assess awareness of depression, knowledge about depression and attitudes to seeking treatment.

Respondents were first asked what they considered the major health problems in Australia at present. The most frequently mentioned were cancer (32 per cent) and heart disease (26 per cent), followed by alcohol and substance misuse (10 per cent), diabetes (8 per cent), infectious diseases (6 per cent) and asthma (5 per cent). Only small proportions mentioned mental health in general (3 per cent), depression (2 per cent) or anxiety/stress/pressure (2 per cent). These figures contrast with the estimates of burden of disease in Australia provided by the Australian Institute of Health and Welfare, which rank mental health as third after cardiovascular disease and cancer, with depression the biggest single contributor within the mental health category (Mathers et al. 1999). However, when respondents were asked to nominate the major mental health problems in Australia, depression was most commonly seen as the major problem (by 39 per cent), followed by anxiety/stress/pressure (18 per cent).

The next section of the survey assessed knowledge about depression. Fifty per cent of respondents could differentiate depression from normal sadness, citing its greater intensity and longer duration. However, 64 per cent underestimated the lifetime risk of depression in the population. Respondents were also asked to rate the effect of several events or life circumstances on depression. They were asked about three events known to increase risk (unemployment, having a serious medical condition, birth of a child), two neutral factors (having a job with lots of responsibility, living in a rural area) and one protective factor (being married). The three risk factors were recognised as such by a large majority but, contrary to the evidence, 55 per cent thought marriage increased risk.

When given a list of potential treatments, the most frequently rated as helpful were support from family and friends (97 per cent), exercise (91 per cent), yoga (87 per cent) and psychological therapies (87 per cent). Antidepressant medications were rated as likely to be helpful by 65 per cent, compared with 59 per cent for St John's wort and 25 per cent for sleeping tablets or sedatives. The higher rating of antidepressants in this survey may have been because the question related to depression rather than to a vignette that did not mention depression. When asked whom they would turn to if they were suffering from depression, the respondents rated family highest (45 per cent), followed by GPs (28 per cent) and friends (15 per cent). When asked about first choice of treatments, respondents indicated a preference for non-pharmacological treatments, such as counselling and support from others.

Young people's understanding

Little research has yet been aimed at determining the attitudes, knowledge and beliefs of young people in relation to depression or other mental illnesses on a large scale. As yet unpublished data (Kelly et al. 2002) from a pilot study of a questionnaire adapted from Jorm et al. (1997b) has shown that the mental health literacy of adolescents may be better in some respects than that of adults. Respondents were offered a vignette of a young woman (Jenny) with signs of depression. Eighty-four per cent identified Jenny's problem as being depression. Of that group, some made more than one diagnosis, with the most common second diagnosis being an eating disorder.

Respondents rated most people and treatments as being helpful. The most helpful were talking to friends (91 per cent), reading about others who had been depressed (85 per cent), getting counselling (86 per cent), talking to family (78 per cent) and then a range of lifestyle treatments. While very few treatments were considered harmful, and few of these were appropriate for treating depression (for example, antipsychotics and tranquillisers), hospitalisation was seen as harmful by more than two-thirds of the respondents. In contrast to their adult counterparts, 68 per cent of the young people felt that antidepressants were helpful. Doctors and teachers were rated lowest, but were still rated as helpful by more than half the respondents.

It is interesting that young people were less optimistic about Jenny's chances of recovery after appropriate professional help. More than half felt that Jenny would recover but would suffer similar problems later. Without help, most felt she would get worse.

Young people also had a good understanding of the causes and risk factors associated with depression. They rated recent traumas such as the death of a family member or close friend, life problems and childhood problems as being the most likely causes, but, like the adults, underestimated genetic factors in depression.

Groups within the community considered at the highest risk of depression were unemployed people, young people, poorer people, girls and early school leavers. Those considered least at risk were older people.

Only around 33 per cent of young people felt that Jenny would suffer discrimination as a result of her problems. Most young people suggested that unkindness or cruelty at the hands of peers would be the most common form of discrimination. When asked about willingness to spend time with a young person with depression, most were happy to spend both social time and schoolwork time with that person.

Similar results to these were found in a study of students in rural South Australia in 1999 (Willcocks 1999).

PROFESSIONAL UNDERSTANDING

The results of the surveys of the public suggest that there is a gap between public and professional understanding of depression. To assess whether this is the case, postal surveys of various professional groups were carried out using a modified version of the questionnaire used in the National Survey of Mental Health Literacy. Surveys were carried out with samples of Australian GPs, psychiatrists and clinical psychologists in 1996 (Jorm et al. 1997a), and with mental health nurses in 1998 (Caldwell and Jorm 2000). There was a general consensus among the GPs, psychiatrists and clinical psychologists about the interventions that are likely to be helpful for the person in the depression vignette. Two-thirds or more of each profession rated the following as likely to be helpful: seeing a GP, psychiatrist or clinical psychologist; antidepressants; counselling; and cognitive behaviour therapy. There are some obvious discrepancies with the results with the public, who tended to favour lifestyle interventions and were predominantly negative about antidepressants.

The gulf between public and professional views may reduce as the public become better informed. Some reciprocal change in professional views is also possible, so that they become closer to those of the public. An analysis of age group differences in healthcare professionals showed that the younger generation of GPs and psychiatrists tended to have views closer to those of the public (Jorm et al. 1997c). Although the younger professionals shared the core beliefs of the older ones about standard interventions for depression, they were also more open to some non-standard interventions. For example, younger GPs were more positive about help from family and friends, telephone counselling, reading self-help books, and courses on relaxation, stress management, meditation or yoga.

There have also been comparisons between the public and various groups of health professionals in their beliefs about outcomes for depression (Caldwell and Jorm 2001; Hugo 2001). In general, healthcare professionals are less optimistic than the public about outcomes after treatment. They are less likely to expect full recovery and more likely to expect relapse. GPs and psychiatrists are more pessimistic than clinical psychologists and mental health nurses. On the other hand, the public tend to be less optimistic about outcomes if professional help is not received, with most expecting the person to get worse or not improve, whereas many professionals expect at least some recovery. In other words, professionals tend to see depression as a condition that often has a relapsing course, but one in which remission may occur even without treatment, while the public are more likely to see treatment as producing long-term cures and no remission without treatment.

Healthcare professionals have also been asked about discrimination against people who have suffered from depression (Caldwell and Jorm 2001). GPs, psychiatrists and mental health nurses were more likely to believe that discrimination would occur than were members of the public. Only clinical psychologists were similar to the public in discrimination beliefs.

IMPROVING PUBLIC UNDERSTANDING

Given the gaps between public and professional understanding, there has been considerable interest in recent years in educating the public about depression and other mental disorders. Various approaches are possible, including universal information campaigns aimed at the whole population, campaigns aimed at subgroups of special interest such as young people, and information programs aimed at interested individuals. Here we describe some approaches that have been used in Australia or New Zealand. Some of these are aimed specifically at depression, whereas others cover mental health more generally, including depression.

General community

In Australia, programs to increase community awareness and understanding have been developed by *beyondblue: the national depression initiative. beyondblue* is a private company set up with funding from the Commonwealth and state governments. One of its aims is to 'reduce the stigma associated with depression by increasing awareness of symptoms, causes and treatments and by promoting the experiences of people whose lives have been affected by the illness'. *beyondblue* has supported a range of activities, including community forums on depression, a workplace-based depression awareness campaign, and extensive media publicity (for example, using prominent sporting, media and political figures to raise awareness).

The Rotary Health Research Fund is another Australian organisation that has campaigned to increase public understanding of mental disorders, including depression. The fund has organised Rotary clubs across Australia to run community forums. These are advertised widely in the local community and involve short talks by a clinician, consumer and carer, followed by audience questions. As of 2002, more than 20 000 people had attended these forums. The fund has also run short community awareness advertisements on television, giving messages to reduce stigma and to promote help-seeking.

While it is possible that these campaigns are having beneficial effects, this is difficult to evaluate. As yet, there are no data monitoring changes in public understanding over time.

Young people

There are various campaigns, most of which have been launched in recent years, aimed at increasing young people's understanding and knowledge of mental disorders. In line with the habits and preferences of young people, many of these campaigns have an Internet component. Most of these campaigns focus on the mental disorders that are most relevant to young people: depression, anxiety, and often psychosis, which often has its onset in late teens or early twenties.

One campaign, MindMatters, describes itself as a whole-school and school community-based approach to mental health (Wyn et al. 2000). Materials focus on such broad areas as improving mental health literacy and resilience to difficulties, understanding grief and loss, community mental health, and a suicide prevention component. MindMatters was developed by the Commonwealth Department of Health and Aged Care in response to the 1996 audit of Mental Health Education in Australian Secondary Schools (Wyn et al. 1996). The package comprises a curriculum pack which can be used flexibly by teachers in different teaching areas, a program of professional development nationwide for teachers and other school professionals, and a website for teachers with interactive forums and further information. Evaluation was carried out in twenty-four pilot schools in 1998 and 1999 by the Hunter Institute of Mental Health (Waring et al. 2000).

The mental health literacy component of MindMatters consists mainly of materials in the section titled 'Understanding mental illness'. This component includes information, fact sheets, worksheets and activities that aim to educate students on mental health issues such as depression, anxiety, psychotic disorders, and eating disorders. There is a section that aims to reduce stigmatising attitudes, and a video that includes interviews with people who have experienced mental illness.

The evaluation of MindMatters was to include ascertaining improvement in knowledge and attitudes around mental illness, but problems with the sample meant this section could not be evaluated effectively.

beyondblue will pilot a project in Australian schools in 2003–2005 titled 'The beyondblue schools research initiative' (Burns et al. 2002). This campaign aims to increase resilience and coping in schools, improve mental health literacy, improve help-seeking attitudes in students and create a school environment that is more responsive to the mental health needs of the students. The project will be piloted in twenty-four schools throughout Australia. Components will include increasing supportive environments, a classroom teaching and learning component, a pathways approach to accessing professional help inside and outside the school, and public forums to increase community awareness of mental health.

Another campaign, focusing on psychosis, bipolar disorder and depression, is the *Compass Project*. The *Compass Project* was developed under the auspices of Orygen Youth Health in Melbourne (formerly MH-SKY – mental health services for kids and youth). The main components are a website with information for young people (<www.getontop.org>) and an information campaign, including television and cinema advertising, and print materials. The aims of the campaign are to reduce stigma and increase knowledge of mental disorders, and to decrease delays in help-seeking for such mental disorders. The program is currently being evaluated in regions of Victoria for eventual use in other regions of Australia.

Interested individuals

One program for individuals, developed in Australia, involves first aid training that is specifically designed to cover mental disorders. Mental Health First Aid is a 12-hour program designed for members of the public or workplaces (Kitchener and Jorm 2002). It covers mental health crisis situations such as suicidal thoughts, panic attacks, exposure to psychological trauma, and acute psychotic behaviour. The course also gives information about major mental disorders, including depression, anxiety, psychosis and substance abuse. An evaluation of the program has shown that participants are better able to recognise disorders, change their beliefs about treatments to become more like those of healthcare professionals, develop more positive attitudes, have increased confidence in providing help, and increase the amount of help they provide to others.

The World Wide Web is becoming a major source of health information for the public and has great potential for improving public understanding of depression. It has been reported that more Internet users search the Web for information on depression than any other condition (Griffiths and Christensen 2002). However, for the Web to have benefits, depression sites must provide high-quality information. Unfortunately, the quality of information and accessibility of many depression sites is poor. A systematic assessment of Australian websites against a range of criteria found that the following sites provide the highest quality of content (Griffiths and Christensen 2002):

- beyondblue <http://www.beyondblue.org.au>
- BluePages <http://bluepages.anu.edu.au>
- CRUfAD <http://www.crufad.unsw.edu.au>
- Infrapsych <http://www.infrapsych.com.au>

Randomised controlled trials of websites are needed to find out if they produce benefits to people suffering from depression. Such trials are under way and results will appear over the next few years.

New Zealand campaigns

In 1997, the Mason Report identified discrimination and stigma as being a major impediment to quality of life for people suffering mental illness in New Zealand (Mason 1996). In response to that report, the New Zealand Ministry for Health developed a campaign called *Like Minds Like Mine/Whakaitia te Whakawhiu i te Tangata*. This campaign consists of a website, <www.likeminds.govt.nz>, and advertising materials in print, on television, and on the radio, and aims to increase people's knowledge of mental illness and accordingly reduce stigma. One feature of the campaign was using well-known New Zealand public figures to illustrate that anyone could develop a mental illness. This campaign had an effect on people's opinions of those suffering with a mental disorder, and people's knowledge of mental disorders. In particular, the campaign increased people's recall of depression as a mental disorder, and this effect was maintained at follow-up (Ackroyd and Wyllie 2002).

In New Zealand, the focus of many campaigns is to reduce the incidence of suicide. A notable campaign is SPINZ (Suicide Prevention Information New Zealand), which focuses mainly on decreasing the youth suicide rate in New Zealand. SPINZ provides information and resources for preventing youth suicide. The main component of SPINZ is the website, <www.spinz.org.nz>, which lists many organisations in New Zealand for mental health assistance.

CONCLUSION

Among both the public and healthcare professionals there is a range of beliefs about depression. However, it is possible to describe a prototypical public or professional view, which clearly shows the contrast in understanding between the two groups. The public underestimates the public health importance of depression, in terms of both prevalence and disease burden. They recognise depression as a mental health problem, but frequently use different terminology from healthcare professionals to describe this disorder. They favour lifestyle and psychological interventions and tend to be negative about medication, whereas healthcare professionals see antidepressant medication, cognitive behaviour therapy and counselling as the most appropriate treatments. The public see depression as primarily arising from stressors in the social environment, but tend to underestimate the importance of personal vulnerability. They believe that depression can be cured with appropriate professional help, but see a poor outcome without professional help. By contrast, professionals tend to see depression as a relapsing condition, even with treatment, but believe that some remission occurs even without treatment. Both the public and healthcare professionals see depression as a stigmatised condition that may result in sufferers being discriminated against, but the healthcare professionals tend to have more negative views than the public.

There has been increasing action to improve public understanding of depression. While this would be expected to lead to gradual improvements in public understanding, there are few data on the issue. There is a need for rigorous evaluation of these community education programs.

REFERENCES

Ackroyd S, Wyllie A (2002) Impacts of National Media Campaign to Counter Stigma and Discrimination Associated with Mental Illness: Survey 4. Report for Ministry of Health. Auckland: Phoenix Research.

Burns J, Patton G, Spence S, Sawyer M, Glover S, Kay D, et al. (2002) Preventing depression in young people: Beyondblue schools research projects. *Australasian Society for Psychiatric Research, Annual Scientific Meeting.*

Caldwell TM, Jorm AF (2000) Mental health nurses' beliefs about interventions for schizophrenia and depression: A comparison with psychiatrists and the public. *Australian and New Zealand Journal of Psychiatry* 34:602-11.

—— (2001) Mental health nurses' beliefs about likely outcomes for people with schizophrenia or depression: A comparison with the public and other healthcare professionals. *Australian and New Zealand Journal of Mental Health Nursing* 10:42-54.

Goldney RD, Fisher LJ, Wilson DH (2001) Mental health literacy: An impediment to the optimum treatment of major depression in the community. *Journal of Affective Disorders* 64:277-84.

Goldney RD, Fisher LJ, Wilson DH, Cheok F (2002) Mental health literacy of those with major depression and suicidal ideation: An impediment to help seeking. *Suicide and Life-Threatening Behavior* 32:394-403.

Griffiths KM, Christensen H (2002) The quality and accessibility of Australian depression sites on the World Wide Web. *Medical Journal of Australia* 176 (10 Suppl):S97-S104.

Highet NJ, Hickie IB, Davenport TA (2002) Monitoring awareness of and attitudes to depression in Australia. *Medical Journal of Australia* 176 (10 Suppl):S63-8.

Hugo M (2001) Mental health professionals' attitudes towards people who have experienced a mental health disorder. *Journal of Psychiatric and Mental Health Nursing* 8:419-25.

Jorm AF, Korten AE, Jacomb PA, Rodgers B, Pollitt P (1997a) Beliefs about the helpfulness of interventions for mental disorders: A comparison of general practitioners, psychiatrists and clinical psychologists. *Australian and New Zealand Journal of Psychiatry* 31:844-51.

Jorm AF, Korten AE, Jacomb PA, Christensen H, Rodgers B, Pollitt P (1997b) 'Mental health literacy': A survey of the public's ability to recognise mental disorders and their beliefs about the effectiveness of treatment. *Medical Journal of Australia* 166:182-6.

Jorm AF, Korten AE, Jacomb PA, Rodgers B, Pollitt P, Christensen H, et al. (1997c) Helpfulness of interventions for mental disorders: Beliefs of health professionals compared with the general public. *British Journal of Psychiatry* 171:233-7.

Kelly CM, Rodgers B, Jorm AF (2002) Unpublished data from the Adolescent Mental Health Literacy Project Phase 2. Canberra: Australian National University, Centre for Mental Health Research.

Kitchener BA, Jorm AF (2002) Mental health first aid training for the public: Evaluation of effects on knowledge, attitudes and helping behavior. *BMC Psychiatry* 2:10.

Mason KHC (1996) Inquiry under s47 of the Health and Disability Services Act 1993 in Respect of Certain Mental Health Services: Report of the Ministerial Inquiry to the Minister of Health Hon. Jenny Shipley. Wellington, NZ: Ministry of Health.

Mathers C, Vos T, Stevenson C (1999) *The Burden of Disease and Injury in Australia.* Canberra: Australian Institute of Health and Welfare.

Parslow RA, Jorm AF (2002) Improving Australians' depression literacy. *Medical Journal of Australia* 177 (7 Suppl):S117-21.

Waring T, Hazell T, Holbrook A, Hazell P (2000) Report of the MindMatters (National Mental Health in Schools Project) Evaluation Project. Vols 1-4. Newcastle, Australia: (MindMatters Evaluation Consortium) Hunter Institute of Mental Health.

Willcocks A (1999) *Mental Health Literacy and Depressive Symptomatology of Adolescents Living in Rural Areas. Adelaide*: Department of Psychology, University of Adelaide.

Wyn J, Cahill H, Holdsworth R, Rowling L, Carson S (2000) MindMatters, a whole-school approach promoting mental health and wellbeing. *Australian and New Zealand Journal of Psychiatry* 34:594-601.

Wyn J, Taylor B, Sheehan M, Harris A, McDonnell E, Holdsworth R, et al. (1996) The Audit of Mental Health Education in Australian Secondary Schools. Commissioned by the Mental Health Branch of the Commonwealth Department of Health and Aged Care. Conducted by the Youth Research Centre and the Centre for Social Health.

CHAPTER 40

MOOD DISORDERS AND THE GLOBAL BURDEN OF DISEASE

Peter R Joyce and
Philip B Mitchell

In 1996, Murray and Lopez, on behalf of the World Health Organization, World Bank and the Harvard School of Public Health, published *The Global Burden of Disease* (Murray and Lopez 1996). For the first time, a comprehensive assessment of the mortality and disability from all diseases, injuries and risk factors was undertaken using transparent and inclusive methodological approaches. In the summary of this landmark study, four major surprises were highlighted, the first of which can be summarised as 'the burden of mental illnesses, such as mood disorders, alcohol and drug dependence and schizophrenia have previously been seriously underestimated by approaches that focus on mortality, rather than disability and mortality'. In the study, the authors developed the DALY (disability adjusted life year) as the primary measure of disease burden. The DALY expresses years of life lost to premature death and years lived with a disability of specified severity and duration. One DALY is thus one lost year of healthy life. The DALY, as a measure of disease burden, makes value judgments on life expectancy. Are years of health life worth more in young adulthood than in late life, are all people equal, and how does one compare years of life lost due to premature death and years of life lived with disabilities of varying severity?

In developed countries, which include Australia and New Zealand, suicide is the ninth leading cause of death and accounts for just over 1 per cent of deaths. However, in 1990, unipolar major depression was the leading cause of disability in the world, and bipolar disorder was the sixth leading cause of disability (with alcohol use fourth and schizophrenia ninth). Using the DALY as the primary measure of disease burden, unipolar major depression was the fourth leading cause of disease burden. In the developed world, for women aged 15–44 years, unipolar major depression was the leading cause of disease burden (about 20 per cent), and bipolar disorder was the fourth leading cause of disease burden (about 4 per cent) (Murray and Lopez 1996).

EPIDEMIOLOGY OF MOOD DISORDERS

The calculation of disease burden (DALYs) requires satisfactory estimates of both mortality and morbidity. For depression and bipolar disorder, the excess mortality is partially due to suicide (see Chapter 37) but is also contributed to by natural causes of death, particularly cardiovascular disease (Carney et al. 2001; Osby et al. 2001; Penninx et al. 2001; Von Ammon Cavanaugh et al. 2001). Estimates of morbidity require understanding of prevalence rates, and of the disability associated with mood disorders.

Over the past 25 years, there has been unprecedented research activity in the psychiatric epidemiology of mood disorders (Weissman et al. 1996; Regier et al. 1998; Joyce 2000). In the early and mid-1980s, the National Institute of Mental Health (NIMH) Epidemiological Catchment Area (ECA) study was completed in the United States (Regier et al. 1984; Weissman et al. 1988) and equivalent studies were undertaken in other countries, including New Zealand (Wells et al. 1989). Then the National Comorbidity Study (NCS) was completed in the United States (Kessler et al. 1994). National psychiatric epidemiology studies have also been completed in Britain (Jenkins et al. 1997) and Australia (Andrews et al. 2001). Across these studies, the current (1 month) prevalence of major depression is typically 3–5 per cent, with a rate of 3.2 per cent in the Australian National Survey of Mental Health and Wellbeing (Wilhelm et al. 2003). Women consistently have higher rates of major depression than men (Weissman et al. 1993; Blazer et al. 1994).

Lifetime rates of major depressive disorders have varied considerably between studies, with lifetime rates as low as 3.7 per cent in the Baltimore site of the NIMH ECA study (Weissman et al. 1988) and 17.1 per cent in the NCS (Blazer et al. 1994), to more than 30 per cent in other community studies (Beautrais et al. 1996). This suggests that lifetime recall of major depression may be problematic, and discrepancies between studies suggest that methodological and interviewing differences are very important. However, the literature has focused more on issues of recall bias (Andrews et al. 1999; Kendler et al. 2001).

Conversely, the lifetime prevalence of bipolar disorder (usually bipolar I and II) has more consistently been estimated at between 1 and 2 per cent (Weissman et al. 1996). The greatest controversies in the epidemiology of bipolar disorder are the prevalences of bipolar spectrum disorders (see Chapter 6), and of childhood onset bipolar disorders (Chapter 30).

REDUCING THE BURDEN

Reducing the disease burden due to mood disorders will require a range of interventions. These include:

- prevention of depression and bipolar disorder
- improvements in treatment-seeking by people with mood disorders
- improvements in the recognition and diagnosis of mood disorders in both primary care and mental health services
- improvements in the delivery of currently available effective treatments
- improvements in the efficacy of current treatments.

Given the substantial genetic contribution to the aetiology and the low prevalence of bipolar disorder, prevention strategies are difficult to envisage. The key prevention issues around bipolar disorder relate to early identification and early intervention in people at high risk. For major depression, some initial studies have been undertaken on the prevention of childhood and adolescent depression, although the findings are not yet sufficiently robust to recommend a more general availability of such interventions (Beardslee and Gladstone 2001). There are also active efforts in preventing suicide, and these usually include improvements in the recognition and treatment of mood disorders (Goldney 1998; Isacsson 2000; Joyce 2001: Chapter 37).

In Chapter 39, Jorm and Kelly highlight how changing the public understanding of mood disorders should influence patterns of appropriate help-seeking behaviour. Campaigns to reduce stigma are also potentially important to changing public perceptions and willingness to seek help. The biggest challenge probably lies in changing the knowledge, understanding and treatment-seeking behaviour of young men, who traditionally are the sector of the population least likely to access health services, especially mental health services.

Hickie and Davenport (Chapter 36) have highlighted the vital role of primary care services to improvements in the recognition and delivery of evidence-based treatments for mood disorders. Mood disorders contribute substantially to the mental health burden in primary care, yet many neither seek treatment nor receive evidence-based treatment (Andrews et al. 2000, 2001). Given that mood disorders are usually chronic or recurrent, how primary care and mental health services are organised may be fundamental to managing these chronic disorders and delivering effective relapse prevention and chronic care services (Davis et al. 1999; Paykel et al. 1999; Katon et al. 2001; Geddes et al. 2003; Lam et al. 2003).

Although our current treatments, including psychotherapeutic, psychopharmacological and physical, are effective, considerable room remains for improvements in efficacy. While half of all depressed patients may respond satisfactorily to a first antidepressant or psychotherapy, that still leaves about half who do not. Some of these will respond to other treatments, such as a change of treatment approach or a second antidepressant; nevertheless, considerable improvement is possible.

Mood disorder research and service delivery is at an interesting crossroads. Developments in neuroscience, molecular genetics, cognitive sciences, psychotherapy, clinical science and epidemiology suggest that major investment in mood disorder research and innovations in service delivery could substantially lower the disease burden due to these common and devastating conditions.

REFERENCES

Andrews G, Anstey K, Brodaty H, Issakidis C, Luscombe G (1999) Recall of depressive episode 25 years previously. *Psychological Medicine* 29:787-91.

Andrews G, Sanderson K, Slade T, Issakidis C (2000) Why does the burden of disease persist? Relating the burden of anxiety and depression to effectiveness of treatment. *Bulletin of the World Health Organization* 78:446-54.

Andrews G, Henderson S, Hall W (2001) Prevalence, comorbidity, disability and service utilisation: Overview of the Australian National Mental Health Survey. *British Journal of Psychiatry* 178:145-53.

Beardslee WR, Gladstone TR (2001) Prevention of childhood depression: Recent findings and future prospects. *Biological Psychiatry* 49:1101-10.

Beautrais AL, Joyce PR, Mulder RT, Fergusson DM, Deavoll BJ, Nightingale SK (1996) Prevalence and comorbidity of mental disorders in persons making serious suicide attempts: A case–control study. *American Journal of Psychiatry* 153:1009-14.

Blazer DG, Kessler RC, McGonagle KA, Swartz MS (1994) The prevalence and distribution of major depression in a national community sample: The national comorbidity survey. *American Journal of Psychiatry* 151:979-86.

Carney RM, Freedland KE, Jaffe AS (2001) Depression as a risk factor for coronary heart disease mortality. *Archives of General Psychiatry* 58:229-30.

Davis JM, Janicak PG, Hogan DM (1999) Mood stabilizers in the prevention of recurrent affective disorders: A meta-analysis. *Acta Psychiatrica Scandinavica* 100:406-17.

Geddes JR, Carney SM, Davies C, Furukawa TA, Kupfer DJ, Frank E, et al. (2003) Relapse prevention with antidepressant drug treatment in depressive disorders: A systematic review. *Lancet* 361:653-61.

Goldney RD (1998) Suicide prevention is possible: A review of recent studies. *Archives of Suicide Research* 4:329-39.

Isacsson G (2000) Suicide prevention – a medical breakthrough? *Acta Psychiatrica Scandinavica* 102:113-17.

Jenkins R, Bebbington P, Brugha T, Farrell M, Gill B, Lewis G, et al. (1997) The National Psychiatric Morbidity surveys of Great Britain – strategy and methods. *Psychological Medicine* 27:765-74.

Joyce PR (2000) Epidemiology of Mood Disorders. In Gelder MG, Lopez-Ibor JJ, Jr, Andreasen NC (eds), *New Oxford Textbook of Psychiatry*, Vol. 1. Oxford: Oxford University Press, pp. 695-701.

—— (2001) Improvements in the recognition and treatment of depression and decreasing suicide rates. *New Zealand Medical Journal* 114:535-6.

Katon W, Rutter C, Ludman EJ, Von Korff M, Lin E, Simon G, et al. (2001) A randomized trial of relapse prevention of depression in primary care. *Archives of General Psychiatry* 58:241-7.

Kendler KS, Gardner CO, Prescott CA (2001) Are there sex differences in the reliability of a lifetime history of major depression and its predictors? *Psychological Medicine* 31:617-25.

Kessler RC, McGonagle KA, Zhao S, Nelson CB, Hughes M, Eshleman S, et al. (1994) Lifetime and 12-month prevalence of DSM-III-R psychiatric disorders in the United States. *Archives of General Psychiatry* 51:8-19.

Lam DH, Watkins ER, Hayward P, Bright J, Wright K, Kerr N, et al. (2003) A randomized controlled study of cognitive therapy for relapse prevention for bipolar affective disorder: Outcome of the first year. *Archives of General Psychiatry* 60:145-52.

Murray CJL, Lopez AD (eds) (1996) *The Global Burden of Disease: A comprehensive assessment of mortality and disability from diseases, injuries, and risk factors in 1990 and projected to 2020*. Cambridge, MA: Harvard University Press on behalf of the World Health Organization and the World Bank.

Osby U, Brandt L, Correia N, Ekbom A, Sparen P (2001) Excess mortality in bipolar and unipolar disorder in Sweden. *Archives of General Psychiatry* 58:844-50.

Paykel ES, Scott J, Teasdale JD, Johnson AL, Garland A, Moore R, et al. (1999) Prevention of relapse in residual depression by cognitive therapy: A controlled trial. *Archives of General Psychiatry* 56:829-35.

Penninx BWJH, Beekman ATF, Honig A, Deeg DJH, Schoevers RA, Van Eijk JTM, et al. (2001) Depression and cardiac mortality: Results from a community-based longitudinal study. *Archives of General Psychiatry* 58:221-7.

Regier DA, Kaelber CT, Rae DS, Farmer ME, Knauper B, Kessler RC, et al. (1998) Limitations of diagnostic criteria and assessment instruments for mental disorders. Implications for research and policy. *Archives of General Psychiatry* 55:109-15.

Regier DA, Myers JK, Kramer M, Robins LN, Blazer DG, Hough RL, et al. (1984) The NIMH Epidemiologic Catchment Area program. Historical context, major objectives, and study population characteristics. *Archives of General Psychiatry* 41:934-41.

Von Ammon Cavanaugh S, Furlanetto LM, Creech SD, Powell LH (2001) Medical illness, past depression, and present depression: A predictive triad for in-hospital mortality. *American Journal of Psychiatry* 158:43-8.

Weissman MM, Bland R, Joyce PR, Newman S, Wells JE, Wittchen HU (1993) Sex differences in rates of depression: Cross-national perspectives. *Journal of Affective Disorders* 29:77-84.

Weissman MM, Leaf PJ, Tischler GL, Blazer DG, Karno M, Bruce ML, et al. (1988) Affective disorders in five United States communities. *Psychological Medicine* 18:141-53.

Weissman MM, Bland RC, Canino GJ, Faravelli C, Greenwald S, Hwu HG, et al. (1996) Cross-national epidemiology of major depression and bipolar disorder. *JAMA* 276:293-9.

Wells JE, Bushnell JA, Hornblow AR, Joyce PR, Oakley-Browne MA (1989) Christchurch Psychiatric Epidemiology Study, Part I: Methodology and lifetime prevalence for specific psychiatric disorders. *Australian and New Zealand Journal of Psychiatry* 23:315-26.

Wilhelm K, Mitchell P, Slade T, Brownhill S, Andrews G (2003) Prevalence and correlates of DSM-IV major depression in an Australian national survey. *Journal of Affective Disorders* 75:155-62.

INDEX

Index compiled by: Russell Brooks